Dendrites

Dendrites

Edited by

Greg Stuart
Australian National University

Nelson Spruston
Northwestern University

Michael Häusser
University College London

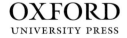
OXFORD
UNIVERSITY PRESS

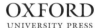

OXFORD

UNIVERSITY PRESS

Great Clarendon Street, Oxford OX2 6DP
Oxford University Press is a department of the University of Oxford.
It furthers the University's objective of excellence in research, scholarship,
and education by publishing worldwide in

Oxford New York

Athens Auckland Bangkok Bogotá Buenos Aires Calcutta
Cape Town Chennai Dar es Salaam Delhi Florence Hong Kong Istanbul
Karachi Kuala Lumpur Madrid Melbourne Mexico City Mumbai
Nairobi Paris São Paulo Singapore Taipei Tokyo Toronto Warsaw
with associated companies in Berlin Ibadan

Oxford is a registered trade mark of Oxford University Press
in the UK and in certain other countries

Published in the United States
by Oxford University Press Inc., New York

© Oxford University Press 1999

The moral rights of the author have been asserted

Database right Oxford University Press (maker)

First published 1999

A catalogue record for this book is available from the British Library.

Library of Congress Cataloguing in Publication Data
Dendrites / edited by Greg Stuart, Nelson Spruston, Michael Hausser.
p. cm.
Includes bibliographical references.
1. Dendrites. I. Stuart, Greg. II. Spruston, Nelson.
III. Hausser, Michael.
[DNLM: 1. Dendrites. WL 102.5 D391 1999]
QP363.D46   1999   573.8′5—dc21   99-39418

ISBN 0 19 850488 8

Typeset by Downdell, Oxford
Printed and bound by
Biddles Ltd, Guildford & King's Lynn

Foreword

By Dan Johnston, Baylor College of Medicine

The vast majority of synapses in the central nervous system terminate on neuronal dendrites. These tree-like structures are responsible for transforming the information received from synapses into a neural code that is then transmitted to other neurons. Dendritic signal processing is fundamental for the learning, memory, and behavior that we all take for granted in our day to day lives. This outstanding book is the first to deal exclusively with the emerging field of neuronal dendrites, and it covers the subject all the way from the molecular to the systems level of analysis. Stuart, Spruston, and Häusser have assembled an impressive group of neuroscientists who present their latest findings on dendrites in a clear and highly readable manner.

We have known about the existence of dendrites since they were first visualized by Camillo Golgi in 1873 using his newly discovered silver stain. Ramòn y Cajal later suggested that dendrites function as the site for input connections from other neurons, and further proposed that information flowed from the dendrites to the soma, and then to the synapse via the axon. Studies of electrical signaling in dendrites began in the 1930s and fueled great debates about whether dendrites were electrically active or passive and about how synaptic inputs were integrated to produce action potentials in the neuron. It is only with recent technical advances, however, that many of the questions about how dendrites work—questions that have intrigued neuroscientists for well over 100 years—can now be addressed experimentally. The methodological advances, which are fully described in this book, include the ability to make patch-clamp recordings from dendritic membranes, to optically image changes in ion concentrations within dendritic spines, and the development of specific molecular probes for identifying and localizing proteins and mRNA in dendrites and for following dendritic development and plasticity.

'Dendrites' is a short and deceptively simple title, yet a book devoted exclusively to neuronal dendrites is long overdue. Our understanding of dendrites has made a quantum jump in the past 10 years, and many of the former debates about dendritic function have been put to rest, only to be replaced by new ones. This book is timely not only because it lays the foundation for our current understanding of the field, but also because it will help to shape the questions that need to be addressed in the future. *Dendrites* will certainly deserve a careful reading by anyone interested in the neuronal basis of cognition

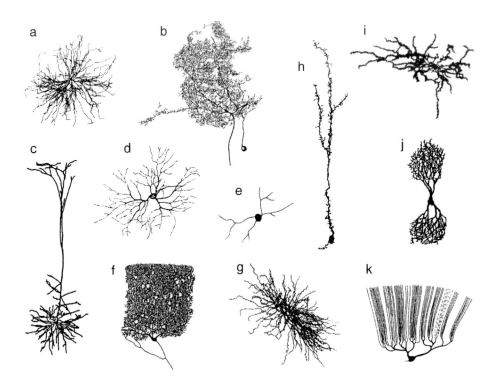

Dendritic trees come in different shapes and sizes. The size of the dendritic tree (largest dimension) is given in brackets. (a) Cat spinal motoneuron (2.6 mm). (b) Locust mesothoracic ganglion spiking interneuron (0.54 mm). (c) Rat neocortical layer 5 pyramidal neuron (1.03 mm). (d) Cat retinal ganglion neuron (0.39 mm). (e) Salamander retinal amacrine neuron (0.16 mm). (f) Human cerebellar Purkinje neuron. (g) Rat thalamic relay neuron (0.35 mm). (h) Mouse olfactory granule neuron (0.26 mm). (i) Rat striatal spiny projection neuron (0.37 mm). (j) Human nucleus of Burdach neuron. (k) Fish Purkinje neuron (0.42 mm). Modified from Mel, B. W. (1994). *Neural Computation*, **6**, 1031–1085.

Preface

It's hard not to get excited about the brain. It is by far the most complex organ in the body, containing more neurons than stars in the Milky Way. It is the seat of consciousness, thought, imagination, emotion, and creativity. It makes us human, and understanding how it works is, perhaps, the ultimate challenge.

This book is about dendrites. For the uninitiated, dendrites form the major receiving part of neurons. It is within these complex, branching structures that the real work of the nervous system takes place. The dendrites of neurons receive thousands of synaptic inputs from other neurons. But dendrites do more than simply collect and funnel these signals to the soma and axon; they shape and integrate these inputs in complex ways.

As is obvious from a quick look at the morphology of different neuronal types (Figure), not all dendrites are alike. Not only do the dendrites of different neurons look different, they also have different functional properties. This heterogeneity is unlikely to have evolved by chance, and presumably plays an essential role in the function of individual neurons within their respective neuronal networks.

Despite being discovered more than 100 years ago, dendrites received little attention until the early 1950s (see Chapter 8). More recently, largely because of technical advances, there has been a resurgence of interest in dendrites, which has led to substantial new information on their properties and role in neuronal function. The main aim of this book, the first of its kind on the subject, is to gather this new information into a single volume covering a wide range of topics on dendrites, from their morphology and development, through to their biochemical, electrical and computational properties.

Our own interest in dendrites dates back to our time as graduate students. All three of us did our PhDs in laboratories with a keen interest in dendrites, and we thank Steve Redman, Dan Johnston and Julian Jack for introducing us to this fascinating subject. Perhaps the main motivation for this book, however, comes from our time together in Bert Sakmann's laboratory, one of the places where the 'new age' of dendritic research began. This area of research is now rapidly expanding, and we expect this book to be one of many to cover the topic. We thank the participating authors for their excellent contributions and hope that this book serves both as a valuable resource and an impetus for further research into the exciting world of dendrites.

Canberra   G. S.
Evanston   N. S.
London   M. H.
March 1999

Contents

Contributors

Hollis T. Cline
Cold Spring Harbor Laboratory, 1 Bungtown Rd., Cold Spring Harbor,
NY 11724, USA
cline@cshl.org

James H. Eberwine
Department of Pharmacology, University of Pennsylvania Medical Center,
36th & Hamilton Walk, Philadelphia, PA 19104, USA
eberwine@pharm.med.upenn.edu

Mark Farrant
Department of Pharmacology, University College London,
Gower Street, London WC1E 6BT, United Kingdom
m.farrant@ucl.ac.uk

John C. Fiala
Department of Neurology, Children's Hospital, Enders 208, 300 Longwood Ave,
Boston, MA 02115, USA
fiala_j@al.tch.harvard.edu

Kristen M. Harris
Department of Neurology, Children's Hospital, Enders 208, 300 Longwood Ave,
Boston, MA 02115, USA
harrisk@al.tch.harvard.edu

Michael Häusser
Department of Physiology, University College London, Gower Street, London
WC1E 6BT, United Kingdom
m.hausser@ucl.ac.uk

Fritjof Helmchen
Biological Computation Research Department, Bell Laboratories, Lucent
Technologies, 600 Mountain Avenue, Murray Hill, NJ 07974, USA
fritjof@physics.bell-labs.com

Gilles Laurent
Division of Biology 139–74, California Institute of Technology, 1201 E California
Blvd, Pasadena, CA 91125, USA
laurentg@its.caltech.edu

Michael London
Department of Neurobiology, Institute of Life Sciences and Center for Neural Computation, Hebrew University, Jerusalem 91904, Israel
mikilon@lobster.ls.huji.ac.il

Jeffrey C. Magee
Neuroscience Center, Louisiana State University Medical Centre, 2020 Gravier St., New Orleans, LA 70112, USA
jmagee@lsumc.edu

Zachary F. Mainen
Cold Spring Harbor Laboratory, 1 Bungtown Rd., Cold Spring Harbor, NY 11724, USA
zach@cshl.org

Bartlett W. Mel
Department of Biomedical Engineering, University of Southern California, Mail Code 1451, Los Angeles, CA 90089, USA
mel@lnc.usc.edu

Zoltan Nusser
Department of Neurology, UCLA School of Medicine, Los Angeles, California 90095–1769, USA
nusser@ucla.edu

Wilfrid Rall
Mathematical Research Branch, NIH, BSA Bldg(350), Bethesda, MD 20892-2690, USA
wilrall@helix.nih.gov

Idan Segev
Department of Neurobiology, Institute of Life Sciences and Center for Neural Computation, Hebrew University, Jerusalem 91904, Israel
idan@lobster.ls.huji.ac.il

R. Angus Silver
Department of Physiology, University College London, Gower Street, London WC1E 6BT, United Kingdom
a.silver@ucl.ac.uk

Nelson Spruston
Dept. Neurobiology and Physiology, Institute for Neuroscience, Northwestern University, 2153 N Campus Drive, Evanston, IL 60208–3520, USA
spruston@nwu.edu

Greg Stuart
Division of Neuroscience, John Curtin School of Medical Research, Mills Road, Australian National University, Canberra, A.C.T. 0200, Australia
Greg.Stuart@anu.edu.au

Catherine S. Woolley
Dept. Neurobiology and Physiology, Northwestern University, 2153 N Campus Drive, Evanston, IL 60208–3520, USA
cwoolley@nwu.edu

Abbreviations and Symbols

4-AP	4-aminopyridine
5HT	5-hydroxytryptamine
AC	adenylate cyclase
A/N	AMPA/NMDA current ratio
Aga IVA	ω-Agatoxin IVA
AHP	after hyperpolarization
AMPA	α-amino-3-hydroxy-5-methyl-4-isoxazolepropionic acid
AP5	2-amino-5-phosphonopentanoic acid
ARC	activity-regulated cDNAs
aRNA	amplified antisense RNA
BAPTA	1,2-bis(2-aminophenoxy)ethane-N, N, N', N'-tetraacetic acid
BDNF	brain-derived neurotrophic factor
BK	big conductance Ca^{2+}-activated K^+ channel
C	membrane capacitance
C/A	commissural/associational
CA1	cornu ammonis (Ammon's horn), subregion 1
CA3	cornu ammonis (Ammon's horn), subregion 3
CaM	calmodulin
CaMKII	calcium calmodulin-dependent protein kinase II
cAMP	cyclic adenosine monophosphate
Ca_L	L-type Ca^{2+} channel
Ca_N	N-type Ca^{2+} channel
Ca_P	P-type Ca^{2+} channel
Ca_R	R-type Ca^{2+} channel
Ca_T	T-type Ca^{2+} channel
CBP	CREB binding protein
Cdc42	member of the Rho family of small GTPases
cDNA	complementary deoxyribonucleic acid
cGMP	cyclic guanosine monophosphate
C_i	ith coefficient of a multi-exponential function
c_m	membrane capacitance per unit length
C_m	specific membrane capacitance
CNQX	6-cyano-7-nitroquinoxaline-2,3-dione
CNS	central nervous system
CNTs	cyclic nucleotides
CPG15	candidate plasticity gene 15
CREB	cAMP response element binding protein
CS	conditioned stimulus
CV	coefficient of variation

d	diameter
D	diffusion coefficient
D_x	diffusion coefficient for ligand x
D_{app}	apparent diffusion coefficient
D_{aqu}	aqueous diffusion coefficient
D_{cyto}	cytosolic diffusion coefficient
DAB	3,3'-diaminobenzidine
DAG	diacylglycerol
DC	direct current
DCMD	descending contralateral motion detector neuron
ddPCR	differential display polymerase chain reaction
DHP	dihydropyridine
DM-Nitrophen	1-(2-nitro-4,5-dimethoxyphenyl)-N, N, N', N'-tetrakis[(oxycarbonyl)methyl]-1,2-ethanediamine
DNA	deoxyribonucleic acid
DR	delayed rectifier
EC_{50}	concentration giving half-maximal response
ECS	electroconvulsive shock
E_{GABA}	reversal potential for GABA-gated currents
eIF-2α	translation initiation factor 2 α
EM	electron microscopy
E_{Na}	equilibrium potential for Na^+
eph	subfamily of receptor tyrosine kinases (ephrins)
EPSC	excitatory postsynaptic current
EPSP	excitatory postsynaptic potential
ER	endoplasmic reticulum
E_{rev}	reversal potential
E–S	EPSP–spike potentiation
E_{syn}	synaptic reversal potential
FMR1	fragile X mental retardation protein 1
$\bar{g}_{K_A}$	maximum K^+ conductance (A type)
$\bar{g}_{K_{DR}}$	maximum K^+ conductance (delayed rectifier)
$\bar{g}_{Na}$	maximum Na^+ conductance
$\bar{g}_{AMPA}$	maximum AMPA conductance
$\bar{g}_{NMDA}$	maximum NMDA conductance
GABA	γ-aminobutyric acid
$GABA_A$	GABA receptor, type A
$GABA_B$	GABA receptor, type B
$GABA_C$	GABA receptor, type C
GAD	glutamic acid decarboxylase
GAP43	growth-associated protein 43
GDP	guanosine diphosphate
GluR	glutamate receptor
GlyR	glycine receptor
G_m	specific membrane conductance
GPI	glycosylphosphatidylinositol
GR	geometric ratio

GRE	glucocorticoid response element binding protein
g_{syn}	synaptic conductance
GTP	guanosine triphosphate
GVIA	ω-conotoxin GVIA
H	hyperpolarization-activated channel
HVA	high-voltage activated
I_{AHP}	slow AHP current
IC_{50}	concentration yielding 50% inhibition
I_{dend}	dendritic membrane current
$I-f$	current–frequency
IF	intermediate filaments
I_h	hyperpolarization-activated current
$I_{input}(x)$	current injected at distance x
IP_3	inositol 1,4,5-trisphosphate
IPSC	inhibitory postsynaptic current
IPSP	inhibitory postsynaptic potential
I_{stim}	stimulus current
I_{th}	current threshold
KA	kainate
K_A	A-type K^+ current
K_B	dissociation constant for buffer B
KC	Kenyon cell
K_D	D-type K^+ current
κ_f	binding ratio of fixed buffer
K_{ir}	inward rectifier K^+ current
κ_m	binding ratio of mobile buffer
k_{off}	dissociation rate
k_{on}	association rate
K_S	sustained (non-inactivating) K^+ current
l	length
L	electrotonic length
L-AP4	L-amino-4-phosphonobutyrate
LGMD	lobula giant motion detector neuron
LGN	lateral geniculate nucleus
LN	local neuron
LPTC	lobula plate tangential cell
LTD	long-term depression
LTP	long-term potentiation
LVA	low-voltage activated
M	molecular weight
MAP	mitogen activated protein kinase
MAP2A	microtubule associated protein 2A
MB	mushroom body
mEPSC	miniature excitatory postsynaptic current
MF	mossy fiber
mGluR	metabotropic glutamate receptor
MHC	major histocompatability antigen

mIPSC	miniature inhibitory postsynaptic current
mPSCs	miniature postsynaptic currents
mRNA	messenger ribonucleic acid
ms	milliseconds
mV	millivolts
NCAM	neural cell adhesion molecule
NMDA	*N*-methyl-D-aspartate
NR	NMDA receptor
NT-3	neurotrophin-3
NT-4/5	neurotrophin-4/neurotrophin-5
NT-6	neurotrophin-6
ODEs	ordinary differential equations
PCR	polymerase chain reaction
PD	pyloric dilator neuron
PDEs	partial differential equations
PKA	protein kinase A
PKC	protein kinase C
PLC	phospholipase C
PN	projection neuron
P_o	channel open probability
$P_{o,max}$	maximal channel open probability (at saturating transmitter concentrations)
PP	perforant path
PSA	polysialic acid
PSC	postsynaptic current
PSD	postsynaptic density
PSP	postsynaptic potential
PTP	post-tetanic potentiation
R	membrane resistance
Rac	member of the Rho family of small GTPases
Rho	a family of small GTPases
r_i	axial resistance per unit length
R_i	intracellular resistivity
r_m	membrane resistance per unit length
R_m	specific membrane resistivity
R_N	input resistance
RNA	ribonucleic acid
RT-PCR	reverse-transcriptase polymerase chain reaction
$R_{x,0}$	transfer resistance (or impedance) between x and 0 (soma)
RyR	ryanodine receptor
SBFI	sodium-binding benzofuran isophthalate
SER	smooth endoplasmic reticulum
SK	small conductance Ca^{2+}-activated K^+ channel
t	time
TAQ	*Thermus aquaticus*
tCaMKII	catalytic subunit of CaMKII
TEA	tetraethylammonium

TPA	tissue plasminogen activator
TPEN	N, N, N', N'-tetrakis-(2-pyridylmethyl)ethylenediamine
TrkA	tyrosine receptor kinase A
TrkB	tyrosine receptor kinase B
TTX	tetrodotoxin
US	unconditioned stimulus
V_{com}	command potential
V_{dend}	dendritic membrane potential
V_e	extracellular potential
V_m	membrane potential
V_{rest}	resting potential
VSCC	voltage-sensitive Ca^{2+} channel
V_{soma}	somatic membrane potential
V_{syn}	synaptic membrane potential
V_{th}	voltage threshold
X	electrotonic distance
x	dendritic location
ZD7288	I_h blocker (Zeneca Pharmaceuticals)
αDTX	α dendrotoxin
λ	space constant
λ_{ch}	chemical length constant (diffusion length)
τ_0	0th (slowest) time constant of a multi-exponential function
τ_{act}	activation time constant
τ_{ch}	chemical time constant
τ_{deact}	deactivation time constant
τ_{decay}	time constant of decaying exponential
τ_i	ith time constant of a multi-exponential function
τ_m	membrane time constant
τ_{rise}	time constant of rising exponential

1

Dendrite structure

John C. Fiala and Kristen M. Harris
Children's Hospital, Boston

Summary

Dendrites are extensions of the cell body of the neuron specialized for receiving and processing the vast majority of excitatory synaptic inputs. Dendrites exhibit enormously diverse forms. In many cases the shape of the dendritic arbor can be related to the mode of connectivity between neurons, with dendrites often ramifying in characteristic spatial domains where they receive specific inputs. At the ultrastructural level, dendrites are distinct from axons and astroglia processes, having a characteristic composition of subcellular organelles. Synapses occur directly on the shaft of some dendrites, but other dendrites have specialized enlargements and protrusions to receive synaptic input. These synaptic specializations also occur in many different forms. The use of serial electron microscopy to obtain detailed quantitative data on these structures has shown that different synaptic specializations have different intracellular organelles and synaptic compositions. Understanding the structural diversity of both dendritic arbors and synaptic specializations will be essential for understanding the intricacies of dendritic function and the contribution dendrites make to mental processes.

Introduction

What is the purpose of dendrites? Why do they exhibit such an overwhelming variety and complexity of shapes? How are their shapes related to neuronal function? Ramón y Cajal posed and, to a remarkable extent, answered these questions 100 years ago in his Histology of the Nervous System (Ramón y Cajal 1995). Ramón y Cajal established that the two types of neuronal processes, axons and dendrites, do not interconnect in anastomotic continuity. Neurons are independent entities. The many dendrites of a neuron receive electrical impulses from the axons of other neurons and conduct this activity to the neuron's own axon for transmission to other cells. This basic tenet is often referred to as the *neuron doctrine*.

Ramon y Cajal also saw that the complexity of dendrites reflects the number of connections that a neuron receives. Consider that a neuron without dendrites, having a roughly spherical cell body, has a very limited surface area for receiving inputs.

Increasing surface area by enlarging the cell body would mean prohibitive increases in cell and brain volume. Dendrites can be thought of as extensions of the cell body which provide increased surface area at much lower cell volumes. For example, 97% of the surface area of a motor neuron (excluding the axon) is dendritic (Ulfhake and Kellerth 1981). The dendrites have 370 000 μm^2 of surface area while occupying only 300 000 μm^3. To provide an equivalent surface, a spherical cell body would be 340 μm in diameter and occupy 20 000 000 μm^3. The fact that 80% of the surface area of proximal dendrites of motor neurons is covered with synapses (Kellerth *et al.* 1979) suggests that this increased surface area is indeed valuable for increasing the number of inputs to a neuron.

Dendrites make relatively local connections as compared with the axon. The axon, emerging either from the soma or a dendrite, can extend to distant targets, up to a meter or more away from the cell body in some cases (e.g. motor neurons and corticospinal projection neurons). Dendrites are rarely longer than 1–2 mm, even in the largest neurons, and are often much smaller (Table 1.1). In many neurons the diameter of dendrites at their origin from the cell body is proportional to the diameter of the cell body (Chen and Wolpaw 1994; Ulfhake and Kellerth 1981). Furthermore, these dendrites are tapered, such that the total length and the number of branches are correlated with the diameter of the proximal segment. Thus, larger neurons typically have both larger perikarya and more extensive dendritic fields (Table 1.1).

Ramon y Cajal argued that phylogenetic differences in specific neuronal morphologies support the relationship between dendritic complexity and number of connections. The complexity of many types of vertebrate neuron, including cerebellar Purkinje cells, cortical pyramidal cells, and mitral cells of the olfactory bulb, increases with increasingly complex nervous systems. These changes are driven both by the need to make more connections and by the need to make connections with additional cell types at specific locations. As expressed by Sholl (1956), it is the *mode of connectivity* between neurons that is the most critical property of their diverse morphologies.

Dendrite arbors

Classification of morphologies is difficult because of the large number of different dendritic arborization patterns in the central nervous system. For this reason, contemporary expositions often fall back on the simple scheme originated by Ramón y Cajal, in which neurons are classified as *unipolar*, *bipolar*, and *multipolar*, based on the number and orientation of processes emanating from the cell body. Ramón y Cajal intended this only as an introduction, however, and developed a detailed classification to differentiate the wide variety of multipolar neurons. A more geometrical classification of dendritic arborizations will be useful for understanding the purposes of this diversity.

The primary contribution of dendrites to the mode of connectivity of a neuron is through their characteristic branching and extension into specific spatial domains (Table 1.2). Axons from particular sources ramify within these domains, such that particular portions of the dendritic arbor receive specific inputs. A further

Table 1.1 Typical dimensions of dendrites for a few types of neuron

Neuron	Average soma diameter (μm)	Number of dendrites at soma	Proximal dendrite diameter (μm)	Number of branch points	Distal dendrite diameter (μm)	Dendrite extent* (μm)	Total dendritic length (μm)
Cerebellar granule cell (cat)	7	4	1	0	0.2–2	15	60
Starburst amacrine cell (rhesus)	9	1	1	40	0.2–2	120	–
Dentate gyrus granule cell (rat)	14	2	3	14	0.5–1	300	3200
CA1 pyramidal cell (rat)	21						11 900
basal dendrites		5	1	30	0.5–1	130	5500
stratum radiatum		1	3	30	0.25–1	110	4100
stratum lacunosum-moleculare				15	0.25–1	500	2300
Cerebellar Purkinje cell (guinea pig)	25	1	3	440	0.8–2.2	200	9100
Principal cell of globus pallidus (human)	33	4	4	12	0.3–0.5	1000	7600
Meynert cell of visual cortex (macaque)	35						15 400
basal dendrites		5	3	–	–	250	10 200
apical dendrites		1	4	15	2–3	1800	5200
Spinal α-motoneuron (cat)	58	11	8	120	0.5–1.5	1100	52 000

* The average distance from the cell body to the tips of the longest dendrites.

Sources: Ito (1984); Mariani (1990); Claiborne et al. (1990); Bannister and Larkman (1995a); Rapp et al. (1994); Palay (1978); Yelnik et al. (1984); Ulfhake and Kellerth (1981)

characteristic of dendritic branching patterns is the extent to which they fill the spatial domain of their arborization (Fig. 1.1). At one extreme, a dendrite connects a single remote target to the rest of the neuron. This is a *selective* arborization. At the other extreme, dendritic branches occupy most of the domain of arborization in a *space-filling* arborization. An example of this is the cerebellar Purkinje cell arbor that synapses with at least half of the parallel fiber axons that pass through it (Napper and Harvey 1991; Palay and Chan-Palay 1974). Most dendritic arborizations lie between the selective and space-filling varieties and are referred to as *sampling* arborizations.

Many approaches have been used to characterize the density of dendritic arborizations (Uylings *et al.* 1975). Branch ordering schemes are frequently used, such as the *centrifugal method* wherein the dendrites emerging from the cell soma are primary, their first branches are secondary and so on, with increasing order until the tips are reached. Alternatively, the *Strahler method* might be used wherein the dendritic tips are all given the order number 1 and then branch numbers are increased sequentially towards the soma. The number of dendrite segments of each order characterizes the amount of branching of the arbor. A simpler scheme is just to count the number of branch points in the entire dendritic arbor. Such schemes

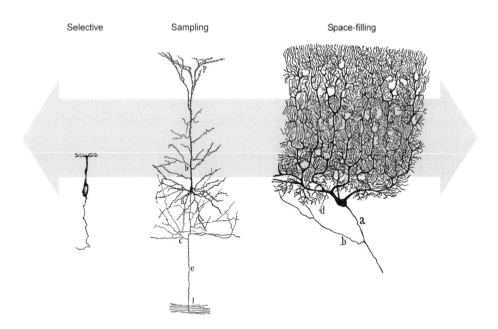

Fig. 1.1   The densities of dendritic arbors lie on a continuum of values. Differences in arbor density reflect differences in connectivity. At one extreme are selective arborizations in which each dendrite connects the cell body to a single remote target. An olfactory sensory cell is used to illustrate this. At the other extreme lie space-filling arborizations in which the dendrites cover a region, as with the cerebellar Purkinje cell. Intermediate arbor densities are referred to as sampling arborizations, as demonstrated by a pyramidal cell from cerebral cortex. (Drawings of neurons from Ramón y Cajal 1995.)

Table 1.2 Some characteristic dendritic arborization patterns

Pattern	Characteristics	Examples
Adendritic	Cell body lacks dendrites	Dorsal root ganglion cells Sympathetic ganglion cells
Spindle radiation	Two dendrites emerge from opposite poles of the cell body and have few branches	Lugaro cells Bipolar cells of cortex
Spherical radiation		
Stellate	Dendrites radiate in all directions from the cell body	Spinal neurons Neurons of subcortical nuclei (e.g. inferior olive, pons, thalamus, striatum) Cerebellar granule cells
Partial	Dendrites radiate from cell body in directions restricted to a part of a sphere	Neurons at edges of 'closed' nuclei (e.g. Clarke's column, inferior olive, vestibular nuclei)
Laminar radiation		
Planar	Dendrites radiate from cell body in all directions within a thin domain	Retinal horizontal cells
Offset	Plane of radial dendrites offset from cell body by one or more stems	Retinal ganglion cells
Multi	Cell has multiple layers of radial dendrites	Retinal amacrine cells

Table 1.2 (*cont.*)

Pattern	Characteristics	Examples
Cylindrical radiation 	Dendrites ramify from a central soma or dendrite in a thick cylindrical (disk-shaped) domain	Pallidal neurons Reticular neurons
Conical radiation 	Dendrites radiate from cell body or apical stem within a cone or paraboloid	Granule cells of dentate gyrus and olfactory bulb Primary dendrites of mitral cells of olfactory bulb Semilunar cells of piriform cortex
Biconical radiation 	Dendrites radiate in opposite directions from the cell body	Bitufted, double bouquet, and pyramidal cells of cerebral cortex Vertical cells of superior colliculus
Fan radiation 	One or a few dendrites radiate from cell body in a flat fan shape	Cerebellar Purkinje cells

provide a sense of how branched a neuron is, but do not indicate the extent to which they fill the space of their arborizations, an important factor when considering their potential for connectivity.

Another measure, *fractal dimension*, can be used to quantify the extent to which an arborization fills its spatial domain. From basic geometry, linear objects have a dimension of 1, planar objects have a dimension of 2, and solid objects, such as a sphere, have a dimension of 3. In addition, there exist objects with non-integer dimensions, often called *fractal* objects, that fill a portion of the space in which they are embedded. Dendritic arbors can be considered fractal on a limited scale (Smith *et al.* 1989). Selective arborizations have fractal dimensions close to unity while space-filling arborizations have fractal dimensions close to the dimension of the geometrical region they occupy. For instance, the fractal dimension of Purkinje cell dendritic arbors that fill the two-dimensional domain in which they ramify, is about 1.8 in mammals. In agreement with Ramón y Cajal's assessment of the phylo-genetic trend in complexity, the fractal dimension of Purkinje cells increases with phylogeny, from a value of 1.13 in the lamprey up to a value of 1.86 in man (Takeda *et al.* 1992).

Sampling arborizations have fractal dimensions greater than 1 but much less than the dimension of the spatial domain in which they arborize. For example retinal ganglion cells, which have essentially planar arbors, have a fractal dimension of approximately 1.5 (Fernandez *et al.* 1994; Wingate *et al.* 1992). To understand how the differences in fractal dimension relate to differences in connectivity, consider that a retinal ganglion cell with a sampling planar arbor covering 25 000 μm^2 receives only 2000 synapses (Sterling 1990), whereas a Purkinje cell with a space-filling planar arbor of 50 000 μm^2 receives 160 000 synapses (Harvey and Napper 1991).

Dendritic complexity can reflect a propensity for a neuron to make contacts with axons from a large number of cells or many connections with the axons of just a few cells. This depends on the axonal arborization pattern and the direction of axons relative to dendrites. For example, parallel fiber axons are orthogonal to the dendritic tree of the Purkinje cell, permitting few synapses per axon (Palay and Chan-Palay 1974). An ascending axon of a granule cell in the plane of the Purkinje arbor, however, makes as many as 17 synapses with a single Purkinje cell (Bower and Woolston 1983; Harvey and Napper 1991). Thus in brain regions where dendrites take on a characteristic orientation, the relative orientation of axons has a significant impact on connectivity.

Table 1.2 illustrates some characteristic dendrite arborization patterns ranging from *adendritic* ganglion cells, which have only a branched axon and no dendrites, to the dense *fan radiations* of cerebellar Purkinje cells. For instance, the slender neurons found throughout the brain can frequently be characterized as having a *spindle radiation*, because two sparsely-branching dendrites emerge from opposite poles of the cell body. The Lugaro cell of cerebellar cortex and the bipolar cell of cerebral cortex are examples of this pattern.

A common arborization pattern in the central nervous system is that of the *spherical radiation* (stellate) cells. These are found throughout the brain and spinal cord, and predominate in non-laminated subcortical nuclei such as the inferior olive, pontine nuclei, striatum, thalamus, etc. In most cases, stellate cells have sampling arborizations with many synapses along the length of each dendritic segment. Many nominally stellate neurons can, on closer inspection, be seen to come in characteristic patterns that are not uniformly spherical radiations. For instance, neurons near the border of a *closed* nucleus extend dendrites into only that part of the sphere that lies within the nucleus (partial spherical radiation; Table 1.2). More generally stellate neurons are often distinguishable by specific characteristics. Although attempts have been made to describe the variety of stellate types in general terms (Ramon-Moliner 1968), classification often comes down to individual characteristics. For example, in the ventral cochlear nucleus there is a unique set of descriptive morphologies:

spherical bushy, globular bushy, stellate, bushy multipolar, elongate, octopus, and giant (Ostapoff *et al.* 1994). These descriptors are not readily applicable to stellate neurons in other areas of the brain.

In some neurons, dendrites radiate in arbitrary directions from the cell body but are restricted to a planar region. This type of *laminar radiation* (Table 1.2) is seen in horizontal cells of the retina (Kolb *et al.* 1994), and in some interneurons of cortex (Parra *et al.* 1988). Dendrites of retinal ganglion cells are laminar radiations offset by an apical stem. Nearly 20 kinds of retinal ganglion cell can be distinguished by their dendritic arborization patterns (Sterling 1990). Three basic types, alpha, beta, and gamma cells (Wingate *et al.* 1992), are easily distinguished physiologically (Fukuda *et al.* 1984). Apparently the pattern of dendritic arborization of these neurons contributes to their physiological differences. The contribution of morphology to physiology is examined in more detail in Chapters 8–10.

Dendritic arbors that are truly stellate do not receive segregated inputs. In other words, the same types of axons contact all parts of the arbor. In brain areas where there are layers of cells and fibers, such as cerebral cortex, dendritic arborizations receive specific sources in specific spatial domains. For example, the arbors of some retinal ganglion cells lie in the outer third of the inner plexiform layer (Sterling 1990). These receive contacts from bipolar cells that respond to light turning off. Other retinal ganglion cells have arbors in the inner two thirds of the inner plexiform layer, receiving contacts from bipolar cells that respond to light turning on. The physiological differences between on- and off-ganglion cells arise in part from differences in their regions of dendritic arborization and sources of input.

Frequently, dendritic arbors ramify into more than one layer to access more than one type of afferent. Such is the case with the many multilaminar forms of retinal amacrine cells. At least 26 different types of amacrine cells can be identified on the basis of their dendritic arborization patterns (Mariani 1990; Kolb *et al.* 1992; MacNeil and Masland 1998). As with ganglion cells, these morphological differences almost certainly denote differences in the computational roles of these neurons, but the functions of most amacrine cell types are not yet known.

In many regions, such as the retina, there is an enormous variety of distinct neuronal shapes, but in other brain regions there appears to be relatively few. One example of the latter is the globus pallidus of primates in which small interneurons are infrequent. Principal components analysis reveals that the large pallidal neurons belong to a single population (Yelnik *et al.* 1984). The dendrites of these neurons fill cylindrical spatial domains approximately 1500×1000 μm in diameter and 250 μm thick (Tables 1.1 and 1.2). These dendritic disks are parallel to the boundaries of the globus pallidus and thus perpendicular to incoming striatal axons, such that each neuron receives a wide distribution of inputs.

Pyramidal cells often extend dendrites into two distinct conical arbors, one apical and one basal. This configuration corresponds to a *biconical radiation* (Table 1.2) and can be characterized by different afferents contacting the basal versus apical domains. Pyramidal cells are a good example of how arborization patterns depend on the cell body location relative to preferred input sources. The length of an apical dendrite of a cortical neuron depends on how far the cell body is from the outermost (e.g. plexiform) layer in which it ramifies its apical tuft. Cells very near the outermost layer usually have no apical stem, because one is not required to reach the appropriate axonal contacts (Ramón y Cajal 1995). The dendritic arbors of pyramidal cells are sampling arborizations (Porter *et al.* 1991). Because the direction of dendrites relative to that of afferent axons varies, pyramidal cells can receive many synapses from a single axon which runs parallel to a dendritic segment or few synapses from axons which traverse its dendrites perpendicularly (Sholl 1956; Sorra and Harris 1993; see also Fig. 1.2b).

Afferents sometimes traverse the apical stem dendrite of pyramidal cells, in which case additional dendritic branches emanate from the apical stem in a *cylindrical radiation*. This occurs, for example, in the large pyramidal cells of hippocampal area CA1 (Fig. 1.2a). Here, the apical tuft arborizes in stratum lacunosum-moleculare and receives perforant path input from entorhinal cortex. The middle arbor in stratum radiatum receives the Schaffer axon collaterals from CA3 pyramidal cells. The basal cone extends into stratum oriens where it receives afferents from a more proximal part of CA3 (Amaral and Witter 1989). A CA1 pyramidal cell can be characterized as having three different spatial domains of dendritic arborization, an apical cone, a basal cone, and a central cylinder, each with different sampling densities. A similar pattern is frequently seen in neocortical pyramidal cells, such as those of visual cortex (Feldman and Peters 1978).

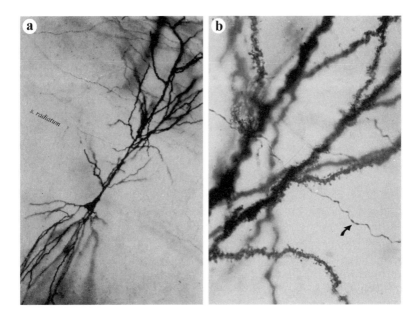

Fig. 1.2 A pyramidal cell from area CA1 of the rat hippocampus silver-impregnated using the Golgi method. This and subsequent figures are from the brains of adult rats. (a) At low magnification the basal and apical dendrites can be seen to ramify into conical domains. Additional dendrites extend obliquely from the apical stem in stratum radiatum. (b) At higher magnification numerous spines can be seen extending from the dendrites. A thinner, non-spiny process (arrow) recognizable as an axon passes nearby.

Table 1.2 summarizes some common arborization patterns but it is far from exhaustive. Just as pyramidal cells can have cylindrical radiations from the apical dendrite, many other arbors can be characterized by elaborations on or combinations of the basic patterns of Table 1.2. For instance, it is common for the apical stem of pyramidal cells in CA1 to bifurcate midway through stratum radiatum, each branch giving rise to an apical tuft (Bannister and Larkman 1995*a*). Similarly, the apical stems in mitral and tufted cells of the olfactory bulb can be branched with a tuft on the end of each branch. Thus, a *branched conical radiation* might be included in Table 1.2. Mitral cells can also exhibit a laminar radiation of secondary dendrites from the soma (Kishi *et al*. 1982). Another example is the giant pyramidal cell referred to as a Betz cell. This cell has an essentially stellate arbor around the cell body and an apical cone ramifying in the outermost layers of cortex (Ramón y Cajal 1995).

It is important to note that dendrites are not completely static structures. Individual dendrites can extend or retract over periods of days to weeks (Purves *et al*. 1986; Stern and Armstrong 1998). Much modern research into the cellular basis of learning and memory has focused on activity-dependent changes in the strength of synapses, an idea as old as the neuron doctrine itself (Tanzi 1893). But Ramón y Cajal thought that synaptic plasticity alone could not explain the slow acquisition and long-term retention of the complex skills of an expert pianist or mathematician (Ramón y Cajal 1995). He suggested that learning also involves the growth of neuronal processes, establishing new communication pathways between neurons and brain regions that were not connected before. Recent research (Chapters 2 and 14) has reawakened interest in the intriguing possibility that continual changes in the dendritic arbor could play an important role in brain function.

Intracellular structure of dendrites

Electron microscopy reveals that the contents of large proximal dendrites are similar to those of the perikaryon from which they arise (Fig. 1.3). Perikaryal organelles such as the Golgi apparatus and the granular (or rough) endoplasmic reticulum extend into the proximal dendrites, reinforcing the view that dendrites are extensions of the cell body. These characteristically perikaryal organelles diminish however, with increasing distance from the cell body and decreasing dendrite diameter.

The cytoskeleton of dendrites is composed of microtubules, neurofilaments, and actin filaments. Microtubules are long, thin structures, approximately 24 nm in diameter, oriented to the longitudinal axis of the dendrite. In regions of the dendrite free from large organelles, they are found in a regular array at a density of $50–150\ \mu m^{-2}$ (Fig. 1.4). Microtubules are typically spaced 80–200 nm apart, except in places where mitochondria or other organelles squeeze in between them. Microtubules are the 'railroad tracks' of the cell and they play an important role in the transport of mitochondria and other organelles (Overly *et al*. 1996).

Axons also contain microtubules, usually with closer spacing than in dendrites. However, the fine processes of glia do not contain microtubules ordered in a regular array. Glial processes are highly irregular, extending protrusions into narrow crevices between axonal and dendritic processes (Fig. 1.4). Axons tend to maintain a

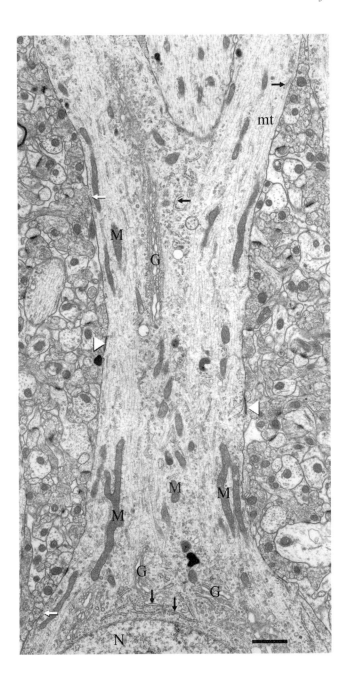

Fig. 1.3 Perikaryal organelles extend into the apical dendrite of a CA1 pyramidal cell to the first branch point. The smaller branch at the right shows fewer of the characteristically perikaryal organelles. Nucleus (N), granular endoplasmic reticulum (black arrows), Golgi apparatus (G), polyribosomes (circled), mitochondria (M), microtubules (mt), hypolemmal endoplasmic reticulum (white arrows), subsurface cisternal junctions of endoplasmic reticulum (white arrow heads). Scale bar: 1 μm.

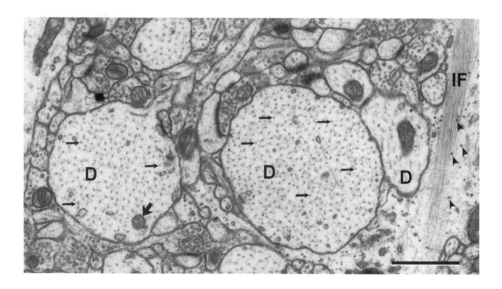

Fig. 1.4   The regular array of microtubules (small arrows) is clearly visible in large dendrites (D) shown in cross-section. A cross-sectioned mitochondrion (large arrow) is visible. A glia process is readily identified by the presence of numerous glycogen granules (arrow heads) and a bundle of intermediate filaments (IF). Scale bar: 1 µm.

consistent, convex cross-sectional shape except where they expand into varicosities containing mitochondria and/or synaptic vesicles. Small dendrites tend to be more irregular in cross-section than axons, while still maintaining convexity compared with glia. The ultrastructure of glia also differs from that of axons and dendrites in that glia characteristically contain glycogen granules and bundles of intermediate filaments (Fig. 1.4).

Smooth endoplasmic reticulum (SER) is an organelle found throughout dendrites which is thought to be involved in the regulation of calcium. SER in aldehyde-fixed brain tissue usually appears as flattened compartments (cisternae) with a clear interior, which are occasionally swollen depending on the state of the tissue or quality of preservation. These cisternae are bounded by a wavy membrane (Fig. 1.5a). Hypolemmal cisternae are those parts of the SER network which lie just beneath the plasmalemma. Often these cisternae form characteristic junctions (Fig. 1.3) that could give access to the extracellular space (Henkart *et al.* 1976). In the three-dimensional view obtained by reconstruction from serial sections (Fig. 1.5b), the cisternae of SER form a continuous reticulum throughout the dendrites (Harris and Stevens 1988, 1989; Martone *et al.* 1993; Spacek and Harris 1997).

Organelles of the early endosomal pathway involved in membrane protein sorting and recycling are common in dendrites. *Recycling endosomes* appear as tubular compartments that are not part of a reticulum (Fig. 1.5a). These can be distinguished from SER by their darker interior, more uniform diameter, and the frequent occurrence of specialized coats at the ends of the tubule. These coated ends might represent sites of budding of recycling vesicles bound for the plasmalemma

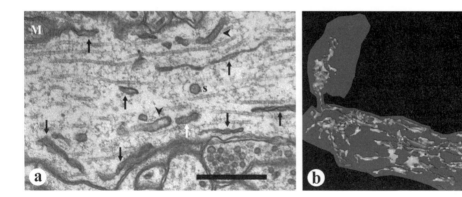

Fig. 1.5 The smooth endoplasmic reticulum (SER) forms a continuous compartment in dendrites. (a) Pieces of SER appear as thin cisternae with wavy membranes (black arrows). SER cisternae can be seen in continuity with the outer membrane of mitochondria (M). (See also Spacek and Lieberman 1980). Endosomal compartments (black arrow heads) are tubes which do not connect in a reticulum throughout the dendrite. These have a uniform diameter and dark, grainy interior. Recycling endosomes frequently have a coated tip at one end (white arrow). The spherical vesicle (s) with its dark interior is related to the endosomal compartments, but it is unclear whether it will merge with or has just budded from a recycling endosome. Scale: 0.5 µm. (b) Three-dimensional reconstruction of the SER in a different dendrite and spine reveals the interconnectivity of the cisternae.

(Bauerfeind *et al.* 1996). *Sorting endosomes* can be identified by the occurrence of similar tubular compartments connected to larger, spherical organelles with interior vesicles (Gruenberg and Maxfield 1995). These spherical compartments mature into *multivesicular bodies*, separate from the sorting endosome, and are transported to the cell body for processing in late endosomes and lysosomes (Parton *et al.* 1992). Thus, multivesicular bodies in dendrites occur alone or in conjunction with the sorting endosome compartments (Fig. 1.6). In three dimensions the latter complex can be seen to emanate many tubular profiles with coated tips (Fig. 1.6b).

Coated pits and vesicles representing the initial step in endocytosis are frequently seen in dendrites (Fig. 1.7a). The cytoplasmic coat is composed of *clathrin* (Brodsky 1988) giving it a distinctive periodic structure recognizable as the same coat found on the tips of early endosomes. Clathrin-coated vesicles uncoat less than a minute after their formation from a coated pit (Fine and Ockleford 1984). For this reason coated vesicles are found only in the vicinity of their locus of generation within the dendrite. Coated vesicles and coated pits occur more frequently in dendrites during development (Altman 1971) and during periods of synaptic remodeling (McWilliams and Lynch 1981).

Ribosomes are sites of protein synthesis within cells. Free ribosomes, those not attached to ER, occur throughout the cytoplasm of dendrites at a very low density compared with the perikaryon. Frequently, they are closely clustered into groups of 3 to 30 (Fig. 1.7b), called *polyribosomes* (Steward and Reeves 1988). Groups of polyribosomes often occur together in dendrites, especially at the branch points. In contrast to dendrites, axons are generally devoid of ribosomes, suggesting that new

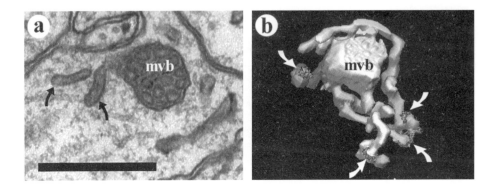

Fig. 1.6 Sorting endosomes form complex structures which include multivesicular bodies. (a) A multivesicular body (mvb) with its connected tubular compartments of sorting endosome (arrows) in a hippocampal pyramidal cell dendrite. Scale: 0.25 μm. (b) Three-dimensional reconstruction of a sorting endosome from a different dendrite. The tubular sorting compartments often end in coated tips (arrows) with the same appearance as in Fig. 1.5(a). The top of the multivesicular body (mvb) is removed to reveal the interior vesicles.

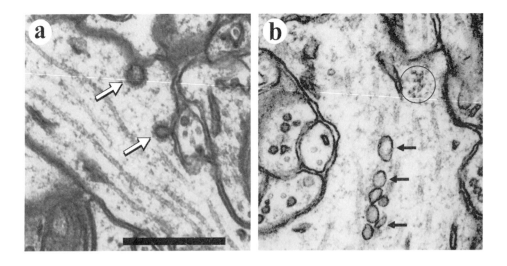

Fig. 1.7 Some other ultrastructural features frequently found in distal dendrites. (a) Clathrin-coated pits (arrows) are the initial step in the endosomal pathway. These pits can form into vesicles destined for recycling endosomes. (b) This section of dendrite contains polyribosomes (circled) and a string of large, clear vesicles (arrows) similar in appearance to strings of vesicles in the Golgi apparatus. Scale: 0.5 μm.

proteins are transported from the cell body rather than manufactured within the axon.

Mitochondria in dendrites are usually elongated and oriented with their long axis parallel to the microtubules. Given their likely roles in calcium signalling and prevention of excitotoxicity (Miller 1998), it is interesting that mitochondria are not distributed uniformly throughout the dendritic arbor. Larger, proximal dendrites have fewer mitochondria per unit of cross-sectional area than thinner distal dendrites (Peters *et al.* 1991). For example, in stratum radiatum of area CA1 mitochondria comprise about 2% of intracellular space in the apical stem dendrites, while filling 13% of the thinnest branches in the apical tuft (Nafstad and Blackstad 1966).

Synaptic specializations of dendrites

Although a dendrite is adjacent to many axons and other dendrites throughout its length, functional connectivity occurs at specialized sites where neurons communicate. These are called *synapses*. 'Synapses' is the plural of synapsis, a term first employed by Foster and Sherrington (Foster 1897). Synapsis means 'connection' (Murray *et al.* 1919), *apropos* for the site of connectivity between neurons. In modern usage, the singular of synapses is usually expressed as *synapse*. Synapses are made on the surface of the dendrite, so called *shaft* synapses, but many synapses lie on specialized enlargements of or protrusions from the dendrites (Table 1.3). Shaft synapses are only 5% of all synapses on the pyramidal cell dendrites in stratum radiatum (Harris *et al.* 1992; Kirov *et al.* 1999).

An example of a synaptic specialization of a dendrite is found in amacrine cells of the retina. The dendrites of AI amacrine cells are not tapered in the same way as motoneurons. They are very thin and have numerous *varicosities* or swellings at contacts with rod bipolar cells (Ellias and Stevens 1980). The varicosities receive synapses from rod bipolar cells. In addition, these varicosities contain synaptic vesicles and make reciprocal synapses on the rod bipolar cells. There are other examples of presynaptic dendrites in the nervous system, such as in granule, mitral and tufted cells of the olfactory bulb, although these do not necessarily have similar varicosities.

Filopodia are another synaptic specialization of dendrites. All neurons exhibit dendritic filopodia transiently during development (Morest 1969). As discussed in Chapter 2, filopodia seem to play a role in synaptogenesis, making numerous nascent synaptic contacts (Fiala *et al.* 1998). Filopodia are rarely seen on dendrites in normal adult brain, perhaps because such long protrusions are not required for establishing new contacts. Adult neuropil is densely packed with axonal boutons, such that only a short dendritic outgrowth is required for a dendrite to encounter a new presynaptic partner.

The most common synaptic specializations of dendrites are *simple spines*. Spines are protrusions from the dendrite of usually no more than 2 μm, often ending in a bulbous head attached to the dendrite by a narrow stalk or neck (Figs 1.2b and 1.8). Simple spines are frequent on the dendrites of cerebral pyramidal cells, striatal neurons, granule cells of the dentate gyrus, cartwheel cells of the dorsal cochlear nucleus, and cerebellar Purkinje cells, to name a few *spiny* neurons. More generally

Table 1.3 Synaptic specializations of dendrites

Pattern	Characteristics	Examples
Varicosity	An enlargement in a thinner dendrite associated with synaptic contacts	Retinal amacrine cells
Filopodium	A long, thin protrusion with a dense actin matrix and few internal organelles	Normally only seen during development
Simple spine		
Sessile	Synaptic protrusions without a neck constriction	
	Stubby spine	Pyramidal cells of cortex
	Crook thorn	Cerebellar dentate nucleus
Pedunculated	Bulbous enlargement at tip	
	Thin spine	Pyramidal cells of cortex
	Mushroom spine	Pyramidal cells of cortex
	Gemmule	Olfactory bulb granule cell
Branched spine	Each branch has a unique presynaptic partner and each branch has the shape characteristics of a simple spine	CA1 pyramidal cells Granule cells of dentate gyrus Cerebellar Purkinje cells
Claw ending	Synaptic protrusions at the tip of the dendrite associated with one or more glomeruli	Granule cells of cerebellar cortex and dorsal cochlear nucleus

Table 1.3   (*cont.*)

Pattern	Characteristics	Examples
Brush ending	Spray of complex dendritic protrusions at the end of dendrite that extends into glomerulus and contains presynaptic elements	Unipolar brush cells of cerebellar cortex and dorsal cochlear nucleus
Thorny excrescence	Densely lobed dendritic protrusion into a glomerulus	Proximal dendrites of CA3 pyramidal cells and dentate gyrus mossy cells
Racemose appendage	Twig-like branched dendritic appendages that contain synaptic varicosities and bulbous tips	Inferior olive Relay cells of lateral geniculate nucleus
Coralline excrescence	Dendritic varicosity extending numerous thin protrusions, velamentous expansions and tendrils	Cerebellar dentate nucleus Lateral vestibular nucleus

neurons are classified as *spiny*, *sparsely spiny*, and *non-spiny* (or *smooth*) according to the density of simple spines on their dendrites (Peters and Jones 1984). Such a classification is complicated by the fact that different dendrites of a given neuron can exhibit widely different spine densities (Feldman and Peters 1978). Even along the length of a dendritic segment, spine densities can vary widely. Nominally non-spiny dendrites often have a few simple spines.

Determining the density of spines on dendrites is difficult because of their small size. With light microscopy, the dendrite obscures spines that lie above or below it in the section such that only the spines extending laterally can be accurately counted. Nor is this problem completely remedied by three-dimensional confocal microscopy. To compensate, many studies have applied correction factors for hidden spines (Bannister and Larkman 1995*b*; Trommald *et al.* 1995). A more accurate estimate of spine density can be obtained by use of serial electron microscopy (EM). By reconstructing cross-sectioned dendrites from EM (Fig. 1.8), all spines, including the shortest, can be counted. In addition, serial EM enables accurate determination of spine dimensions as described below.

When the spine density on the dendrites of CA1 pyramidal cells is estimated, different values are obtained for different regions of the arbor. Spines are most dense on the lateral branches of the apical stem in stratum radiatum where they average about 3 μm^{-1} of dendrite as measured by both serial EM (Harris *et al.* 1992) and by light microscopy with correction (Bannister and Larkman 1995*b*; Trommald *et al.* 1995). On the dendrites of the apical and basal cones there are 1.4 spines μm^{-1} and 2.4 spines μm^{-1}, respectively (Bannister and Larkman 1995*b*). In total, CA1 pyramidal cells have $\sim$30 000 spines, with 50% located in stratum radiatum and 40% in stratum oriens. By comparison, pyramidal cells of visual cortex are much less spiny. Total counts of only 15 000 spines are obtained for large pyramidal cells in visual cortex, with a maximum density of 1.5 spines μm^{-1} (Larkman 1991). Much higher spine densities (7.2 spines μm^{-1}) are found on certain neostriatal neurons (Graveland *et al.* 1985). The spiniest neuron in the brain might be the cerebellar

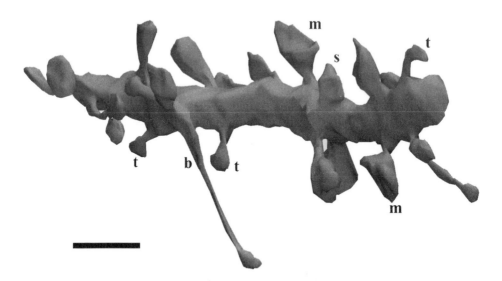

Fig. 1.8 This segment of spiny dendrite from stratum radiatum of area CA1 was reconstructed from 71 serial section electron micrographs (Harris and Stevens 1989). The 7-μm segment has 17 simple spines and three branched spines for a total of 23 spine heads. In evidence are stubby (s), thin (t), and mushroom (m) spine shapes. Although this view of the dendrite was carefully chosen, it is apparent that obtaining an accurate spine count would be difficult by light microscopy. Only one of the branched spines (b) can be observed from this viewpoint. Scale: 1 μm.

Purkinje cell, with spine densities reaching as much as 15 spines μm^{-1} (Harris and Stevens 1988). There are so many spines on spiny neurons that they contribute substantially to the surface area of the cell. In the case of the CA1 pyramidal cell, spines contribute nearly half of the dendritic surface area (Bannister and Larkman 1995*b*).

Occasionally, two or more simple spines share a common stalk. These are called *branched spines* (Table 1.3). The individual branches exhibit the same range of morphologies as simple spines (Fig. 1.8) and rarely synapse with the same bouton (Harris and Stevens 1988; Trommald and Hullenberg 1997; Sorra *et al.* 1998). Branched spines occur infrequently on spiny neurons, being only 2% of all dendritic protrusions on CA1 pyramidal cells (Harris *et al.* 1992) or dentate granule cells (Trommald and Hullenberg 1997). Apparently, branched spines are formed by accidental proximity of spine origins. This is a rare event because spine origins have a non-random tendency to separate (Trommald *et al.* 1995; Ward *et al.* 1995). Branched spines are more frequent on dendrites with higher spine densities, such as Purkinje cell dendrites where approximately 6% of spines are branched (Harris and Stevens 1988). Likewise, higher spine densities lead to larger numbers of branches per occurrence. Up to 5 branches have been found on cerebellar Purkinje cells (Harris and Stevens 1988) whereas CA1 branched spines rarely have more than two branches (Sorra *et al.* 1998).

When large axon terminals interact with dendrites, they often do so in synaptic complexes called glomeruli. Dendrites extend complex, multilobed protrusions into these glomeruli to make large areas of synaptic contact, thereby strengthening the efficacy of the connection between the neurons. A simple example is the *claw endings* of the dendrites of granule cells of cerebellar cortex, which make several synapses with a mossy fiber axon terminal (Eccles *et al.* 1967). Another type of specialized dendritic ending associated with some cerebellar glomeruli is the brush endings of unipolar brush cells (Table 1.3). These multilobed protrusions have a unique appearance which may be related to the fact that they are presynaptic to the claw endings of cerebellar granule cells and postsynaptic to mossy fiber rosettes (Mugnaini *et al.* 1994).

In hippocampus, another type of mossy fiber with large boutons makes contact on the *thorny excrescences* of CA3 pyramidal cells. CA3 pyramidal cells have large numbers of simple spines, but 90% of the dendritic protrusions on the proximal apical dendrite of pyramidal cells are thorny excrescences (Chicurel and Harris 1992). The complexity of these thorny excrescences varies, with some having many lobes and others having just a few. Three-dimensional reconstructions have been obtained of excrescences with as many as 16 lobes, all of which synapse with a single giant mossy fiber bouton. The density of lobes in thorny excrescences often gives them the appearance of a bunch of grapes (Hama *et al.* 1994). A more sparsely lobed appearance characterizes the *racemose appendages* seen in inferior olive (Ruigrok *et al.* 1990) and lateral reticular nucleus (Hrycyshyn and Flumerfelt 1981).

A final example, that by no means exhausts the kinds of synaptic specializations of dendrites, is the *coralline excrescences* found on dendrites of the small neurons of the cerebellar and vestibular nuclei. These complex varicosities have numerous synaptic protrusions (Chan-Palay 1977) and sometimes thin tendrils similar in appearance to filopodia (Morest 1969; Sotelo and Angaut 1973). This appearance of filopodia, in adult animals, lead to the suggestion that these coralline excrescences represent growth processes of dendrites.

Like the dendrites themselves, dendritic synaptic specializations are not static structures (Chapter 14). In cases where they have been studied by time-lapse microscopy (Dailey and Smith 1996; Dunaevsky *et al.* 1998; Fischer *et al.* 1998), they seem to be highly motile structures. The heads of simple pedunculated spines seem to be in constant motion, continually changing shape, and swaying on their necks. Recent data support the idea that spines extend and retract under the influence of changes in activity (Kirov and Harris 1998), possibly with a time-course of just a few minutes (Halpain *et al.* 1998; Engert and Bonhoeffer 1999; Maletic *et al.* 1999).

Shapes of simple spines

The diversity of structure in synaptic specializations of dendrites is most effectively studied with serial EM. This methodology has been used most extensively to study simple spines on spiny neurons. In the mature brain simple spines vary greatly in size (Table 1.4), with volumes ranging from less than 0.01 μm^3 to more than 1.5 μm^3. Simple spines of different sizes and shapes can be neighbors on the same parent dendrite (Harris and Kater 1994), and occasionally form synapses with the same presynaptic bouton (Sorra and Harris 1993). These observations suggest that dendritic synaptic specializations are unique units that are not determined uniformly by cell type or presynaptic partner.

In pyramidal cells, two principal types of simple spine can be distinguished: *sessile* and *pedunculated* (Jones and Powell 1969). Sessile spines do not have a substantial neck constriction (Fig. 1.8). Sessile spines are often called *stubby* spines (Peters and Kaiserman-Abramof 1970), especially when the length of the spine is less than or equal to its width (Harris *et al.* 1992). The bulbous head of pedunculated spines attaches to the dendrite through a thin stalk or neck. Among pedunculated spines, two varieties are commonly distinguished. *Thin* spines are those with a small head (Fig. 1.8). Large-headed spines, those with a spine head diameter greater than 0.6 μm, are called *mushroom* spines (Fig. 1.8).

Not all spiny neurons have the same distribution of spine shapes as pyramidal cells (Fig. 1.9). For example, spines on the tertiary dendrites of cerebellar Purkinje cells constitute a single morphological class with head diameters similar to thin spines on pyramidal cells and neck diameters similar to those of mushroom spines (Spacek and Hartmann 1983). In other spiny neurons there is a continuum of spine shapes, with clear stubby, thin, and mushroom varieties but many spines intermediate between these shapes. For instance, some mushroom spines have very long necks, whereas some thin spines have rather large heads. This makes distinct shape classes difficult to distinguish (Trommald and Hullenberg 1997; Wilson *et al.* 1983). Still, the majority of simple spines have a thin shape (Graveland *et al.* 1985; Harris *et al.* 1992; Peters and Kaiserman-Abramof 1970).

Additional types of simple spines are found on specific neurons. One example is the bent sessile spines in cerebellar dentate nucleus called *crook thorns* (Chan-Palay 1977). The granule cells of the olfactory bulb have particularly large pedunculated spines sometimes referred to as *gemmules*. These spines can be 5 μm long, with heads 1–2 μm in diameter (Cameron *et al.* 1991).

Table 1.4 Dimensions of simple spines on spiny neurons

Neuron	Total length (µm)	Neck diameter (µm)	Neck length (µm)	Total volume (µm^3)	Total surface area (µm^2)	PSD area (µm^2)	PSD/head area ratio
Cerebellar Purkinje cell	0.7–3.0	0.1–0.3	0.1–2	0.06–0.2	0.7–2	0.04–0.4	0.17 ± 0.09
CA1 pyramidal cell	0.2–2	0.04–0.5	0.1–2	0.004–0.6	0.1–4	0.01–0.5	0.12 ± 0.06
Visual cortex pyramidal cell	0.5–3	0.07–0.5	–	0.02–0.8	0.5–5	0.02–0.7	0.10 ± 0.04
Neostriatal spiny neuron	–	0.1–0.3	0.6–2	0.04–0.3	0.6–3	0.02–0.3	0.125
Dentate gyrus granule cell	0.2–2	0.05–0.5	0.03–0.9	0.003–0.2	0.1–3	0.003–0.2	–

Sources: Harris and Stevens (1988); Harris and Stevens (1989); Spacek and Hartman (1983); Wilson et al. (1983); Trommald and Hullenberg (1997).

a

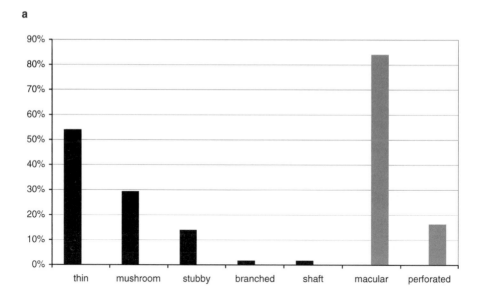

b

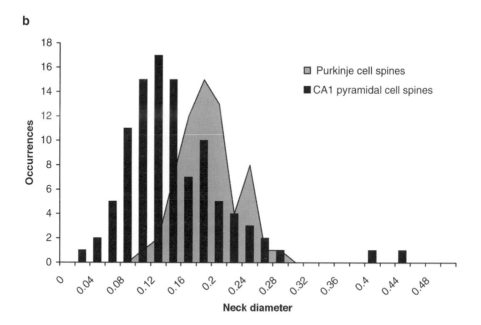

Fig. 1.9 The distribution of simple spine shapes as determined by three-dimensional reconstruction. (a) Spines with a thin shape are most frequent in stratum radiatum of area CA1. These spines tend to have macular synapses (see text), the most common synapse shape. (b) Measured neck diameters show a skewed distribution, with CA1 pyramidal cell spine necks tending to be thinner than those of spines from cerebellar Purkinje cell tertiary dendrites.

The separation of simple spines into thin-necked and thick-necked varieties might be functionally relevant because the presence of a neck constriction can serve to isolate the spine head compartment from the dendrite (Holmes 1990; Koch and Zador 1993; Svoboda *et al.* 1996). The distribution of spine neck diameters on most spiny neurons does not follow a normal distribution (Fig. 1.9b). Rather, the distribution is skewed toward larger neck sizes (Trommald and Hullenberg 1997; Wilson *et al.* 1983). This, and the fact that cerebellar spines have spine neck dimensions similar to thick-necked spines on pyramidal cells (Spacek and Hartmann 1983), suggest the possibility of a functionally distinct thick-necked spine class.

Simple spines occasionally have even smaller protrusions that extend into the interior of surrounding structures such as boutons or glia. These *spinules* are surrounded by invaginations of apposed membrane often with a clathrin-like coat visible on the cytoplasmic side at the tip of the invagination (Fig. 1.10). Spinules in the hippocampus originate from all parts of the spine surface, often at the edges of synapses (Westrum and Blackstad 1962; Tarrant and Routtenberg 1977; Sorra *et al.* 1998). Although the function of spinules is not known, it might involve bulk membrane recycling, because spinules are increased after intense stimulation (Applegate and Landfield 1988). Similar structures are found on other types of synaptic specializations, such as on the claw endings of cerebellar granule cells (Eccles *et al.* 1967) and on the lobes of thorny excrescences (Chicurel and Harris 1992).

Intracellular structure of synaptic specializations

The diversity of shapes of synaptic specializations is accompanied by a diversity in intracellular composition. The size of a synaptic specialization seems to be a factor in its composition. Small dendritic protrusions such as simple spines rarely contain

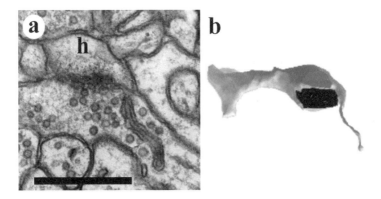

Fig. 1.10   A thin spine from stratum radiatum with a long spinule extending from the edge of the synapse. (a) The spinule extends from the head of the spine (h) into the presynaptic bouton. Scale: 0.5 μm. (b) Three-dimensional reconstruction of the entire spine with the area of synaptic contact shown in black.

microtubules. Simple spines have actin-based cytoskeletons that can facilitate rapid, calcium-induced changes in spine structure (Fifkova 1985; Fischer *et al.* 1998) or spine loss (Halpain *et al.* 1998). Similarly, microtubules are absent from filopodia even though they are present in the dendrites from which they arise. Occasionally, microtubules contribute to the cytoskeletons of larger synaptic specializations such as thorny excrescences (Chicurel and Harris 1992; Ebner and Colonnier 1975).

Another major difference between large and small synaptic specializations is the presence of mitochondria. Filopodia and simple spines rarely contain mitochondria. An exception is the large spines of olfactory bulb granule cells that often have mitochondria in the head. Because these spines make reciprocal synapses on mitral cell dendrites, it has been suggested that the presence of mitochondria might be related to presynaptic function (Cameron *et al.* 1991). Other specializations with presynaptic functions such as the varicosities of AI amacrine cells and the brush endings of unipolar brush cells likewise contain numerous mitochondria. However, thorny excrescences and claw endings are not presynaptic and they can also contain a mitochondrion in the head of a protrusion. The larger synaptic specializations of the relay cells of lateral geniculate nucleus also contain many mitochondria without having a presynaptic function (Wilson *et al.* 1984).

Most synaptic specializations also contain SER (Figs 1.5 and 1.11). These cisternae are continuous with the reticulum in the dendrite. Thin spines and filopodia contain relatively little SER. In claw endings of cerebellar granule cells, each mitochondrion is surrounded by a single cistern of SER. Larger spines contain larger amounts of SER that often becomes laminated into a characteristic appearance (Fig. 1.11) called the *spine apparatus* (Gray 1959). Mushroom spines and gemmules frequently contain spine apparati, as do the thorny excrescences of area CA3.

Smooth and coated vesicles, endosomes, and polyribosomes also occur in synaptic specializations (Fig. 1.11; see also Spacek and Harris 1997). However the complement of organelles in each instance is unique, suggesting local regulation of subcellular functions, possibly in response to different levels of neuronal activity. In dentate granule cells, as many as 80% of polyribosome clusters in dendrites lie within or at the base of spines, while only 12% of spines have these polyribosome clusters (Steward *et al.* 1996). In hippocampal area CA1, serial EM analyses reveal that more than 50% of spines have some polyribosomes (Harris and Spacek 1995). A similarly high frequency was found in the lobes of thorny excrescences using serial EM (Chicurel and Harris 1992), suggesting that polyribosomes are more common in synaptic specializations than is obvious through single section analysis.

The synapses on synaptic specializations have also been extensively examined with EM. Most synapses in the brain are chemical synapses. This is the principal type of synapse found on the synaptic specializations of dendrites. A chemical synapse consists of apposed membranes separated by a gap called the *synaptic cleft* (Fig. 1.12). Neurotransmitters released from synaptic vesicles on the presynaptic side of the cleft diffuse across the cleft to activate receptors in the postsynaptic membrane. The presynaptic element is usually a varicosity or end bulb of an axon, called a *bouton*.

In aldehyde-fixed tissue, several different types of chemical synapse can be distinguished based on the size and shape of the presynaptic vesicles and the form of the perisynaptic structures (Peters and Palay 1996). Two principal types are

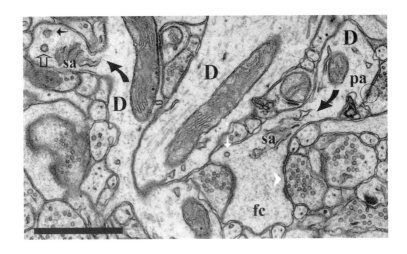

Fig. 1.11 Simple spines contain a unique complement of organelles. Dendrites (D) from stratum radiatum give rise to large spines (large arrows). The spines contain mainly a darker, floccular cytoplasm (fc) consistent with a denser actin matrix. The spines contain a specialization of SER called the spine apparatus (sa). A further extension of SER can be seen in one spine (small arrow). This spine also contains a spherical vesicle (open arrow). The other large spine contains a smaller clear profile (white arrow) that can be seen to be a tubule, perhaps endosomal, in cross-section by examining adjacent serial sections. The bouton presynaptic to this spine wraps around the spine head so that the synapse appears on both sides in this section. The postsynaptic density has a gap, or perforation, on one side (white arrow head). Also visible in this section is a puncta adhaerens junction (pa; see text) next to a symmetric synapse. Scale: 1 μm.

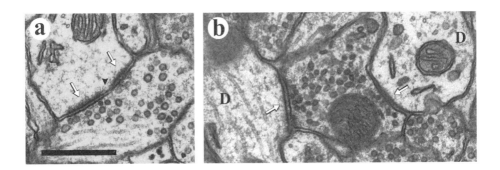

Fig. 1.12 The two most common types of synapse seen in the brain are asymmetrical and symmetrical types with small vesicles. (a) The asymmetrical synapse is characterized by a thick postsynaptic density (arrows) and small, round vesicles presynaptically. This synapse, located on a stubby protrusion, has a perforation (arrow head). (b) The symmetrical synapse is characterized by equal densities pre- and postsynaptically, and small, flattened vesicles presynaptically. This bouton makes two symmetrical synapses (arrows) on the shafts of two different dendrites (D). Scale: 0.5 μm.

commonly referred to as *asymmetric* and *symmetric* synapses. Asymmetric synapses are characterized by round presynaptic vesicles ~ 30–50 nm in diameter and a *postsynaptic density* (Fig. 1.12a). The postsynaptic density (PSD) is a densely stained structure that contains numerous receptors, structural proteins, and signaling molecules that are important for synaptic transmission and plasticity (Kennedy 1997). Symmetric synapses have a much thinner postsynaptic density, matched by an equal density on the presynaptic side (Fig. 1.12b). In addition, many of the presynaptic vesicles at symmetric synapses appear flattened rather than round. Asymmetric synapses are usually excitatory and contain the neurotransmitter glutamate. In contrast, symmetric synapses usually contain the inhibitory neuro-transmitters GABA or glycine, and often neuromodulatory peptides.

In visual cortex 84% of synapses are asymmetric and 16% are symmetric (Beaulieu and Colonnier 1985). Most of the asymmetric synapses (79%) occur on dendritic spines; 21% occur on dendrite shafts, and very few (0.1%) are found on cell bodies. The inhibitory synapses show a different pattern. Most (62%) are found on dendrite shafts; 31% occur on dendritic spines, and 7% occur on cell bodies. Thus, symmetric synapses are only 7% of all dendritic spine synapses, but 93% of all soma synapses in this brain region.

Simple spines typically have a single asymmetric synapse located on the spine head. Occasionally spines have a second synapse, usually on the spine neck (Spacek and Hartmann 1983). The second synapse can be either symmetric or asymmetric (Jones and Powell 1969). In neostriatum, approximately 8% of spines receive a second symmetric synapse (Wilson *et al.* 1983). The striatal neurons that make reciprocal connections with substantia nigra have an additional 39% of their spines contacted by a different (probably dopaminergic) type of symmetric synapse containing large, pleomorphic vesicles (Freund *et al.* 1984).

Glomeruli often contain inhibitory axons in addition to the primary excitatory terminals. Thus it is common for synaptic specializations that project into glomeruli to receive multiple types of synaptic contact. For example, the racemose append-ages of inferior olivary neurons receive both excitatory and inhibitory synapses (De Zeeuw *et al.* 1990).

When viewed in three dimensions, synapses can be seen to exhibit size-dependent variations in morphology (Spacek and Hartmann 1983). Small synapses, like those on the heads of thin spines, are typically *macular* (Fig. 1.9), consisting of a single round region without holes (Fig. 1.13). Larger synaptic junctions often have interior regions devoid of pre- and postsynaptic density. These synapses can be U-shaped, annular, or exhibit multiple holes, and are often called *perforated* synapses. In some cases, a contact between a single bouton and a dendrite is composed of two or more disjoint synaptic regions. This type of perforated synapse is sometimes referred to as a *segmented*, or multifocal, synapse (Geinisman *et al.* 1987).

Macular and perforated synapses are found on simple spines as well as on the shafts of dendrites. When located on spines, the synaptic area occupies approxi-mately 10% of the surface area of the spine head (Spacek and Hartmann 1983). This relationship between synapse and spine area is consistent over different spine morphologies and neuron types. This relationship seems to hold for more compli-cated synaptic specializations also, such as the thorny excrescences of CA3 (Chicurel and Harris 1992). Spine surface area, spine volume, SER volume, bouton volume,

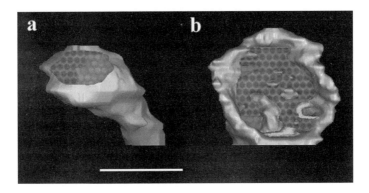

Fig. 1.13 Three-dimensional reconstruction of perforated and macular synapses. (a) The region with dark circles (left) indicates the synaptic area of a macular synapse. This is adjacent to a large puncta adhaerens junction (light circles; right) between the spine and the presynaptic bouton. (b) A perforated synapse (dark circles) has places in the interior of the synaptic region which are non-synaptic, seen as islands of gray spine head within the synapse. Puncta adhaerentia are also present (light circles; lower and upper left). Scale: 1 μm.

and number of synaptic vesicles are all highly correlated with synapse size (Harris and Stevens 1988, 1989; Harris and Sultan 1995). Thus, smaller thin spines have smaller synapses, which tend to be macular. Larger mushroom spines have larger synapses, which tend to be perforated (Harris and Stevens 1989; Harris *et al.* 1992).

It has been suggested that synapse perforations might be related to synaptic plasticity, representing a state of enhanced efficacy or an intermediate stage in a process of synapse proliferation through splitting (Jones and Harris 1995). Spinous synapses do not appear to split, however (Sorra *et al.* 1998). Instead, perforations might be related to the excess membrane inserted during synaptic vesicle fusion prior to bulk endocytosis (Shupliakov *et al.* 1997). Many aspects of the synaptic anatomy, such as the number of synaptic vesicles, the frequency and appearance of membrane recycling components, and the curvature of the synapse, might be related to functional state (Van Harreveld and Trubatch 1975; Applegate and Landfield 1988).

Cell-adhesion junctions, sometimes referred to as *puncta adhaerentia* (Figs 1.11 and 1.13), are occasionally located at the edges of the PSDs of simple spines (Spacek and Harris 1998). These junctions contain a different set of structural and signaling molecules from those in the PSD (Fannon and Colman 1996; Fields and Ito 1997). Puncta might also modulate synaptic efficacy because their disassembly and re-assembly might be needed for synaptic plasticity (Luthl *et al.* 1994; Muller *et al.* 1996; Tang *et al.* 1996).

Finally, synapses differ in the extent to which they are surrounded by glial processes. In cerebellar cortex, nearly all spine synapses are completely ensheathed by the Bergmann astroglial processes (Spacek 1985). In contrast, only 58% of hippocampal synapses have even partial astroglial ensheathment (Ventura and Harris 1999), comparable with cortical spine synapses (Spacek 1985). Thus many, but certainly not all synapses have astrocytic processes at their perimeter, whereby neurotransmitter could be detected and spillover between neighboring synapses limited (Bergles and Jahr 1997; Diamond *et al.* 1998; Luscher *et al.* 1998). An important question is whether the amount of astrocytic ensheathment is regulated by activity, such that astrocytic processes grow to synapses where glutamate is escaping from the synaptic cleft (Cornell-Bell *et al.* 1990).

Concluding remarks

A hundred years after Ramón y Cajal, the intricacies of the relationship between structure and function in neurons are still being discovered. The pattern of dendritic arborization is clearly related to connectivity, but also seems to contribute to dendritic computation, particularly when the dendrite is endowed with active mechanisms (Shepherd 1998). Similarly, the synaptic specializations extended by dendrites contribute significantly to connectivity. They enable thin dendrites to reach multiple axons such that larger numbers of synapses interdigitate in a relatively small brain volume. However, they probably have additional functions related to neuronal computation and learning (Shepherd 1996). The enormous diversity in the structure, composition, and plasticity of dendrites and their synaptic specializations suggests that the functional contributions of these structures to mind and brain are enormously diverse.

Acknowledgements

Thanks to Marcia Feinberg and Karen Szumowski for assistance with the figures. Thanks also to Betsy Velasquez for assistance with the bibliographic material. Contributions to some three-dimensional reconstructions were made by Josef Spacek and Rachel Ventura. This work was supported by NIH grants NS21184, NS33574, Human Brain Project (HBP) grant R01 MH/DA 57351 (KMH) and MR center grant P30-HD18655 (Dr. Joseph Volpe, PI). The HBP research is funded jointly by NIMH, NIDA, and NASA.

References

Altman, J. (1971). Coated vesicles and synaptogenesis. A developmental study in the cerebellar cortex of the rat. *Brain Research*, **30**, 311–22.

Amaral, D. G. and Witter, M. P. (1989). The three-dimensional organization of the hippocampal formation: a review of anatomical data. *Neuroscience*, **31**, 571–91.

Applegate, M. D. and Landfield, P. W. (1988). Synaptic vesicle redistribution during hippocampal frequency potentiation and depression in young and aged rats. *Journal of Neuroscience*, **8**, 1096–111.

Bannister, N. J. and Larkman, A. U. (1995a). Dendritic morphology of CA1 pyramidal neurones from the rat hippocampus: I. Branching patterns. *Journal of Comparative Neurology*, **360**, 150–60.

Bannister, N. J. and Larkman, A. U. (1995b). Dendritic morphology of CA1 pyramidal neurones from the rat hippocampus: II. Spine distributions. *Journal of Comparative Neurology*, **360**, 161–71.

Bauerfeind, R., Galli, T., and De Camilli, P. (1996). Molecular mechanisms in synaptic vesicle recycling. *Journal of Neurocytology*, **25**, 701–15.

Beaulieu, C. and Colonnier, M. (1985). A laminar analysis of the number of round-asymmetrical and flat-symmetrical synapses on spines, dendritic trunks, and cell bodies in area 17 of the cat. *Journal of Comparative Neurology*, **231**, 180–89.

Bergles, D. E. and Jahr, C. E. (1997). Synaptic activation of glutamate transporters in hippocampal astrocytes. *Neuron*, **19**, 1297–308.

Bower, J. M. and Woolston, D. C. (1983). Congruence of spatial organization of tactile projections to granule cell and Purkinje cell layers of cerebellar hemispheres of the albino rat: vertical organization of cerebellar cortex. *Journal of Neurophysiology*, **99**, 745–66.

Brodsky, F. M. (1988). Living with clathrin: its role in intracellular membrane traffic. *Science*, **242**, 1396–402.

Cameron, H. A., Kaliszewski, C. K., and Greer, C. A. (1991). Organization of mitochondria in olfactory bulb granule cell dendritic spines. *Synapse*, **8**, 107–118.

Chan-Palay, V. (1977). *Cerebellar dentate nucleus: organization, cytology, and transmitters*. Springer, Berlin.

Chen, X. Y. and Wolpaw, J. R. (1994). Triceps surae motoneuron morphology in the rat: a quantitative light microscopic study. *Journal of Comparative Neurology*, **343**, 143–57.

Chicurel, M. E. and Harris, K. M. (1992). Three-dimensional analysis of the structure and composition of CA3 branched dendritic spines and their synaptic relationships with mossy fiber boutons in the rat hippocampus. *Journal of Comparative Neurology*, **325**, 169–82.

Claiborne, B. J., Amaral, D. G., and Cowan, W. M. (1990). Quantitative, three-dimensional analysis of granule cell dendrites in the rat dentate gyrus. *Journal of Comparative Neurology*, **302**, 206–19.

Cornell-Bell, A. H., Thomas, P. G., and Smith, S. J. (1990). The excitatory neurotransmitter glutamate causes filopodia formation in cultured hippocampal astrocytes. *Glia*, **3**, 322–34.

Dailey, M. E. and Smith, S. J. (1996). The dynamics of dendritic structure in developing hippocampal slices. *Journal of Neuroscience*, **16**, 2983–94.

De Zeeuw, C. I., Ruigrok, T. J., Holstege, J. C., Jansen, H. G., and Voogd, J. (1990). Intracellular labeling of neurons in the medial accessory olive of the cat: II. Ultrastructure of dendritic spines and their GABAergic innervation. *Journal of Comparative Neurology*, **300**, 478–94.

Diamond, J. S., Bergles, D. E., and Jahr, C. E. (1998). Glutamate release monitored with astrocyte transporter currents during LTP. *Neuron*, **21**, 425–33.

Dunaevsky, A., Heintz, N., Mason, C. A., and Yuste, R. (1998). Two-photon imaging of dendritic spines of cerebellar and cortical cells transfected with GFP. *Society for Neuroscience Abstracts* **24**, 790.

Ebner, F. F. and Colonnier, M. (1975). Synaptic patterns in the visual cortex of turtle: an electron microscopic study. *Journal of Comparative Neurology*, **160**, 51–80.

Eccles, J. C., Ito, M., and Szentagothai, J. (1967). *The cerebellum as a neuronal machine*. Springer, New York.

Ellias, S. A. and Stevens, J. K. (1980). The dendritic varicosity: a mechanism for electrically isolating the dendrites of cat retinal amacrine cells? *Brain Research*, **196**, 365–72.

Engert, F. and Bonhoeffer, T. (1999). Dendritic spine changes associated with hippocampal long-term synaptic plasticity. *Nature*, **399**, 66–70.

Fannon, A. M. and Colman, D. R. (1996). A model for central synaptic junctional complex formation based on the differential adhesive specificities of the cadherins. *Neuron*, **17**, 423–434.

Feldman, M. L. and Peters, A. (1978). The forms of non-pyramidal neurons in the visual cortex of the rat. *Journal of Comparative Neurology*, **179**, 761–94.

Fernandez, E., Eldred, W. D., Ammermuller, J., Block, A., Von Bloh, W., and Kolb, H. (1994). Complexity and scaling properties of amacrine, ganglion, horizontal, and bipolar cells in the turtle retina. *Journal of Comparative Neurology*, **347**, 397–408.

Fiala, J. C., Feinberg, M., Popov, V. and Harris, K. M. (1998). Synaptogenesis via dendritic filopodia in developing hippocampal area CA1. *Journal of Neuroscience*, **18**, 8900–11.

Fields, R. D. and Ito, K. (1997). Neural cell adhesion molecule in activity-dependent development and synaptic plasticity. *Trends in Neurosciences*, **19**, 473–80.

Fifkova, E. (1985). Actin in the nervous system. *Brain Research*, **9**, 187–215.

Fine, R. E. and Ockleford, C. D. (1984). Supramolecular cytology of coated vesicles. *International Review of Cytology*, **91**, 1–43.

Fischer, M., Kaech, S., Knutti, D., and Matus, A. (1998). Rapid actin-based plasticity in dendritic spines. *Neuron*, **20**, 847–54.

Foster, M. (1897). *A textbook of physiology*, (17th edn). p. 929. MacMillan, New York.

Freund, T. F., Powell, J. F., and Smith, A. D. (1984). Tyrosine hydroxylase-immunoreactive boutons in synaptic contact with identified striatonigral neurons, with particular reference to dendritic spines. *Neuroscience*, **13**, 1189–215.

Fukuda, Y., Hsiao, C. F., Watanabe, M., and Ito, H. (1984). Morphological correlates of physiologically identified Y-, X-, and W-cells in cat retina. *Journal of Neurophysiology*, **52**, 999–1013.

Geinisman, Y., Morrell, F., De Toledo-Morrell, L. (1987). Axospinous synapses with segmented postsynaptic densities: a morphologically distinct synaptic subtype contributing to the number of profiles of 'perforated' synapses visualized in random sections. *Brain Research* **423**, 179–88.

Graveland, G. A., Williams, R. S., and Difiglia, M. (1985). A Golgi study of the human neostriatum: neurons and afferent fibers. *Journal of Comparative Neurology*, **234**, 317–33.

Gray, E. G. (1959). Axo-somatic and axo-dendritic synapses of the cerebral cortex: an electron microscope study. *Journal of Anatomy (London)*, **93**, 420–33.

Gruenberg, J. and Maxfield, F. R. (1995). Membrane transport in the endocytic pathway. *Current Opinion in Cell Biology*, 7, 552–63.

Halpain, S., Hipolito, A., and Saffer, L. (1998). Regulation of F-actin stability in dendritic spines by glutamate receptors and calcineurin. *Journal of Neuroscience*, **18**, 9835–44.

Hama, K., Arii, T., and Kosaka, T. (1994). Three-dimensional organization of neuronal and glial processes: high voltage electron microscopy. *Microscopy Research Technique*, **29**, 357–67.

Harris, K. M. and Kater, S. B. (1994). Dendritic spines: Cellular specializations imparting both stability and flexibility to synaptic function. *Annual Review of Neuroscience*, **17**, 341–71.

Harris, K. M. and Spacek, J. (1995). Three-dimensional organization of SER and other organelles in dendritic spines of rat hippocampus (CA1). *Society for Neuroscience Abstracts*, **21**, p. 594.

Harris, K. M. and Stevens, J. K. (1988). Dendritic spines of rat cerebellar Purkinje cells: Serial electron microscopy with reference to their biophysical characteristics. *Journal of Neuroscience*, **8**, 4455–69.

Harris, K. M. and Stevens, J. K. (1989). Dendritic spines of CA1 pyramidal cells in the rat hippocampus: serial electron microscopy with reference to their biophysical characteristics. *Journal of Neuroscience*, **9**, 2982–97.

Harris, K. M. and Sultan, P. (1995). Variation in the number, location, and size of synaptic vesicles provides an anatomical basis for the nonuniform probability of release at hippocampal CA1 synapses. *Neuropharmacology*, **34**, 1387–95.

Harris, K. M., Jensen, F. E., and Tsao, B. (1992). Three-dimensional structure of dendritic spines and synapses in rat hippocampus (CA1) at postnatal day 15 and adult ages: implications for the maturation of synaptic physiology and long-term potentiation. *Journal of Neuroscience*, **12**, 2685–705.

Harvey, R. J. and Napper, R. M. A. (1991). Quantitative studies on the mammalian cerebellum. *Progress in Neurobiology*, **36**, 437–63.

Henkart, M., Landis, D. M. D., and Reese, T. S. (1976). Similarity of junctions between plasma membranes and endoplasmic reticulum in muscle and neurons. *Journal of Cell Biology*, **70**, 338–47.

Holmes, W. R. (1990). Is the function of dendritic spines to concentrate calcium? *Brain Research*, **519**, 338–42.

Hrycyshyn, A. W. and Flumerfelt, B. A. (1981). Cytology and synaptology of the lateral reticular nucleus of the cat. *Journal of Comparative Neurology*, **197**, 459–75.

Ito, M. (1984). *The cerebellum and neural control*. Raven Press, New York.

Jones, D. G. and Harris, R. J. (1995). An analysis of contemporary morphological concepts of synaptic remodeling in the CNS: perforated synapses revisited. *Reviews in the Neurosciences*, **6**, 177–219.

Jones, E. G. and Powell, T. P. S. (1969). Morphological variations in the dendritic spines of the neocortex. *Journal of Cell Science*, **5**, 509–29.

Kellerth, J. O., Berthold, C. H., and Conradi, S. (1979). Electron microscopic studies of serially sectioned cat spinal alpha-motoneurons. III. Motoneurons innervating fast-twitch (type FR) units of the gastrocnemius muscle. *Journal of Comparative Neurology*, **184**, 755–67.

Kennedy, M. B. (1997). The postsynaptic density at glutamatergic synapses. *Trends in Neurosciences* **20**, 264–8.

Kirov, S. A. and Harris, K. M. (1998). Blocking synaptic transmission in adult rat hippocampal slices induces spine-like protrusions. *Society for Neuroscience Abstracts*, **24**, 274.

Kirov, S. A., Sorra, K. E., and Harris, K. M. (1999). Slices have more synapses than perfusion-fixed hippocampus from both young and mature rats. *Journal of Neuroscience*, **19**, 2876–86.

Kishi, K., Mori, K., and Tazawa, Y. (1982). Three-dimensional analysis of dendritic trees of mitral cells in the rabbit olfactory bulb. *Neuroscience Letters*, **28**, 127–32.

Koch, C. and Zador, A. (1993). The function of dendritic spines: devices subserving biochemical rather than electrical compartmentalization. *Journal of Neuroscience*, **13**, 413–22.

Kolb, H., Linberg, K. A., and Fisher, S. K. (1992). Neurons of the human retina: a Golgi study. *Journal of Comparative Neurology*, **318**, 147–87. .

Kolb, H., Fernandez, E., Schouten, J., Ahnelt, P., Linberg, K. A., and Fisher, S. K. (1994). Are there three types of horizontal cell in the human retina? *Journal of Comparative Neurology*, **343**, 370–86.

Larkman, A. V. (1991). Dendritic morphology of pyramidal neurones of the visual cortex of the rat. II. Spine distributions. *Journal of Comparative Neurology*, **306**, 332–43.

Luscher, C., Malenka, R. C., and Nicoll, R. A. (1998). Monitoring glutamate release during LTP with glial transporter currents. *Neuron*, **21**, 435–41.

Luthl, A., Laurent, J. P., Figurov, A., Muller, D., and Schachner, M. (1994). Hippocampal long-term potentiation and neural cell adhesion molecules L1 and NCAM. *Nature*, **372**, 777–9.

MacNeil, M. A. and Masland, R. H. (1998). Extreme diversity among amacrine cells: implications for function. *Neuron*, **20**, (5), 971–82.

Maletic-Savatic, M., Malinow, R., and Svoboda, K. (1999). Rapid dendritic morphogenesis in CA1 hippocampal dendrites induced by synaptic activity. *Science*, **283**, 1923–7.

Mariani, A. P. (1990). Amacrine cells of the rhesus monkey retina. *Journal of Comparative Neurology*, **301**, 382–400.

Martone, M. E., Zhang, Y., Simpliciano, V. M., Carragher, B. O., and Ellisman, M. H. (1993). Three-dimensional visualization of the smooth endoplasmic reticulum in Purkinje cell dendrites. *Journal of Neuroscience*, **13**, 4636–46.

McWilliams, J. R. and Lynch, G. (1981). Sprouting in the hippocampus is accompanied by an increase in coated vesicles. *Brain Research*, **211**, 158–64.

Miller, R. J. (1998). Mitochondria—the Kraken wakes! *Trends in Neurosciences*, **21**, 95–7.

Morest, D. K. (1969). The growth of dendrites in the mammalian brain. *Zeitschrift für Anatomie und Entwickelungsgeschichte*, **128**, 290–317.

Mugnaini, E., Floris, A., and Wright-Goss, M. (1994). Extraordinary synapses of the unipolar brush cell: an electron microscopic study in the rat cerebellum. *Synapse*, **16**, 284–311.

Muller, D., Wang, C., Skibo, G., Toni, N., Cremer, H., Calaora, V., *et al.* (1996). PSA–NCAM is required for activity-induced synaptic plasticity. *Neuron*, **17**, 413–22.

Murray, J. A. H., Bradley, H., Craigie, W. A., and Onions, C. T. (eds.) (1919). *A new English dictionary on historical principles*. Clarendon Press, Oxford.

Nafstad, P. H. J. and Blackstad, T. W. (1966). Distribution of mitochondria in pyramidal cells and boutons in hippocampal cortex. *Zeitschrift für Zellforschung und Mikroskopische Anatomie*, **73**, 234–45.

Ostapoff, E. M., Feng, J. J., and Morest, D. K. (1994). A physiological and structural study of neuron types in the cochlear nucleus. II. Neuron types and their structural correlation with response properties. *Journal of Comparative Neurology*, **346**, 19–42.

Overly, C. C., Rieff, H. I., and Hollenbeck, P. J. (1996). Organelle motility and metabolism in axons vs dendrites of cultured hippocampal neurons. *Journal of Cell Science*, **109**, 971–80.

Palay, S. L. (1978). The Meynert cell, an unusual cortical pyramidal cell. In *Architectonics of the Cerebral Cortex*, (ed. M. A. B. Brazier and H. Petsche), pp. 31–42. Raven Press, New York.

Palay, S. L. and Chan-Palay, V. (1974). *Cerebellar cortex: cytology and organization*. Springer-Verlag, New York.

Parra, P., Gulyas, A. I., and Miles, R. (1998). How many subtypes of inhibitory cells in the hippocampus? *Neuron*, **20**, 983–93.

Parton, R. G., Simons, K., and Dotti, C. G. (1992). Axonal and dendritic endocytic pathways in cultured neurons. *Journal of Cell Biology*, **119**, 123–37.

Peters, A. and Jones, E. G. (ed.) (1984). *Cerebral cortex. Vol. 1: Cellular components of the cerebral cortex*. Plenum Press, New York.

Peters, A. and Kaiserman-Abramof, I. R. (1970). The small pyramidal neuron of the rat cerebral cortex. The perikaryon, dendrites and spines. *American Journal of Anatomy*, **127**, 321–56.

Peters, A. and Palay, S. L. (1996). The morphology of synapses. *Journal of Neurocytology*, **25**, 687–700.

Peters, A., Palay, S. L., and Webster, H. De F. (1991). *The fine structure of the nervous system*. Oxford University Press, New York.

Porter, R., Ghosh, S., Lange, G. D., and Smith, T. G. Jr. (1991). A fractal analysis of pyramidal neurons in mammalian motor cortex. *Neuroscience Letters*, **130**, 112–16.

Purves, D., Hadley, R. D., and Voyvodic, J. T. (1986). Dynamic changes in the dendritic geometry of individual neurons visualized over periods of up to three months in the superior cervical ganglion of living mice. *Journal of Neuroscience*, **6**, 1051–60.

Ramón y Cajal, S. (1995). *Histology of the nervous system of man and vertebrates*. (trans. N. Swanson and L. W. Swanson) Oxford University Press, New York. (Originally published: *Histologie du systeme nerveux de l'homme et des vertebres*. (trans. L. Azoulay), Paris, 1909–11.

Ramon-Moliner, E. (1968). The morphology of dendrites. In *The structure and function of nervous tissue*, Vol. I (ed. G. H. Bourne), pp. 205–67. Academic Press, New York.

Rapp, M., Segev, I., Yarom, Y. (1994). Physiology, morphology and detailed passive models of guinea-pig cerebellar Purkinje cells. *Journal of Physiology*, **474**, 101–18.

Ruigrok, T. J. H., De Zeeuw, C. I., Van Der Burg, J., and Voogd, J. (1990). Intracellular labeling of neurons in the medial accessory olive of the cat: I. Physiology and light microscopy. *Journal of Comparative Neurology*, **300**, 462–77.

Scholl, D. A. (1956). *The organization of the cerebral cortex*. Wiley, New York.

Shepherd, G. M. (1996). The dendritic spine: a multifunctional integrative unit. *Journal of Neurophysiology*, **75**, 2197–210.

Shepherd, G. M. (1998). Information processing in dendrites. In *Fundamental neuroscience*, (ed. M. J. Zigmond, F. E. Bloom, S. C. Landis, J. L. Roberts, and L. R. Squire), pp. 363–88. Academic Press, New York.

Shupliakov, O., Low, P., Grabs, D., Gad, H., Chen, H., David, *et al.* (1997). Synaptic vesicle endocytosis impaired by disruption of dynamin-SH3 domain interactions. *Science*, **276**, 259–63.

Smith, T. G., Marks, W. B., Lange, G. D., Sheriff, W. H., and Neale, E. A. (1989). A fractal analysis of cell images. *Journal of Neuroscience Methods*, **27**, 173–80.

Sorra, K. E., Fiala, J. C., and Harris, K. M. (1998). Critical assessment of the involvement of perforations, spinules, and spine branching in hippocampal synapse formation. *Journal of Comparative Neurology*, **398**, 225–40.

Sorra, K. E. and Harris, K. M. (1993). Occurrence and three-dimensional structure of multiple synapses between individual radiatum axons and their target pyramidal cells in hippocampal area CA1. *Journal of Neuroscience*, **13**, 3736–48.

Sotelo, C. and Angaut, P. (1973). The fine structure of the cerebellar central nuclei in the cat. I. Neurons and neuroglial cells. *Experimental Brain Research*, **16**, 410–30.

Spacek, J. (1985). Three-dimensional analysis of dendritic spines. III. Glial sheath. *Anatomy and Embryology*, **171**, 245–52.

Spacek, J. and Harris, K. M. (1997). Three-dimensional organization of smooth endoplasmic reticulum in hippocampal CA1 dendrites and dendritic spines of the immature and mature rat. *Journal of Neuroscience*, **17**, 190–203.

Spacek, J. and Harris, K. M. (1998). Three-dimensional organization of cell adhesion junctions at synapses and dendritic spines in area CA1 of the rat hippocampus. *Journal of Comparative Neurology*, **393**, 58–68.

Spacek, J. and Hartmann, M. (1983). Three-dimensional analysis of dendritic spines. I. Quantitative observations related to dendritic spine and synaptic morphology in cerebral and cerebellar cortices. *Anatomy Embryology*, **167**, 289–310.

Spacek, J. and Lieberman, A. R. (1980). Relationships between mitochondrial outer membranes and agranular reticulum in nervous tissue: ultrastructural observations and a new interpretation. *Journal of Cell Science*, **46**, 129–47.

Sterling, P. (1990). Retina. In *The synaptic organization of the brain*. (3rd edn). (ed. G. M. Shepherd), pp. 170–215. Oxford University Press, New York.

Stern, J. E. and Armstrong, W. E. (1998). Reorganization of the dendritic trees of oxytocin and vasopressin neurons of the rat supraoptic nucleus during lactation. *Journal of Neuroscience*, **18**, 841–53.

Steward, O. and Reeves, T. M. (1988). Protein-synthetic machinery beneath postsynaptic sites on CNS neurons: association between polyribosomes and other organelles at the synaptic site. *Journal of Neuroscience*, **8**, 176–84.

Steward, O., Falk, P. M., and Torre, E. R. (1996). Ultrastructural basis for gene expression at the synapse: synapse-associated polyribosome complexes. *Journal of Neurocytology*, **25**, 717–34.

Svoboda, K., Tank, D. W., and Denk, W. (1996). Direct measurement of coupling between dendritic spines and shafts. *Science*, **272**, 716–19.

Takeda, T., Ishikawa, A., Ohtomo, K., Kobayashi, Y., and Matsuoka, T. (1992). Fractal dimension of dendritic tree of cerebellar Purkinje cell during onto- and phylogenetic development. *Neuroscience Research*, **13**, 19–31.

Tang, L., Hung, C. P., and Schuman, E. M. (1996). Role of cadherin molecules in synaptic plasticity in the adult rat hippocampus. *Society for Neuroscience* Abstracts, **22**, 332.

Tanzi, E. (1893). I Fatti e le induzioni nell'odierna istologia del sistema nervoso. *Riv Sperim Freniatria Med Leg*, **19**, 419–72.

Tarrant, S. B. and Routtenberg, A. (1977). The synaptic spinule in the dendritic spine: electron microscopic study of the hippocampal dentate gyrus. *Tissue and Cell*, **9**, 461–73.

Trommald, M. and Hullenberg, G. (1997). Dimensions and density of dendritic spines from rat dentate granule cells based on reconstructions from serial electron micrographs. *Journal of Comparative Neurology*, **377**, 15–28.

Trommald, M., Jensen, V., and Andersen, P. (1995). Analysis of dendritic spines in rat CA1 pyramidal cells intracellularly filled with a fluorescent dye. *Journal of Comparative Neurology*, **353**, 260–74.

Ulfhake, B. and Kellerth, J. O. (1981). A quantitative light microscopic study of the dendrites of cat spinal alpha-motoneurons after intracellular staining with horseradish peroxidase. *Journal of Comparative Neurology*, 202, 571–83.

Uylings, H. B. M., Smit, G. J., and Veltman, W. A. N. (1975). Ordering methods in quantitative analysis of branching structures of dendritic trees. In *Physiology and pathology of dendrites* (ed. G. W. Kreutzberg), *Advances in Neurology*, **12**, 247–54.

Van Harreveld, A. and Trubatch, J. (1975). Synaptic changes in frog brain after stimulation with potassium chloride. *Journal of Neurocytology*, **4**, 33–46.

Ventura, R. and Harris, K. M. (1999). Three-dimensional relationships between hippocampal synapses and astrocytes. *Journal of Neuroscience*, (in press.)

Ward, R., Moreau, B., Marchand, M.-J., and Garenc, C. (1995). A note on the distribution of dendritic spines. *Journal für Hirnforschung*, **36**, 519–22.

Westrum, L. E. and Blackstad, T. (1962). An electron microscope study of the stratum radiatum of the rat hippocampus (regio superior, CA1) with particular emphasis on synaptology. *Journal of Comparative Neurology*, **119**, 281–309.

Wilson, C. J., Groves, P. M., Kitai, S. T., and Linder, J. C. (1983). Three-dimensional structure of dendritic spines in the rat neostriatum. *Journal of Neuroscience*, **3**, 383–98.

Wilson, J. R., Friedlander, M. J., and Sherman, S. M. (1984). Fine structural morphology of identified X- and Y-cells in the cat's lateral geniculate nucleus. *Proceedings of the Royal Society of London B*, **221**, 411–36.

Wingate, R. J., Fitzgibbon, T., and Thompson, I. D. (1992). Lucifer yellow, retrograde tracers, and fractal analysis characterize adult ferret retinal ganglion cells. *Journal of Comparative Neurology*, **323**, 449–74.

Yelnik, J., Percheron, G., and Francois, C. (1984). A Golgi analysis of the primate globus pallidus. II. Quantitative morphology and spatial orientation of dendritic arborizations. *Journal of Comparative Neurology*, **227**, 200–13.

2

Development of Dendrites

Hollis T. Cline
Cold Spring Harbor Laboratory

Summary

Neurons can be categorized according to structural and functional properties, which are reproducible from animal to animal. The factors controlling the acquisition of these features have been a topic of research for centuries. As methods develop to enable more detailed analysis of the development of dendritic structure and function, the consensus view has shifted from the idea that dendritic development is governed by intrinsic programs to the idea that dendritic structure and function develops as part of a continual dynamic process that balances the effects of neuronal activity, growth-promoting and growth-inhibiting proteins, and homeostatic mechanisms. An important realization is that, precisely contrary to the old view, dendrites develop as part of a neural circuit, and constant feedback and feedforward mechanisms operate during the development of circuits to ensure that they will function in the developing and adult animal. The demonstration that synaptic activity, activity-regulated proteins and activity-induced genes influence dendrite growth provides strong support for a model of interactive regulation of dendrite development.

Introduction

Dendritic arbor development is severely impaired in several developmental disorders. Purpura demonstrated that dendritic arbors of cortical neurons of children with mental retardation are significantly smaller than normal and spine density is reduced (Purpura 1975). Children with Fragile X, and mutant mouse models of the disease, have deformed dendritic arbors and spine disgenesis (Comery *et al.* 1997). Several neurotoxins, such as lead, impair brain function and dendrite development (Pettit and LeBoutillier 1979). These studies indicate the severity of the consequences of abnormal dendrite development and motivate research toward an understanding of the mechanisms regulating the normal and abnormal development of dendritic structure and function.

Twenty years ago the general consensus was that dendritic arbor development was regulated by intrinsic mechanisms, although several studies provided data which might now be interpreted as providing support for the idea that input activity participates in controlling dendrite development. For instance, Mason (1983) examined dendritic arbor development in the lateral geniculate nucleus (LGN) of early postnatal kittens and found that the afferents and dendrites develop in parallel. Although she concluded from this that there was little evidence for afferent influence of dendritic development, LGN neurons are responsive to retinal input at E39 (Shatz and Kirkwood 1983), at the earliest stages of dendritic arbor development. Comparable studies in visual cortex demonstrated that dendritic arbor elaboration also overlaps with the period of afferent invasion of the cortical layers. Based on an apparently similar temporal overlap as seen in the LGN, Zec and Tieman concluded that dendritic arbor development might depend on activity, although the early emergence of dendrites was probably independent of afferent activity (Zec and Tieman 1994). This chapter will review some of the abundant data collected in an effort to understand the mechanisms regulating dendritic development.

Glutamate function in the developing brain

Glutamate is the most prevalent excitatory neurotransmitter in the brain. Glutamate receptors fall into two general classes—metabotropic and ionotropic (see Chapters 4 and 5). The ionotropic glutamate receptors are named for the agonists which they bind preferentially—α-amino-3-hydroxy-5-methyl-4-isoxazolepropionic acid (AMPA), kainate, and N-methyl-D-aspartate (NMDA; Hollman and Heinemann 1994). Molecular analysis of the receptors indicates that the different classes are comprised of distinct subsets of subunits which form heteromultimers. The AMPA-type receptors mediate fast excitatory synaptic transmission (see Chapter 5), whereas the kainate receptors seem to be involved in synaptic transmission only in special circumstances at certain synapses. The NMDA receptor is a voltage and ligand-dependent receptor which conducts calcium. On the basis of these properties, the NMDA receptor is capable of detecting synchronous activity of multiple inputs, or input activity which is correlated with postsynaptic activity (see Chapter 13). This correlated activity is then signaled to the postsynaptic neuron as a rise in intracellular calcium. The properties of glutamate receptors have been reviewed extensively elsewhere (Hollman and Heinemann 1994).

Development of glutamatergic synaptic responses

Activity-dependent regulation of synaptic physiology during brain development has been documented in several recent papers. In adult brain, glutamatergic synaptic responses are usually mediated by activation of both NMDA- and AMPA-type glutamate receptors. Glutamatergic synaptic transmission undergoes a developmental transition from immature synapses mediated predominantly by NMDA receptors, to mature synapses mediated by mixed NMDA and AMPA receptors. This can be expressed as an increase in the ratio of AMPA receptor-mediated current to NMDA receptor-mediated current (A/N ratio) or an increase in synaptic strength with maturation (Isaac *et al.* 1997; Durand *et al.* 1996; Liao and Malinow 1996; Wu *et al.* 1996; Li and Zhuo 1998; Zhang *et al.* 1998). The transition from weaker, low

A/N synapses to strong, high A/N synapses seems to be a general phenomenon because it has been observed in a variety of experimental systems during development (Isaac *et al.* 1997; Durand *et al.* 1996; Liao and Malinow 1996; Wu *et al.* 1996; Li and Zhuo 1998; Zhang *et al.* 1998) and during such diverse forms of plasticity as hippocampal and cortical long-term potentiation (Liao *et al.* 1995; Durand *et al.* 1996; Isaac *et al.* 1997) and prism-induced shifts in central visual projections of the barn owl (Feldman *et al.* 1996; Feldman and Knudsen 1997, 1998). Recent studies have also demonstrated that the developmental increase in strength of glutamatergic synaptic transmission is activity and NMDA receptor-dependent (Isaac *et al.* 1997; Durand *et al.* 1996; Liao and Malinow 1996; Wu *et al.* 1996; Li and Zhuo 1998; Zhang *et al.* 1998), akin to long-term potentiation of synaptic transmission in the adult hippocampus. In addition to the electrophysiological studies just cited, the shift in A/N ratio has also been detected by immuno-electron microscopy (Petralia *et al.* 1999), where synapses with only NMDA receptors were seen in early postnatal rodent hippocampus, while synapses with both NMDA and AMPA receptors were only seen at synapses in older animals.

In vivo imaging of dendritic arbor elaboration

In vivo imaging of optic tectal neurons in intact albino Xenopus tadpoles enables direct observation of the structural dynamics that occur during dendritic arbor formation. High-resolution confocal time-lapse images of single DiI-labeled neurons in the Xenopus optic tectum were imaged at daily intervals over a period of 5–6 days (Fig. 2.1). During this period their synaptic responses mature from relatively weak, low AMPA/NMDA synapses to stronger, high AMPA/NMDA synapses. The imaging studies reveals that tectal cell development can be categorized into three stages (Fig. 2.2). During stage 1, neurons differentiate from neuroepithelial progenitors and projection neurons extend their efferent axon.

Stage 2 neurons, which are in the rapid phase of growth, are morphologically simple and show dramatic rearrangements in the dendritic arbor over 2-h intervals, and even over 10-min periods. The rearrangements include addition of new branches, complete retraction of branches, and both extension or shortening of branches which were present in the previous observation. Slightly more branch additions than retractions occur over 6 h, which accounts for the net increase in arbor elaboration over longer periods. Branches are added at any point along a parent dendrite, not just at growing branch tips. This type of neuronal growth, called backbranching, has previously been shown for axon arbor elaboration (Harris *et al.* 1987; O'Rourke *et al.* 1994). Arbors show a coordinated increase in branch length and branch tips, indicating that dendritic arbors do not develop first by extending long branches which subsequently add side branches.

Time-lapse imaging of morphologically complex, stage 3 neurons indicates that they have slower growth rates and fewer dendritic branch rearrangements (Figs 2.3 and 2.4). They continue to exhibit modest dynamics rearrangements in their branch tips, consistent with their continued elaboration during later stages of development (Lázár 1973). Dendritic arbor stabilization, seen in morphologically complex neurons, is due to a decreased rate of branch retractions, consistent with the

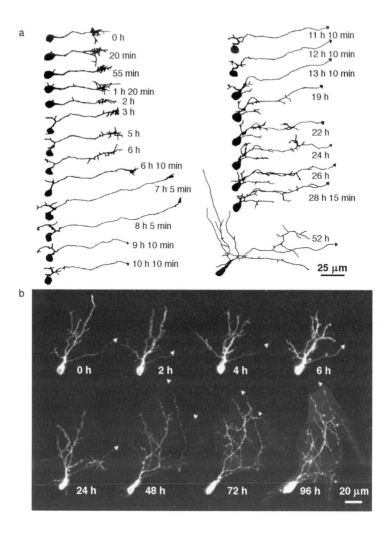

Fig. 2.1   Time-lapse *in vivo* images of DiI-labeled optic tectal neurons collected at the time-points specified. (a) Drawings of an immature neuron as it extends its efferent axon. The axon is tipped with a large dynamic growth cone. When the axon exits the tectum, the dendritic arbor begins to elaborate. (b) Images of a neuron whose dendritic arbor grows rapidly over the next few days. The photomontage shows 3D reconstructions of confocal optical sections.

stabilization of a synaptic contact and the branch supporting it and a decreased rate of branch additions.

Activity-dependent development of dendritic arbor structure

The potential regulatory role of neuronal activity in dendritic arbor development has been a controversial area. Although there is consensus that afferent activity patterns

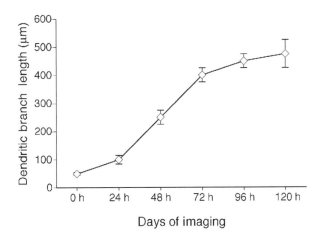

Fig. 2.2   Change in dendritic branch length over 6 days *in vivo*. Dendritic growth rate is initially slow as the neuron extends the axon. The dendritic arbor then grows rapidly for a period of 2–3 days, after which dendritic growth rate slows.

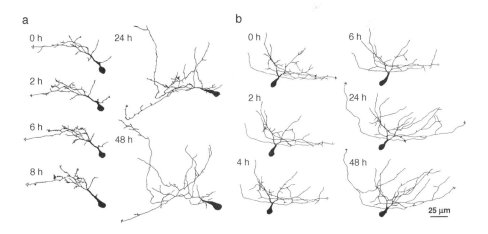

Fig. 2.3   Dendritic arbors are dynamic in rapidly growing neurons and more stable in complex neurons. Drawings of a rapidly growing (stage 2) neuron (a) and a more stable stage 3 neuron (b) collected at the time-points specified. Compare the dendritic dynamics at short observation intervals and the rapid increase in branch length over each day of imaging in the stage 2 neuron with the stage 3 neuron. Scale bar in (b) applies also to (a).

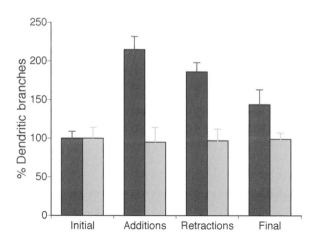

Fig. 2.4 Dendritic arbor stability increases with neuronal maturity. Data from neurons imaged at 2-h intervals over a 6-h period were analyzed to test whether dynamic rearrangements of rapidly growing stage 2 neurons are greater than the slower-growing stage 3 neurons. Initial and final branch numbers, cumulative branch additions and retractions in stage 2 (black bars) and stage 3 (gray bars) neurons over the 6-h observation period graphed relative to initial branch tip number. Note that the relative rates of branch additions and retractions of stage 3 neurons is half that in stage 2 neurons.

control both the projection site and morphology of afferent axons and the strength of neuronal connections (Constantine-Paton *et al.* 1990; Shatz 1990; Fields and Nelson 1992; Antonini and Stryker 1993), there is no consensus on the effect of afferent activity on dendritic arbor development. The dendritic fields of neurons in many regions of the brain are oriented toward their afferent inputs (Greenough and Chang 1988; Katz and Constantine-Paton 1988; Katz *et al.* 1989; Schweitzer 1991; Kossel *et al.* 1995), probably because of either directed growth or stabilization of dendrites by afferents. In dissociated cell cultures, afferents seem to operate locally to sculpt the dendritic arbor (Mattson *et al.* 1988; Kossel *et al.* 1997). Time-lapse images of developing axons and dendrites in cultured hippocampal slices suggest that contacts between pre- and postsynaptic elements stabilize dendritic branches (Dailey and Smith 1996; Ziv and Smith 1996). Manipulations of excitatory or inhibitory transmitter systems in brain slice preparations and *in vivo* lead to changes in dendritic arbor development (Kalb 1994; Vogel and Prittie 1995; McAllister *et al.* 1996; Sanes and Hafidi 1996; Rajan and Cline 1998); these studies have not, however, yielded a consensus on the role of activity in regulating dendritic arbor development.

Multiple types of neuronal activity could contribute to the activity-dependent regulation of dendritic arbor structure and function. Early after differentiation, neurons have long-lasting calcium-dependent action potentials. Later, voltage-dependent sodium channels are expressed and enable fast action potentials in response to depolarization to threshold. Immature neurons and astrocytes throughout the brain can be electrically coupled so that ionic changes in one cell can spread rapidly to neighboring cells (Yuste *et al.* 1992, 1995). Ionic changes can spread as waves through the tissue, as in retina (Meister *et al.* 1991) and hippo-campus (Strata *et al.* 1997). Within the retina, waves of activity may be required to determine receptor field properties (Sernagor and Grzywacz 1996) and might function to establish topographic projections in the CNS (Penn *et al.* 1998). Similarly in the hippocampus or cortex, waves of activity may establish organized projections from one brain region to another (Strata *et al.* 1997). These waves of activity are transient during development and occur during the period of afferent ingrowth, synaptogenesis and dendritic arbor formation.

Several studies indicate that blocking synaptic activity (Kalb 1994; Vogel and Prittie 1995) or sensory deprivation (Wiesel and Hubel 1963; Feng and Rogowski 1980; Constantine-Paton and Ferrari-Eastman 1981; Parks 1981; Trune 1982; Lund *et al.* 1991) during development can prevent normal elaboration of dendritic arbors. Other studies show that denervation after synapse formation results in dendritic atrophy (Valverde 1968; Benes *et al.* 1977; Deitch and Rubel 1984), supporting a role for afferent activity in maintaining dendritic structure. A third group of studies demonstrates that dendrites are more elaborate in regions where synaptic inputs may be greater in number or more correlated in their activity patterns (Harris and Woolsey 1981; Katz and Constantine-Paton 1988; Katz *et al.* 1989; Kossel *et al.* 1995). Other reports come to the opposite conclusion, that blocking NMDA receptors can increase dendritic growth and spine density (Rocha and Sur 1995; McAllister *et al.* 1996). Finally, several studies conclude that mechanisms controlling dendritic develop-ment are not influenced by synaptic activity (Goodman and Model 1990; Wong *et al.* 1991; Dalva *et al.* 1994; Kossel *et al.* 1997) although some of the data do show changes in spine density (Wong *et al.* 1991; Dalva *et al.* 1994; Kossel *et al.* 1997).

Ion-channel activity, which can in turn affect synaptic transmission or responses to it, can also affect dendritic arbor development. For instance, potassium channels, which regulate neuronal excitability, are required for dendritic arbor development *in vivo* (Jones *et al.* 1995). Recent studies in which potassium-channel subunits have been knocked out in mice show defects in synaptic plasticity, learning and memory (Silva *et al.* 1998). As in many such experiments, it is likely that a single manipulation results in multiple primary, secondary, tertiary, etc. changes in brain function.

Glutamatergic synaptic activity and the development of dendritic structure

One reason for the range in data on the effect of glutamate receptor blockade on dendritic arbor development might be the time of the manipulation relative to maturation of glutamatergic synaptic responses. This possibility has been tested in optic tectal neurons, for which the pattern of electrophysiological and morpho-logical maturation is known (Wu *et al.* 1996; Wu and Cline 1998), by examining whether dendritic arbor development is more sensitive to glutamate receptor blockade in immature neurons with low A/N ratios than in more mature neurons with higher A/N ratios. Dendritic arbor growth was severely impaired by NMDA receptor blockade early during development of the arbor when glutamatergic synapses were mediated principally by NMDA receptors. More mature neurons were less sensitive to either NMDA or AMPA receptor blockade than immature neurons

(Rajan and Cline 1998). These data indicate that more mature neurons with strong synaptic inputs (i.e. high A/N synapses) have more stable dendritic arbors than younger neurons with weaker inputs (i.e. low A/N synapses).

The differential effects of blocking NMDA and AMPA receptors on the initial formation of the dendritic arbor might reflect the relative preponderance of NMDA receptor-mediated synaptic transmission compared with AMPA receptor-mediated synaptic transmission in young neurons (Wu *et al.* 1996), the postulated neuro-trophic role for extrasynaptic NMDA receptors in newly differentiated neurons (Blanton *et al.* 1990; LoTurco *et al.* 1991), and the developmentally regulated change in subunit composition of the NMDA receptor in developing neurons (Monyer *et al.* 1992). As also seen in other systems, NMDA receptor-mediated currents in younger neurons from caudal tectum have slower decay kinetics than more mature neurons (Cline *et al.* 1997). Prolonged calcium influx through these receptors could result in significantly greater changes in intracellular calcium concentration than might result indirectly from AMPA receptor-mediated depolarizations. It is likely that the spatial and temporal changes in intracellular calcium concentrations directly regulate the cellular mechanisms controlling cytoskeletal stability and branching dynamics (Kater and Mills 1991; Lankford *et al.* 1996). As neurons mature, their dendritic structure becomes less dynamic and their AMPA receptor-mediated synaptic trans-mission increases. Consistent with this shift in AMPA/NMDA ratio, the AMPA antagonist 6-cyano-7-nitroquinoxaline-2,3-dione (CNQX) has a greater effect on dendritic morphology as neurons mature.

It is interesting to note that blocking glutamate receptor activity has a significantly different outcome for more complex neurons compared with simpler neurons. In complex neurons, blocking glutamate receptors leads to a net decrease in total dendritic branch length, suggesting that synaptic activity is required not only to promote branch additions and branch-length extensions, as in younger neurons, but also to maintain branches already present at the start of the experiment. This suggests that synaptic activity can recruit growth-promoting mechanisms in younger neurons which might not be available for activation in more mature neurons. These data further indicate that the same pharmacological manipulation, in this case blocking glutamate receptors, can have a very different influence on dendritic morphology depending on the developmental state of the neurons. The different effects of activity blockers on dendritic development reported in the literature might reflect the different developmental stage of neurons when the experiments were performed, not only with respect to the AMPA/NMDA ratio, but also other cellular elements that jointly control morphological development.

The NMDA antagonist D-2-amino-5-phosphonovaleric acid (AP5) can alter branch dynamics and branch-length extensions while TTX has no detectable influence on these parameters. Such a selective influence of NMDA receptor activity on neurite outgrowth has also been reported in cultured Xenopus tectal neurons (Lin and Constantine-Paton 1998). These data indicate that NMDA receptor activity can influence dendritic arbor development independently of the generation of sodium-dependent action potentials in tectal neurons. This suggests that spontaneous release of transmitter and miniature postsynaptic currents (mPSCs), which occur in the presence of TTX are sufficient to affect dendritic arbor growth. The relatively high affinity of NMDA receptors for glutamate in developing tissue (Kutsewada *et al.*

1992), and the delayed expression of glutamate transporters during development (Ullensvang *et al.* 1997) provide the conditions for low levels of spontaneously released glutamate to activate NMDA receptors even in the absence of action potential activity. Another recent report indicates that spontaneous mPSCs mediated by AMPA receptors are sufficient to maintain spines (McKinney *et al.* 1999). Recent demonstration of a metabotropic action of AMPA receptor (Hayashi *et al.* 1999) suggests that such a pathway might also be activated by NMDA receptor.

Spines, the sites of excitatory synapses, seem to be particularly sensitive to changes in afferent activity, neurotrophins and steroid hormones. During development of the visual system, spine density increases with eye opening (Lund *et al.* 1991; Sutton and Brunso-Bechtold 1991); this seems, however, to be a transient increase in spine density followed by a developmental decrease in spine density. Spine density decreases with reduced synaptic input (Lund *et al.* 1991) and increases when animals are reared in enriched environments (Turner and Greenough 1985; see Chapter 14). Once again, however, the response of spines to experimental manipulations does not fit into a simple scheme of increased activity leading to increased spine density. Spine density decreases in visual cortical neurons with monocular deprivation, but not with binocular deprivation (Lund *et al.* 1991), suggesting some comparison of activity levels contributes to the regulation of spine density. TTX increases spine density in developing LGN neurons (Dalva *et al.* 1994) and retinal ganglion cells (Wong *et al.* 1991), possibly by preventing the spine retraction that normally occurs during development. Blocking the NMDA type of glutamate receptor also increases spine density (Rocha and Sur 1995). Time-lapse imaging of spine formation in cultured hippocampal slices indicates that afferent activity increases spine formation by an NMDA receptor-dependent mechanism (Maletic-Savatic *et al.* 1999). It seems likely that in more mature neurons, with complex dendritic arbors, the principal activity dependent means of modulating dendritic structural plasticity is through modulation of the density and morphology of spines, rather than relatively large-scale changes in dendritic arbor structure that occur at earlier stages of dendritic arbor development (see Chapter 14 for further discussion of these issues).

Structural dynamics and synaptic strength

Does the strength of synaptic inputs influence dendritic arbor development? The higher growth rate and rapid structural dynamics of stage 2 neurons correlate with the relatively weak retinotectal inputs, whereas the slower growth rate and stable dendritic structure of stage 3 neurons correlate with the stronger synaptic inputs these more mature neurons receive. These data suggest that stronger synaptic inputs stabilize the dendritic arbor and that weaker inputs, with lower AMPA/NMDA ratios, enable the dendritic arbor to undergo greater rearrangements. Greater dendritic dynamics are correlated with a faster arbor growth rate, suggesting some relationship between high rates of branch additions and retractions and net growth of the arbor. *In vivo*, where AMPA receptor function is a delayed aspect of synaptic maturation (Isaac *et al.* 1997; Durand *et al.* 1996; Liao and Malinow 1996; Wu *et al.* 1996), dendritic arbors probably remain dynamic until increased synaptic strength promotes their stabilization.

Inherent in the model that synaptic strength regulates dendritic arbor development, is the idea that branches supporting weaker synaptic inputs remain dynamic even in mature neurons. Indeed, recordings from mature neurons in rostral tectum show that they continue to have some synapses mediated principally by NMDA receptors (Wu *et al.* 1996) and fine branch dynamics are still observed in stage 3 neurons imaged at 2-h intervals. Furthermore, this hypothesis predicts that modifying synaptic strength will lead to corresponding changes in branch dynamics. In support of this idea, increasing synaptic strength by expressing calcium calmodulin-dependent protein kinase II (CaMKII) in tectal neurons reduced dendritic dynamics (Wu *et al.* 1996; Wu and Cline 1998). The developmental decrease in arbor dynamics with neuronal maturation is comparable with the reduced dynamics seen with expression of a truncated, constitutively active form of CaMKII (tCaMKII; Wu and Cline 1998). This supports the conclusion that the developmental increase in tectal cell CaMKII expression provides neurons with a mechanism to translate strong synaptic input into stable dendritic structure. The interplay between glutamate receptor activity, CaMKII, and as yet undefined downstream effectors which control cytoskeletal assembly and disassembly remain an area of active research effort. Recent evidence that glutamate receptor activity and CaMKII can activate a pathway involving regulation of actin cytoskeletal dynamics by a RasGTPase (SynGap; Chen *et al.* 1998; Kim *et al.* 1998) suggests a mechanism by which dendrite dynamics can be locally controlled by synaptic activity.

A developmental decrease in dendritic branch dynamics has been observed in hippocampal slice cultures (Dailey and Smith 1996) and dissociated hippocampal neuronal cultures (Ziv and Smith 1996). Using dissociated hippocampal neuronal cultures, in which the presence of synapses was assessed by uptake of FM 4-64 into presynaptic sites, Ziv and Smith demonstrated that FM 4-64-labeled presynaptic sites were associated with persistent dendritic branches compared with the dynamic dendritic branches which were apparently without presynaptic contact (Ziv and Smith 1996). Although Ziv and Smith concluded that synaptogenesis stabilizes dendritic branches, other data (Rajan and Cline 1998; Wu and Cline 1998) indicate that it is more likely the addition of AMPA receptor, and the increased synaptic strength that comes about with the addition of these receptors, that specifically promotes dendritic arbor stability, rather than synaptogenesis *per se*.

It would be interesting to see whether experimental conditions which result in reorganization of sensory projections and a recapitulation of the developmental program of synaptic maturation, as seen in the prism-shifted visual projection of the barn owl (Feldman *et al.* 1996; Feldman and Knudsen 1997, 1998) also result in an increase in structural dynamics of those neurons with increased NMDA receptor-mediated responses.

Afferents inputs and dendritic arbor refinement

The dendritic arbors of many neurons are highly polarized, with the arbor extending toward the afferents. *In vivo* imaging of tectal neurons demonstrates clear regionalized arbor elaboration and regionalized retractions. Such localized branch elaboration might reflect the trophic effect of inputs on dendritic arbor growth and over time would be expected to result in a polarized dendritic arbor. A trophic effect of afferents has been convincingly demonstrated in the auditory system where different afferents terminate on different portions of the dendritic arbor in neurons in nucleus laminaris. Deafferentation of specific afferents leads to selective atrophy of the corresponding part of the dendritic arbor (Gray *et al.* 1982; Smith *et al.* 1983). Katz and Constantine-Paton previously noted a rostral bias in dendritic arbor elaboration in tectal neurons from postmetamorphic *Rana pipiens* and suggested that it might be because of a trophic influence of retinal afferents (Katz and Constantine-Paton 1988).

In vivo imaging of dendritic growth indicates that glutamatergic synaptic activity promotes the initial development of the dendritic arbor by increasing rates of branch tip additions and increasing elongation of existing branch tips. Once the dendritic arbor has formed, synaptic activity is required to stabilize and maintain dendritic arbor structure; this is consistent with studies demonstrating that the loss of afferent activity leads to dendritic atrophy (Valverde 1968; Benes *et al.* 1977; Deitch and Rubel 1984). During the phase of rapid dendritic growth, a local decrease in excitatory input to developing tectal cell dendrites might reduce local dendritic elaboration, while a local increase in afferent activity might promote local growth. Reduced branch elongation in AP5-treated simple neurons indicates that synaptic inputs on to major branch tips of the dendritic arbor stabilize those structures and are required to maintain branch length. Synaptic inputs can also increase the stability of the rapidly growing dendritic arbor by reducing rates of branch-tip retractions in young neurons.

Such a developmental influence of synaptic inputs on dendritic arbor development might underlie the directed dendritic arborization seen in several systems: Optic tectal neurons from frogs have a rostro-caudal bias in the dendritic arbor. Neurons from dually-innervated frog optic tectum (Katz and Constantine-Paton 1988) and cat cortex (Kossel *et al.* 1995) exhibit a preference to arborize dendrites within eye-specific stripes. The stratification of retinal ganglion cells dendrites requires glutamate receptor activity (Bodnarenko and Chalupa 1993). Finally, synaptic inputs might control the selective pruning of dendritic branch tips seen in cortical Layer 5 pyramidal neurons (Koester and O'Leary 1992) and oriented dendritic elaboration in barrel cortical neurons (Harris and Woolsey 1981). Time-lapse images of dendritic spine dynamics in hippocampal pyramidal neurons from cultured slices also support a model in which synaptic inputs stabilize spines during synaptogenesis (Dailey and Smith 1996; Ziv and Smith 1996).

Branch retraction also plays an important role in refinement of dendritic arbor structure. In rat visual cortex, layer 5 pyramidal neurons project either to the ipsilateral superior colliculus or to the contralateral cortex via the corpus callosum. Before postnatal day 3 (P3), layer 5 pyramidal neurons are morphologically indistinguishable, with tufted apical dendrites reaching into layer 1. The corticocortical layer 5 pyramidal neurons acquire their mature phenotype by retraction of the tufted apical dendrites (Koester and O'Leary 1992; Kasper *et al.* 1994). Similarly, in the barrel fields of the somatosensory cortex, two processes are involved in the generation of oriented dendritic arbors—selective maintenance and extension of branches that arise from the internally-oriented side of the soma and selective retraction of branches that arise from the septum-oriented side of the soma (Greenough and Chang 1988). *In vivo* imaging shows that dendrites are constantly adding and retracting branches even in neurons with complex dendritic arbors (Rajan and Cline 1998; Wu and Cline 1998).

GABA function in the developing CNS

GABA is the principal inhibitory neurotransmitter in the adult brain. It acts at two classes of receptors, the ionotropic $GABA_A$ and $GABA_C$ receptors and the metabotropic $GABA_B$ receptor. $GABA_A$ receptors are located postsynaptically, are permeable to Cl^- and sensitive to bicuculline and picrotoxin (see Chapter 5). $GABA_B$ receptors are G-protein coupled receptors which are located both pre- and postsynaptically (Alger and Nicoll 1982; Chapter 4). Presynaptic $GABA_B$ receptors inhibit transmitter release (Fukuda *et al.* 1993; Gaiarsa *et al.* 1995). Postsynaptic $GABA_B$ receptors inhibit neuronal activity by activating K^+ channels. $GABA_C$ receptors are postsynaptic, chloride-permeable receptors which are sensitive to picrotoxin, but insensitive to bicuculline (Martina *et al.* 1995). $GABA_C$ receptors have been reported in the retinas of many species (Lukasiewicz and Shields 1998), in chick and frog optic tectum and the rodent central visual pathway (Martina *et al.* 1995; Nistri and Sivilotti 1995).

GABA seems to play several different roles during early embryogenesis and during the development of the nervous system, including the regulation of cell proliferation, differentiation, neuronal migration, and growth-cone guidance (Lauder 1993; Schousboe and Redburn 1995; Fukura *et al.* 1996). Once synapses do form, GABA again seems to play multiple roles, initially as a depolarizing transmitter, and then, as neurons develop mature Cl^- transport mechanisms, as a hyperpolarizing transmitter. Many of the early effects of GABA seem to be a result of the activation of $GABA_A$ receptors. Presynaptic $GABA_B$ receptors are functional and can reduce transmitter release early in development; postsynaptic $GABA_B$-receptor function has not, however, been detected until later stages in CNS development (Fukuda *et al.* 1993; Gaiarsa *et al.* 1995).

Until recently it was thought that GABAergic synaptic responses were not present in neonatal brain. Inhibitory postsynaptic responses reportedly developed after excitatory responses in mammalian brain and do not become fully functional until late in development (Berardi and Morrone 1984; Komatsu and Iwakiri 1991; Luhmann and Prince 1991; Burgard and Hablitz 1993; Agmon *et al.* 1996; Shi *et al.* 1997). More recent work indicates that activation of $GABA_A$ receptors depolarizes immature neurons and increases calcium influx through voltage-dependent calcium channels in many neuronal cell types (Zhang *et al.* 1991; Wang *et al.* 1994a; Owens *et al.* 1996; Rohrbough and Spitzer 1996; Ben-Ari *et al.* 1997; Leinekugel *et al.* 1997; Schwartz *et al.* 1998). During early stages of dendrite development GABA might depolarize neurons which have a high fraction of synapses with pure NMDA synapses. In so doing, the GABA-mediated depolarization might enable, by removal of the voltage-dependent Mg^{2+} block of NMDA receptors, the addition of AMPA receptors to silent synapses. In support of this idea, Leinekugel *et al.* (1997) recently demonstrated that depolarizing $GABA_A$ receptors cooperates with NMDA receptor activity in early postnatal hippocampal neurons to increase action potential activity and cause the generation and synchronization of giant depolarizing potentials.

The magnitude and direction of current flow in response to GABA receptor activation depends on the resting membrane potential (V_{rest}) of the neuron relative to the reversal potential for GABA-gated currents (E_{GABA}). Immature neurons might have more depolarized E_{GABA} than more mature neurons. Such a developmental shift in E_{GABA} has been observed in cortical and hippocampal neurons (Luhmann and Prince 1991; Zhang *et al.* 1991; Agmon *et al.* 1996; Owens *et al.* 1996) in which early postnatal neurons have E_{GABA} up to 25 mV more positive than neurons from more mature animals.

Development of GABAergic neurons

Considerable effort has been devoted toward understanding the biochemistry and molecular biology of GABAergic neuronal development. In mammalian cortex and hippocampus, GABAergic interneurons become postmitotic well before pyramidal or granule neurons (Ben-Ari *et al.* 1994). As development proceeds, GABA-ergic neurons form a heterogeneous group of cells characterized by variable morphologies, content of other neuroactive substances and laminar distribution (Hendry and Jones 1986; Antal 1991). Expression of peptide transmitters, which colocalize with GABA, develops relatively late (Hendry and Jones 1986; Debski and Constantine-Paton 1993). GABA immunoreactivity is reduced in somatosensory and visual cortices by deprivation paradigms (Hendry and Jones 1986; Warren *et al.* 1989; Kossut *et al.* 1991). The activity-dependent control of GABA expression seems to be regulated through brain-derived neurotrophic factor (BDNF; Mizuno *et al.* 1994; Widmer and Hefti 1994; Marty *et al.* 1996; Rutherford *et al.* 1997), the synthesis and release of which is also activity-regulated. Several studies have reported that the numbers of GABA-immunoreactive cells decrease during normal development (Berki *et al.* 1995; Kotak *et al.* 1998) or that distinct populations of cells transiently express GABA during early stages of development (Micheva and Beaulieu 1995). In Xenopus spinal cord, differentiation of GABAergic neurons is activity-regulated and in particular depends on calcium levels (Spitzer *et al.* 1993).

The expression of individual ionotropic GABA receptor subunits also seems to be regulated during development (Laurie *et al.* 1992; Fritschy *et al.* 1994) and by neuronal activity (Mower *et al.* 1988; Hendry *et al.* 1990; Huntsman *et al.* 1994). The different subunit composition of GABA receptors might result in different electro-physiological properties (Verdoorn *et al.* 1990; Xiang *et al.* 1998).

Several studies suggest that there might be some fundamental differences in the regulation of the morphological development of projection neurons compared with interneurons. For instance, the axon arbors of GABAergic interneurons elaborate extensively within the hippocampus while the axons of pyramidal neurons are still short (Ben-Ari *et al.* 1994). Although CaMKII activity regulates dendritic arbor stability in Xenopus tectal projection neurons (Wu and Cline 1998; Zou and Cline 1999), the morphological development of GABA-ergic interneurons is unaffected by CaMKII activity (Zou and Cline 1999), consistent with observations that GABA-ergic neurons do not express CaMKII (Benson *et al.* 1991). In addition, the activity-regulated protein CPG15 promotes dendritic arbor elaboration selectively in projection neurons, without any apparent effect on interneuronal development (Nedivi *et al.* 1998). In mammalian tissue, interneurons express a different range of cell-surface antigens which could influence their development (Hockfield and Kalb 1993; Benson *et al.* 1998). These studies suggest that axonal and dendritic arbor development of interneurons and projection neurons might be regulated differently.

Regulation of dendritic arbor elaboration by GABA

Exposure of cultured neurons to bicuculline for 3 days dwarfs neurite outgrowth, leading to the suggestion that GABA acts trophically to promote dendritic arbor growth (Barbin *et al.* 1993). Another study reported that GABA can either increase or reduce neurite outgrowth depending on the culture conditions (Michler 1990). A careful examination of multiple interacting factors demonstrated that in hippocampal cultures, GABA$_A$ receptor agonists increase interneuron dendritic arbor development in cultures of young neurons (in which GABA acts as a depolarizing transmitter) indirectly by increasing BDNF expression and release from nearby non-GABAergic neurons. BDNF then promotes development of the GABA-ergic interneurons. As neurons mature, and GABA becomes hyperpolarizing, GABA$_A$-receptor activation now inhibits dendritic arbor elaboration, again due to an indirect effect on the paracrine function of BDNF (Marty *et al.* 1996). This intimate interaction between BDNF and GABA-ergic neuronal development has also been shown *in vivo*. In transgenic mice which prematurely express BDNF, GABA-ergic inhibition develops early, which in turn has multiple effects on brain function (Huang *et al.* 1999) including synaptic connectivity and neuronal plasticity. This study highlights the importance of interacting factors operating in brain development. For instance, infusion of BDNF disrupts the formation of ocular dominance columns (Cabelli *et al.* 1995), possibly via its action on GABAergic inhibition.

Activity-regulated proteins and dendritic development

The signal transduction mechanisms linking glutamate receptor activity to modification in synaptic strength and neuronal structure are not yet clear. Considerable effort has been devoted toward understanding calcium-dependent events, because transient increases in cytosolic calcium follow synaptic activity. Calcium is known to affect synaptic physiology and neuronal growth by triggering calcium-dependent proteins, such as calcium calmodulin-dependent protein kinase II (CaMKII), protein kinase C (PKC), protein kinase A (PKA) and other Ca dependent pathways.

   CaMKII is a multifunctional kinase, located in both pre- and postsynaptic neurons throughout the brain. Presynaptic CaMKII activity controls neurotransmitter release (Llinas *et al.* 1991) and might regulate presynaptic plasticity (Chapman *et al.* 1995). In postsynaptic neurons, CaMKII is a major constituent of the postsynaptic density (PSD; Kennedy *et al.* 1983) where it can influence synaptic plasticity by phosphorylating AMPA receptors (McGlade-McCulloh *et al.* 1992), cytoskeletal proteins (Schulman 1993), or other proteins potentially involved in synaptic plasticity (Scott and Soderling 1992; Schulman and Hanson 1993; Mayford *et al.* 1996*b*; Omkumar *et al.* 1996; Kennedy 1997; Chen *et al.* 1998; Kennedy 1998; Kim *et al.* 1998; Zhang *et al.* 1999).

CaMKII has been implicated in several forms of neural plasticity such as learning and memory in mice (Silva *et al.* 1992*a,b*; Mayford *et al.* 1996*a*; Giese *et al.* 1998) and fruit flies (Griffith *et al.* 1993), experience-dependent plasticity in the adult barrel cortex (Glazewski *et al.* 1996) and synaptic plasticity (Malenka *et al.* 1989; Malinow *et al.* 1989). In *Drosophila*, blocking CaMKII activity by expressing an inhibitory peptide increased neuronal growth at the neuromuscular junction (Wang *et al.* 1994*b*). Mutant mice lacking αCaMKII have defects in developmental visual system plasticity (Gordon *et al.* 1996). αCaMKII expression is developmentally regulated (Kelly *et al.* 1987; Braun and Schulman 1995; Wu and Cline 1998), such that its expression correlates with times of synapse maturation and dendritic arbor stabilization. Postsynaptic CaMKII activity promotes the morphological and synaptic maturation of the optic tectal neurons (Figs 2.5 and 2.6) (Wu *et al.* 1996; Wu and Cline 1998) and presynaptic retinal axons (Zou and Cline 1996*a,b*). These studies indicate that CaMKII-dependent pathways play a role in activity-dependent functional and structural plasticity during development.

Activity-dependent circuit formation

The development of dendrite structure and function clearly has bearing on the development of neural circuits. The conservation across species of the developmental shift from pure NMDA receptor synapses to synapses with AMPA and NMDA receptors suggests this transition might play an important functional role in circuit formation. Correlated afferent activity patterns operating via NMDA receptor—and CaMKII-dependent mechanisms—might control synaptic strength and the stabilization of neuronal structure during the development of organized projections from one brain region to another. In the developing retinotectal system, retinal axon arbor structure is constantly changing in living tadpoles during a period of map refinement as the axons rapidly add and retract branches (Witte *et al.* 1996). Clusters of synaptic vesicle proteins, marking putative presynaptic sites, are located on the transient branches, suggesting that they are capable of forming synapses with tectal neurons (Pinches and Cline 1998). During refinement of the topographic projection these branches might form pure NMDA trial synapses which test for coactivity with other inputs converging on the same postsynaptic tectal cell (Cline *et al.* 1997). Pure NMDA synapses can detect convergent coactive activity because they conduct current only when the postsynaptic neuron is simultaneously depolarized (Nowak *et al.* 1984), for instance by converging co-active inputs. At early stages of development of tectal neurons, this synaptic input promotes dendritic arbor growth. Later, when neurons express αCaMKII, coactive synaptic inputs have a different effect on neuronal growth and synaptic physiology. Under these conditions, calcium influx through NMDA receptors can activate CaMKII (Fukunaga *et al.* 1992). Increased CaMKII activity then promotes the addition of functional AMPA receptors to

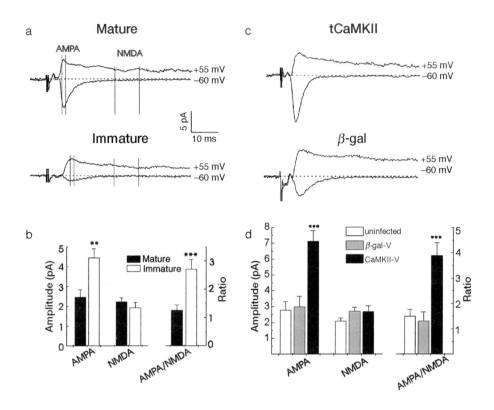

Fig. 2.5 Developmental increase in the AMPA component is promoted by CaMKII expression. (a) The amplitude of the AMPA component recorded at −60 mV is greater in mature neurons (top) than in immature neurons (bottom). The amplitude of the NMDA component does not change with development. Averaged traces of evoked retinotectal synaptic currents following a minimal stimulation protocol. (b) Quantification of the amplitudes of the AMPA and NMDA components and their ratio during normal development. Mature neurons express CaMKII, but immature neurons do not. (c) Expression of the catalytic subunit of CaMKII (tCaMKII) in immature tectal neurons increases the amplitude of the AMPA component, but not the NMDA component in retinotectal evoked synaptic currents. (d) Quantification of the amplitudes of the AMPA and NMDA components. Control neurons from animals expressing β-galactosidase (β -gal) are comparable with neurons from uninfected control animals. (Modified from Wu *et al.* 1996.)

synapses (Wu *et al.* 1996). Increased CaMKII activity also stabilizes the dendritic arbor structure by reducing the rates of branch additions and retractions (Wu and Cline 1998). In this way afferent activity patterns can coordinately control synaptic strength and structural plasticity through CaMKII-dependent mechanisms. Trial synapses which are not coactive with other inputs on the postsynaptic neuron would not activate NMDA receptors and the sequence of events of calcium influx, CaMKII activity, increased AMPA receptor function and branch stabilization would not occur. Consequently these trial synapses would not be stabilized and would retract. Because the trial synapses are thought to be silent unless their activity is correlated

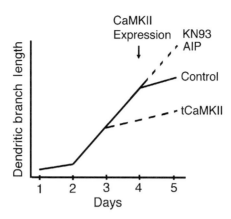

Fig. 2.6 Summary of the effects of CaMKII on dendritic arbor development. During normal development CaMKII expression correlates with the time when dendritic arbor growth rate slows in mature neurons. Premature expression of catalytic subunit of CaMKII (tCaMKII) with a viral vector slows arbor growth rate and stabilizes dendritic branch dynamics. Blocking endogenous CaMKII, either with the antagonist KN93 or by viral expression of the peptide inhibitor AIP, maintain neurons in the rapid growth phase.

with other input activity, retinal afferents could test for sites where coactive inputs also terminate during the refinement of the topographic projection, without degrading information transfer (Cline *et al.* 1997). When the trial synapses are coactive, they will increase AMPA receptor-mediated synaptic responses and so begin to contribute to the transfer of topographically organized visual information.

Activity-induced genes and dendritic growth

Neuronal activity can also influence the development of dendritic structure and function by inducing genes whose protein products in turn have an impact on dendritic function. Screening performed by several laboratories to identify activity-induced genes successfully revealed a large pool of candidate plasticity genes (Nedivi *et al.* 1993; Qian *et al.* 1993; Yamagata *et al.* 1993). Many of the genes identified by these unbiased screens were previously known to be regulated by activity, such as the transcription factor zif268, and potential downstream effector proteins such as GAP43, CaMKII, glutamic acid decarboxylase, and neurotrophins. Other induced genes were previously known, but their induction by activity had been unrecognized, such as class 1 major histocompatibility antigen (MHC1), and tissue plasminogen activator (tPA) (Reviewed by Nedivi 1999). Many known activity-induced genes have functions related to structural remodeling. This suggests that a significant fraction of the remainder of candidate plasticity genes will also have functions related to neuronal structure.

A large fraction of the pool of activity-induced genes were unidentified—novel genes at the time of the screening. Identification of the candidate plasticity genes was the first step toward determining a potential function in structural and functional plasticity. The large pool of candidate plasticity genes was then subjected to secondary screening in an attempt to identify those whose expression is regulated during development and is also induced by a physiological stimulus, with the idea that such a subset of activity-regulated genes might play a role in experience-dependent structural plasticity. Subsequent analysis of the functions of activity-induced genes, such as Arc, Homer, Narp and CPG15 in neuronal plasticity have revealed multiple mechanisms by which activity can have an impact on neuronal function.

Candidate plasticity gene 15 (CPG15) is an example of a novel activity-induced gene which was subsequently demonstrated to have both structural and functional effects on dendritic development (Naeve *et al.* 1997; Nedivi *et al.* 1997; Haas *et al.* 1998). Sequence analysis of the CPG15 cDNA predicted a small, secreted protein bound to the extracellular surface of the cell through a glycosylphosphatidylinositol (GPI) linkage. The gene and protein are highly conserved from Xenopus to human. The potential function of CPG15 *in vivo* has been examined most thoroughly in Xenopus, although studies have also been conducted in rat and cat (Nedivi 1999). Each system has its particular advantages and has revealed different aspects of CPG15 function. In Xenopus, CPG15 protein is expressed in the retinal ganglion cells, where it is enriched in their axons within the tectal neuropil. CPG15 is expressed widely in the brain, including optic tectal neurons. The potential function of CPG15 in dendritic arbor development has been examined with time-lapse images of single optic tectal neurons from living Xenopus tadpoles over periods of 3 days. Combining *in vivo* imaging with vaccinia virus-mediated gene transfer shows that CPG15 functions as a membrane-bound growth-promoting molecule. In addition to promoting dendritic arbor elaboration, CPG15 expression enhances the strength of retinotectal synaptic transmission and promotes the maturation of glutamatergic synapses (Haas *et al.* 1998). CPG15 enhances dendritic arbor growth *in vivo,* selectively in projection neurons (Fig. 2.7), but has no effect on dendritic development in interneurons. This again indicates that the regulation of interneuron dendritic development is controlled differently from that of projection neurons, perhaps by different molecular participants.

CPG15, a protein linked to the membrane by a glycosylphosphatidylinositol (GPI) linkage, controls growth of neighboring neurons through an intercellular signaling mechanism. Viral expression of a truncated form of CPG15, lacking the GPI consensus sequence, inhibits dendritic arbor growth in tectal neurons and blocks the normal maturational program of glutamatergic synapses. This indicates that the GPI link is necessary for CPG15 function. These data further indicate that expression of soluble CPG15 interferes with the function of endogenous CPG15.

The mechanism by which CPG15 promotes dendritic arbor development is not yet clear. Exposure of cultured neurons to CPG15 induces BDNF (Naeve *et al.* 1997). This, together with the observation that CPG15 acts in a non-cell autonomous fashion, suggests that it might trigger additional gene transcription by interacting with a membrane-bound receptor. Although CPG15 is a novel gene, the proteins most similar to it are ligands of the eph subfamily of receptor tyrosine kinases (ephrins). Two of the ephrins, ephrin-A2 and ephrin-A5 are anchored to the membrane by a GPI-linkage, similar to CPG15. Recent data suggest that in addition

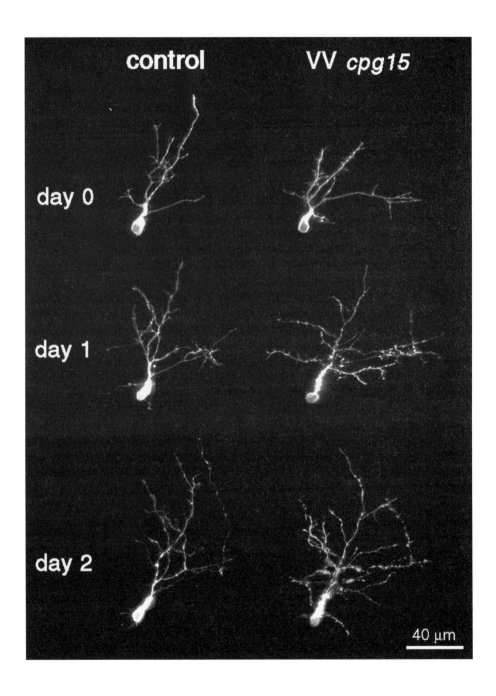

Fig. 2.7 CPG15, an activity-induced protein, increases dendritic arbor elaboration. Single DiI-labeled neurons were imaged over 3 days *in vivo* either in control animals or in animals virally expressing CPG15. CPG15 increases dendritic growth rate and complexity.

to their function as guidance molecules for topographic mapping of retinotectal projections (Cheng and Flanagan 1994; Drescher *et al.* 1995; Nakamoto *et al.* 1996), the membrane-bound ephrins may also play a role in learning and memory, as well as their cellular correlate, long-term potentiation.

These findings suggest the existence of a new class of activity-regulated growth-promoting proteins, which by virtue of being membrane-bound, might enable exquisite spatial and temporal control of neuronal growth.

Neurotrophins

Neurotrophins comprise a family of at least five structurally related proteins, nerve growth factor (NGF), brain-derived neurotrophic factor (BDNF), neurotrophin-3 (NT-3), neurotrophin-4/neurotrophin-5 (NT-4/5) and neurotrophin-6 (NT-6). Neurotrophins exert their function through binding and activation of receptor tyrosine kinases (reviewed by Lewin and Barde 1996). Their role in promoting dendritic arbor elaboration *in vivo* was demonstrated originally for neurons from the peripheral nervous system (Purves *et al.* 1988). Neurotrophins can also function within the CNS to regulate dendritic arbor development (McAllister *et al.* 1995), spine density (Shimada *et al.* 1998) and synaptic transmission (Lewin and Barde 1996).

Neurotrophins and their receptors are expressed within the CNS. Their expression levels and distribution vary with development (Allendoerfer *et al.* 1994; Cohen-Cory and Fraser 1994). Neurotrophin gene expression is strongly induced by neuronal activity (Gall and Isackson 1989; Ernfors *et al.* 1991; Castren *et al.* 1992, 1993; Cabell and Audesirk 1993) and neurotrophins may be released from dendrites in response to activity (Blochl and Thoenen 1995). These data suggest that neurotrophin synthesis and release might be regulated by activity and by extension, neurotrophin mediated control of dendritic development is indirectly controlled by neuronal activity. Despite its appeal, direct and convincing evidence for this scenario *in vivo* is not yet available.

A vast literature has documented the effects of neurotrophins applied to neuronal structure in dissociated cell culture (Lewin and Barde 1996). Exposure of cortical slice cultures to neurotrophins can increase or reduce dendritic arbor elaboration in a cell-type specific manner (McAllister *et al.* 1995). The action of neurotrophins on dendritic arbor development is quite complex. Different neurotrophins can either promote or diminish dendritic arbor growth in subsets of neurons; different neuro-trophins can also affect either apical or basal dendrites preferentially (McAllister *et al.* 1995, 1997). The response of dendritic arbors to neurotrophin application in slice culture also depends on glutamate-receptor activity in the culture—blocking glutamate receptor activity with AP5 or CNQX blocks dendritic arbor elaboration in either the presence or absence of applied neurotrophins (McAllister *et al.* 1996).

One source of the complexity of the effects of neurotrophins on dendritic arbor development has to do with sorting out the sites of action of the neurotrophins. One example of this issue was mentioned above, in which GABA$_A$-receptor activity affects dendritic arbor development indirectly by regulating neurotrophin synthesis and release from pyramidal neurons. The interplay between excitatory activity, BDNF and the regulation of inhibition controls the levels of excitability within the network (Rutherford *et al.* 1997); this in turn can modulate dendritic structure. The effects of neurotrophins in dendritic arbor development *in vivo* are also likely mediated through multiple intracellular and intercellular pathways.

As the functions of more activity-induced genes are discovered, studies of their unique and overlapping functions will enhance our understanding of mechanisms that control development of dendrite structure and function, and their modification by activity.

Regulation of dendritic development: other mechanisms

GTPases and Neuronal Growth

Several recent studies (Luo *et al.* 1994, 1997; Sone 1997; Zipkin *et al.* 1997; Builluart *et al.* 1998; D'Adamo *et al.* 1998; Kaufmann *et al.* 1998; Steven *et al.* 1998) suggest that the Rho family of small GTPases, including Rho, Rac and Cdc42, might play a role in early neuronal development. GTPases are widely expressed in the developing brain. In addition to their roles in cell proliferation and migration, the RhoA GTPases are essential for neuronal development in *C. elegans*, Drosophila, rodents and humans (Luo *et al.* 1994, 1997; Sone 1997; Zipkin *et al.* 1997; Builluart *et al.* 1998; D'Adamo *et al.* 1998; Kaufmann *et al.* 1998; Steven *et al.* 1998). In humans, defects in GTPase signaling have recently been identified as the genetic basis of some forms of mental retardation (Builluart *et al.* 1998; D'Adamo *et al.* 1998), which is characterized by striking deficits in dendritic arbor development (Purpura 1975). The pathophysiology of Huntington's disease, an autosomal dominant neurodegenerative disorder associated with dendritic structural abnormalities and degeneration, might also involve errors in GTPase signaling pathways (Colomer *et al.* 1997).

The Rho GTPases, including Rho, Rac and Cdc42 were first identified as being required for establishment of polarity and budding in yeast (Van Aelst and D'Souza-Schorey 1997; Hall 1998) and by analogy, these highly conserved proteins may regulate polarity and branching in neurons. Extensive studies in cell culture have established an interaction between the Rho GTPases and the cytoskeleton (Van Aelst and D'Souza-Schorey 1997; Hall 1998). According to studies in neuronal cell lines (Tigyi *et al.* 1996; Kozma *et al.* 1997; Threadgill *et al.* 1997; Van Leeuwen *et al.* 1997), the three RhoA GTPases, Rac, Rho and Cdc42 play distinct roles in regulating cytoskeletal stability. Rho increases process retraction; Cdc42 and Rac increase process extension. Numerous effector proteins downstream of the GTPases have been identified which probably mediate the multiple cellular effects of the signaling pathways (Luo *et al.* 1997; Van Aelst and D'Souza-Schorey 1997; Hall 1998).

GTPases act as molecular switches—when they bind GTP, they activate downstream effectors, and when they bind GDP, they do not activate effectors. The general idea of the signaling pathway is that an extracellular signal acting through a transmembrane receptor activates proteins called GTPase exchange factors (GEFs). The GEFs catalyze the exchange of GDP for GTP required for GTPase activation. Active GTPases can then send at least two types of downstream signal. One is a local signal which modifies the actin cytoskeleton, microtubules (Cook *et al.* 1998) and intermediate filaments (Sin *et al.* 1998). The second pathway, mediated by specific downstream effectors, activates gene transcription (reviewed by Van Aelst and D'Souza-Schorey 1997).

In Drosophila, Rac is required for axonal but not dendritic outgrowth and targeting (Luo *et al.* 1994; Sone 1997; Kaufmann *et al.* 1998). In contrast, Cdc42 seems to be required for both axonal and dendritic development in some Drosophila neurons (Luo *et al.* 1994). Transgenic mice expressing the constitutively active Rac are ataxic and their Purkinje cells have deficient axonal growth but an abundance of abnormal dendritic 'mini' spines (Luo *et al.* 1997). These differences between the responses of axonal and dendritic compartments of the same neuron to the same experimental manipulation could be because of different downstream effector pathways in dendrites and axons.

The potential function of Rho in CNS development has not yet been examined *in vivo*; in neuronal cell culture, however, Rho activity appears to increase neurite retraction (Gebbink *et al.* 1997; Kozma *et al.* 1997; Hall 1998; Sin *et al.* 1998). Alternately, Rho might operate to effectively prevent branch initiation and extension (Tigyi *et al.* 1996), however increased process outgrowth has been observed in cultured cortical neurons transfected with active Rho (Threadgill *et al.* 1997).

Although there is no direct evidence for a connection between GTPase signaling pathways and regulation by synaptic activity, there are several hints that these signaling pathways can cross, which could in turn have bearing on mechanisms of dendritic arbor development. Cdc42 is induced in the brain after activity (Gong *et al.* 1996), as is rheb, a ras-related protein (Yamagata *et al.* 1994). The RhoA GTPases can regulate cell—cell contacts through presentation and clustering of cadherins and integrins on the cell surface (Hall 1998), which can have a direct effect on dendritic process outgrowth. The recent evidence that cadherins can function in synapse stabilization (Fannon and Colman 1996) suggests an intriguing connection between GTPases and synaptogenesis. Disruption of the actin cytoskeleton results in redistribution of glutamate receptors (Allison *et al.* 1998), suggesting that mechanisms responsible for maintaining the integrity of the cortical actin cytoskeleton, such as those involving GTPases, might regulate synaptogenesis, synaptic maintenance and dendritic arbor morphology. Additional hints of an interaction between GTPase signal-transduction pathways and those concerning synaptic activity come from studies demonstrating that some proteins involved in GTPase signaling are concentrated in postsynaptic densities (Kennedy 1998). Furthermore, GTPases, Rac1 and Cdc42 modulate voltage-dependent Ca^{2+} currents in neuronal cell culture (Wilk-Blaszczak *et al.* 1997), suggesting multiple potential pathways by which GTPases might influence morphological and physiological development of dendrites.

Concluding remarks

Multiple factors interact to accomplish the development of dendrite structure and function. Recent studies which address the mechanisms regulating dendritic development using multidisciplinary approaches have provided considerable insight into the complex contributions of feedforward and feedback systems in controlling circuit formation. It now seems that, rather than being controlled by intrinsic factors, dendrite development is primarily controlled by activity. Activity can take many forms, from waves of calcium spreading through gap junctions to spontaneous release of transmitter which can act metabotropically at receptors. It also seems that the tools we have traditionally used to test for the role of activity in brain development have failed us. They do not block all mechanisms that can be regulated by activity. Again, the observations that spontaneous levels of transmitter release are sufficient to maintain dendritic spine density (McKinney *et al.* 1999) and that AMPA receptor binding of glutamate can activate non-receptor tyrosine kinase (Hayashi *et al.* 1999) are particularly sobering examples of new found activity-dependent mechanisms that are not sensitive to the traditional activity blocker, TTX. Experiments in the intact animal have also taught us that many redundant mechanisms work hard to generate a functional nervous system. When we manipulate a single protein in this complex system, the cells and the circuit call into action a variety of counteracting mechanisms which operate to compensate for the insult. These counteracting, homeostatic mechanisms are also fundamental to brain development.

References

Agmon, A., Hollrigel, G., and O'Dowd, D. (1996). Functional GABAergic synaptic connection in neonatal mouse barrel cortex. *Journal of Neuroscience*, **16**, 4684–95.

Alger, B. E. and Nicoll, R. A. (1982). Pharmacological evidence for two kinds of GABA receptor on rat hippocampal pyramidal cells studied *in vitro*. *Journal of Physiology (Lond)*, **328**, 125–41.

Allendoerfer, K. L., Cabelli, R. J., Escandon, E., Kaplan, D. R., Nikolics, K., and Shatz, C. J. (1994). Regulation of neurotrophin receptors during the maturation of the mammalian visual system. *Journal of Neuroscience*, **14**, 1795–811.

Allison, D. W., Gelfand, V. I., Spector, I., and Craig, A. M. (1998). Role of actin in anchoring postsynaptic receptors in cultured hippocampal neurons: differential attachment of NMDA versus AMPA receptors. *Journal of Neuroscience*, **18**, 2423–36.

Antal, M. (1991). Distribution of GABA immunoreactivity in the optic tectum of the frog: a light and electron microscopic study. *Neuroscience*, **42**, 879–91.

Antonini, A. and Stryker, M. P. (1993). Rapid remodeling of axonal arbors in the visual cortex. *Science*, **260**, 1819–21.

Barbin, G., Pollard, H., Gaiarsa, J., and Ari, Y. B. (1993). Involvement of GABA$_A$ receptors in the outgrowth of cultured hippocampal neurons. *Neuroscience Letters*, **152**, 150–4.

Ben-Ari, Y., Tseeb, V., Raggozzino, D., Khazipov, R., and Gaiarsa, J. L. (1994). γ-Amino-butyric acid (GABA): a fast excitatory transmitter which may regulate the development of hippocampal neurones in early postnatal life. *Progress in Brain Research*, **102**, 261–73.

Ben-Ari, Y., Khazipov, R., Leinekugel, X., Caillard, O., and Gaiarsa, J.-L. (1997). GABA$_A$, NMDA and AMPA receptors: a developmentally regulated 'menage a trois'. *Trends in Neuroscience*, **20**, 523–9.

Benes, F., Parks, T., and Rubel, E. (1977). Rapid dendritic atrophy following deafferentation, an EM morphometric analysis. *Brain Research*, **122**, 1–13.

Benson, D., Isaacson, P., Hendry, S., and Jones, T. (1991). Differential gene expression for glutamic acid decarboxylase and type II calcium-calmodulin-dependent protein kinase in basal ganglia, thalamus, and hypothalamus of the monkey. *Journal of Neuroscience*, **11**, 1540–64.

Benson, D., Yoshihara, Y., and Mori, K. (1998). Polarized distribution and cell type-specific localization of telencephalin, and intercellular adhesion molecule. *Journal of Neuroscience Research*, **52**, 43–53.

Berardi, N. and Morrone, M. (1984). Development of γ-aminobutyric acid mediated inhibition of x cells of the cat lateral geniculate nucleus. *Journal of Physiology (Lond)*, **357**, 525–37.

Berki, A., O'Donovan, M., and Antal, M. (1995). Developmental expression of glycine immunoreactivity and its colocalization with GABA in the embryonic chick lumbosacral spinal cord. *Journal of Comparative Neurology*, **362**, 583–96.

Blanton, M. G., LoTurco, J. J., and Kriegstein, A. (1990). Endogenous neurotransmitter activates *N*-methyl-D-aspartate receptors on differentiating neurons in embryonic cortex. *Proceedings of the National Academy of Science USA*, **87**, 8027–30.

Blochl, A. and Thoenen, H. (1995). Characterization of nerve growth factor (NGF) release from hippocampal neurons: evidence for a constitutive and an unconventional sodium-dependent regulated pathway. *European Journal of Neuroscience*, **7**, 1220–8.

Bodnarenko, S. R. and Chalupa, L. M. (1993). Stratification of On and OFF dendrites depends on glutamate-mediated afferent activity in the developing retina. *Nature*, **364**, 144–6.

Braun, A. P. and Schulman, H. (1995). The multifunctional calcium/calmodulin dependent protein kinase: from form to function. *Annual Review of Physiology*, **57**, 417–45.

Builluart, P., Bienvenu, T., Ronce, N., des Portes, V., Vinet, M. C., Zemni, R., *et al.* (1998). Oligophrenin-1 encodes a rhoGAP protein involved in X-linked mental retardation. *Nature*, **392**, 823–6.

Burgard, E. and Hablitz, J. (1993). Developmental changes in NMDA and non-NMDA receptor-mediated synaptic potentials in rat neocortex. *Journal of Neurophysiology*, **69**, 230–40.

Cabell, L. and Audesirk, G. (1993). Effects of selective inhibition of protein kinase C, cyclic AMP-dependent protein kinase, and Ca^{2+}/calmodulin-dependent protein kinase on neurite development in cultured rat hippocampal neurons. *International Journal of Developmental Neuroscience*, **11**, 357–68.

Cabelli, R. J., Andreas, H., and Shatz, C. J. (1995). Inhibition of ocular dominance column formation by infusion of NT-4/5 or BDNF. *Science*, **267**, 1662–6.

Castren, E., Zafra, F., Thoenen, H., and Lindholm, D. (1992). Light regulates expression of brain-derived neurotrophic factor mRNA in rat visual cortex. *Proceedings of the National Academy of Science USA*, **89**, 9444–8.

Castren, E., Pitkanen, M., Sirvio, J., Parsadanian, A., Lindholm, D., Thoenen, H., *et al.* (1993). The induction of LTP increases BDNF and NGF mRNA but decreases NT-3 mRNA in the dentate gyrus. *Neuroreport*, **4**, 895–8.

Chapman, P. F., Frenguelli, B. G., Smith, A., Chen, C.-H., and Silva, A. (1995). The α-Ca^{2+}/calmodulin kinase II: a bidirectional modulator of presynaptic plasticity. *Neuron*, **14**, 591–7.

Chen, H.-J., Rojas-Soto, M., Oguni, A., and Kennedy, M. B. (1998). A synaptic Ras-GTPase activating protein (p135 SynGAP) inhibited by CaM kinase II. *Neuron*, **20**, 895–904.

Cheng, H.-J. and Flanagan, J. G. (1994). Identification and cloning of ELF-1, a developmentally expressed ligand for the Mek4 and Sek receptor tyrosine kinases. *Cell*, **79**, 157–68.

Cline, H. T., Wu, G.-Y., and Malinow, R. (1997). *In vivo* development of neuronal structure and function. *Cold Spring Harbor Symposium Quant. Biol.*, **61**, 95–104.

Cohen-Cory, S. and Fraser, S. E. (1994). BDNF in the development of the visual system of Xenopus. *Neuron*, **12**, 747–61.

Colomer, V., Engelender, S., Sharp, A. H., Duan, K., Cooper, J. K., Lanahan, A., *et al.* (1997). Huntingtin-associated protein 1 (HAP1) binds to a Trio-like polypeptide, with a rac1 guanine nucleotide exchange factor domain. *Human Molecular Genetics*, **6**, 1519–25.

Comery, T. A., Harris, J. B., Willems, P. J., Oostra, B. A., Irwin, S. A., Weiler, I. J. *et al.* (1997). Abnormal dendritic spines in fragile X knockout mice: maturation and pruning deficits. *Proceedings of the National Academy of Science USA*, **94**, 5401–4.

Constantine-Paton, M. and Ferrari-Eastman, P. (1981). Topographic and morphometric effects of bilateral embryonic eye removal on the optic tectum and nucleus isthmus of the leopard frog. *Journal of Comparative Neurology* **196**, 645–61.

Constantine-Paton, M., Cline, H. T., and Debski, E. A. (1990). Patterned activity, synaptic convergence and the NMDA receptor in developing visual pathways. *Annual Review of Neuroscience*, **13**, 129–54.

Cook, T. A., Nagasaki, T., and Gundersen, G. G. (1998). Rho guanosine triphosphatase mediates the selective stabilization of microtubules induced by lysophosphatidic acid. *Journal of Cell Biology*, **141**, 175–85.

D'Adamo, P., Menegon, A., Lo, N. C., Grasso, M., Gulisano, M., Tamanini, F. *et al.* (1998). Mutations in GDI1 are responsible for X-linked non-specific mental retardation *Nature Genetics* **19**, 134–9.

Dailey, M. E. and Smith, S. J. (1996). The dynamics of dendritic structure in developing hippocampal slices. *Journal of Neuroscience*, **16**, 2983–94.

Dalva, M. B., Ghosh, A., and Shatz, C. J. (1994). Independent control of dendritic and axonal form in the developing lateral geniculate nucleus. *Journal of Neuroscience*, **14**, 3588–602.

Debski, E. A. and Constantine-Paton, M. (1993). The development of non-retinal afferent projections to the frog optic tectum and the substance P immunoreactivity of tectal connections. *Developmental Brain Research*, **72**, 21–39.

Deitch, J. S. and Rubel, E. W. (1984). Afferent influences on brain stem auditory nuclei of the chicken: time course and specificity of dendritic atrophy following deafferentation. *Journal of Comparative Neurology*, **229**, 66–79.

Drescher, U., Kremoser, C., Handwerker, C., Loschinger, J., Noda, M., and Bonhoeffer, F. (1995). *In vitro* guidance of retinal ganglion cell axons by RAGS, a 25 kDa tectal protein related to ligands for Eph receptor tyrosine kinases. *Cell*, **82**, 359–70.

Durand, G. M., Kovalchuk, Y., and Konnerth, A. (1996). Long-term potentiation and functional synapse induction in developing hippocampus. *Nature*, **381**, 71–5.

Ernfors, P., Bengzon, J., Kokaia, Z., Persson, H., and Lindvall, O. (1991). Increased levels of messenger RNAs for neurotrophic factors in the brain during kindling epileptogenesis. *Neuron*, **7**, 165–76.

Fannon, A. M. and Colman, D. R. (1996). A model for central synaptic junctional complex formation based on the differential adhesive specificities of the cadherins. *Neuron*, **17**, 423–34.

Feldman, D. E. and Knudsen, E. I. (1997). An anatomical basis for visual calibration of the auditory space map in the barn owl's midbrain. *Journal of Neuroscience*, **17**, 6820–37.

Feldman, D. E. and Knudsen, E. I. (1998). Pharmacological specialization of learned auditory responses in the inferior colliculus of the barn owl. *Journal of Neuroscience*, **18**, 3073–87.

Feldman, D. E., Brainard, M. S., and Knudsen, E. I. (1996). Newly learned auditory responses mediated by NMDA receptors in the owl inferior colliculus. *Science*, **271**, 525–8.

Feng, A. and Rogowski, B. (1980). Effects of monaural and binaural occlusion on the morphology of neurons in the medial superior olivary nucleus of the rat. *Brain Research*, **189**, 530–4.

Fields, R. D. and Nelson, P. G. (1992). Activity-dependent development of the vertebrate nervous system. *International Review of Neurobiology*, **34**, 133–214.

Fritschy, J.-M., Paysan, J., Enna, A., and Mohler, H. (1994). Switch in the expression of rat GABA$_A$-receptor subtypes during postnatal development: an immunohistochemical study. *Journal of Neuroscience*, **14**, 5302–24.

Fukuda, A., Mody, I., and Prince, D. (1993). Differential ontogenesis of presynaptic and postsynaptic GABA$_B$ inhibition in rat somatosensory cortex. *Journal of Neurophysiology*, **70**, 448–52.

Fukunaga, K., Solderling, T. R., and Miyamoto, E. (1992). Activation of Ca^{++}/calmodulin-dependent protein kinase II and protein kinase C by glutamate in cultured rat hippocampal neurons. *Journal of Biological Chemistry*, **267**, 22527–33.

Fukura, H., Komiya, Y., and Igarashi, M. (1996). Signaling pathway downstream of GABA$_A$ receptor in the growth cone. *Journal of Neurochemistry*, **67**, 1426–34.

Gaiarsa, J., McLean, H., Congar, P., Leinekugel, X., Khazipov, R., Tseeb, V. *et al.* (1995). Postnatal maturation of gamma-aminobutyric acid A and B-mediated inhibition in the CA3 hippocampal region of the rat. *Journal of Neurobiology*, **26**, 339–49.

Gall, C. M. and Isackson, P. J. (1989). Limbic seizures increase neuronal production of messenger RNA for nerve growth factor. *Science*, **245**, 758–61.

Gebbink, M. F., Kranenburg, O., Poland, M., van, H. F., Houssa, B., and Moolenaar, W. H. (1997). Identification of a novel, putative Rho-specific GDP/GTP exchange factor and a RhoA-binding protein: control of neuronal morphology. *Journal of Cell Biology*, **137**, 1603–13.

Giese, K. P., Fedorov, N. B., Filipkowski, R. K., and Silva, A. J. (1998). Autophosphorylation at Thr286 of the alpha calcium-calmodulin kinase II in LTP and learning. *Science*, **279**, 870–3.

Glazewski, S., Chen, C.-M., Silva, A., and Fox, K. (1996). Requirement for α-CaMKII in experience-dependent plasticity of the barrel cortex. *Science*, **272**, 421–3.

Gong, T. W., Hegeman, A. D., Shin, J. J., Adler, H. J., Raphael, Y., and Lomax, M. I. (1996). Identification of genes expressed after noise exposure in the chick basilar papilla. *Hearing Research*, **96**, 20–32.

Goodman, L. A. and Model, P. G. (1990). Eliminating afferent impulse activity does not alter the dendritic branching of the amphibian mauthner cell. *Journal of Neurobiology*, **21**, 283–94.

Gordon, J. A., Cioffi, D., Silva, A. J., and Stryker, M. P. (1996). Deficient plasticity in the primary visual cortex of α-calcium/calmodulin-dependent protein kinase II mutant mice. *Neuron*, **17**, 491–9.

Gray, L., Smith, Z., and Rubel, E. W. (1982). Developmental and experimental changes in dendritic symmetry in n. laminaris of the chick. *Brain Research*, **244**, 360–4.

Greenough, W. T. and Chang, F.-L. F. (1988). Dendritic pattern formation involves both oriented regression and oriented growth in the barrels of mouse somatosensory cortex. *Developmental Brain Research*, **43**, 148–52.

Griffith, L. C., Verselis, L. M., Aitken, K. M., Kyriacou, C. P., Danho, W., and Greenspan, R. J. (1993). Inhibition of calcium/calmodulin-dependent protein kinase in Drosophila disrupts behavioral plasticity. *Neuron*, **10**, 501–9.

Haas, K., Nedivi, E., Malinow, R., and Cline, H. T. (1998). Expression of the activity-induced gene, CPG15, promotes maturation of retinotectal synapses. *Society for Neuroscience Abstracts*, **24**, 1038.

Hall, A. (1998). Rho GTPases and the actin cytoskeleton. *Science*, **279**, 509–14.

Harris, R. and Woolsey, T. (1981). Dendritic plasticity in mouse barrel cortex following postnatal vibrissa follicle damage. *Journal of Comparative Neurology* **196**, 357–76.

Harris, W. A., Holt, C. E., and Bonhoeffer, F. (1987). Retinal axons with and without their somata, growing to and arborizing in the tectum of Xenopus embryos: a time-lapse video study of single fibres *in vivo*. *Development*, **101**, 123–33.

Hayashi, T., Umemori, H., Mishina, M., and Yamamoto, T. (1999). The AMPA receptor interacts with and signals through the protein tyrosine kinase Lyn. *Nature*, **397**, 72–6.

Hendry, S. and Jones, E. (1986). Reduction in number of immunostained GABAergic neurones in deprived-eye dominance columns of monkey area 17. *Nature*, **320**, 750–3.

Hendry, S., Fuchs, J., deBlas, A., and Jones, E. (1990). Distribution and plasticity of immunocytochemically localized GABA$_A$ receptors in adult monkey visual cortex. *Journal of Neuroscience*, **10**, 2438–50.

Hockfield, S. and Kalb, R. G. (1993). Activity-dependent structural changes during neuronal development. *Current Opinion in Neurobiology*, **3**, 87–92.

Hollman, M. and Heinemann, S. (1994). Cloned glutamate receptors. *Annual Review of Neuroscience*, **17**, 31–108.

Huang, Z. J., Kirkwood, A., Pizzorusso, T., Porcciatti, V., Bear, M. F., Maffei, L., and Tonegawa, S. (1999). Precocious development of visual cortical inhibition and visual acuity in transgenic mice overexpressing BDNF in postnatal forebrain. *Cell*. (In press.)

Huntsman, M., Isackson, P., and Jones, E. (1994). Lamina-specific expression and activity-dependent regulation of seven GABA_A receptor subunit mRNAs in monkey visual cortex. *Journal of Neuroscience*, **14**, 2236–59.

Isaac, J. T., Crair, M. C., Nicoll, R. A., and Malenka, R. C. (1997). Silent synapses during development of thalamocortical inputs. *Neuron*, **18**, 1–20.

Jones, S. M., Hofmann, A. D., Lieber, J. L., and Ribera, A. B. (1995). Overexpression of potassium channel RNA: *in vivo* development rescues neurons from suppression of morphological differentiation *in vitro*. *Journal of Neuroscience*, **15**, 2867–74.

Kalb, R. G. (1994). Regulation of motor neuron dendrite growth by NMDA receptor activation. *Development*, **120**, 3063–71.

Kasper, E. M., Lubke, J., Larkman, A. U., and Blakemore, C. (1994). Pyramidal neurons in layer 5 of the rat visual cortex. III. Differential maturation of axon targeting, dendritic morphology, and electrophysiological properties. *Journal of Comparative Neurology*, **339**, 495–518.

Kater, S. B. and Mills, L. R. (1991). Regulation of growth cone behavior by calcium. *Journal of Neuroscience*, **11**, 891–9.

Katz, L. C. and Constantine-Paton, M. (1988). Relationships between segregated afferents and postsynaptic neurons in the optic tectum of three-eyed frogs. *Journal of Neuroscience*, **8**, 3160–80.

Katz, L., Gilbert, C., and Wiesel, T. (1989). Local circuits and ocular dominance columns in monkey striate cortex. *Journal of Neuroscience*, **9**, 1389–99.

Kaufmann, N., Wills, Z. P., and Van, V. D. (1998). Drosophila Rac1 controls motor axon guidance. *Development*, **125**, 453–61.

Kelly, P. T., Shields, S., Conway, K., Yip, R., and Burgin, K. (1987). Developmental changes in calmodulin-kinase II activity at brain synaptic junctions: alterations in holoenzyme composition. *Journal of Neurochem*, **49**, 1927–40.

Kennedy, M. B. (1997). The postsynaptic density at glutamatergic synapses. *Trends in Neuroscience*, **20**, 264–8.

Kennedy, M. B. (1998). Signal transduction molecules at the glutamatergic postsynaptic membrane. *Brain Research Reviews*, **26**, 243–57.

Kennedy, M. B., McGuinness, T., and Greengard, P. (1983). A calcium/calmodulin dependent protein kinase from mammalian brain that phosphorylates synapsin I: partial purification and characterization. *Journal of Neuroscience*, **3**, 818–31.

Kim, J. H., Liao, D., Lau, L.-F., and Huganir, R. L. (1998). SynGAP: a synaptic RasGAP that associates with the PSD-95/SAP90 protein family. *Neuron*, **20**, 683–91.

Koester, S. E. and O'Leary, D. D. M. (1992). Functional classes of cortical projection neurons develop dendritic distinctions by class-specific sculpting of an early common pattern. *The Journal of Neuroscience*, **12**, 1382–93.

Komatsu, Y. and Iwakiri, M. (1991). Postnatal development of neuronal connections in cat visual cortex studied by intracellular recording in slice preparation. *Brain Research*, **540**, 14–24.

Kossel, A., Lowel, S., and Bolz, J. (1995). Relationships between dendritic fields and functional architecture in striate cortex of normal and visually deprived cats. *Journal of Neuroscience*, **15**, 3913–26.

Kossel, A., Williams, C., Schweizer, M., and Kater, S. (1997). Afferent innervation influences the development of dendritic branches and spines via both activity-dependent and non-activity-dependent mechanisms. *Journal of Neuroscience*, **17**, 6314–24.

Kossut, M., Stewart, M. G., Siucinska, E., Bourne, R. C., and Gabbot, P. L. A. (1991). Loss of γ-aminobutyric acid (GABA) immunoreactivity from mouse first somatosensory cortex following neonatal, but not adult, denervation. *Brain Research*, **538**, 161–71.

Kotak, V., Korada, S., Schwartz, I., and Sanes, D. (1998). A developmental shift from GABAergic to glycinergic transmission in the central auditory system. *Journal of Neuroscience*, **18**, 4646–55.

Kozma, R., Sarner, S., Ahmed, S., and Lim, L. (1997). Rho family GTPases and neuronal growth cone remodelling: relationship between increased complexity induced by Cdc42Hs, Rac1, and acetylcholine and collapse induced by RhoA and lysophosphatidic acid. *Molecular and Cell Biology*, **17**, 1201–11.

Kutsewada, T., Kashiwabuchi, T., Mori, H., Sakimura, K., Kushiya, E., Araki, K., et al. (1992). Molecular diversity of the NMDA receptor channel. *Nature*, **358**, 36–41.

Lankford, K., Kenney, A., and Kocsis, J. (1996). Cellular mechanisms regulating neurite initiation. *Progress in Brain Research*, **108**, 55–81.

Lauder, J. M. (1993). Neurotransmitters as growth regulatory signals: role of receptors and second messengers. *Trends in Neuroscience*, **16**, 233–9.

Laurie, D., Wisden, W., and Seeburg, P. (1992). The distribution of thirteen GABA$_A$ receptor subunit mRNAs in the rat brain. III. Embryonic and postnatal development. *Journal of Neuroscience*, **12**, 4151–72.

Lázár, G. (1973). The development of the optic tectum in Xenopus laevis: a golgi study. *Journal of Anatomy*, **116**, 347–55.

Leinekugel, X., Medina, I., Khalilov, I., Ben-Ari, Y., and Khazipov, R. (1997). Ca^2 oscillations mediated by the synergistic excitatory actions of GABA$_A$ and NMDA receptors in the neonatal hippocampus. *Neuron*, **18**, 243–55.

Lewin, G. R. and Barde, Y. A. (1996). Physiology of the neurotrophins. *Annual Review of Neuroscience*, **19**, 289–317.

Li, P. and Zhuo, M. (1998). Silent glutamatergic synapses and nociception in mammalian spinal cord. *Nature*, **393**, 695–8.

Liao, D. and Malinow, R. (1996). Deficiency in induction but not expression of LTP in hippocampal slices from young rats. *Learning and Memory*, **3**, 138–49.

Lin, S.-Y. and Constantine-Paton, M. (1998). Suppression of sprouting: an early function of NMDA receptors in the absence of AMPA/KA receptor activity. *Journal of Neuroscience*, **18**, 3725–37.

Llinas, R., Gruner, J. A., Sugimori, M., McGuinness, T. L., and Greengard, P. (1991). Regulation by synapsin I and Ca^{2+}-calmodulin-dependent protein kinase II of the transmitter release in squid giant synapse. *Journal of Physiology (Lond)*, **436**, 257–82.

LoTurco, J. J., Blanton, M. G., and Kriegstein, A. R. (1991). Initial expression and endogenous activation of NMDA channels in early neocortical development. *Journal of Neuroscience*, **11**, 792–9.

Luhmann, H. and Prince, D. (1991). Postnatal maturation of the GABAergic system in rat neocortex. *Journal of Neurophysiology*, **65**, 247–63.

Lukasiewicz, P. D. and Shields, C. R. (1998). A diversity of GABA receptors in the retina. *Seminars in Cellular and Developmental Biology*, **9**, 293–99.

Lund, J. S., Holbach, S. M., and Chung, W.-W. (1991). Postnatal development of thalamic recipient neurons in the monkey striate cortex: II. Influence of afferent driving on spine acquisition and dendritic growth of layer 4c spiny stellate neurons. *Journal of Comparative Neurology*, **309**, 129–40.

Luo, L., Liao, Y. J., Jan, L. Y., and Jan, Y. N. (1994). Distinct morphogenetic functions of similar small GTPases: Drosophila Drac1 is involved in axonal outgrowth and myoblast fusion. *Genes and Development*, **8**, 1787–802.

Luo, L., Jan, L. Y., and Jan, Y. N. (1997). Rho family GTP-binding proteins in growth cone signalling. *Current Opinion in Neurobiology*, **7**, 81–6.

Malenka, R. C., Kauer, J. A., Perkel, D. J., Mauk, M. D., Kelly, P. T., Nicoll, R. A., et al. (1989). An essential role for postsynaptic calmodulin and protein kinase activity in long-term potentiation. *Nature*, **340**, 554–7.

Maletic-Savatic, M., Malinow, R., and Svoboda, K. (1999). Rapid dendritic morphogenesis in CA1 hippocampal dendrites induced by synaptic activity. *Science*, **283**, 1923–7.

Malinow, R., Schulman, H., and Tsien, R. W. (1989). Inhibition of postsynaptic PKC or CaMKII blocks induction but not expression of LTP. *Science*, **245**, 862–6.

Martina, M., Strata, F., and Cherubini, R. (1995). Whole cell and single channel properties of a new GABA receptor transiently expressed in the hippocampus. *Journal of Neurophysiology*, **73**, 902–6.

Marty, S., Berninger, B., Carroll, P., and Thoenen, H. (1996). GABAergic stimulation regulates the phenotype of hippocampal interneurons through the regulation of brain-derived neurotrophic factor. *Neuron*, **16**, 565–70.

Mason, C. A. (1983). Postnatal maturation of neurons in the cat's lateral geniculate nucleus. *Journal of Comparative Neurology*, **217**, 458–69.

Mattson, M. P., Hunter, A. T., and Kater, S. B. (1988). Neurite outgrowth in individual neurons of a neuronal population is differentially regulated by calcium and cyclic AMP. *Journal of Neuroscience*, **8**, 1704–11.

Mayford, M., Bach, M. E., Huang, Y.-Y., Wang, L., Hawkins, R. D., and Kandel, E. R. (1996*a*). Control of memory formation through regulated expression of a CaMKII transgene. *Science*, **274**, 1678–83.

Mayford, M., Bach, M. E., and Kandel, E. (1996*b*). CaMKII function in the nervous system explored from a genetic perspective. *Cold Spring Harbor Symposium Quantitative Biology*, **61**, 219–24.

McAllister, A. K., Lo, D. C., and Katz, L. C. (1995). Neurotrophins regulate dendritic growth in developing visual cortex. *Neuron*, **15**, 791–803.

McAllister, A. K., Katz, L. C., and Lo, D. C. (1996). Neurotrophin regulation of cortical dendritic growth requires activity. *Neuron*, **17**, 1057–64.

McAllister, A. K., Katz, L. C., and Lo, D. C. (1997). Opposing roles for endogenous BDNF and NT-3 in regulating cortical dendritic growth. *Neuron*, **18**, 767–78.

McGlade-McCulloh, E., Yamamoto, H., Tan, S.-E., Brickey, D. A., and Soderling, T. R. (1992). Phosphorylation and regulation of glutamate receptors by calcium/calmodulin-dependent protein kinase II. *Nature*, **362**, 640–2.

McKinney, R. A., Capogna, M., Durr, R., Gahwiler, B. H., and Thompson, S. M. (1999). Miniature synaptic events maintain dendritic spines via AMPA receptor activation. *Nature Neuroscience*, **2**, 44–9.

Meister, M., Wong, R. O., Baylor, D. A., and Shatz, C. J. (1991). Synchronous bursts of action potentials in ganglion cells of the developing mammalian retina. *Science*, **252**, 939–43.

Micheva, and Beaulieu, C. (1995). Postnatal development of GABA neurons in the rat somatosensory barrel cortex: a quantitative study. *European Journal of Neuroscience*, **7**, 419–30.

Michler, A. (1990). Involvement of GABA receptors in the regulation of neurite growth in cultured embryonic chick tectum. *International Journal of Developmental Neuroscience*, **8**, 463–72.

Mizuno, K., Carhahan, J., and Nawa, H. (1994). Brain-derived neurotrophic factor promotes differentiation of striatal GABAergic neurons. *Developmental Biology*, **165**, 243–56.

Monyer, H., Sprengel, R., Schoepfer, R., Herb, A., Higuchi, M., Lomeli, H., *et al.* (1992). Heteromeric NMDA receptors: molecular and functional distinction of subtypes. *Science*, **256**, 1217–21.

Mower, G., Rustad, R., and White, W. (1988). Quantitative comparisons of gamma-aminobutyric acid neurons and receptors in the visual cortex of normal and dark-reared cats. *Journal of Comparative Neurology*, **272**, 293–302.

Naeve, G. S., Ramakrishnan, M., Rainer, K., Hevroni, D., Citri, Y., and Theill, L. E. (1997). Neuritin: a gene induced by neural activity and neurotrophins that promotes neuritogenesis. *Proceedings of the National Academy of Sciences USA*, **94**, 2648–53.

Nakamoto, M., Cheng, H.-J., Friedman, G. C., McLaughlin, T., Hansen, M. J., Yoon, C. H. *et al.* (1996). Topographically specific effects of ELF-1 on retinal axon guidance *in vitro* and retinal axon mapping *in vivo*. *Cell*, **86**, 755–66.

Nedivi, E. (1999). Molecular analysis of developmental plasticity in neocortex. *Journal of Neurobiology*. (In press.)

Nedivi, E., Hevroni, D., Naot, D., Israeli, D., and Citri, Y. (1993). Numerous candidate plasticity-related genes revealed by differential cDNA cloning. *Nature*, **363**, 718–22.

Nedivi, E., Wu, G.-Y., and Cline, H. T. (1997). cpg15, A candidate plasticity-related gene involved in dendritic arbor growth. *Society for Neuroscience Abstracts*, **23**, 607.

Nedivi, E., Wu, G. Y., and Cline, H. T. (1998). Promotion of dendritic growth by CPG15, an activity-induced signaling molecule. *Science*, **281**, 1863–6.

Nistri, A. and Sivilotti, L. (1995). An unusual effect of γ-aminobutyric acid on synaptic transmission of frog tectal neurones *in vitro*. *British Journal of Pharmacology*, **85**, 917–21.

Nowak, L., Bregestovski, P., Ascher, P., Herbert, A., and Provchiantz, A. (1984). Magnesium gates glutamate-activated channels in mouse central neurons. *Nature*, **307**, 462–5.

O'Rourke, N. A., Cline, H. T., and Fraser, S E. (1994). Rapid remodeling of retinal arbors in the tectum with and without blockade of synaptic transmission. *Neuron*, **12**, 921–34.

Omkumar, R. V., Kiely, M. J., Rosenstein, A. J., Min, K. T., and Kennedy, M. B. (1996). Identification of a phosphorylation site for calcium/calmodulin-dependent protein kinase II in the NR2B subunit of the *N*-methyl-D-aspartate receptor. *Journal of Biological Chemistry*, **271**, 31670–8.

Owens, D., Boyce, L., Davis, M., and Kriegstein, A. (1996). Excitatory GABA responses in embryonic and neonatal cortical slices demonstrated by gramicidin perforated-patch recordings and calcium imaging. *Journal of Neuroscience*, **16**, 6414–23.

Parks, T. (1981). Changes in the length and organization of nucleus laminaris dendrites after unilateral otocyst ablation in chick embryos. *Journal of Comparative Neurology*, **202**, 47–57.

Penn, A. A., Riquelme, P. A., Feller, M. B., and Shatz, C. J. (1998). Competition in retino-geniculate patterning driven by spontaneous activity. *Science*, **279**, 2108–12.

Petralia, R. S., Esteban, J. A., Wang, Y.-X., Partridge, J. G., Zhao, H.-M., Wenthold, R. J., *et al.* (1999). Selective acquisition of AMPA receptors during postnatal development suggest a molecular basis for silent synapses. *Nature Neuroscience*, **2**, 31–6.

Pettit, T. L. and LeBoutillier, J. C. (1979). Effects of lead exposure during development on neocortical dendritic and synaptic structure. *Experimental Neurology*, **64**, 482–92.

Pinches, E. A. and Cline, H. T. (1998). Distribution of synaptic vesicle proteins within single retinotectal axons of Xenopus tadpoles. *Journal of Neurobiology*, **35**, 426–34.

Purpura, D. P. (1975). Dendritic differentiation in human cerebral cortex: normal and aberrant developmental patterns. *Advances in Neurology*, **12**, 91–134.

Purves, D., Snider, W. D., and Voyvodic, J. T. (1988). Trophic regulation of nerve cell morphology and innervation in the autonomic nervous system. *Nature*, **336**, 123–8.

Qian, Z., Gilbert, M. E., Colicos, M. A., Kandel, E. R., and Kuhl, D. (1993). Tissue-plasminogen activator is induced as an immediate-early gene during seizure, kindling and long-term potentiation. *Nature*, **361**, 453–7.

Rajan, I. and Cline, H. T. (1998). Glutamate receptor activity is required for normal development of tectal cell dendrites *in vivo*. *Journal of Neuroscience*, **18**, 7836–46.

Rocha, M. and Sur, M. (1995). Rapid acquisition of dendritic spines by visual thalamic neurons after blockade of *N*-methyl-D-aspartate receptors. *Proceedings of the National Academy of Sciences USA*, **92**, 8026–30.

Rohrbough, J. and Spitzer, N. (1996). Regulation of intracellular Cl⁻ levels by Na⁺-dependent Cl⁻ cotransport distinguishes depolarizing from hyperpolarizing GABA$_A$ receptor-mediated responses in spinal neurons. *Journal of Neuroscience*, **16**, 82–91.

Rutherford, L., DeWan, A., Lauer, H., and Turrigiano, G. (1997). Brain-derived neurotrophic factor mediates the activity-dependent regulation of inhibition in neocortical cultures. *Journal of Neuroscience*, **17**, 4527–35.

Sanes, D. H. and Hafidi, A. (1996). Glycinergic transmission regulates dendrite size in organotypic culture. *Journal of Neurobiology*, **31**, 503–11.

Schousboe, A. and Redburn, D. A. (1995). Modulatory actions of gamma aminobutyric acid (GABA) on GABA type A receptor subunit expression and function. *Journal of Neuroscience Research*, **41**, 1–7.

Schulman, H. (1993). The multifunctional Ca^{2+}/calmodulin-dependent protein kinases. *Current Opinion in Cell Biology*, **5**, 247–53.

Schulman, H. and Hanson, P. I. (1993). Multifunctional Ca^{2+}/calmodulin-dependent protein kinase. *Neurochemistry Research*, **18**, 65–77.

Schwartz, T., Rabinowitz, D., Unni, V., Kumar, V., Smetters, D., Tsiola, A., *et al.* (1998). Networks of coactive neurons in developing layer 1. *Neuron*, **20**, 541–52.

Schweitzer, L. (1991). Morphometric analysis of developing neuronal geometry in the dorsal cochlear nucleus of the hamster. *Developmental Brain Research*, **59**, 39–47.

Scott, J. D. and Soderling, T. R. (1992). Serine/threonine protein kinases. *Current Opinion in Neurobiology* **1992**, 289–95.

Sernagor, E. and Grzywacz, N. M. (1996). Influence of spontaneous activity and visual experience on developing retinal receptive fields. *Current Biology*, **6**, 1503–8.

Shatz, C. J. (1990). Impulse activity and the patterning of connections during CNS development. *Neuron*, **5**, 745–56.

Shatz, C. J. and Kirkwood, P. A. (1983). Prenatal development of functional connections in the cat's retinogeniculate pathway. *Journal of Neuroscience*, **4**, 1378–97.

Shi, J., Aamodt, S., and Constantine-Paton, M. (1997). Temporal correlations between functional and molecular changes in NMDA receptors and GABA neurotransmission in the superior colliculus. *Journal of Neuroscience*, **17**, 6264–76.

Shimada, A., Mason, C. A., and Morrison, M. E. (1998). TrkB signaling modulates spine density and morphology independent of dendrite structure in cultured neonatal Purkinje cells. *Journal of Neuroscience*, **18**, 8559–70.

Silva, A. J., Paylor, R., Wehner, J. M., and Tonegawa, S. (1992*a*). Impaired spatial learning in alpha-calcium-calmodulin kinase II mutant mice. *Science*, **257**, 206–11.

Silva, A. J., Wang, Y., Paylor, R., Wehner, J. M., Stevens, C. F., and Tonegawa, S. (1992*b*). Alpha calcium/calmodulin kinase II mutant mice: deficient long-term potentiation and impaired spatial learning. *Cold Spring Harbor Symposium Quantitative Biology*, **57**, 527–39.

Silva, A. J., Giese, K. P., Fedorov, N. B., Frankland, P. W., and Kogan, J. H. (1998). Molecular, cellular, and neuroanatomical substrates of place learning. *Neurobiology of Learning and Memory*, **1**, 44–61.

Sin, W. C., Chen, X. Q., Leung, T., and Lim, L. (1998). RhoA-binding kinase alpha translocation is facilitated by the collapse of the vimentin intermediate filament network. *Molecular and Cellular Biology*, **18**, 6325–39.

Smith, Z. D. J., Gray, L., and Rubel, E. W. (1983). Afferent influences on brainstem auditory nuclei in the chicken: n. laminaris dendritic length following monaural conductive hearing loss. *Journal of Comparative Neurology*, **220**, 199–205.

Sone, M. (1997). Still life, a protein in synaptic terminals of Drosophila homologous to GDP–GTP exchangers. *Science*, **275**, 1405.

Spitzer, N. C., Debaca, R. C., Allen, K. A., and Holliday, J. (1993). Calcium dependence of differentiation of GABA immunoreactivity in spinal neurons. *Journal of Comparative Neurology*, **337**, 168–75.

Steven, R., Kubiseski, T. J., Zheng, H., Kulkarni, S., Mancillas, J., Ruiz, M. A., *et al.* (1998). UNC-73 activates the Rac GTPase and is required for cell and growth cone migrations in C. elegans. *Cell*, **92**, 785–95.

Strata, F., Atzori, M., Molnar, M., Ugolini, G., Tempia, F., and Cherubini, E. (1997). A pacemaker current in dye-coupled hilar interneurons contributes to the generation of giant GABAergic potentials in developing hippocampus. *Journal of Neuroscience*, **17**, 1435–46.

Sutton, J. K. and Brunso-Bechtold, J. K. (1991). A Golgi study of dendritic development in the dorsal lateral geniculate nucleus of normal ferrets. *Journal of Comparative Neurology*, **309**, 71–85.

Threadgill, R., Bobb, K., and Ghosh, A. (1997). Regulation of dendritic growth and remodeling by Rho, Rac, and Cdc42. *Neuron* **19**, 625–34.

Tigyi, G., Fischer, D. J., Sebok, A., Yang, C., Dyer, D. L., and Miledi, R. (1996). Lyso-phosphatidic acid-induced neurite retraction in PC12 cells: control by phosphoinositide-Ca^{2+} signaling and Rho. *Journal of Neurochemistry*, **66**, 537–48.

Trune, D. (1982). Influence of neonatal cochlear removal on development of mouse cochlear nucleus: II. Dendritic morphometry of its neurons. *Journal of Comparative Neurology*, **209**, 425–34.

Turner, A. M. and Greenough, W. T. (1985). Differential rearing effects on rat visual cortex synapses: I. Synaptic and neuronal density and synapses per neuron. *Brain Research*, **329** 195–203.

Ullensvang, K., Lehre, K. P., Storm-Mathisen, J., and Danbolt, N. C. (1997). Differential developmental expression of the two rat brain glutamate transporter proteins GLAST and GLT. *European Journal of Neuroscience*, **9**, 1646–55.

Valverde, F. (1968). Structural changes in the area striata of the mouse after enucleation. *Experimental Brain Research*, **5**, 274–92.

Van Aelst, L. and D'Souza-Schorey, C. (1997). Rho GTPases and signaling networks. *Genes and Development*, **11**, 2295–322.

Van Leeuwen, F. N., Kain, H. E., Kammen, R. A., Michiels, F., Kranenburg, O. W., and Collard, J. G. (1997). The guanine nucleotide exchange factor Tiam1 affects neuronal morphology; opposing roles for the small GTPases Rac and Rho. *Journal of Cell Biology*, **139**, 797–807.

Verdoorn, T. A., Draguhn, A., Ymer, S., Seeburg, P. H., and Sakmann, B. (1990). Functional properties of recombinant rat GABAA receptors depend upon subunit composition. *Neuron*, **4**, 919–28.

Vogel, M. W. and Prittie, J. (1995). Purkinje cell dendritic arbors in chick embryos following chronic treatment with an *N*-methyl-D-Aspartate receptor antagonist. *Journal of Neurobiology*, **26**, 537–52.

Wang, J., Reichling, D. B., Kyrozis, A., and MacDermott, A. B. (1994*a*). Developmental loss of GABA- and glycine-induced depolarization and Ca^{2+} transients in embryonic rat dorsal horn neurons in culture. *European Journal of Neuroscience*, **6**, 1275–80.

Wang, J., Renger, J. J., Griffith, L. C., Greenspan, R. J., and Wu, C. (1994*b*). Concomitant alterations of physiological and developmental plasticity in Drosophila CaM kinase II-inhibited synapses. *Neuron*, **13**, 1373–84.

Warren, R., Tremblay, N., and Dykes, R. W. (1989). Quantitative study of glutamic acid decarboxylase-immunoreactive neurons and cytochrome oxidase activity in normal and partially deafferented rat hindlimb somatosensory cortex. *Journal of Comparative Neurology*, **228**, 583–92.

Weisel, T. N. and Hubel, D. H. (1963). Effects of visual deprivation on morphology and physiology of cells in the cat's lateral geniculate body. *Journal of Neurophysiology*, **26**, 978–93.

Widmer, H. R. and Hefti, F. (1994). Stimulation of GABAergic neuron differentiation by NT-4/5 in cultures of rat cerebral cortex. *Developmental Brain Res*, **80**, 279–84.

Wilk-Blaszczak, M., Singer, W. D., Quill, T., Miller, B., Frost, J. A., Sternweis, P. C., *et al.* (1997). The monomeric G-proteins Rac1 and/or Cdc42 are required for the inhibition of voltage-dependent calcium current by bradykinin. *Journal of Neuroscience*, **17**, 4094–100.

Witte, S., Stier, H., and Cline, H. T. (1996). *In vivo* observations of timecourse and distribution of morphological dynamics in xenopus retinotectal axon arbors. *Journal of Neurobiology*, **31**, 219–34.

Wong, R. O. L., Herrman, K., and Shatz, C. J. (1991). Remodelling of retinal ganglion cell dendrites in the absence of action potential activity. *Journal of Neurobiology*, **22**, 685–97.

Wu, G.-Y. and Cline, H. T. (1998). Stabilization of dendritic arbor structure *in vivo* by CaMKII. *Science*, **279**, 222–6.

Wu, G.-Y., Malinow, R., and Cline, H. T. (1996). Maturation of a central glutamatergic synapse. *Science*, **274**, 972–6.

Xiang, Z., Huguenard, J., and Prince, D. (1998). GABA$_A$ receptor-mediated currents in inter-neurons and pyramidal cells of rat visual cortex. *Journal of Physiology (Lond)*, **506**, 715–30.

Yamagata, K., Andreasson, K. I., Kaufmann, W. E., Barnes, C. A., and Worley, P. F. (1993). Expression of a mitogen-inducible cyclooxygenase in brain neurons: regulation by synaptic activity and glucocorticoids. *Neuron*, **11**, 371–86.

Yamagata, K., Sanders, L. K., Kaufmann, W. E., Yee, W., Barnes, C. A., Nathans, D., *et al.* (1994). *rheb*, a growth factor- and activity-regulated gene, encodes a novel ras-related protein. *Journal of Biological Chemistry*, **269**, 16333–9.

Yuste, R., Peinado, A., and Katz, L. C. (1992). Neuronal domains in developing neocortex. *Science*, **257**, 665–9.

Yuste, R., Nelson, D. A., Rubin, W. W., and Katz, L. C. (1995). Neuronal domains in developing neocortex: mechanisms of coactivation. *Neuron*, **14**, 7–17.

Zec, N. and Tieman, S. B. (1994). Development of the dendritic fields of layer 3 pyramidal cells in the kitten's visual cortex. *Journal of Comparative Neurology*, **339**, 288–300.

Zhang, L., Spigelman, I., and Carlen, P. (1991). Development of GABA-mediated, chloride-dependent inhibition in CA1 pyramidal neurones of immature rat hippocampal slices. *Journal of Physiology*, **444**, 25–49.

Zhang, L. L., Tao, H. W., Holt, C. E., Harris, W. A., and Poo, M.-M. (1998). A critical window for cooperation and competition among developing retinotectal synapses. *Nature*, **395**, 37–44.

Zhang, W., Vazquez, L., Apperson, M., and Kennedy, M. B. (1999). Citron binds to PSD-95 at glutamatergic synapses on inhibitory neurons in the hippocampus. *Journal of Neuroscience*, **19**, 96–108.

Zipkin, I. D., Kindt, R. M., and Kenyon, C. J. (1997). Role of a new Rho family member in cell migration and axon guidance in *C. elegans. Cell*, **90**, 883–94.

Ziv, N. E. and Smith, S. J. (1996). Evidence for a role of dendritic filopodia in synaptogenesis and spine formation. *Neuron*, **17**, 91–102.

Zou, D.-J. and Cline, H. T. (1999). Coordinated regulation of retinal axon and tectal cell growth by endogenous CaMKII *in vivo. Journal of Neuroscience*, **19**, (in press).

Zou, D.-J. and Cline, H. T. (1996*a*). Control of retinotectal axon arbor growth by postsynaptic CaMKII. In *Progress in brain research. neuronal development and plasticity*, (ed. R. R. Mize and R. S. Erzurumlu). Elsevier, Amsterdam.

Zou, D.-J. and Cline, H. T. (1996*b*). Expression of constitutively active Ca^{2+}/calmodulin-dependent protein kinase in target tissue modifies presynaptic axon arbor growth. *Neuron*, **16**, 529–39.

3

Dendritic localization of mRNAs and local protein synthesis

James H. Eberwine
University of Pennsylvania Medical School

Summary

RNA was first found to be present in neuronal dendrites over 30 years ago. Until recently little progress had been made in understanding the role of dendritic localization of mRNA in neuronal functioning. New discoveries have revealed:

(1) that many mRNAs are unevenly distributed throughout dendrites;

(2) that mRNA transport to dendrites can be regulated; and

(3) that regulated protein synthesis can occur in dendrites.

These data reveal a complex system for modulation of the protein composition of individual synapses that in turn enables exquisite specification of synaptic responsiveness to pre- and postsynaptic modulation.

Introduction

Neurons have an exquisite morphology that is necessary to their proper functioning. The cell soma is clearly defined by the cell membrane and contains the nucleus. Branching out from the soma are multiple processes called dendrites and a single axon. The somatodendritic domain of a rat hippocampal neuron in primary culture is visible in Fig. 3.1 in which these domains are immunohistochemically stained for the microtubule-associated protein (MAP2A) which partitions into these neuronal structures. Each of these subcellular structures serve distinct cellular roles. Dendrites receive neurochemical signals from presynaptic neurons through the activation of receptors, channels and/or transporters. Such activation causes a postsynaptic response in the dendrite resulting in a variety of biochemical changes including influx of Ca^{2+}, the generation of action potentials and stimulation of phosphorylation. The role of dendrites in facilitating various cellular physiologies is well documented. In particular it is clear that there is a postsynaptic component of long-term potentiation (LTP) where the change in electrophysiological responsiveness that occurs at synapses in response to LTP is thought to reflect biochemical changes in the postsynaptic dendrite.

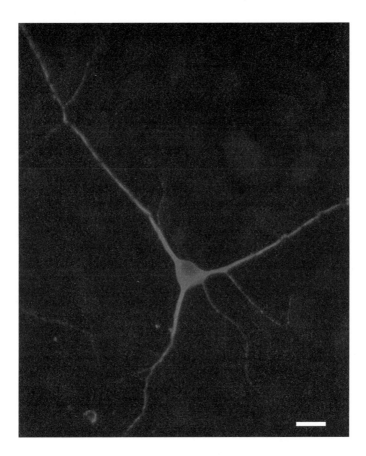

Fig. 3.1 Map2A immunohistochemical staining of a rat hippocampal pyramidal cell. Primary cultures of rat hippocampal cells (Buchhalter and Dichter 1991) were immunostained with an antibody that recognizes the MAP2A protein. A secondary antibody labeled with Cy3 was used for antigen visualization. Distinct from the neuron a faint background can be observed corresponding to the glial cells in the culture. The length of the scale bar corresponds to 10 μm.

Dendrites usually extend hundreds of micrometers away from the soma (up to 2 mm in some adult neurons; see Chapter 1), so the question arises as to what biochemical changes are occurring at the synapse and do they require modulation from the cell soma? If cell soma regulation is required, how does it happen in a fast enough manner to elicit a rapid synaptic response and how can such a signal be specifically directed to a particular synapse? This is a particularly vexing question because of the immense number and diversity of synapses on the dendrites of any individual neuron, with each synapse potentially containing different abundances of various synaptic proteins. This problem can be simplified to the question of how does an individual synapse change in response to activation? There are several ways in which this could happen including:

(1) the local post-translational modification of proteins, thus altering their function;
(2) movement of proteins in and out of the synaptic region, thus changing the functional protein repertoire; or
(3) local synthesis of proteins within this synaptic region that would function locally.

Much time could be spent discussing the evidence for each of these possibilities but for the sake of brevity only the implications of local protein synthesis will be discussed in detail in this chapter. A necessary prerequisite for local protein synthesis in the dendrites of neurons is the presence of mRNAs and the protein synthetic machinery within these structures.

Evidence for mRNA localization in neuronal dendrites

Over the last 30 years evidence has accumulated that mRNAs are localized in neuronal dendrites. Indeed the identification of the repertoire of dendritically localized mRNAs has increased significantly in the last five years. This is in part because of the increased sensitivity of methods of mRNA detection. The mRNAs present in dendrites encode proteins that fall into several functional classes including structural proteins (MAP2), enzymes (CaMKII), nitric oxide synthase, growth factors (netrin, BDNF, NT3), growth factor receptors (TrkA and TrkB), ligand-gated ion channels (glutamate, GABA, glycine), voltage-gated ion channels (Ca^{2+} channels), and even transcription factors such as cAMP response element binding protein (CREB; see Garner *et al.* 1988; Burgin *et al.* 1990; Miyashiro *et al.* 1994; Crino and Eberwine 1996; Racca *et al.* 1997; Crino *et al.* 1998). The wide diversity of proteins encoded by dendritically localized mRNAs suggests that if these mRNAs are locally translated then they might play important and wide-ranging regulatory roles in dendrites. It is important to note that even though these mRNAs are present in dendrites they are also present in higher abundance in the cell soma. No mRNA has been identified that is so enriched in the dendrites that the somatic contribution of mRNA translation products would be minimal compared with that synthesized in the dendrites. This is an important point to consider in that the dendritic and somatic compartments of the neuron should be viewed as a gradient of regulatory potential wherein the concentration of mRNA in either compartment is related to its potential for translation. Somatic protein synthesis contributes mostly to somatic function but also to distal dendritic function and *vice versa*; proteins synthesized in dendrites likely contribute most significantly to dendritic function but probably have a regulatory influence on the cell soma. This latter idea will be presented in more detail later when the potential role of dendritically localized CREB mRNA is discussed.

Initially, mRNA localization to dendrites was assayed by the technique of *in situ* hybridization (Eberwine *et al.* 1994). This methodology utilizes a labeled antisense probe to hybridize to the corresponding mRNA, with subsequent microscopy to visualize the cellular region in which the labeled probe hybridized. This methodology was used successfully to localize MAP2 and calmodulin dependent protein kinase II (CaMKII) mRNAs to dendrites (Garner *et al.* 1988; Burgin *et al.* 1990). An *in situ* hybridization result showing MAP2A mRNA in neuronal cell soma and dendrites is shown in Fig. 3.2. These dendritic mRNAs are in relatively high abundance and can easily be visualized with *in situ* hybridization methodologies. In the early papers describing the localization of these mRNAs the probe was labeled with ^{3}H, which has low-energy alpha particle emission, hence the localization had to be visualized with emulsion autoradiography. The low-energy emission enabled very specific localization to be visualized but often required several weeks of emulsion exposure. The advent of ^{35}S- and ^{33}P-labeled probes that are low beta-particle emitters significantly reduced the exposure time. Furthermore, probe preparation procedures utilizing digoxigenin as a label with sensitive digoxigenin detection methods eliminated the need for autoradiography making *in situ* hybridization procedures easier to use and significantly faster. Such methods have been used to localize several mRNAs to dendrites including those for activity-regulated cDNAs (ARC) and glycine receptors (Lyford *et al.* 1995; Racca *et al.* 1997).

The advantage of *in situ* hybridization detection of mRNAs is the clear visualization of mRNAs in dendrites. Disadvantages include the lack of sensitivity of the methodology and the inability to localize simultaneously more than 2–3 different mRNAs in a single section. This limitation in the number of detectable mRNAs is because of the limited number of commercially available labels that can be used to label probes. This problem was overcome by the use of two different nucleic acid amplification methodologies to amplify the mRNA complement of individual dendrites to an analyzable quantity (Miyashiro *et al.* 1994). In these studies primary cultures of rat hippocampal neurons were utilized as the source of dendrites. To insure that only dendritic mRNA was amplified individual dendrites were mechanically severed from their cognate cell somata by utilizing a patch pipette as a scalpel. The severed dendrite was aspirated into a patch pipette containing the reagents necessary for conversion of the mRNA into cDNA. This single-stranded cDNA was further manipulated to produce a double-stranded cDNA that could be either linearly amplified with the T7 bacteriophage-derived T7 RNA polymerase in the RNA amplification (aRNA) procedure (Van Gelder *et al.* 1990; Eberwine *et al.* 1992) or exponentially amplified using TAQ polymerase (thermus aquaticus polymerase) in the differential display polymerase chain reaction (ddPCR; Liang and Pardee 1992). These studies showed that there was a large complement of mRNAs present in individual dendrites. Indeed on the basis of estimates generated in my laboratory, of the 10 000 different mRNAs thought to be present in the cell soma, approximately 500 different mRNAs are probably present in dendrites. Cloning and identification of many of these mRNAs has rapidly progressed proving the dendritic localization of several known and novel mRNAs, including those for the glutamate and GABA receptors. Also the Miyashiro study showed, importantly, that the mRNA composition of an individual dendrite could differ from that of other dendrites. This suggests that there is a differential targeting of 'targetable' mRNAs to individual dendrites.

Possible mRNA targeting mechanisms

The presence of mRNAs in dendrites raises the question of how these mRNAs make their way from the cell soma to the dendrite. An obvious mechanism for the

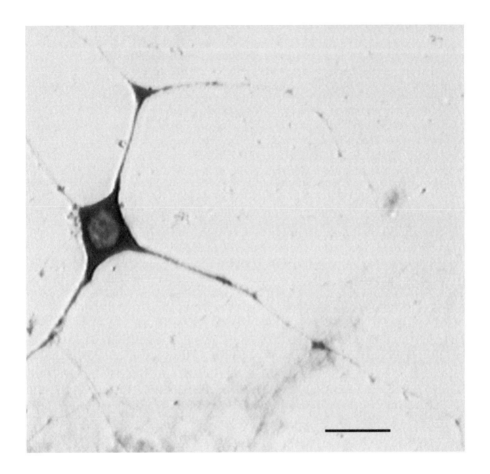

Fig. 3.2 Subcellular localization of MAP2A mRNA determined by *in situ* hybridization. A MAP2A antisense cRNA probe containing digoxigenin-labeled nucleotides was hybridized to the mRNA present in this fixed neuron. The digoxigenin-labeled cRNA was detected by a secondary antibody coupled to peroxidase followed by visualization with 3,3′-diaminobenzidine (DAB). The perinuclear localization of MAP2A mRNA is readily apparent, as is the dendritic subcellular localization. The length of the scale bar corresponds to 10 μm.

movement of mRNAs into dendrites is through passive diffusion, where the mRNA just flows to the dendrites as part of the gradient of mRNA distribution throughout the cellular cytoplasm. This mechanism seems unlikely for a number of reasons. If diffusion was the mechanism for mRNA transport then one would expect all mRNAs to diffuse in a similar manner, hence all mRNAs that are present in the cell soma would also be present in dendrites. This is not supported by data showing that many mRNAs are only present in the cell soma and are excluded from dendrites. One interpretation of this result that would be consistent with passive diffusion is that there might be a mechanism by which mRNAs are blocked from transport into the dendrite, or in other words, there may be a 'gate' at the junction of the dendrite and cell soma that stops passage of most mRNAs and allows only a select few to diffuse through. This seems unlikely because it is difficult to envision how such a gating mechanism could be selective in actively inhibiting dendritic localization of 1000s of somatically localized mRNAs.

A more likely mechanism for transport of mRNAs into the dendrite is through the association of RNAs with specific chaperone proteins binding and transporting mRNA to dendrites. In the Drosophila embryo and Xenopus oocyte model systems, RNA-binding proteins have been shown to bind to selective mRNAs and facilitate their transport to different regions of the developing tissue. In these systems the association of RNA-binding proteins with the transported mRNA is through binding of the protein to a primary sequence contained within, and a secondary/ tertiary structure formed by, the mRNAs. The specific interaction of RNA-binding proteins with mRNA structural characteristics provides a mechanism by which selective mRNAs (only those containing a particular sequence/structure) can be transported. To date no specific mRNA dendritic targeting sequence has been found for a mammalian mRNA but there is evidence that one might exist in the CaMKII mRNA (Mayford *et al.* 1996). Indeed it is interesting to speculate that there are a large variety of RNA-binding proteins each of which binds to selective classes of mRNAs, i.e. those with the appropriate mRNA sequence/structure. While this mRNA sequence/structure might define those particular mRNAs that are targeted to dendrites, it might also be responsible for association of specific mRNAs with particular synapses where the RNA–RNA-binding protein complex could dock, thus providing a mechanism for differential localization of mRNAs within a dendrite. In the same vein, it is reasonable to speculate that a shared mRNA sequence/structure could dictate the co-regulation of translation of these mRNAs.

Regulated mRNA transport to dendrites

Regardless of the mechanism of mRNA transport, data are accumulating that show that the transport of mRNAs to dendritic sites can be regulated. For example; electroconvulsive shock (ECS) stimulates the transport of activity-regulated cDNA (ARC) mRNA to dendrites (Lyford *et al.* 1995). There is also a concomitant increase in cell soma levels of ARC mRNA. The influence of ECS on mRNA localization is selective because MAP2A mRNA levels in the dendrite are not altered by ECS.

There is also evidence of regulated mRNA transport into dendrites during neuronal development. In the dendritic growth cones of cultured hippocampal pyramidal cells several mRNAs have been detected (Crino and Eberwine 1996). Among these mRNAs there are three whose abundances are reduced in response to treatment of the cultures with the Ca^{2+} ionophore A23187, including the mRNA encoding a high-affinity nerve-growth-factor receptor (Trk-A). This suggests that there is a calcium component to the transport of at least a subclass of the dendritically targeted mRNAs. Additionally, this study showed that there was a developmental time-course to the presence of these mRNAs in the maturing dendrite, as this was dependent on the time in culture.

These studies suggest that synaptic modulation and local dendritic environment might dictate which mRNAs are localized to specific dendrites or even to sub-dendritic synaptic domains.

RNA in axons

Data have been published showing RNAs in the axon of particular types of neuron. The number of axonal mRNAs is quite limited, with the best examples being vasopressin mRNA in the axons of the magnocellular neurons of the hypothalamus, BC1 RNA in these same axons, and olfactory receptor mRNAs in the axons of neurons whose cell bodies are in the olfactory epithelium (Mohr *et al.* 1991; Tiedge *et al.* 1993; Trembleau *et al.* 1994; Wang *et al.* 1998) Interestingly, there is no evidence for translational machinery in axons, hence the role of mRNAs in axons is unclear. Presuming that these RNAs cannot be translated in axons, these RNAs, which are highly charged, might serve as carrier molecules for other molecules such as proteins, moving them down the axon or potentially as ion sinks to neutralize counter-ion charge. It is unlikely (although not impossible) that these axonally localized mRNA are secreted. Because so little is known about the biology associated with the localization of mRNAs in axons this topic will not be discussed in any greater detail in this chapter.

Evidence proving protein synthesis in dendrites

The presence of mRNAs in synaptic regions suggests that these mRNAs can be locally translated in dendrites, possibly for local function. Protein translation is a complicated process involving the coordinated activity of hundreds of proteins and mRNAs. A hallmark of protein synthetic capacity is the presence of ribosomes that provide the structural scaffolding on which proteins are synthesized. Briefly protein synthesis occurs in a multi-step process in which initiation factor proteins initially interact with a small subunit ribosome (Rhoads 1993). Next a mRNA can interact with this complex forming the initiation complex. A large ribosome subunit will bind to the initiation complex followed by movement of the large and small ribosome complex along the mRNA synthesizing protein from the 5′-end of the mRNA towards the 3′-end (N-terminal to C-terminal). Multiple ribosomes can interact with an individual mRNA, each synthesizing protein independently. This multi-ribosome–mRNA complex is called a polysome.

The first clear indication that protein synthesis might occur in dendrites was electron microscopic identification of ribosomes in dendrites (Bodian 1965; Steward and Levy 1982). Indeed, these landmark studies identified ribosomes and polysomes in dendritic regions at the base of dendritic spines (see Chapter 1). These polysomes exist in the cytoplasm and correspond to the class of polysomes involved in synthesizing cytoplasmic proteins.

Further evidence that dendritic protein synthesis can occur came from the immunohistochemical localization of proteins involved in the translation process in this cellular compartment (Rao and Steward 1991; Teidge and Brosius 1996; Steward and Reeves 1988). Since ribosomes can be visualized in dendrites, it is reasonable to expect to find ribosome structural proteins within dendrites. Indeed, ribosomal P proteins and other ribosome associate proteins have been found by several groups in the dendritic region. Perhaps more interesting are some of the other translation proteins such as the initiation and elongation factors. These proteins, which can freely diffuse in the cytoplasm, associate with the ribosomal mRNA complex to aid in formation of the initiation complex and actual elongation of proteins. The presence of these proteins in dendrites suggests, but does not prove, that the ribosomal complexes are biologically active. Interestingly there are two additional observations that bear on the presence of initiation factors in the dendrite. There is strong evidence showing that NMDA receptor activation will stimulate the phosphorylation of eIF-2α, one of the translation initiation factors, within the dendritic compartment. Phosphorylation is necessary for activation of this initiation factor so that translation can proceed (Scheetz *et al.* 1997). Also the mRNA for eIF-2α has been found in rat hippocampal neuronal dendrites, suggesting that eIF-2α can be locally synthesized in the dendrite at times of translational need (Miyashiro *et al.* 1994).

More recently proteins associated with the translation of integral membrane proteins have also been localized in the dendrites (Tiedge and Brosius 1996; Gardiol *et al.* 1999). These proteins range from those required for docking of the pre-sequence of secreted proteins with the rough endoplasmic reticulum to antigens associated with the Golgi complex. The presence of these proteins in dendrites raises the interesting possibility that integral membrane proteins might be synthesized in dendritic regions. If this is possible then it is conceivable that the neurotransmitter repertoire underneath particular synapses might be altered by local protein synthesis in response to specific types of presynaptic input. This would reconcile the dendritic localization of the mRNAs for integral membrane proteins such as the glutamate and GABA receptors (Miyashiro *et al.* 1994; Crino *et al.* 1996; Gardiol *et al.* 1999) with a potential role in synaptic physiology or plasticity (Chapters 5 and 13). These data also are important for understanding the new evidence suggesting that membrane fusion of postsynaptic constituents with the postsynaptic membrane must occur to initiate and maintain LTP. (Lledo *et al.* 1998). If functional integral membrane proteins such as glutamate receptors can be produced in dendrites, it is conceivable that their insertion into the membrane (possibly by fusion of Golgi vesicles containing glutamate receptor with the postsynaptic membrane) might be important for maintaining agonist-induced potentiation of synaptic regions.

In addition to these dendritic constituent characterization papers there is an abundance of functional data strongly supporting the idea of local protein synthesis in dendrites. Among the first such functional studies were radioactive amino acid incorporation studies in isolated dendrites. Briefly dendrites are incubated with radiolabeled amino acids and protein synthesis is detected in emulsion autoradiography of these severed processes (Torre and Steward 1992). Various controls must be done for these experiments to be interpretable, including use of protein synthesis inhibitors to show the requirement of protein synthesis for generation of an autoradiographic signal. A more quantitative approach utilizing isolated synaptoneurosomes has allowed a quantitative determination of changes in protein synthesis in dendritic compartments as a result of neurotransmitter stimulation (Weiler and Greenough 1993). Synaptoneurosomes are the membrane/vesicle fraction of a cell or tissue homogenate. In the Weiler and Greenough studies synaptoneurosomes are derived from hippocampal or cortical tissue isolated from rats treated with various neuromodulators. These are the first studies suggesting that protein synthesis can be altered in response to neurotransmitter modulation.

Formal molecular proof of local protein synthesis came from studies utilizing translation of epitope-tagged mRNAs as markers of translation (Crino and Eberwine 1996). In these experiments a reporter cDNA encoding glutathione synthase kinase was engineered to contain an in-frame c-myc epitope at the C-terminus of the coding region of the mRNA. mRNA was made from this cDNA construct and coated with lipids to facilitate membrane fusion. The lipid-coated mRNA was sprayed on to the individual severed dendrites using a patch pipette to deliver the reagents. The c-myc epitope is immunohistochemically detectable only if the reporter mRNA is translated. A schematic diagram of this assay is shown in Fig. 3.3. In these studies basal protein synthesis was undetectable but stimulation of isolated dendrites with the growth factors BDNF or NT-3 stimulated protein synthesis and facilitated the visualization of the locally synthesized c-myc epitope. The presence of c-myc immunoreactivity clearly proved the concept of local protein synthesis in dendrites. This assay has broad applicability and is currently being used by a number of investigators to examine the biochemistry of local protein synthesis in dendrites. These studies built upon the pioneering work of Kang and Schuman (1996) who showed that BDNF or NT-3 stimulation of synaptic plasticity required local dendritic protein synthesis.

Hypothesis for short-loop regulation of synaptic physiology by local protein synthesis

The existence of a panoply of mRNAs that differs between dendrites (Miyashiro *et al.* 1994), and the capacity of dendrites to synthesize proteins suggest that the dendritic protein composition might be altered by synaptic stimulation. Indeed, using the synaptoneurosome preparation Greenough and colleagues have shown that metabotropic glutamate receptor activation of dendritic areas will stimulate local protein synthesis (Weiler *et al.* 1994). Recently they have shown that the mRNA for FMR1 protein is one of these glutamate responsive mRNAs (Weiler *et al.* 1997). FMR1 protein is deficient in a neurological disease called Fragile-X syndrome. FMR1 protein is present in synaptic areas of normal neurons, but is absent from these sites in the neurons of humans who suffer from Fragile-X syndrome and in those of FMR1 knockout mice. Interestingly, the FMR1 protein is thought to be an RNA-binding protein that can complex with ribosomal RNAs to alter the translational efficiency of polysomes. This suggests the intriguing hypothesis that glutamate activation of metabotropic receptors might alter the translational capacity of a synapse by directly modulating the synthesis of translational regulatory RNA-binding proteins. Indeed in unpublished work we have cloned several additional mRNAs containing sequences that suggest that they encode candidate RNA-binding proteins from individual dendrites; this further supports a local role for many RNA-binding proteins in modulation of synaptic translational capacity. A schematic diagram of this proposed short-loop regulatory pathway for modulation of dendritic function is shown in Fig. 3.4.

Another facet of this hypothesis is the presence of mRNA and protein for the translation initiation factor, eIF-2α in dendrites, suggesting that altered local translation of eIF-2α mRNA might impact upon the initiation of protein synthesis.

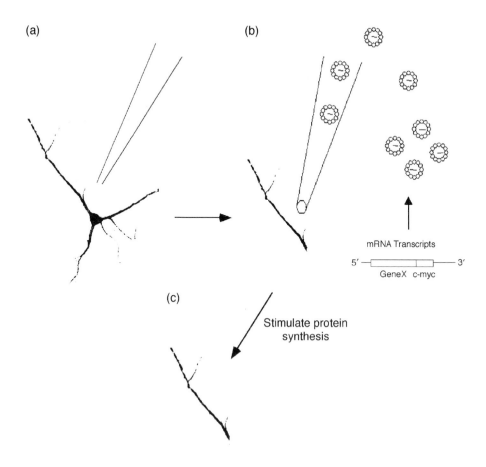

Fig. 3.3 Schematic diagram of single dendrite mRNA transfection assay. (a) A patch pipette is used to sever the dendrite mechanically from the cell soma in primary cultures of hippocampal neurons. The cell soma is aspirated into the pipette and discarded. (b) A second larger patch pipette is filled with lipid-coated mRNA containing the protein-coding region for any gene (GeneX) extended at its 3′-end with a c-myc epitope. This is sprayed on to the severed dendrite. After dendrite transfection, protein synthesis is stimulated and if the fusion mRNA is translated then c-myc immunoreactivity will be detected in the isolated dendrite as depicted in (c).

Possible role of dendritic protein synthesis in converting synaptic stimulation into neuronal response

The possible influence of dendritic protein synthesis on the local synaptic environment is readily apparent. Less clear cut is whether dendritic protein synthesis can influence generalized cellular functioning. Insight into this issue was recently

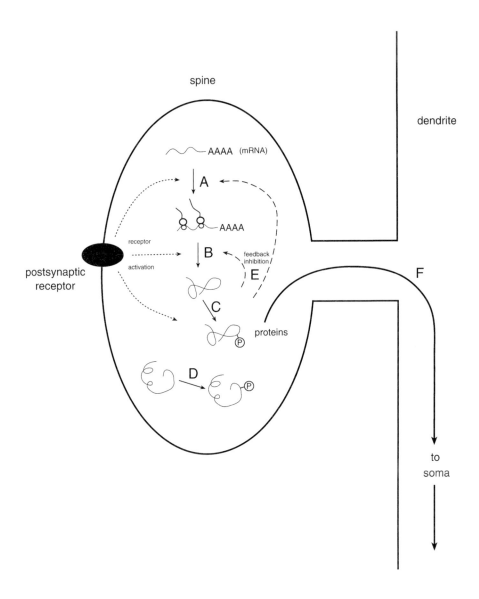

Fig. 3.4 Short regulatory loop in dendrites. This schematic diagram shows how pre-synaptic stimulation of a dendritic spine might alter various synaptic biological processes. Postsynaptic receptor activation might stimulate protein translation on dendritic mRNA (A and B) and local post-translational modification (e.g. phosphorylation, P) of proteins synthesized in the dendrite (C) or the soma (D). These newly synthesized and/or modified proteins might then exert feedback inhibition of the translation process to limit local protein synthesis (E). Proteins synthesized and/or modified in the synapse might be translocated from the dendritic spine back to the cell soma (F) where they might affect a generalized cellular function. This short regulatory loop should afford rapid and specific dendritic responsiveness to various presynaptic stimuli.

provided by the recent discovery of transcription factor mRNAs in neuronal dendrites (Crino *et al.* 1998). In these studies both mRNA and protein for cAMP response element binding protein (CREB) was found in dendrites. This unexpected result is quite curious, since transcription factors function to regulate transcription of genes in the nucleus. To investigate the physiological role of dendritically localized CREB mRNA, CREB mRNA was shown to be translated into protein in the dendrite (using the assay schematized in Fig. 3.3). Further, microdiffusion into the dendrites of fluorescence-tagged CREB protein showed that CREB protein can move from dendrites through the cell soma into the nucleus. This suggested that the dendritically synthesized CREB could find its way to the nucleus where it might function to alter the transcription of genes. Past studies of CREB have shown that CREB activation of gene transcription requires phosphorylation of Ser[133] on the CREB protein. Using an antibody that recognizes phospho-Ser[133] CREB it was shown that CREB could be phosphorylated in the dendritic domain. Before these studies it had been thought that phosphorylation of dendritic CREB occurred exclusively in the nucleus. Together, these studies suggest that synaptic stimulation can elicit dendritic production of transcription factors that can alter nuclear gene transcription. These data have generated a novel hypothesis for a dendritic signaling pathway called dendritic imprinting. This hypothesis suggests that the synthesis and modification of transcription factors in dendrites bypasses the previous signaling pathways where activation of signal transduction pathways converged on the nucleus resulting in phosphorylation of CREB localized in the nucleus. The converging of signaling pathways on nuclear CREB results in the integration of signaling events and loss of synaptic specificity of signaling. Dendritically synthesized and modified CREB would enable specific dendritic signals to generate functional CREB independently of other signaling events. However, it is unlikely that the small amount of CREB made in the dendrites would have much of a signaling effect when compared with the large amount of nuclear CREB. Since we know that CREB can be phosphorylated in the dendrite, it is reasonable to hypothesize that dendritic CREB is distinctly post-translationally modified when compared with nuclear CREB. In particular there are several possible phosphorylation sites on CREB and it is conceivable that specific types of synaptic stimulation could produce specific phosphorylation patterns on CREB that would differentially regulate gene transcription. This remains to be proven. A schematic diagram illustrating the potential contribution of dendritically synthesized CREB to neuronal function is presented in Fig. 3.5.

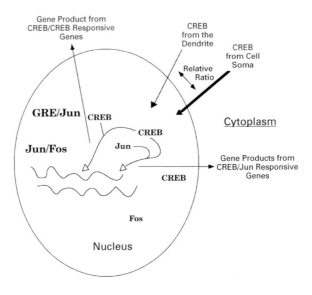

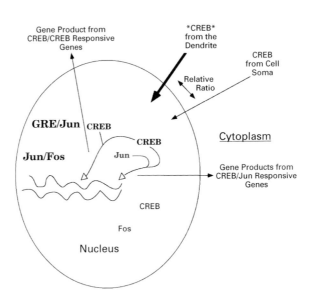

Fig. 3.5 Dendritic imprinting of the nucleus. This schematic diagram illustrates how the small amount of dendritically localized CREB protein might influence postsynaptic gene transcription. In the top diagram, if the CREB protein has the same post-translational modifications as the somatically synthesized CREB then there will be little contribution of dendritically localized CREB to the overall transcription of CREB-regulated genes. In the bottom diagram, the possibility that dendritic CREB has post-translational modifications (such as a distinct phosphorylation pattern, etc.) that would distinguish it from somatic CREB is presented in context of its potential influence on the relative ratio of CREB-containing transcription factor dimers in the nucleus. GRE is the glucocorticoid response element binding protein while Jun and Fos are other transcription factors.

Concluding remarks

It should be clear from this brief review that localization of mRNAs to dendrites might have profound physiological consequences for dendritic and cellular functioning. The dendritic synthesis of proteins from these localized mRNAs might alter the local synaptic environment, dendritic translational capacity and general cellular functioning. One important facet of such specificity of subcellular functioning is how the signaling inputs from this subcellular region can be 'kept in check' or controlled within the cellular context (Martin *et al.* 1997; Schuman 1997). There are at least two mechanisms through which this could be accommodated. Briefly, once a synaptic signal is received and processed by the cell soma a cellular response to the signaling synapse could be:

(1) very specific and targeted for transport only to that particular synapse; or

(2) transported to all synapses with the signaling synapse responding while other synapses do not.

The first hypothesis seems unlikely given the number of synapses that would have to be specifically modulated by the cell and the need for such a synaptic modulatory function to be very rapid. The second hypothesis of a generalized cellular response (Pozzo-Miller *et al.* 1997) resulting in a specific synaptic modulation should be viewed in context of the nature of the postsynaptic modifications initiated by presynaptic stimulation of individual synaptic areas. Once a stimulus is processed in a synapse the synaptic environment is altered by a combination of local translation and local protein modification. These changes might alter the ability of a synapse to respond to both presynaptic stimulation, as well as retrograde modulation from the cognate cell body. In other words, it is probable that specific signals do not have to be generated within the cell soma to modulate individual synapses, but rather this is locally controlled by specific protein synthesis and/or post-translational modification (this idea is depicted schematically in Fig. 3.6). This is an expansion of the idea put forth by Frey and Morris (1998), in which they argue that the specific targeting of proteins from the cell soma to activated synapses occurs through prior synaptic tagging of these activated synapses, creating an appropriate 'docking site' for the targeted proteins.

Cellular regulation mediated through synapses is a complicated process requiring the interplay of many cellular constituents. With the estimated number of synapses on any individual neuron often being many tens of thousands, the individual and integrated functioning of these synapses by dendritic local protein synthesis and bidirectional signaling between synapses and the soma is likely to be more important to proper neuronal functioning than previously thought.

Acknowledgements

This work was supported by NIH grants AG9900 and MH58561. Jennifer Phillips kindly contributed Figs 1 and 2. Qian Chen's help with figure preparation is also appreciated. Janet Estee Kacharmina generously provided a critical reading of this manuscript.

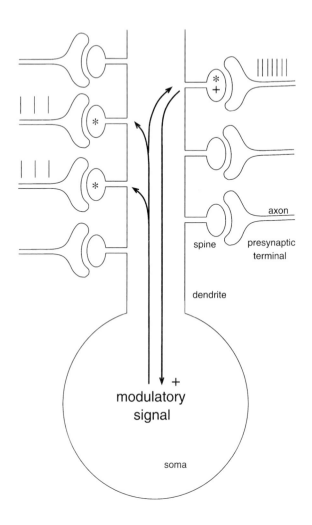

Fig. 3.6 Synaptic specification as modified by local protein synthesis. Schematic diagram showing that presynaptic input (action potentials indicated by vertical lines above presynaptic axons) might result in the production of a 'tag' (*), which renders the synapse specifically responsive to modulatory signals transported from the soma to the dendrites. In some cases the modulatory signal in the soma might be constitutively produced, whereas in other cases it may be stimulated by a signal (+) produced at active synapses (perhaps a subset of those synapses expressing the tag, shown here schematically as the synapse which received a higher frequency presynaptic input). See Frey and Morris (1998) for a description of evidence that such a system might operate in long-term potentiation.

References

Bodian, D. (1965). A suggestive relationship of nerve cell RNA with specific synaptic sites. *Proceedings of the National Academy of Sciences USA*, **53**, 418–25.

Buchhalter, J. and Dichter, M. (1991). Electrophysiologic comparison of pyramidal and stellate nonpyramidal neurons in dissociated hippocampal cell cultures of rat hippocampus. *Brain Research Bulletin*, **26**, 333–8.

Burgin, K. E., Waxham, M. N., Rickling, S., Westgate, S. A., Mobley, W. C., and Kelly, P. T. (1990). *In situ* hybridization histochemistry of Ca^{++}/calmodulin-dependent protein kinase in developing rat brain. *Journal of Neuroscience*, **10**, 1788–98.

Crino, P. and Eberwine, J. (1996). Molecular characterization of the dendritic growth cone: regulated mRNA transport and local protein synthesis. *Neuron*, **17**, 1173–11.

Crino, P., Khodakhah, K., Becker, K., Ginsberg, S., Hemby, S., and Eberwine, J. (1998). Presence and phosphorylation of transcription factors in dendrites. *Proceedings of the National Academy of Sciences USA*, **95**, 2313–18.

Eberwine, J., Yeh, H., Miyashiro, K., Cao, Y., Nair, S., Finnell, R., *et al.* (1992). Analysis of gene expression in single live neurons. *Proceedings of the National Academy of Sciences USA*, **89**, 3010–14.

Eberwine, J., Valentino, K., and Barchas, J. (ed.) (1994). *In situ hybridization in neurobiology*. Oxford University Press, New York.

Frey, A. and Morris, C. (1998). Synaptic tagging: implications for late maintenance of hippocampal long-term potentiation. *Trends in Neuroscience* **21**, 181–8.

Gardiol, A., Racca, C., and Triller, A. (1999). Dendritic and postsynaptic protein synthetic machinery. *Journal of Neuroscience*, **19**, 168–79.

Garner, C., Tucker, R., and Matus, A. (1988). Selective localization of messenger RNA for cytoskeletal protein MAP2 in dendrites. *Nature*, **336**, 374–7.

Kang, H. and Schuman, E. (1996). A requirement for local protein synthesis in neurotrophin-induced hippocampal synaptic plasticity. *Science*, **273**, 1402–6.

Liang, P. and Pardee, A. (1992). Differential display of eukaryotic messenger RNA by means of the polymerase chain reaction. *Science*, **257**, 967–71.

Lledo, P., Zhang, X., Sudhof, T., Malenka, R., and Nicoll, R. (1998). Postsynaptic membrane fusion and long-term potentiation. *Science*, **279**, 399–403.

Lyford, G., Yamagata, K., Kaufmann, W., Barnes, C., Copeland, N., Gilbert, D., *et al.* (1995). Arc, a growth factor and activity regulated gene, encodes a novel cytoskeleton-associated protein that is enriched in neuronal dendrites. *Neuron*, **14**, 433–45.

Martin, K., Casadio, A., Zhu, H., Rose, J., Chen, M., Bailey, C., and Kandel, E. (1997). Synapse-specific long-term facilitation of aplysia sensory to motor synapses: a function to local protein synthesis in memory storage, *Cell*, **91**, 927–38.

Mayford, M., Baranes, D., Podsypanina, K., and Kandel, E. (1996). The 3'-untranslated region of CaMKII is a *cis*-acting signal for the localization and translation of mRNA in dendrites. *Proceedings of the National Academy of Sciences USA*, **93**, 13250–5.

Miyashiro, K., Dichter, M., and Eberwine, J. (1994). On the nature and distribution of mRNAs in hippocampal neurites: implications for neuronal functioning. *Proceedings of the National Academy of Sciences USA*, **91**, 10800–4.

Mohr, E., Fehr, S., and Richter, D. (1991). Axonal transport of neuropeptide encoding mRNAs within the hypothalamo-hypophyseal tract of rats. *European Molecular Biology Organization Journal*, **10**, 2419–24.

Pozzo-Miller, L., Pivovarova, B., Leapman, R., Buchanan, R., Reese, T., and Andrews, B. (1997). Activity-dependent calcium sequestration in dendrites of hippocampal neurons in brain slices. *Journal of Neuroscience*, **17**, 8729–38.

Racca, C., Gardiol, A., and Triller, A. (1997). Dendritic and postsynaptic localizations of glycine receptor a subunit mRNAs. *Journal of Neuroscience*, **17**, 1691–700.

Rao, A. and Steward, O. (1991). Evidence that protein constituents of the postsynaptic membrane specializations are locally synthesized: analysis of proteins synthesized within synaptosome. *Journal of Neuroscience*, **11**, 2881–95.

Rhoads, R. (1993). Regulation of eukaryotic protein synthesis by initiation factors. *Journal of Biological Chemistry*, **268**, 3017–3020.

Scheetz, A., Niarn, A., and Constantine-Paton, M. (1997). *N*-methyl-D-aspartate receptor activation and visual activity induce elongation factor-2 phosphorylation in amphibian tecta: a role for NMDA receptors in controlling protein synthesis. *Proceedings of the National Academy of Sciences*, **94**, 14770–5.

Schuman, E. (1997). Synapse specificity and long-term information storage. *Neuron*, **18**, 339–42.

Steward, O. and Levy, W. (1982). Preferential localization of polyribosomes under the base of dendritic spines in granule cells of the dentate gyrus. *Journal of Neuroscience*, **2**, 284–91.

Steward, O. and Reeves, T. (1988). Protein-synthetic machinery beneath postsynaptic sites on CNS neurons: association between polyribosomes and other organelles at the synaptic site. *Journal of Neuroscience*, **8**, 176–84.

Tiedge, H. and Brosius, J. (1996). Translational machinery in dendrites of hippocampal neurons in culture. *Journal of Neuroscience*, **16**, 7171–81.

Tiedge, H., Zhou, A., Thorn, N., and Brosius, J. (1993). Transport of BC1 RNA in hypothalamo-neurohypophyseal axons. *Journal of Neuroscience*, **13**, 4214–19.

Torre, E. R. and Steward, O. (1992). Demonstration of local protein synthesis within dendrites using a new cell culture system that permits the isolation of living axons and dendrites from their cell bodies. *Journal of Neuroscience*, **12**, 762–72.

Trembleau, A., Morales, M., and Bloom, F. (1994). Aggregation of vasopressin mRNA in a subset of axonal swelling of the median eminence and posterior pituitary: light and electron microscopic evidence. *Journal of Neuroscience*, **14**, 39–53.

Van Gelder, R., von Zastrow, M., Yool, A., Dement, W., Barchas, J., and Eberwine, J. (1990). Amplified RNA (aRNA) synthesized from limited quantities of heterogeneous cDNA. *Proceedings of the National Academy of Sciences USA*, **87**, 1663–7.

Wang, F., Nemes, A., Mendelsohn, M., and Axel, R. (1998). Odorant receptors govern the formation of a precise topographic map. *Cell*, **93**, 47–60.

Weiler, I. J. and Greenough, W. (1993). Metabotropic glutamate receptors trigger postsynaptic protein synthesis. *Proceedings of the National Academy of Sciences USA*, **90**, 7168–71.

Weiler, I. J., Wang, X., and Greenough, W. T. (1994). Synapse-activated protein synthesis as a possible mechanism of plastic neural change. *Progress in Brain Research*, **100**, 189–94.

Weiler, I. J., Irwin, S., Klintsova, A., Spencer, C., Brazelton, A., Miyashiro, K., et al. (1997). Fragile X mental retardation protein is translated near synapses in response to neurotransmitter activation. *Proceedings of the National Academy of Sciences USA*, **94**, 5395–400.

4

Subcellular distribution of neurotransmitter receptors and voltage-gated ion channels

Zoltan Nusser

UCLA School of Medicine

Summary

This chapter describes the subcellular distribution of transmitter- and voltage-activated channels in neurons in the CNS as detected with specific antibodies at the light and electron microscopic level. These studies reveal that ionotropic glutamate, $GABA_A$ and glycine receptors are concentrated at glutamatergic, GABAergic and glycinergic synapses, respectively, and also present at lower densities in the extra-synaptic plasma membrane. The number and density of synaptic receptors can be regulated, allowing an input-specific fine-tuning of the postsynaptic response. Group I metabotropic glutamate receptors are excluded from postsynaptic specializations at glutamatergic synapses. Presynaptic group II and III metabotropic glutamate and $GABA_B$ receptors are found on both GABAergic and glutamatergic terminals, implicating a possible role of trans-synaptic diffusion of both GABA and glutamate in neuronal information processing. Relatively little is known about the precise subcellular distribution and densities of voltage-gated Na^+, Ca^{2+} or K^+ channels in the dendrites of central neurons. Some information, however, is available. For example, certain K^+ channels are selective enriched on cerebellar basket cell axons and Na^+ channels are concentrated at the nodes of Ranvier of myelinated axons.

Introduction

Several approaches have been used to study the subcellular distribution of ligand- and voltage-gated ion channels in the CNS. I shall provide a short overview of different techniques, highlighting their advantages and disadvantages for revealing the precise origin of these proteins. Electron microscopic autoradiography has been used to study the subcellular distribution of nicotinic acetylcholine receptors using high-affinity $[^{125}I]\alpha$-bungarotoxin and that of Na^+ channels with $[^{125}I]\alpha$-scorpion toxin. This method has also been successfully used to determine the density of these channels at the neuromuscular junction. With this method, however, only proteins with known high-affinity ligands/toxins can be studied. Furthermore, it is most of the time impossible to distinguish between different receptor/channel subtypes using autoradiography. Immunocytochemistry with selective antibodies overcomes some of these limitations. Visualization of antigen–antibody complexes with fluorescent-coupled secondary antibodies (fluorescent method) is widely used and has several advantages. The fluorescent method has high sensitivity, the co-localization of several antigens can be performed simultaneously, and this method produces a non-diffusable marker allowing the quantitative comparison of different antigenic sites. However, fluorescent reactions can only be analysed at the light microscopic level, and even if confocal microscopy is applied, the low spatial resolution (>0.2 µm) of this method is its greatest limitation. The most widely used electron microscopic immunocytochemical method uses enzymatic reactions to visualize the antibody–antigen complexes (peroxidase method). This method has high sensitivity and correlated light and electron microscopy can easily be performed. In addition, the immunoperoxidase method provides reliable information about whether the origin of the reaction is pre- or postsynaptic, whether the epitope(s), recognized by the antibody, is (are) located on the intra- or extracellular face of the plasma membrane, and for certain epitopes whether the antigen is associated with endomembranes. However, due to the diffusable nature of the peroxidase reaction end product, this method is not suitable for synaptic localization of epitopes and quantitative comparisons between distinct subcellular compartments cannot be made. Using non-diffusable markers (e.g. gold particles; immunogold method) and reacting the surface of resin-embedded tissue (postembedding reactions) allows the identification of the site of the reaction with a resolution of ~ 20 nm. This method employs particulate markers, which are quantifiable. Furthermore, since the surface of the electron microscopic sections is directly in contact with the antibodies, there is no difference between the exposed tissue elements in their access to antibodies, making quantitative comparisons between two antigenic sites possible. Thus, the post-embedding immunogold method seems to be the most appropriate approach for high-resolution, quantitative localization of cell surface molecules.

Subcellular distribution of ionotropic glutamate receptors

The major excitatory neurotransmitter in the mammalian CNS is glutamate. This transmitter is mainly released from presynaptic axon terminals onto the cell bodies and dendrites of neurons where it exerts its influence through the activation of ion channel forming (ionotropic) and G-protein coupled (metabotropic) receptors. A large variety of both ionotropic and metabotropic glutamate receptors (GluRs) has recently been identified with pharmacological and molecular techniques (reviewed by Seeburg 1993; Hollmann and Heinemann 1994; Nakanishi 1994; Pin and Duvoisin 1995). Ionotropic GluRs can be grouped into three categories; α-amino-3-hydroxy-5-methyl-4-isoxazolepropionate (AMPA), kainate and *N*-methyl-D-aspartate (NMDA)-type GluRs according to their agonist selectivity and sequence homology. Four subunits (GluR1–4 or GluRA–D) of the AMPA-type GluRs, five subunits (GluR5–7, KA1 and KA2) of the kainate-type GluRs and six subunits (NR1, NR2A-D and NR3) of the NMDA-type GluRs have been discovered, creating dozens of homo- and heteromultimeric assemblies with distinct kinetic and pharmacological properties. The molecular complexity of GluRs is further increased by post-translational modifications such as alternative splicing and RNA editing (reviewed by Seeburg 1996), which affect several functional properties of these channels (e.g. receptor deactivation and desensitization). Clearly, the distribution and the molecular make-up of GluRs is fundamentally important in determining the effect of synaptically released glutamate. In addition, their precise location in relation to the site of transmitter release will also have a profound influence on the postsynaptic response.

AMPA receptors

It has long been assumed that AMPA receptors are concentrated at the postsynaptic specialization of glutamatergic synapses. This followed from the fast onset and rise times of postsynaptic AMPA receptor-mediated responses (see Chapter 5) although these receptors have a relatively low affinity for glutamate (Patneau and Mayer 1990). In patch-clamp recordings, AMPA receptors were also found on extra-synaptic somatic and dendritic membranes (see Chapter 5). Since light microscopic autoradiographic studies do not have the resolution to distinguish synaptic and extrasynaptic receptors, the precise distribution and relative densities of GluRs on the surface of nerve cells remained elusive before the first high-resolution immunocytochemical studies were carried out. The cloning of ionotropic GluR subunits initiated the production of several subunit-selective antibodies that were used in immunohistochemical studies to determine the regional, cellular and subcellular distribution of AMPA receptors (Blackstone *et al.* 1992; Petralia and Wenthold 1992; Molnar *et al.* 1993; Baude *et al.* 1994). Using immunoperoxidase methods, these studies conclusively identified AMPA receptors in the Golgi apparatus, endoplasmic reticulum and on the extrasynaptic plasma membranes of hippocampal and cerebellar neurons. Peroxidase reaction end-products have also been found on postsynaptic specializations of asymmetrical (excitatory) synapses, but a possible secondary deposition after diffusion could not be excluded (Nusser and Somogyi 1997). Furthermore, relative receptor densities at distinct subcellular compartments could not be determined with immunoperoxidase methods. The first convincing evidence for the clustering of AMPA receptors at synaptic sites came from high-resolution immunogold localization (Nusser *et al.* 1994; Baude *et al.* 1995; Phend *et al.* 1995; Kharazia *et al.* 1996; Matsubara *et al.* 1996; Rubio and Wenthold 1997; Nusser *et al.* 1998*a*) and immunofluorescence (Craig *et al.* 1993, 1994; Richmond *et al.* 1996) studies. Craig *et al.* (1994) have demonstrated that in cultured hippocampal neurones GluR1 subunit immunofluorescent puncta were associated with glutamatergic terminals, whereas no AMPA receptor immunoreactivity was found postsynaptic to glutamic acid decarboxylase-immunopositive terminals. Similarly, an enrichment of immunogold particles for AMPA receptor subunits was found at asymmetrical synapses in the cerebellum, hippocampus, neocortex, and brain stem, whereas symmetrical synapses between GABAergic terminals and somata and dendrites were immunonegative (Nusser *et al.* 1994; Baude *et al.* 1995; Phend *et al.* 1995; Matsubara *et al.* 1996). Immunoparticles were found to have either a uniform distribution within the synaptic specialization (Nusser *et al.* 1994) or to be less concentrated at the center of the synapse (Matsubara *et al.* 1996; Kharazia and Weinberg 1997).

Recent studies addressed two fundamentally important questions regarding the cell-surface distribution of GluRs. First, as most nerve cells express several GluR subtypes and receive glutamatergic inputs from functionally distinct sources, the question arises whether every synapse expresses all receptor subtypes or whether different receptors are employed by distinct glutamatergic inputs. Rubio and Wenthold (1997) have chosen the fusiform cells of the dorsal cochlear nucleus to study the distribution of AMPA receptors, because these cells express several GluR subtypes and receive glutamatergic inputs from parallel fibers on their apical dendrites, and from auditory fibers on their basal dendrites. The GluR2 subunit was found at both parallel and auditory fiber synapses with approximately the same density, whereas the GluR4 subunit was only detectable at auditory synapses on the basal dendrites. A similar differential distribution was found for the 1α subtype of the metabotropic GluR. These results demonstrate that on a single cell, distinct glutamatergic inputs can act through different receptor subtypes, contributing to the fulfilment of input-specific functional requirements. Secondly, the amount of receptors also plays an important role in the postsynaptic response to the released transmitter. To investigate if every glutamatergic synapse on the surface of a nerve cell contains the same amount of AMPA receptors or if synaptic AMPA receptor number could vary, Nusser *et al.* (1998*a*) have studied the quantitative pattern of AMPA receptor expression in the rat hippocampus using electron microscopic immunogold localization. Pyramidal cells in the CA3 area receive glutamatergic inputs from commissural/associational (C/A) fibers in strata oriens and radiatum, from mossy fibers in stratum lucidum and from entorhinal fibers in stratum laconosum-moleculare. Thus, the amount, density and variability of synaptic AMPA receptors could be compared at these functionally distinct glutamatergic synapses. Every mossy synapse on pyramidal cell complex spines was found to be immunopositive for AMPA receptors. AMPA receptors in these synapses had a non-Gaussian, positively skewed distribution with a coefficient of variation (CV = mean/standard deviation) of ~ 0.8. In contrast, the distribution of AMPA receptor content at C/A synapses on pyramidal cell spines had a much larger variability ($CV \sim 1.9$) and approximately 15% of the synapses were immunonegative. As there was a positive, linear correlation between the gold particle number and synaptic area of mossy synapses, and the variability in the particle number was similar to that of synaptic areas, a uniform AMPA receptor density was predicted at these synapses. A similar uniform density was found for synaptic $GABA_A$ receptors, allowing the synaptic area to be used to predict the relative receptor content of synapses (see the section on the Subcellular distribution of $GABA_A$ receptors). In contrast, there was a much larger variability in the particle number ($CV = 1.9$) than in the area of C/A synapses on pyramidal cell spines ($CV = 0.9$), suggesting that AMPA receptor density is not uniform and, therefore, the synaptic area cannot be used to predict the relative receptor content at these synapses. Furthermore, the mean number of AMPA receptors at mossy synapses was ~ 4 times higher than that at C/A synapses. These results establish that the amount and variability in synaptic AMPA receptors depends on the identity of the presynaptic input. To test the extent to which postsynaptic cells influence receptor expression, the AMPA receptor content of C/A synapses were compared between pyramidal cell spines and GABAergic interneurone dendrites in the stratum radiatum. Every C/A synapse on an interneuron dendrite contained immunoreactive AMPA receptors. They had a Gaussian distribution with a relatively small variability ($CV \sim 0.5$) and contained on average 4 times as many receptors as C/A synapses on pyramidal cell spines. As the quantitative pattern of AMPA receptor expression is very different in two distinct cell types innervated by a common afferent, it can be concluded that the amount of AMPA receptor at a given glutamatergic synapse is governed by both pre- and postsynaptic elements (Nusser *et al.* 1998*a*).

The following view of the subcellular distribution of AMPA receptors emerges from high-resolution localization studies. Receptors are concentrated at glutamatergic synaptic junctions with an abrupt decrease in their density at the edge of the postsynaptic specialization. The molecular makeup and the number of synaptic AMPA receptors are determined by both pre- and postsynaptic factors such that functionally distinct glutamatergic connections display characteristic patterns of receptor expression. Albeit at a lower density, AMPA receptors are also found on the extrasynaptic plasma membranes of the somata, dendritic shafts and spines, but never on membranes postsynaptic to GABAergic terminals. Furthermore, there is no evidence for the presence of AMPA-type GluRs in axons. Intracellularly, AMPA receptors are associated with the endoplasmic reticulum, Golgi apparatus, multi-vesicular bodies and the spine apparatus.

Kainate receptors

The recent development of AMPA and kainate receptor selective agonists and antagonists (reviewed by Bleakman and Lodge 1998) initiated several studies examining the role of kainate receptors in the CNS (Castillo *et al.* 1997; Lerma *et al.* 1997; Vignes and Collingridge 1997). It has been demonstrated that kainate receptor-mediated responses could be evoked in CA3 pyramidal cells by stimulating mossy fibers (Castillo *et al.* 1997; Vignes and Collingridge 1997) in agreement with the very high density of kainate binding sites in the stratum lucidum of the CA3 area (Cotman *et al.* 1987). However, a single stimulus was not sufficient to evoke a kainate receptor-mediated excitatory postsynaptic current (EPSC) in CA3 pyramidal cells, suggesting that these receptors may be present extrasynaptically, rather than being concentrated at postsynaptic densities. In contrast, a single stimulus is sufficient to evoke kainate mediated EPSCs on GABAergic interneurons (Frerking *et al.* 1998), indicating that the precise location of these receptors may be cell type dependent. Electron microscopic localization of the GluR6/7 and KA2 subunits with the immunoperoxidase method indicates that, in the hippocampus and neocortex, the majority of immunoreactive kainate receptors were present intracellularly in pyramidal cells (Huntley *et al.* 1994; Petralia *et al.* 1994*a*). However, similar intense cytoplasmic labeling was obtained for NMDA receptor subunits with conventional immunoperoxidase methods, which could be dramatically reduced by antigen-retrieval procedures (see Fritschy *et al.* 1998; Watanabe *et al.* 1998). Thus, it remains to be determined whether such antigen-retrieval procedures would also reduce the intensity of cytoplasmic kainate receptor immunostaining. Furthermore, as discussed above, the immunoperoxidase method is not appropriate for determining the synaptic enrichment of receptors. Presently, these receptors have not been localized with a non-diffusable marker, and consequently their relative densities and precise location in relation to the transmitter release site remain unknown. Interestingly, fish and chick kainate binding proteins, which are highly homologous to mammalian kainate receptor subunits (Hollmann and Heinemann 1994), have been found at high density on cerebellar Bergmann glial membranes (Somogyi *et al.* 1990). As these glial processes tightly surround Purkinje cell spines, the location of kainate binding proteins, and perhaps the kainate receptors in mammals, suggests an important role in buffering synaptically released glutamate. High-resolution localization studies of the kainate receptors are needed in the mammalian CNS to shed light onto their precise location, relative densities and input specific distribution, to further our understanding of their role in influencing neuronal excitability.

NMDA receptors

NMDA receptors have been the focus of intense scientific research since the late seventies as they are fundamentally important in neuronal development, in sensory perception, learning, and memory formation; and in the pathogenesis of various CNS disorders. Since the development of the first NMDA receptor specific agonists and antagonists and the cloning of NMDA receptor subunits, physiologist, behavioral neuroscientist, and molecular biologist have joined forces to gain more insight into the role of NMDA receptors in various CNS functions and dysfunctions. As for all molecules, it is also true for the NMDA receptors, that for the understanding of their role it is essential to determine their precise subcellular location and their densities in distinct subcellular compartments. The regional and cellular distribution of NMDA receptors have been extensively studied with autoradiography (reviewed by Cotman *et al.* 1987), *in situ* hybridization histochemistry (Watanabe *et al.* 1993; Conti *et al.* 1994; Monyer *et al.* 1994), single cell RT-PCR (Flint *et al.* 1997), and immunohistochemical methods (Aoki *et al.* 1994; Huntley *et al.* 1994; Petralia *et al.* 1994b; Siegel *et al.* 1994; Wenzel *et al.* 1997; Fritschy *et al.* 1998; Watanabe *et al.* 1998). Using conventional immunocytochemical techniques, NMDA receptors were found mainly postsynaptically, but their presynaptic presence has also been indicated (Siegel *et al.* 1994). Furthermore, several studies have concluded that a very significant proportion of the immunoreactive NMDA receptors were present intracellularly in the somata and primary dendrites of nerve cells (Huntley *et al.* 1994; Petralia *et al.* 1994b; Siegel *et al.* 1994). Two recent studies (Fritschy *et al.* 1998; Watanabe *et al.* 1998) have used independent antigen-retrieval methods to re-examine the subcellular distribution of several NMDA receptor subunits. These studies found that either microwave irradiation or protease digestion dramatically reduced the strong intracellular labeling obtained with conventional methods. This allowed presumably synaptic NMDA receptors to be visualized, as strong punctate labeling of the hippocampal neuropile became apparent. Thus, it seems that most of the NMDA receptors are on the surface of nerve cells concentrated presumably at synaptic junctions. Indeed, electron microscopic immunogold localization of the NR1 (Kharazia *et al.* 1996; Somogyi *et al.* 1998) and NR2A/B (Ottersen and Landsend 1997) subunits revealed an enrichment of gold particles at asymmetrical synaptic junctions on cortical and hippocampal pyramidal cell spines. Furthermore, Kharazia *et al.* (1996) provided the first direct evidence for the co-localization of AMPA and NMDA receptors (Fig. 4.1) at individual glutamatergic synapses of neocortical pyramidal cell spines. These studies provide convincing evidence for the synaptic concentration of NMDA receptors in some glutamatergic synaptic junctions, but several important questions regarding the qualitative and quantitative pattern of synaptic NMDA receptor expression remained unanswered. Fritschy *et al.* (1998) and Watanabe *et al.* (1998) have addressed the issue whether functionally distinct glutamatergic synapses can have different subsets of NMDA receptors. In the strata oriens and radiatum of the hippocampal CA3 area, strong immunoreactive puncta for the NR1, NR2A and NR2B subunits were found, whereas in the stratum lucidum only NR1 and NR2A subunits could be detected. These results indicate that the NMDA receptor composition of C/A synapses on CA3 pyramidal cell spines includes the NR1, NR2A, and NR2B subunits, but that of mossy fiber synapses is NR1/NR2A. It is thus no coincidence that the functional properties of C/A and mossy fiber connections to CA3 pyramidal cells differ greatly, and that they express different forms of synaptic plasticity (reviewed by Nicoll and Malenka 1995). The identification of distinct molecular fingerprints, such as the differential NR2B subunit expression as well as the different amount of AMPA receptors (Nusser *et al.* 1998*a*), for these functionally distinct connections will help us predicting the functional properties and types of plasticity of other glutamatergic connections in the brain.

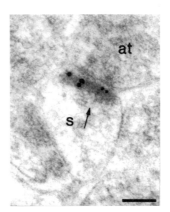

Fig. 4.1 Electron microscopic demonstration of the co-localization of AMPA (large particles; GluR1–4 subunits) and NMDA (small particles; NR1/NR2A subunits) receptors in an asymmetrical synapse (arrow) made by an axon terminal (at) with a pyramidal cell spine (s) in the hippocampal CA1 area. Postembedding immunogold reaction on Lowicryl-resin embedded tissue. Scale bar: 0.2 μm. This figure was kindly prepared by Peter Somogyi. Many thank to Drs Elek Molnar (GluR1–4) and Hannah Monyer (NR2A) for kindly providing the antibodies.

Subcellular distribution of GABA$_A$ receptors

In most brain regions, there is a large diversity in GABA-releasing neurons, which is presumably essential for the fulfilment of their complex functional roles. These include the synchronization of neuronal oscillations, the regulation of the active backpropagation of action potentials into the dendrites, inhibition of dendritic Ca^{2+} electrogenesis, or shunting excitatory synaptic inputs (reviewed by Freund and Buzsaki 1996). Most of these diverse actions are achieved through the activation of ionotropic GABA$_A$ receptors. GABA$_A$ receptors are formed from pentameric assemblies of structurally distinct subunits. To date, nineteen different subunit genes have been identified (α_{1-6}, β_{1-4}, γ_{1-3}, δ, ε, π and ρ_{1-3}), allowing hundreds of thousands of possible subunit combinations. Alternative splicing of some of these genes further increases functional and structural diversity (reviewed by Macdonald and Olsen 1994; Sieghart 1995; Stephenson 1995). For example, the affinity of different receptor subtypes for GABA may vary fifty-fold. Receptor subtypes also influence the rate of deactivation and desensitization upon the prolonged presence of agonist (see Chapter 5). The regulation of GABA$_A$ receptors by protein phosphory-lation also depends on the subunit composition (Moss and Smart 1996). Furthermore, several clinically important drugs, such as the anxiolytic, anticonvulsant, sedative-hypnotic benzodiazepines, some anxiogenic, convulsant β-carbolines, some depressant barbiturates, some anxiolytic, anticonvulsant and hypnotic steroids produce their effects through interacting with GABA$_A$ receptors (reviewed by Sieghart 1995). GABAergic mechanisms and the action of the above mentioned clinically important drugs cannot be fully understood without the identification of:

(a) which GABA$_A$ receptor subtypes exist in the CNS (see Barnard *et al.* 1998);

(b) how do they behave upon functionally relevant activation (see Chapter 5); and

(c) their location and relative abundance at regional, cellular, and subcellular levels.

The regional and cellular distribution of GABA$_A$ receptor subunits have been extensively studied with autoradiography (reviewed by Wamsley and Palacios 1984), *in situ* hybridization histochemistry (Persohn *et al.* 1992; Wisden *et al.* 1992), and immunohistochemistry (Turner *et al.* 1993; Fritschy and Mohler 1995). Several aspects of the subcellular distribution of GABA$_A$ receptor subunits have been revealed by immunofluorescence (Bohlhalter *et al.* 1994; Craig *et al.* 1994; Gao and Fritschy 1994; Koulen *et al.* 1996; Fritschy *et al.* 1998) and electron microscopic immunocytochemical studies (Richards *et al.* 1987; Somogyi *et al.* 1989; Hansen *et al.* 1991; Nusser *et al.* 1995, 1996b, 1997, 1998b,c; Todd *et al.* 1996). These receptors are concentrated at synapses opposite to GABA releasing terminals (Fig. 4.2) and are also present at lower densities on the extrasynaptic plasma membranes of nerve cells. It is interesting to note that so far not a single example has been found where GABA$_A$ receptors are not found extrasynaptically. Nusser *et al.* (1995) have examined the relative densities of synaptic and extrasynaptic GABA$_A$ receptors on the surface of cerebellar granule cells and found that GABA$_A$ receptors are approximately 200 times enriched in GABAergic synaptic junctions. As only a small fraction of the surface of a nerve cell is covered by GABAergic synapses, the amount of extrasynaptic receptors may exceed those found synaptically. Indeed, it

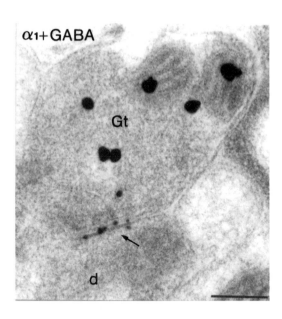

Fig. 4.2 Electron micrograph of freeze-substituted, Lowicryl resin-embedded ultra-thin section showing the enrichment of immunoreactive GABA$_A$ receptor α1 subunits (small particles) in a symmetrical synaptic junction (arrow) made by a GABA immunopositive cerebellar Golgi cell terminal (Gt; enrichment of large particles) with a granule cell dendrite (d). Scale bar: 0.2 µm (Adapted from Nusser *et al.* 1995)

was estimated that more than 50% of all surface GABA$_A$ receptors are located at extrasynaptic sites on granule cells, indicating that extrasynaptic receptors should not be neglected. The fraction of extrasynaptic receptors may be cell-type specific and may depend on the amount of tonic inhibition required (see below and Brickley *et al.* 1996; Rossi and Hamann 1998). Intracellular organelles such as somatic/proximal dendritic endoplasmic reticulum and Golgi apparatus also contain immunoreactive GABA$_A$ receptors (Somogyi *et al.* 1989), consistent with their somatic/proximal dendritic synthesis. When the distribution of GABA$_A$ receptors has been examined in different brain regions, no immunoreactivity for GABA$_A$ receptors could be detected at glutamatergic synapses. However, one should be cautious with this generalization, as an enrichment of the α6, β2/3 and γ2 subunits was found at glutamatergic mossy fiber to granule cell synapses in the cerebellum (Nusser *et al.* 1996*a*, 1998*b*). The functional role of these receptors at glutamatergic synapses is unknown. It seems to be a general rule that if a nerve cell expresses a given ionotropic GABA$_A$ or glutamate receptor in some of its synapses, the same receptor will also be present on the extrasynaptic plasma membrane at a lower density (but see Zamanillo *et al.* 1999). Is the converse also true? Namely, if a nerve cell expresses a receptor subtype extrasynaptically is it always going to be also concentrated at some synapses? To examine this question, electron microscopic immunogold localization of all major GABA$_A$ receptor subunits (α1, α6, β2, β3, γ2 and δ) expressed by cerebellar granule cells was carried out (Nusser *et al.*

1998*b*). The α1, α6, β2/3 and γ2 subunits were found to be concentrated at GABAergic Golgi synapses and were also present in the extrasynaptic membrane at a lower concentration. In contrast, immunoparticles for the δ subunit could not be detected at synaptic junctions, although they were abundantly present in the extrasynaptic dendritic and somatic membranes (Fig. 4.3). The exclusive extra-synaptic location of the δ subunit-containing receptors together with their kinetic properties suggest that tonic inhibition (Brickley *et al.* 1996) could be mainly mediated by *extrasynaptic* δ subunit-containing receptors, whereas phasic inhibition is due to the activation of *synaptic* γ2 subunit-containing receptors.

Analogous to the multiple glutamatergic innervation of neurons, most nerve cells in the CNS also receive GABAergic input from several distinct sources and express multiple GABA$_A$ receptor subtypes. To examine whether every receptor subtype is concentrated at every GABAergic synapse on a single cell or selective synaptic targeting of distinct subtypes exists, the subcellular distribution of α1 and α2 subunits was compared in hippocampal pyramidal cells (Nusser *et al.* 1996*b*). Immunogold particles for the α1 subunit were found at most GABAergic synapses on somata, axon initial segments, and dendrites of CA1 pyramidal cells, whereas immuno-reactive α2 subunits were located only in a subset of somatic and dendritic synapses, but in all of the axon initial segments synapses. Subsequently, Fritschy *et al.* (1998) have also found the same synaptic segregation of α1 and α2 subunit-containing receptors with an immunofluorescence approach. In addition, they demonstrated

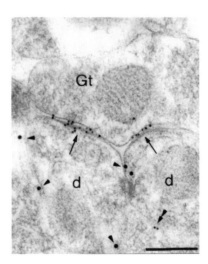

Fig. 4.3 Synapses (arrows) made by a cerebellar Golgi cell terminal (Gt) with granule cell dendrites (d) show an enrichment of the β2/3 subunits (small particles), but do not contain particles for the δ subunit (large particles) of the GABA$_A$ receptor. Immunoparticles for the δ subunit (single arrowheads) at the extrasynaptic dendritic membranes demonstrate that the method is sensitive enough to visualize this subunit. Note that immunoparticles for the β2/3 subunits are also associated with the extrasynaptic dendritic membranes (e.g. double arrowheads). Scale bar: 0.2 μm (Adapted from Nusser *et al.* 1998*b*)

that the same principle also applies for principal cells in all parts of the hippocampal formation (e.g., CA3 area, dentate gyrus) and in the neocortex. Koulen *et al.* (1996) have arrived at a very similar conclusion after examining the precise subcellular distribution of the $\alpha 1$, $\alpha 2$, and $\alpha 3$ subunits on retinal alpha ganglion cells. They found that these different α subunits were concentrated at distinct sites, providing further evidence for an input-selective segregation of distinct GABA_A receptor subtypes on the surface on central neurons.

In addition to qualitative differences in the GABA_A receptor content of different GABAergic synapses on individual nerve cells, it is also important to know whether every GABAergic synapse contains the same amount of receptors. As in most nerve cells the distribution of tetrodotoxin-resistant, miniature inhibitory postsynaptic current (mIPSC) amplitudes is not Gaussian, but positively skewed, suggesting that different synapses may contain different numbers of receptors (reviewed by Mody *et al.* 1994). However, several other interpretations have been put forward (reviewed by Frerking and Wilson 1996). To investigate the variability in postsynaptic GABA_A receptor number, whole-cell patch-clamp recordings of mIPSCs were combined with quantitative immunogold localization of synaptic GABA_A receptors in cerebellar molecular layer interneurons (Nusser *et al.* 1997). Every anatomically defined symmetrical somatic and dendritic synapse contained gold particles for GABA_A receptors. Gold particle number showed a large variability ($CV \approx 0.8$; range: 6–184 gold/synapse) between synapses and had a non-Gaussian, skewed distribution. Gold particle number and synapse size had very similar distributions with almost identical variability, indicating a uniform receptor density between synapses. Indeed, there was a very significant positive linear correlation between the area and immuno-reactive receptor content of synapses. As the synaptic receptor number and the size of mIPSCs had very similar distributions and variabilities, it has been concluded that the major contributor to the variability in quantal amplitude is the variation in the postsynaptic receptor number at different synapses. As the mean number of gold particles was 56 at these GABAergic synapses, and the calculated mean number of functional receptors was 140, the number of functional receptors represented by a single gold particle (*scaling factor* ~ 2.5) could be calculated. The determination of this scaling factor allowed the calculation of the lowest (~ 15) and the largest (~ 500) number of receptors per synapse within the population and the computation of the receptor density (~ 1250 receptors μm^{-2}) at these GABAergic synapses. Interestingly, GABA_A receptor density was found to be uniform also at GABAergic synapses on cerebellar Purkinje cells (Somogyi *et al.* 1998), as well as on hippocampal granule cells (Nusser *et al.* 1998c). However, the receptor density varied across cell types. Moreover, even two different compartments of a single cell type, such as the soma versus axon initial segments of hippocampal granule cells could have different receptor densities (500 compared with 850 receptors μm^{-2}, respectively). These overall density values are an order of magnitude lower than those of the nicotinic acetylcholine receptors at the neuromuscular junction (> 8000 receptors μm^{-2}; Fertuck and Salpeter 1974). Thus, GABA_A receptor packing density is not maximal, supporting the view that postsynaptic receptors are arranged in small 'microclusters' which are separated by receptor-free spaces (Mody *et al.* 1994; Nusser *et al.* 1997). Indeed, immunoparticles tend to be unevenly distributed within a synaptic junction, and clustering of particles was observed in GABAergic synapses of cerebellar interneurones (Nusser *et al.* 1997), Purkinje cells (Somogyi *et al.* 1996) as well as hippocampal granule cells (Nusser *et al.* 1998*c*).

Synapses are not static, but several physiological and pathological conditions could result in dynamic and sometimes long-lasting changes in the synaptic connections between nerve cells. Changes may take place:

(a) presynaptically by altering the probability and dynamics of transmitter release; or

(b) postsynaptically by altering the properties and/or the quantity of receptors; or

(c) the number of transmitter release sites between two nerve cells could also be modified.

Nusser *et al.* (1998*c*) have addressed the question whether the change in quantal size (Otis *et al.* 1994) following an experimental model of temporal lobe epilepsy (kindling) can be attributed to a change in the number of postsynaptic GABA$_A$ receptors. Quantal analysis of evoked IPSCs in hippocampal granule cells revealed a 66% increase in the quantal size after kindling, which resulted directly from a 75% increase in the number of synaptic GABA$_A$ receptors as determined by quantitative immunogold localization (Nusser *et al.* 1998*c*). The augmented receptor number was the consequence of an enlargement in the area of the synapses ($\sim 30\%$) as well as an enhanced receptor density ($\sim 35\%$). Interestingly, evidence was also found for a presynaptic change. The quantal content was reduced by $\sim 40\%$ and the size of the presynaptic boutons increased by an average of $\sim 75\%$. Unfortunately, it could not be determined whether the reduction in quantal content was the direct consequence of the large presynaptic boutons or due to the changes in the properties and/or the quantity of presynaptic receptors or channels. In spite of the uncertainties in the mechanisms, these results are compatible with the existence of a synaptic homeostasis (Davis and Goodman 1998), which would operate to keep the net weight of all connections relatively constant (Turrigiano *et al.* 1998).

Subcellular distribution of glycine receptors

The neurotransmitter glycine, together with GABA, plays an essential role in regulating neuronal excitability in the brain stem and in the spinal cord. The action of glycine is mediated by heteromultimeric glycine receptors (GlyR), which display relatively high homology to GABA$_A$ receptors. In addition, both receptors are permeable to Cl^- and HCO_3^- ions. Similarly to GluR and GABA$_A$ receptors, GlyR heterogeneity is created by multiple genes encoding for GlyR subunits and alternative splicing of mRNAs (reviewed by Betz 1991; Kuhse *et al.* 1995). Interestingly, GlyRs co-purify with a 93-kDa peripheral membrane protein (gephyrin), which is essential for their synaptic clustering (Kirsch *et al.* 1993). The regional, cellular and subcellular distribution of GlyRs and gephyrin have been extensively studied using ligand binding (Probst *et al.* 1986), *in situ* hybridization histochemistry (Malosio *et al.* 1991) and immunohistochemistry (Triller *et al.* 1985, 1991; van den Pol and Gorcs 1988; Bohlhalter *et al.* 1994; Sassoe-Pognetto *et al.* 1995; Koulen *et al.* 1996; Todd *et al.* 1996). The subcellular distribution of gephyrin and GlyRs was first studied by Triller *et al.* (1985) using monoclonal antibodies in rat spinal cord.

Punctate immunofluorescent labeling on the surface of neurones suggested the synaptic location of both GlyRs and gephyrin, which was verified by electron microscopic immunogold localization. The synaptic enrichment of gephyrin and GlyRs has been confirmed by other studies and their co-localization was also demonstrated at synaptic sites (Bechade *et al.* 1996; Todd *et al.* 1996). In the late eighties and early nineties, the presence of gephyrin was interpreted as a good indicator for the enrichment of GlyRs, however, recent studies showed that this is not always the case. In the retina, Sassoe-Pognetto *et al.* (1995) have demonstrated that GABA$_A$ and GlyRs were not co-localized, but gephyrin was present at some GABAergic synapses together with the $\alpha 2$ subunit of the GABA$_A$ receptor, suggesting that gephyrin may also play a role in the clustering of postsynaptic GABA$_A$ receptors. Indeed, an elegant study by Essricht *et al.* (1998) has shown the loss of synaptic clustering of gephyrin in cultured cortical neurones from GABA$_A$ $\gamma 2$ subunit deficient mice, where synaptic GABA$_A$ receptors were also missing. Furthermore, inhibiting gephyrin expression caused the loss of synaptic GABA$_A$ receptor clusters in control hippocampal cells, demonstrating the essential role of gephyrin in the synaptic clustering of GABA$_A$ receptors. In contrast, gephyrin and the GlyR $\alpha 1$ subunit showed a completely overlapping distribution in the spinal cord (Todd *et al.* 1996), suggesting that here the presence of gephyrin is a reliable indicator for GlyRs. The co-localization of gephyrin and GABA$_A$ receptor subunits has also been shown in some junctions postsynaptic to axon terminals containing both GABA and glycine (Bohlhalter *et al.* 1994; Todd *et al.* 1996). The co-release of these two neurotransmitters from a single terminal has recently been established functionally and synaptic currents mediated by both GABA$_A$ and GlyRs have been demonstrated (Jonas *et al.* 1998). It is important to note that, even in spinal cord neurons, not every symmetrical synaptic junction contains GABA$_A$ and GlyRs together. Some synapses displayed immunoreactivity for either GlyRs or GABA$_A$ receptors alone opposite to axon terminals containing high labeling for only glycine or GABA, respectively (Todd *et al.* 1996). These results demonstrate the complexity of the cell surface distribution of GlyRs, the consequences of which are at present unknown but is presumably of great importance.

Subcellular distribution of metabotropic glutamate receptors

The role of glutamate acting through G-protein coupled metabotropic GluRs (mGluRs) is not as widely studied as that through ionotropic receptors. However, several elegant studies have recently demonstrated the essential involvement of mGluRs in olfactory information processing, signal transduction in the retina, and in cerebellum-related functions such as motor learning (reviewed by Nakanishi 1994). It has also been shown that distinct mGluR subtypes are responsible for these diverse functions. So far, eight mGluR subtypes have been identified (mGluR1–8) several of which exist in alternatively spliced variants (reviewed by Nakanishi 1994; Pin and Duvoisin 1995). Metabotropic GluRs can be grouped into three categories according to their agonist selectivity, sequence homology, and signal transduction mechanisms. Group I mGluRs (mGluR1 and 5) stimulate phosphatidylinositol hydrolysis and intracellular Ca^{2+} release and their most potent agonist is quisqualate.

Group II mGluRs consist of mGluR2 and mGluR3, they are negatively coupled to cAMP formation and are most potently activated by LY354740 and DCG-IV. Finally, group III mGluRs (mGluR4, mGluR6–8) also inhibit the formation of cAMP in heterologous expression systems and are selectively activated by L-amino-4-phosphonobutyrate (L-AP4; reviewed by Pin and Duvoisin 1995). Physiological studies suggested the presence of mGluRs postsynaptically on various cell types (e.g. both glutamatergic and GABAergic neurones), as well as presynaptically on glutamatergic and GABAergic axons. Establishing the subcellular distribution of mGluRs is essential in order to identify the subtypes involved in different CNS functions and to predict conditions under which they will be activated. Furthermore, possible effector mechanisms can also be predicted from the fine spatial co-existence of mGluRs with possible effector molecules (e.g. voltage- or ligand-gated channels).

A widespread distribution of group I mGluRs has been found in the CNS by several studies using *in situ* hybridization and immunohistochemistry (see Wada *et al.* 1998 and references therein). In hippocampal, cortical, spinal cord, hypothalamic, striatal, and cerebellar neurones, immunoreactivity for mGluR1 and 5 has been detected postsynaptically on somata, dendritic shafts and dendritic spines, but no detectable level of reactivity was observed on presynaptic axon terminals (Martin *et al.* 1992; Baude *et al.* 1993; Shigemoto *et al.* 1993; Vidnyanszky *et al.* 1994; van den Pol *et al.* 1995; Lujan *et al.* 1996, 1997; Koulen *et al.* 1997; Negyessy *et al.* 1997). Using immunoperoxidase methods at the electron microscopic level, several studies (Martin *et al.* 1992; van den Pol *et al.* 1995) detected peroxidase reaction end product on postsynaptic specializations of asymmetrical synapses, similarly to that found for ionotropic GluRs. In contrast, no immunoreactive group I mGluR was detected in the main body of glutamatergic synaptic specializations with three different immunogold methods, but gold particles were readily observed in peri- and extra-synaptic positions (Fig. 4.4; Baude *et al.* 1993; Nusser *et al.* 1994; Lujan *et al.* 1996). The density of immunogold particles for mGluR1 and 5 decreased as a function of distance from the edge of the postsynaptic specialization (Lujan *et al.* 1997). The segregation of ionotropic and metabotropic GluRs has been shown at individual synapses using double-labeling (Nusser *et al.* 1994). Gold particles labeling AMPA receptors were concentrated in synaptic junctions made by cerebellar parallel fibers with Purkinje cell spines, whereas gold particles for mGluR1α were distributed outside the synaptic specialization, suggesting that different temporal patterns of presynaptic activity may be required for their activation. Indeed, it has been shown that type I mGluR-mediated postsynaptic responses in Purkinje cells could only be evoked by high frequency stimulation of parallel fibers (Batchelor *et al.* 1994; Tempia *et al.* 1998), whereas a single stimulus is sufficient to evoke AMPA receptor-mediated responses. These results show that the pattern of presynaptic activity required for the synaptic activation of mGluR1 can be predicted from the location of the receptor in relation to the transmitter release site. As mentioned previously, Rubio and Wenthold (1997) have found that mGluR1 was not associated with every glutamatergic synapse on the surface of fusiform cells in the cochlear nucleus, but was selectively associated with auditory synapses in the basal dendrites. The synapse specific segregation of mGluRs provides further evidence for the complexity and the highly regulated cell surface distribution of neurotransmitter receptors, including those coupled to G-proteins.

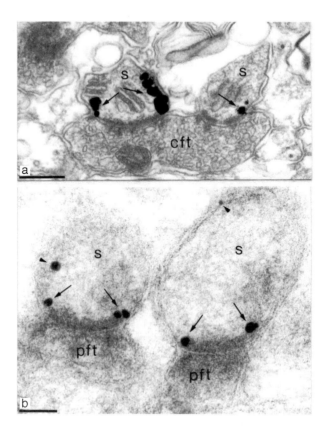

Fig. 4.4 The 1α subtype of the mGluR is concentrated outside the synaptic specializations of asymmetrical synapses in perisynaptic (arrows) and extrasynaptic (arrowheads) positions. (a) Gold particles (arrows) are excluded from the postsynaptic specializations made by a climbing fiber terminal (cft) with Purkinje cell spines (s). Pre-embedding immunogold method. (b) No labeling of the postsynaptic densities between parallel fiber terminals (pft) and spines (s) could be detected using the postembedding immunogold method on freeze-substituted and Lowicryl resin-embedded tissue. Scale bars: (a) 0.2 μm; (b) 0.1 μm (Adapted from Nusser and Somogyi 1997).

In the hippocampus and neocortex, mGluR2 is mainly present presynaptically (Petralia *et al.* 1996; Shigemoto *et al.* 1997), whereas in other brain regions such as the olfactory bulb and the cerebellum, mGluR2 is both pre- and postsynaptic (Hayashi *et al.* 1993; Ohishi *et al.* 1994). The other member of group II mGluRs, mGluR3, is mainly found on glial processes (Shigemoto *et al.* 1997), where its functional role has not been identified. High-resolution localization of mGluR2 on the surface of cerebellar Golgi cells revealed its presence on axons, somata, and dendrites (Ohishi *et al.* 1994; Lujan *et al.* 1997). GABAergic Golgi cell axons were strongly immunopositive, but very little labeling was present in presynaptic specializations. The rest of the terminal, pre-terminal membranes, and small diameter axons were strongly labeled. A very similar distribution of mGluR2 was found in the hippocampus on mossy and entorhinal fibers (Shigemoto *et al.* 1997), indicating that this pattern is a general feature of its distribution. On the dendrites of Golgi cells, immunogold particles for mGluR2 were not associated with glutamatergic synapses, as demonstrated by a detailed quantification, showing that the distribution of gold particles in relation to glutamatergic synapses was not different from a random distribution (Lujan *et al.* 1997). This cell surface distribution of mGluR2 is in sharp contrast to that of group I mGluRs and ionotropic GluRs. The apparently random distribution of postsynaptic mGluR2 on Golgi cell dendrites indicates that these receptors may not be directly activated by synaptically released glutamate, but they may fine-tune Golgi cell excitability as a function of the ambient glutamate level.

Most of the group III mGluRs (mGluR4, 7, and 8) are distributed throughout the CNS (Ohishi *et al.* 1995), whereas mGluR6 is only present in retinal bipolar cells, where its functional role has been extensively studied (Masu *et al.* 1995). Subcellular distribution of mGluR4 and 8 has been studied in the hippocampus, cerebellum, and piriform cortex where these receptors were mainly present on presynaptic axon terminals (Kinoshita *et al.* 1996, 1998; Shigemoto *et al.* 1997; Wada *et al.* 1998). Although, in most brain regions mGluR7 is also a presynaptic receptor (Shigemoto *et al.* 1996, 1997; Wada *et al.* 1998), Brandstatter *et al.* (1996) have detected mGluR7 immunoreactivity both pre- and postsynaptically in the retina. Presynaptic group II and III mGluRs occupy different parts of the axon (Fig. 4.5). As mentioned above, mGluR2 is mainly present in pre-terminal axons, whereas group III mGluRs are restricted to the presynaptic specialization of axon terminals, i.e. to the site of synaptic vesicle fusion (Shigemoto *et al.* 1996, 1997). These results imply that group II and III mGluRs may be activated differentially and they may use different effector mechanisms to influence transmitter release. Interestingly, the enrichment of type III mGluRs at the release site is not exclusive for glutamatergic terminals, as their concentration in the presynaptic specialization of GABAergic terminals has also been demonstrated (Shigemoto *et al.* 1997; Kinoshita *et al.* 1998).

A single cortical or hippocampal pyramidal cell contacts several thousand postsynaptic cells with a very extensive axonal arbor. Heterogeneity in the transmitter release probability has been suggested at different terminals of the same axon (Markram *et al.* 1998). This raises the question whether every axon terminal contains the same amount of presynaptic receptor or whether different amounts of receptor may be present at distinct terminals. Shigemoto *et al.* (1996) have studied the distribution of mGluR7a in the hippocampus and found that a single axon can express different amounts of mGluR7a depending on the postsynaptic target. Namely, when CA3 pyramidal axons contacted other pyramidal cell spines very few if any immunogold particles were present in the presynaptic specialization. However, when the same axon made a synapse on mGluR1α/somatostatin/GABA immunopositive cells, a high density of presynaptic mGluR7a was detected at the release site. The most conspicuous example of the target-cell-specific segregation of mGluR7a arose from the discovery that when a single bouton made a synaptic contact to a somatostatin cell dendrite, the release site contained a high density of mGluR7a labeling, whereas another release site in the same bouton that contacted a pyramidal cell spine contained no label for mGluR7a (Shigemoto *et al.* 1996). An almost identical conclusion was reached in the retina, where Brandstatter *et al.* (1996) have

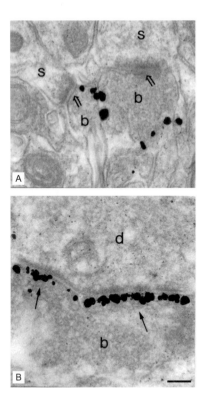

Fig. 4.5 Segregation of group II (mGluR2/3) and group III (mGluR7a) metabotropic GluRs on glutamatergic axon terminals in the rat hippocampus. (A) Gold particles for mGluR2/3 are present at the extrasynaptic membranes of axon terminals (b) making immunonegative synapses (open arrows) with spines (s) of pyramidal cells. (B) Immunogold particles for mGluR7a are concentrated at the presynaptic specializations of asymmetrical synapses (arrows) made by a bouton (b) with an interneurone dendrite (d). Pre-embedding silver intensified immunogold reactions. (a) and (b) at the same magnification. Scale bar: 0.2 μm. This figure was kindly prepared by Prof. Ryuichi Shigemoto.

discovered the target-specific segregation of mGluR7 at bipolar cell ribbon synapses. The apparently complete segregation of mGluR7 between two release sites of a single bouton suggests that coupling of the receptor to its effector is likely to be spatially restricted, and probably membrane delimited. It seems that this target-specific segregation of presynaptic receptors may be a general principle of their organization, because the same phenomenon has been reported (Shigemoto *et al.* 1997) for other mGluRs such as mGluR4a, mGluR7b and mGluR8.

Subcellular distribution of GABA_B receptors

As most neurotransmitter in the CNS, GABA also act through G-protein coupled receptors (GABA_B). These receptors influence neuronal excitability and neurotransmitter release through the regulation of various Ca^{2+} and K^+ channels via both membrane delimited pathways and pathways involving second messengers (reviewed by Bonanno and Raiteri 1993; Bowery 1993). $GABA_B$ receptors have been identified with physiological and pharmacological tools on presynaptic GABA- and glutamatergic axons and postsynaptically on various cell types (reviewed by Thompson 1994; Misgeld *et al.* 1995). Recent pharmacological (reviewed by Bonanno and Raiteri 1993) and cloning studies (Kaupmann *et al.* 1997, 1998) identified pharmacological and structural heterogeneities of $GABA_B$ receptors, raising the possibility that different $GABA_B$ receptor subtypes are responsible for the fulfilment of different functional requirements. Our understanding of the role of $GABA_B$ receptor diversity will be greatly improved by establishing the cell-surface distribution of distinct $GABA_B$ receptor subtypes.

Despite the fact that the first $GABA_B$ receptor subtype ($GABA_BR1$) has been cloned only very recently (Kaupmann *et al.* 1997), three studies have already used subtype-selective antibodies to investigate the subcellular distribution of $GABA_BR1$ and $GABA_BR2$. Koulen *et al.* (1998) have found that $GABA_BR1$ is present both pre- and postsynaptically in rat retina. Immunoreactive $GABA_BR1$ was found presynaptically in horizontal cell processes and in amacrine cells, whereas immunoreactivity for the same receptor subtype was also present postsynaptically on amacrine and ganglion cells. $GABA_B$ receptors on GABAergic horizontal and amacrine cell terminals may function as autoreceptors to reduce the probability of GABA release upon their activation. As Koulen *et al.* (1998) have applied an immunoperoxidase method to study the subcellular distribution of $GABA_BR1$, it was not possible to draw strong conclusions about the synaptic concentration and the subsynaptic distribution of this receptor. Nevertheless, $GABA_B$ receptors could be demonstrated extrasynaptically far away from synapses. The extrasynaptic presence of $GABA_BR1$ was also found by Fritschy *et al.* (1999) using electron microscopic immunoperoxidase localization in the cerebellum. Kaupmann *et al.* (1998) have chosen an electron microscopic immunogold method to study the precise subcellular and subsynaptic distribution of $GABA_BR1$ and $GABA_BR2$ in the cerebellum. Surprisingly, the most intense labeling in the cerebellum was on Purkinje cell spines postsynaptic to glutamatergic parallel fiber terminals, where gold particles were mainly outside the synaptic junctions in perisynaptic and extrasynaptic positions. Immunoreactivity for both receptor subtypes was also found on glutamatergic parallel fiber terminals. The intriguing locations of $GABA_B$ receptors on presynaptic glutamatergic terminals and on postsynaptic spines receiving glutamatergic inputs open new perspectives on GABAergic neurotransmission.

Subcellular distribution of voltage-gated ion channels

The way in which nerve cells respond to spatio-temporally-dispersed synaptic inputs depends, to a large extent, on the properties, subcellular distribution, and densities of voltage-gated ion channels (see Chapters 6, 9, and 10). How cellular neurophysiology contributed to our knowledge of the functional and pharmacological properties of voltage-gated ion channels (Na^+, K^+, and Ca^{2+}) and their subcellular distribution is extensively discussed in Chapter 6. Furthermore, as the functional and structural heterogeneities of Na$^+$, K$^+$, and Ca^{2+} channels have been reviewed extensively elsewhere (Hille 1992), in the next sections, I shall only discuss recent results obtained with different anatomical approaches, regarding the subcellular distribution of voltage-gated K$^+$, Na$^+$, and Ca^{2+} channels.

Voltage-gated K$^+$ channels

Potassium channels comprise the most diverse class of voltage-gated ion channels. Dozens of distinct subunits have been identified (reviewed by Pongs 1992), creating a large number of homo- and heteromultimeric assemblies with distinct functional and pharmacological properties (Hille 1992). Several studies have reported that different K$^+$ channel subunits have unique, but sometimes, overlapping patterns of expression in the CNS (Wang *et al.* 1994; Veh *et al.* 1995). Not only do different cell types express a unique set of K$^+$ channel subunits, but the subcellular distribution of a certain subunit is also cell type dependent (McNamara *et al.* 1993; Sheng *et al.* 1994; Wang *et al.* 1994; Veh *et al.* 1995). For example, in cerebellar basket cells the Kv1.2 subunit is exclusively present on axons, which is in contrast with the immunostaining for the same subunit of somata and dendrites of cerebellar Purkinje and olfactory mitral cells. Furthermore, when the distribution of several subunits was compared on cerebellar basket cell axons with high-resolution immunocytochemistry, Laube *et al.* (1996) have found that the Kv1.1 and Kv1.2 subunits were predominantly localized to septate-like junctions, whereas the Kv3.4 subunit was not concentrated in these junctions but was rather uniformly present on the axonal membrane, comprising the cerebellar Pinceau. None of these subunits was found on the axon collaterals of basket cells, which contacted the somata and proximal dendrites of Purkinje cells, demonstrating a highly regulated subcellular distribution of K$^+$ channels on the surface of a nerve cell. As the Pinceau is a highly specialized structure of basket cell axons surrounding Purkinje cell axon initial segments and such a structure is only present in the cerebellum, it is difficult to generalize from this distribution to that of K$^+$ channels present on other, more conventional, types of axon. Specifically, it will be interesting to see whether K$^+$ channels are present in preterminal axons or in axon terminals and if they are located in axon terminals whether they are concentrated at the site of transmitter release.

Much less is known about the precise distribution of K$^+$ channels on the somato-dendritic compartments of nerve cells. Several studies reported somatic and dendritic staining of several cell types (Sheng *et al.* 1994; Wang *et al.* 1994; Veh *et al.* 1995), but it remains to be determined whether such labeling corresponds to channels present in the plasma membrane or in the cytoplasm. Alonso and Widmer (1997) have addressed this question in the supraoptic nucleus of the hypothalamus, where immunoreactivity for the Kv4.2 subunit outlined the somata of magnocellular neurons. They verified the postsynaptic location of the immunoreactivity with electron microscopy, and found that the immunoperoxidase reaction end product was associated with the plasma membrane and with postsynaptic specializations. As mentioned previously, due to the diffusable nature of the marker, a possible secondary deposition of the reaction end product on the postsynaptic densities could not be excluded. Further experiments with non-diffusable markers will shed light onto the precise distribution of dendritic K$^+$ channels in relation to transmitter release sites and quantitative localizations will help us to determine the densities of K^+ channels at distinct subcellular compartments of the axo-somato-dendritic plasma membranes.

Voltage-gated Na^+ channels

The subcellular distribution of Na^+ channels has been studied in various cell types using fluorescently and radioactively labeled high-affinity toxins (Angelides *et al.* 1988; Boudier *et al.* 1992) and immunocytochemistry (Wollner and Catterall 1986; Devor *et al.* 1993; Dugandzija-Novakovic *et al.* 1995). The highest density of labeling for Na^+ channels was found in the axolemma at the nodes of Ranvier of myelinated axons (reviewed by Black *et al.* 1990), supporting classical views of the axonal distribution of Na^+ channels and their role in action potential propagation. The presence of Na^+ channels on axon-initial segments and on the somato-dendritic plasma membranes has also been reported using fluorescent toxins (Angelides *et al.* 1988) or immunocytochemistry (Laube *et al.* 1996). Angelides *et al.* (1988) have found a 5–10 times higher density of Na^+ channels on axon initial segments than on somata of cultured spinal cord neurones. Similarly, Wollner and Catterall (1986) have found that the axon hillocks of retinal ganglion cells contained a high intensity of labeling whereas the cell bodies were devoid of stain. The determination of the precise distribution and densities of Na^+ channels at different compartments of the dendritic tree will greatly contribute to our understanding of how active dendritic processes participate in the integration of input signals (Chapter 10).

Voltage-gated Ca^{2+} channels

So far six different Ca^{2+} channels have been described according to their functional and pharmacological properties (L, N, P, Q, R, and T). The underlying molecular heterogeneity has also been identified by molecular cloning, revealing a large variety of subunits (α_1, β, $\alpha_2\delta$, and γ; reviewed by Snutch and Reiners 1992; Birnbaumer *et al.* 1994). The regional and cellular distribution of several subunits has been studied using radiolabeled toxin binding, *in situ* hybridization and immunohisto-chemistry. Some information also exists regarding the subcellular distribution of several α_1 subunits. The α_{1A} subunit-containing channels have properties similar to the P/Q-type channels and are mainly present in axon terminals and in some dendritic shafts (Westenbroek *et al.* 1995). A very similar distribution has been reported for the α_{1B} subunit-containing channels (Westenbroek *et al.* 1992; Day *et al.* 1996), which have properties similar to the N-type Ca^{2+} channels. Class C and D α_1 subunits, encoding L-type channels, and the α_{1E} subunit, making R-type channels, have been exclusively found on somato-dendritic compartments throughout the brain with light microscopic immunohistochemistry (Hell *et al.* 1993; Day *et al.* 1996). It is important to note however, that none of these subunits has been localized at the electron microscopic level with particulate markers. Thus, several important questions remain to be determined, such as, how much of the somatic/dendritic immunolabeling found at the light microscopic level corresponds to intracytoplasmic or to surface channels. Are the channels uniformly distributed on the somato-dendritic surface of nerve cells or do different compartments have distinct channel densities? What is the precise distribution of these channels in relation to inhibitory and excitatory synapses? Revealing the answers to some of these questions, I believe, will help us to understand the role of these channels in dendritic integration and information processing.

Concluding remarks

High-resolution localization studies revealed several important principles in the organization of amino acid neurotransmitter receptors on the surface of central neurones. The segregation of distinct GABA and glutamate receptor subtypes to functionally different synapses, the subsynaptic segregation of ionotropic and metabotropic GluRs, the exclusive extrasynaptic presence of certain receptors, the input-specific regulation of the number and density of pre- and postsynaptic receptors comprise just a few examples of the previously unexpected complexity in the cell-surface distribution of receptors. Combined molecular, morphological and functional studies will establish the mechanisms for and the functional consequences of this highly specialized distribution of receptors. Furthermore, similar high-resolution, quantitative studies will be required in order to determine the organizational principles of the distribution of voltage-gated channels on the somato-dendritic surface of central neurons.

Acknowledgements

I would like to thank Drs Istvan Mody, Ryuichi Shigemoto and Peter Somogyi for their comments on the manuscript and Drs Peter Somogyi and Ryuichi Shigemoto for kindly preparing Figs 4.1 and 4.5, respectively. ZN is supported by a Wellcome Prize Travelling Research Fellowship.

References

Alonso, G. and Widmer, H. (1997). Clustering of KV4.2 potassium channels in postsynaptic membrane of rat supraoptic neurons: an ultrastructural study. *Neuroscience*, **77**, 617–21.

Angelides, K. J., Elmer, L. W., Loftus, D., and Elson, E. (1988). Distribution and lateral mobility of voltage-dependent sodium channels in neurons. *Journal of Cell Biology*, **106**, 1911–25.

Aoki, C., Venkatesan, C., Go, C. G., Mong, J. A., and Dawson, T. M. (1994). Cellular and subcellular localization of NMDA-R1 subunit immunoreactivity in the visual cortex of adult and neonatal rats. *Journal of Neuroscience*, **14**, 5202–22.

Barnard, E. A., Skolnick, P., Olsen, R. W., Mohler, H., Sieghart, W., Biggio, G., *et al.* (1998). International union of pharmacology. XV. Subtypes of γ-aminobutyric acid$_A$ receptors: classification on the basis of subunit structure and receptor function. *Pharmacological Reviews*, **50**, 291–313.

Batchelor, A. M., Madge, D. J., and Garthwaite, J. (1994). Synaptic activation of metabotropic glutamate receptors in the parallel fiber-Purkinje cell pathway in rat cerebellar slices. *Neuroscience*, **63**, 911–15.

Baude, A., Nusser, Z., Roberts, J. D. B., Mulvihill, E., McIlhinney, R. A. J., and Somogyi, P. (1993). The metabotropic glutamate receptor (mGluR1α) is concentrated at perisynaptic membrane of neuronal subpopulations as detected by immunogold reaction. *Neuron*, **11**, 771–87.

Baude, A., Molnar, E., Latawiec, D., McIlhinney, R. A. J., and Somogyi, P. (1994). Synaptic and nonsynaptic localization of the GluR1 subunit of the AMPA-type excitatory amino acid receptor in the rat cerebellum. *Journal of Neuroscience*, **14**, 2830–43.

Baude, A., Nusser, Z., Molnar, E., McIlhinney, R. A. J., and Somogyi, P. (1995). High-resolution immunogold localization of AMPA type glutamate receptor subunits at synaptic and non-synaptic sites in rat hippocampus. *Neuroscience*, **69**, 1031–55.

Bechade, C., Colin, I., Kirsch, J., Betz, H., and Triller, A. (1996). Expression of glycine receptor α subunits and gephyrin in cultured spinal neurons. *European Journal of Neuroscience*, **8**, 429–35.

Betz, H. (1991). Glycine receptors: heterogeneous and widespread in the mammalian brain. *Trends in Neurosciences*, **14**, 458–61.

Birnbaumer, L., Campbell, K. P., Catterall, W. A., Harpold, M. M., Hofmann, F., Horne, W. A., *et al.* (1994). The naming of voltage-gated calcium channels. *Neuron*, **13**, 505–6.

Black, J. A., Kocsis, J. D., and Waxman, S. G. (1990). Ion channel organization of the myelinated fiber. *Trends in Neurosciences*, **13**, 48–54.

Blackstone, C. D., Moss, S. J., Martin, L. J., Levey, A. I., Price, D. L., and Huganir, R. L. (1992). Biochemical characterization and localization of a non-N-methyl-D-aspartate glutamate receptor in rat brain. *Journal of Neurochemistry*, **58**, 1118–26.

Bleakman, D. and Lodge, D. (1998). Neuropharmacology of AMPA and kainate receptors. *Neuropharmacology*, **37**, 1187–204.

Bohlhalter, S., Mohler, H., and Fritschy, J.-M. (1994). Inhibitory neurotransmission in rat spinal cord: co-localization of glycine- and GABA_A-receptors at GABAergic synaptic contacts demonstrated by triple immunofluorescence staining. *Brain Research*, **642**, 59–69.

Bonanno, G. and Raiteri, M. (1993). Multiple GABA_B receptors. *Trends in Pharmacological Sciences*, **14**, 259–61.

Boudier, J. L., Le Treut, T., and Jover, E. (1992). Autoradiographic localization of voltage-dependent sodium channels on the mouse neuromuscular junction using ^{125}I-α scorpion toxin. II. Sodium distribution on postsynaptic membranes. *Journal of Neuroscience*, **12**, 454–66.

Bowery, N. G. (1993). GABA_B receptor pharmacology. *Annual Review in Pharmacology and Toxicology*, **33**, 109–47.

Brandstatter, J. H., Koulen, P., Kuhn, R., van der Putten, H., and Wassle, H. (1996). Compartmental localization of a metabotropic glutamate receptor (mGluR7): two different active sites at a retinal synapse. *Journal of Neuroscience*, **16**, 4749–56.

Brickley, S. G., Cull-Candy, S. G., and Farrant, M. (1996). Development of a tonic form of synaptic inhibition in rat cerebellar granule cells resulting from persistent activation of GABA_A receptors. *Journal of Physiology (London)*, **497**, 753–9.

Castillo, P. E., Malenka, R. C., and Nicoll, R. A. (1997). Kainate receptors mediate a slow postsynaptic current in hippocampal CA3 neurons. *Nature*, **388**, 182–6.

Conti, F., Minelli, A., Molnar, M., and Brecha, N. C. (1994). Cellular localization and laminar distribution of NMDAR1 mRNA in the rat cerebral cortex. *Journal of Comparative Neurology*, **343**, 554–65.

Cotman, C. W., Monaghan, D. T., Ottersen, O. P., and Storm-Mathisen, J. (1987). Anatomical organization of excitatory amino acid receptors and their pathways. *Trends in Neurosciences*, **10**, 273–80.

Craig, A. M., Blackstone, C. D., Huganir, R. L., and Banker, G. (1993). The distribution of glutamate receptors in cultured rat hippocampal neurons: postsynaptic clustering of AMPA-selective subunits. *Neuron*, **10**, 1055–68.

Craig, A. M., Blackstone, C. D., Huganir, R. L., and Banker, G. (1994). Selective clustering of glutamate and γ-aminobutyric acid receptors opposite terminals releasing the corresponding neurotransmitters. *Proceedings of the National Academy of Sciences USA*, **91**, 12373–7.

Davis, G. W. and Goodman, C. S. (1998). Synapse-specific control of synaptic efficacy at the terminals of a single neuron. *Nature*, **392**, 82–6.

Day, N. C., Shaw, P. J., McCormack, A. L., Craig, P. J., Smith, W., Beattie, R., *et al.* (1996). Distribution of α_{1A}, α_{1B} and α_{1E} voltage-dependent calcium channel subunits in the human hippocampus and parahippocampal gyrus. *Neuroscience*, **71**, 1013–24.

Devor, M., Govrin-Lippmann, R., and Angelides, K. (1993). Na^+ channel immunolocalization in peripheral mammalian axons and changes following nerve injury and neuroma formation. *Journal of Neuroscience*, **13**, 1976–92.

Dugandzija-Novakovic, S., Koszowski, A. G., Levinson, S. R., and Shrager, P. (1995). Clustering of Na^+ channels and node of Ranvier formation in remyelinating axons. *Journal of Neuroscience*, **15**, 492–503.

Essricht, C., Lorez, M., Benson, J. A., Fritschy, J.-M., and Luscher, B. (1998). Postsynaptic clustering of major $GABA_A$ receptor subtypes requires the γ2 subunit and gephyrin. *Nature Neuroscience*, **1**, 563–71.

Fertuck, H. C. and Salpeter, M. M. (1974). Localization of acetylcholine receptor by ^{125}I-labeled α bungarotoxin binding at mouse motor endplates. *Proceedings of the National Academy of Sciences USA*, **71**, 1376–78.

Flint, A. C., Maisch, U. S., Weishaupt, J. H., Kriegstein, A. R., and Monyer, H. (1997). NR2A subunit expression shortens NMDA receptor synaptic currents in developing neocortex. *Journal of Neuroscience*, **17**, 2469–76.

Frerking, M. and Wilson, M. (1996). Saturation of postsynaptic receptors at central synapses? *Current Opinions in Neurobiology*, **6**, 395–403.

Frerking, M., Malenka, R. C., and Nicoll, R. A. (1998). Synaptic activation of kainate receptors on hippocampal interneurons. *Nature Neuroscience*, **1**, 479–86.

Freund, T. F. and Buzsaki, G. (1996). Interneurons of the hippocampus. *Hippocampus*, **6**, 347–470.

Fritschy, J.-M. and Mohler, H. (1995). $GABA_A$-receptor heterogeneity in the adult rat brain: differential regional and cellular distribution of seven major subunits. *Journal of Comparative Neurology*, **359**, 154–94.

Fritschy, J.-M., Weinmann, O., Wenzel, A., and Benke, D. (1998). Synapse-specific localization of NMDA and $GABA_A$ receptor subunits revealed by antigen-retrieval immunohistochemistry. *Journal of Comparative Neurology*, **390**, 194–210.

Fritschy, J.-M., Meskenaite, V., Weinmann, O., Honer, M., Benke, D., and Mohler, H. (1999). $GABA_B$-receptor splice variants GB1a and GB1b in rat brain: developmental regulation, cellular distribution and extrasynaptic localization. *European Journal of Neuroscience*, **11**, 761–8.

Gao, B. and Fritschy, J. M. (1994). Selective allocation of $GABA_A$ receptors containing the α1 subunit to neurochemically distinct subpopulations of rat hippocampal interneurons. *European Journal of Neuroscience*, **6**, 837–53.

Hansen, G. H., Belhage, B., and Schousboe, A. (1991). Effect of a GABA agonist on the expression and distribution of $GABA_A$ receptors in the plasma membrane of cultured cerebellar granule cells: an immunocytochemical study. *Neuroscience Letters*, **124**, 162–5.

Hayashi, Y., Momiyama, A., Takahashi, T., Ohishi, H., Ogawa-Meguro, R., Shigemoto, R., *et al.* (1993). Role of a metabotropic glutamate receptor in synaptic modulation in the accessory olfactory bulb. *Nature*, **366**, 687–90.

Hell, J. W., Westenbroek, R. E., Warner, C., Ahlijanian, M. K., Prystay, W., Gilbert, M. M., *et al.* (1993). Identification and differential subcellular localization of the neuronal class C and class D L-type calcium channel α1 subunits. *Journal of Cell Biology*, **123**, 949–62.

Hille, B. (1992). *Ionic channels of excitable membranes* (2nd edn). Sinauer, Sunderland, Massachusetts.

Hollmann, M. and Heinemann, S. (1994). Cloned glutamate receptors. *Annual Review of Neuroscience*, **17**, 31–108.

Huntley, G. W., Vickers, J. C., and Morrison, J. H. (1994). Cellular and synaptic localization of NMDA and non-NMDA receptor subunits in neocortex: organizational features related to cortical circuitry, function and disease. *Trends in Neurosciences*, **17**, 536–43.

Jonas, P., Bischofberger, J., and Sandkuhler, J. (1998). Corelease of two fast neurotransmitters at a central synapse. *Science*, **281**, 419–24.

Kaupmann, K., Huggel, K., Heid, J., Flor, P. J., Bischoff, S., Mickel, S. J., *et al.* (1997). Expression cloning of $GABA_B$ receptors uncovers similarity to metabotropic glutamate receptors. *Nature*, **386**, 239–46.

Kaupmann, K., Malitschek, B., Schuler, V., Heid, J., Froestl, W., Beck, P., *et al.* (1998). $GABA_B$ receptor subtypes assemble into functional heteromeric complexes. *Nature*, **396**, 683–7.

Kharazia, V. N. and Weinberg, R. J. (1997). Tangential synaptic distribution of NMDA and AMPA receptors in rat neocortex. *Neuroscience Letters*, **238**, 41–4.

Kharazia, V. N., Phend, K. D., Rustioni, A., and Weinberg, R. J. (1996). EM colocalization of AMPA and NMDA receptor subunits at synapses in rat cerebral cortex. *Neuroscience Letters*, **210**, 37–40.

Kinoshita, A., Ohishi, H., Nomura, S., Shigemoto, R., Nakanishi, S., and Mizuno, N. (1996). Presynaptic localization of a metabotropic glutamate receptor, mGluR4a, in the cerebellar cortex: a light and electron microscope study in the rat. *Neuroscience Letters*, **207**, 199–202.

Kinoshita, A., Shigemoto, R., Ohishi, H., van der Putten, H., and Mizuno, N. (1998). Immunohistochemical localization of metabotropic glutamate receptors, mGluR7a and mGluR7b, in the central nervous system of the adult rat and mouse: a light and electron microscopic study. *Journal of Comparative Neurology*, **393**, 332–52.

Kirsch, J., Wolters, I., Triller, A., and Betz, H. (1993). Gephyrin antisense oligonucleotides prevent glycine receptor clustering in spinal neurons. *Nature*, **366**, 745–8.

Koulen, P., Sassoe-Pognetto, M., Grunert, U., and Wassle, H. (1996). Selective clustering of $GABA_A$ and glycine receptors in the mammalian retina. *Journal of Neuroscience*, **16**, 2127–40.

Koulen, P., Kuhn, R., Wassle, H., and Brandstatter, J. H. (1997). Group I metabotropic glutamate receptors mGluR1α and mGluR5a: localization in both synaptic layers of the rat retina. *Journal of Neuroscience*, **17**, 2200–11.

Koulen, P., Malitschek, B., Kuhn, R., Bettler, B., Wassle, H., and Brandstatter, J. H. (1998). Presynaptic and postsynaptic localization of $GABA_B$ receptors in neurons of the rat retina. *European Journal of Neuroscience*, **10**, 1446–56.

Kuhse, J., Betz, H., and Kirsch, J. (1995). The inhibitory glycine receptor: architecture, synaptic localization and molecular pathology of a postsynaptic ion-channel complex. *Current Opinions in Neurobiology*, **5**, 318–23.

Laube, G., Roper, J., Pitt, J. C., Sewing, S., Kistner, U., Garner, C. C., *et al.* (1996). Ultrastructural localization of Shaker-related potassium channel subunits and synapse-associated protein 90 to septate-like junctions in rat cerebellar Pinceaux. *Molecular Brain Research*, **42**, 51–61.

Lerma, J., Morales, M., Vicente, M. A., and Herreras, O. (1997). Glutamate receptors of the kainate type and synaptic transmission. *Trends in Neurosciences*, **20**, 9–12.

Lujan, R., Nusser, Z., Roberts, J. D. B., Shigemoto, R., and Somogyi, P. (1996). Perisynaptic location of metabotropic glutamate receptors mGluR1 and mGluR5 on dendrites and dendritic spines in the rat hippocampus. *European Journal of Neuroscience*, **8**, 1488–500.

Lujan, R., Roberts, J. D. B., Shigemoto, R., Ohishi, H., and Somogyi, P. (1997). Differential plasma membrane distribution of metabotropic glutamate receptors mGluR1α, mGluR2 and mGluR5, relative to neurotransmitter release sites. *Journal of Chemical Neuroanatomy*, **13**, 219–41.

Macdonald, R. L. and Olsen, R. W. (1994). GABA$_A$ receptor channels. *Annual Review of Neuroscience*, **17**, 569–602.

Malosio, M.-L., Marqueze-Pouey, B., Kuhse, J., and Betz, H. (1991). Widespread expression of glycine receptor subunit mRNAs in the adult and developing rat brain. *EMBO Journal*, **10**, 2401–9.

Markram, H., Wang, Y., and Tsodyks, M. (1998). Differential signaling via the same axon of neocortical pyramidal neurons. *Proceedings of the National Academy of Sciences USA*, **95**, 5323–8.

Martin, L. J., Blackstone, C. D., Huganir, R. L., and Price, D. L. (1992). Cellular localization of a metabotropic glutamate receptor in rat brain. *Neuron*, **9**, 259–70.

Masu, M., Iwakabe, H., Tagawa, Y., Miyoshi, T., Yamashita, M., Fukuda, Y., *et al.* (1995). Specific deficit of the ON response in visual transmission by targeted disruption of the mGluR6 gene. *Cell*, **80**, 757–65.

Matsubara, A., Laake, J. H., Davanger, S., Usami, S., and Ottersen, O. P. (1996). Organization of AMPA receptor subunits at a glutamate synapse: a quantitative immunogold analysis of hair cell synapses in the rat organ of Corti. *Journal of Neuroscience*, **16**, 4457–67.

McNamara, N. M. C., Muniz, Z. M., Wilkin, G. P., and Dolly, J. O. (1993). Prominent location of a K$^+$ channel containing the a subunit Kv1.2 in the basket cell nerve terminals of rat cerebellum. *Neuroscience*, **57**, 1039–45.

Misgeld, U., Bijak, M., and Jarolimek, W. (1995). A physiological role for GABA$_B$ receptors and the effects of baclofen in the mammalian central nervous system. *Progress in Neurobiology*, **46**, 423–62.

Mody, I., De Koninck, Y., Otis, T. S., and Soltesz, I. (1994). Bridging the cleft at GABA synapses in the brain. *Trends in Neurosciences*, **17**, 517–25.

Molnar, E., Baude, A., Richmond, S. A., Patel, P. B., Somogyi, P., and McIlhinney, R. A. J. (1993). Biochemical and immunocytochemical characterization of antipeptide antibodies to a cloned GluR1 glutamate receptor subunit: cellular and subcellular distribution in the rat forebrain. *Neuroscience*, **53**, 307–26.

Monyer, H., Burnashev, N., Laurie, D. J., Sakmann, B., and Seeburg, P. H. (1994). Developmental and regional expression in the rat brain and functional properties of four NMDA receptors. *Neuron*, **12**, 529–40.

Moss, S. J. and Smart, T. G. (1996). Modulation of amino acid-gated ion channels by protein phosphorylation. *International Review in Neurobiology*, **39**, 1–52.

Nakanishi, S. (1994). Metabotropic glutamate receptors: synaptic transmission, modulation, and plasticity. *Neuron*, **13**, 1031–7.

Negyessy, L., Vidnyanszky, Z., Kuhn, R., Knopfel, T., Gorcs, T. J., and Hamori, J. (1997). Light and electron microscopic demonstration of mGluR5 metabotropic glutamate receptor immunoreactive neuronal elements in the rat cerebellar cortex. *Journal of Comparative Neurology*, **385**, 641–50.

Nicoll, R. A. and Malenka, R. C. (1995). Contrasting properties of two forms of long-term potentiation in the hippocampus. *Nature*, **377**, 115–18.

Nusser, Z. and Somogyi, P. (1997). Compartmentalized distribution of GABA$_A$ and glutamate receptors in relation to transmitter release sites on the surface of cerebellar neurones. In *The cerebellum: from structure to control. Progress in brain research, No. 114*, (ed. C. I. de Zeeuw, P. Strata, and J. Voogd), pp. 109–27, Elsevier, Amsterdam.

Nusser, Z., Mulvihill, E., Streit, P., and Somogyi, P. (1994). Subsynaptic segregation of metabotropic and ionotropic glutamate receptors as revealed by immunogold localization. *Neuroscience*, **61**, 421–7.

Nusser, Z., Roberts, J. D. B., Baude, A., Richards, J. G., and Somogyi, P. (1995). Relative densities of synaptic and extrasynaptic GABA$_A$ receptors on cerebellar granule cells as determined by a quantitative immunogold method. *Journal of Neuroscience*, **15**, 2948–60.

Nusser, Z., Sieghart, W., Stephenson, F. A., and Somogyi, P. (1996*a*). The α6 subunit of the GABA$_A$ receptor is concentrated in both inhibitory and excitatory synapses on cerebellar granule cells. *Journal of Neuroscience*, **16**, 103–14.

Nusser, Z., Sieghart, W., Benke, D., Fritschy, J.-M., and Somogyi, P. (1996*b*). Differential synaptic localization of two major γ-aminobutyric acid type A receptor α subunits on hippocampal pyramidal cells. *Proceedings of the National Academy of Sciences USA*, **93**, 11939–44.

Nusser, Z., Cull-Candy, S. G., and Farrant, M. (1997). Differences in synaptic GABA$_A$ receptor number underlie variation in GABA mini amplitude. *Neuron*, **19**, 697–709.

Nusser, Z., Lujan, R., Laube, G., Roberts, J. D. B., Molnar, E., and Somogyi, P. (1998*a*). Cell type and pathway dependence of synaptic AMPA receptor number and variability in the hippocampus. *Neuron*, **21**, 545–59.

Nusser, Z., Sieghart, W., and Somogyi, P. (1998*b*). Segregation of different GABA$_A$ receptors to synaptic and extrasynaptic membranes of cerebellar granule cells. *Journal of Neuroscience*, **18**, 1693–703.

Nusser, Z., Hajos, N., Somogyi, P., and Mody, I. (1998*c*). Increased number of synaptic GABA$_A$ receptors underlies potentiation at hippocampal inhibitory synapses. *Nature*, **395**, 172–7.

Ohishi, H., Ogawa-Meguro, R., Shigemoto, R., Kaneko, T., Nakanishi, S., and Mizuno, N. (1994). Immunohistochemical localization of metabotropic glutamate receptors, mGluR2 and mGluR3, in rat cerebellar cortex. *Neuron*, **13**, 55–66.

Ohishi, H., Akazawa, C., Shigemoto, R., Nakanishi, S., and Mizuno, N. (1995). Distribution of the mRNAs for l-2-amino-4-phosphonobutyrate-sensitive metabotropic glutamate receptors, mGluR4 and mGluR7, in the rat brain. *Journal of Comparative Neurology*, **360**, 555–70.

Otis, T. S., De Korninck, Y., and Mody, I. (1994). Lasting potentiation of inhibition is associated with an increased number of γ-aminobutyric acid type A receptors activated during miniature inhibitory postsynaptic currents. *Proceedings of the National Academy of Sciences USA*, **91**, 7698–702.

Ottersen, O. P. and Landsend, A. S. (1997). Organization of glutamate receptors at the synapse. *European Journal of Neuroscience*, **9**, 2219–24.

Patneau, D. K. and Mayer, M. L. (1990). Structure–activity relationships for amino acid transmitter candidates acting at *N*-methyl-D-Aspartate and quisqualate receptors. *Journal of Neuroscience*, **10**, 2385–99.

Persohn, E., Malherbe, P., and Richards, J. G. (1992). Comparative molecular neuroanatomy of cloned GABA$_A$ receptor subunits in the rat CNS. *Journal of Comparative Neurology*, **326**, 193–216.

Petralia, R. S. and Wenthold, R. J. (1992). Light and electron immunocytochemical localization of AMPA-selective glutamate receptors in the rat brain. *Journal of Comparative Neurology*, **318**, 329–54.

Petralia, R. S., Wang, Y. X., and Wenthold, R. J. (1994*a*). Histological and ultra-structural localization of the kainate receptor subunits, KA2 and GluR6/7, in the rat nervous system using selective antipeptide antibodies. *Journal of Comparative Neurology*, **349**, 85–110.

Petralia, R. S., Wang, Y. X., and Wenthold, R. J. (1994*b*). The NMDA receptor subunits NR2A and NR2B show histological and ultrastructural localization patterns similar to those of NR1. *Journal of Neuroscience*, **14**, 6102–20.

Petralia, R. S., Wang, Y. X., Niedzielski, A. S., and Wenthold, R. J. (1996). The metabotropic glutamate receptors, mGluR2 and mGluR3, show unique postsynaptic, presynaptic and glial localizations. *Neuroscience*, **71**, 949–76.

Phend, K. D., Rustioni, A., and Weinberg, R. J. (1995). An osmium-free method of Epon embedment that preserves both ultrastructure and antigenicity for post-embedding immunocytochemistry. *Journal of Histochemistry and Cytochemistry*, **43**, 283–92.

Pin, J. P. and Duvoisin, R. (1995). The metabotropic glutamate receptors: structure and functions. *Neuropharmacology*, **34**, 1–26.

Pongs, O. (1992). Molecular biology of voltage-dependent potassium channels. *Physiological Reviews*, **72**, S69–S88.

Probst, A., Cortes, R., and Palacios, J. M. (1986). The distribution of glycine receptors in the human brain. A light microscopic autoradiographic study using [^{3}H]strychnine. *Neuroscience*, **17**, 11–35.

Richards, J. G., Schoch, P., Haring, P., Takacs, B., and Mohler, H. (1987). Resolving GABA$_A$/benzodiazepine receptors: cellular and subcellular localization in the CNS with monoclonal antibodies. *Journal of Neuroscience*, **7**, 1866–86.

Richmond, S. A., Irving, A. J., Molnar, E., McIlhinney, R. A., Michelangeli, F., Henley, J. M., *et al.* (1996). Localization of the glutamate receptor subunit GluR1 on the surface of living and within cultured hippocampal neurons. *Neuroscience*, **75**, 69–82.

Rossi, D. J. and Hamann, M. (1998). Spillover-mediated transmission at inhibitory synapses promoted by high affinity α6 subunit GABA$_A$ receptors and glomerular geometry. *Neuron*, **20**, 783–95.

Rubio, M. E. and Wenthold, R. J. (1997). Glutamate receptors are selectively targeted to postsynaptic sites in neurons. *Neuron*, **18**, 939–50.

Sassoe-Pognetto, M., Kirsch, J., Grunert, U., Greferath, U., Fritschy, J.-M., Mohler, H., *et al.* (1995). Colocalization of gephyrin and GABA$_A$-receptor subunits in the rat retina. *Journal of Comparative Neurology*, **356**, 1–14.

Seeburg, P. H. (1993). The molecular biology of mammalian glutamate receptor channels. *Trends in Neurosciences*, **16**, 359–65.

Seeburg, P. H. (1996). The role of RNA editing in controlling glutamate receptor channel properties. *Journal of Neurochemistry*, **66**, 1–5.

Sheng, M., Tsaur, M. L., Jan, Y. N., and Jan, L. Y. (1994). Contrasting subcellular localization of the Kv1.2 K$^+$ channel subunit in different neurons of rat brain. *Journal of Neuroscience*, **14**, 2408–17.

Shigemoto, R., Nomura, S., Ohishi, H., Sugihara, H., Nakanishi, S., and Mizuno, N. (1993). Immunohistochemical localization of a metabotropic glutamate receptor, mGluR5, in the rat brain. *Neuroscience Letters*, **163**, 53–7.

Shigemoto, R., Kulik, A., Roberts, J. D. B., Ohishi, H., Nusser, Z., Kaneko, T., *et al.* (1996). Target-cell-specific concentration of a metabotropic glutamate receptor in the presynaptic active zone. *Nature*, **381**, 523–5.

Shigemoto, R., Kinoshita, A., Wada, E., Nomura, S., Ohishi, H., Takada, M., *et al.* (1997). Differential presynaptic localization of metabotropic glutamate receptor subtypes in the rat hippocampus. *Journal of Neuroscience*, **17**, 7503–22.

Siegel, S. J., Brose, N., Janssen, W. G., Gasic, G. P., Jahn, R., Heinemann, S. F., *et al.* (1994). Regional, cellular, and ultrastructural distribution of N-methyl-D-aspartate receptor subunit 1 in monkey hippocampus. *Proceedings of the National Academy of Sciences USA*, **91**, 564–8.

Sieghart, W. (1995). Structure and pharmacology of γ-aminobutyric acid$_A$ receptor subtypes. *Pharmacological Reviews*, **47**, 181–234.

Snutch, T. P. and Reiner, P. B. (1992). Ca^{2+} channels: diversity of form and function. *Current Opinions in Neurobiology*, **2**, 247–53.

Somogyi, P., Takagi, H., Richards, J. G., and Mohler, H. (1989). Subcellular localization of benzodiazepine/GABA$_A$ receptors in the cerebellum of rat, cat, and monkey using monoclonal antibodies. *Journal of Neuroscience*, **9**, 2197–209.

Somogyi, P., Eshhar, N., Teichberg, V. I., and Roberts, J. D. B. (1990). Subcellular localization of a putative kainate receptor in bergmann glial cells using a monoclonal antibody in the chick and fish cerebellar cortex. *Neuroscience*, **35**, 9–30.

Somogyi, P., Fritschy, J.-M., Benke, D., Roberts, J. D. B., and Sieghart, W. (1996). The γ2 subunit of the GABA$_A$ receptor is concentrated in synaptic junctions containing the α1 and β2/3 subunits in hippocampus, cerebellum and globus pallidus. *Neuropharmacology*, **35**, 1425–44.

Somogyi, P., Nusser, Z., Roberts, J. D. B., and Lujan, R. (1998). Precision and variability in the placement of pre- and postsynaptic receptors in relation to neurotransmitter release sites. In *Central synapses: quantal mechanisms and plasticity*, Human Frontier Science Program Workshop No. 4, (ed. D. S. Faber, H. Korn, S. J. Redman, S. M. Thompson, and J. S. Altman), pp. 82–93. HFSP, Strasbourg.

Stephenson, F. A. (1995). The $GABA_A$ receptors. *Biochemical Journal*, **310**, 1–9.

Tempia, F., Miniaci, M. C., Anchisi, D., and Strata, P. (1998). Postsynaptic current mediated by metabotropic glutamate receptors in cerebellar Purkinje cells. *Journal of Neurophysiology*, **80**, 520–8.

Thompson, S. M. (1994). Modulation of inhibitory synaptic transmission in the hippocampus. *Progress in Neurobiology*, **42**, 575–609.

Todd, A. J., Watt, C., Spike, R. C., and Sieghart, W. (1996). Colocalization of GABA, glycine, and their receptors at synapses in the rat spinal cord. *Journal of Neuroscience*, **16**, 974–82.

Triller, A., Cluzeaud, F., Pfeiffer, F., Betz, H., and Korn, H. (1985). Distribution of glycine receptors at central synapses: an immunoelectron microscopy study. *Journal of Cell Biology*, **101**, 683–8.

Triller, A., Seitanidou, T., Franksson, O., and Korn, H. (1991). Use of confocal microscope for the cellular analysis of the glycine synaptic receptor. *Journal of Receptor Research*, **11**, 347–57.

Turner, J. D., Bodewitz, G., Thompson, C. L., and Stephenson, F. A. (1993). Immunohistochemical mapping of γ-aminobutyric acid type-A receptor α subunits in rat central nervous system. In *Anxiolytic β-carbolines: from molecular biology to the clinic.* (ed. D. N. Stephens), pp. 29–49. Springer, Berlin.

Turrigiano, G. G., Leslie, K. R., Desai, N. S., Rutherford, L. C., and Nelson, S. B. (1998). Activity-dependent scaling of quantal amplitude in neocortical neurons. *Nature*, **391**, 892–6.

van den Pol, A. N. and Gorcs, T. (1988). Glycine and glycine receptor immunoreactivity in brain and spinal cord. *Journal of Neuroscience*, **8**, 472–92.

van den Pol, A. N., Romano, C., and Ghosh, P. (1995). Metabotropic glutamate receptor mGluR5 subcellular distribution and developmental expression in hypothalamus. *Journal of Comparative Neurology*, **362**, 134–50.

Veh, R. W., Lichtinghagen, R., Sewing, S., Wunder, F., Grumbach, I. M., and Pongs, O. (1995). Immunohistochemical localization of five members of the Kv1 channel subunits: contrasting subcellular locations and neuron-specific co- localizations in rat brain. *European Journal of Neuroscience*, **7**, 2189–205.

Vidnyanszky, Z., Hamori, J., Negyessy, L., Ruegg, D., Knopfel, T., Kuhn, R., *et al.* (1994). Cellular and subcellular localization of the mGluR5a metabotropic glutamate receptor in rat spinal cord. *Neuroreport*, **6**, 209–13.

Vignes, M. and Collingridge, G. L. (1997). The synaptic activation of kainate receptors. *Nature*, **388**, 179–82.

Wada, E., Shigemoto, R., Kinoshita, A., Ohishi, H., and Mizuno, N. (1998). Metabotropic glutamate receptor subtypes in axon terminals of projection fibers from the main and accessory olfactory bulbs: a light and electron microscopic immunohistochemical study in the rat. *Journal of Comparative Neurology*, **393**, 493–504.

Wamsley, J. K. and Palacios, J. M. (1984). Amino acid and benzodiazepine receptors, In *Handbook of chemical neuroanatomy*, No. 3, (ed. A. Bjorklund, T. Hokfelt, and M. J. Kuhr), pp. 352–385. Elsevier, Amsterdam.

Wang, H., Kunkel, D. D., Schwartzkroin, P. A., and Tempel, B. L. (1994). Localization of Kv1.1 and Kv1.2, two K^+ channel proteins, to synaptic terminals, somata, and dendrites in the mouse brain. *Journal of Neuroscience*, **14**, 4588–99.

Watanabe, M., Inoue, Y., Sakimura, K., and Mishina, M. (1993). Distinct distributions of five *N*-methyl-D-aspartate receptor channel subunit mRNAs in the forebrain. *Journal of Comparative Neurology*, **338**, 377–90.

Watanabe, M., Fukaya, M., Sakimura, K., Manabe, T., Mishina, M., and Inoue, Y. (1998). Selective scarcity of NMDA receptor channel subunits in the stratum lucidum (mossy fiber-recipient layer) of the mouse hippocampal CA3 subfield. *European Journal of Neuroscience*, **10**, 478–87.

Wenzel, A., Benke, D., Mohler, H., and Fritschy, J. M. (1997). *N*-Methyl-D-aspartate receptors containing the NR2D subunit in the retina are selectively expressed in rod bipolar cells. *Neuroscience*, **78**, 1105–12.

Westenbroek, R. E., Hell, J. W., Warner, C., Dubel, S. J., Snutch, T. P., and Catterall, W. A. (1992). Biochemical properties and subcellular distribution of an N-type calcium channel α_1 subunit. *Neuron*, **9**, 1099–115.

Westenbroek, R. E., Sakurai, T., Elliott, E. M., Hell, J. W., Starr, T. V., Snutch, T. P., *et al.* (1995). Immunochemical identification and subcellular distribution of the α_{1A} subunits of brain calcium channels. *Journal of Neuroscience*, **15**, 6403–18.

Wisden, W., Laurie, D. J., Monyer, H., and Seeburg, P. H. (1992). The distribution of 13 $GABA_A$ receptor subunit mRNAs in the rat brain. I. Telencephalon, diencephalon, mesencephalon. *Journal of Neuroscience*, **12**, 1040–62.

Wollner, D. A. and Catterall, W. A. (1986). Localization of sodium channels in axon hillocks and initial segments of retinal ganglion cells. *Proceedings of the National Academy of Sciences USA*, **83**, 8424–8.

Zamanillo, D., Sprengel, R., Hvalby, O., Jensen, V., Burnashev, N., Rozov, A., *et al.* (1999). Importance of AMPA receptors for hippocampal synaptic plasticity but not for spatial learning. *Science*, **284**, 1805–11.

5

Neurotransmitter-gated ion channels in dendrites

R. Angus Silver and Mark Farrant
University College London

Summary

Both fast excitatory and inhibitory synaptic transmission in the CNS involve the activation of ionotropic receptors. These receptors are found throughout the neuronal membrane but are concentrated at synaptic junctions, the majority of which are located on dendrites remote from the soma. An understanding of synaptic transmission requires detailed knowledge of the properties of transmitter-gated channels and their behavior at the synapse. Obtaining such knowledge is difficult due to the inaccessibility of the synapse and the remoteness of most synapses from the typical recording site at the soma. In this chapter, we will discuss what has been learned from various new approaches for investigating the functional properties of synapses. We focus on synapses using glutamate or γ-aminobutyric acid (GABA) as a transmitter, as these represent the vast majority of CNS synapses. The picture emerging from these studies is that synapses display remarkable diversity in their properties, perhaps reflecting different functional roles played by individual synapses at different dendritic locations.

Introduction

For anyone interested in the processing of information within the CNS, the functional behavior of synapses and their underlying ion channels represent key targets for investigation. The majority of synaptic inputs onto a neuron are located on dendrites. While dendrites clearly provide the necessary basis for many of the complex integrative properties of neurons, they represent a challenge to experimentalists, as most synaptic receptors are both physically and electrically distant from the soma. This inaccessibility makes direct recording from the synaptic membrane virtually impossible, while cable filtering and the activation or inactivation of voltage-gated channels in dendrites can distort the synaptic signal recorded at the soma (Rall and Segev 1985; Major 1993; Spruston *et al.* 1993; Häusser and Roth 1997a; see Chapters 6, 9, and 10). Even under conditions where voltage clamp is near perfect (Silver *et al.* 1992, 1996*b*,*c*; Clark *et al.* 1997; Brickley *et al.* 1999) extracting quantitative information about the postsynaptic channels from synaptic currents is not without its difficulties (Traynelis *et al.* 1993; DeKoninck and Mody 1994; Silver *et al.* 1996*b*).

Many studies have attempted to circumvent these problems by assuming that somatic receptors, which are largely extrasynaptic but more readily accessible to the patch-clamp technique, are representative of those at the synapse (e.g. Lester *et al.* 1990; Colquhoun *et al.* 1992; Hestrin 1992; Raman and Trussell 1992; Jonas *et al.* 1993; Trussell *et al.* 1993; Jones and Westbrook 1995; Silver *et al.* 1996*a*). However, there is now a growing body of evidence that, for some types of receptor on some cells, this assumption may not be valid. Quantitative immunoreceptor labeling (see Chapter 4) as well as electrophysiological studies (Stocca and Vicini 1998; Tóth and McBain 1998; Brickley *et al.* 1999) have demonstrated that receptors with different subunit compositions can be targeted to different locations on the cell surface. In addition to the possible heterogeneous subunit composition of receptors at different sites, the local synaptic environment may also influence both the microscopic and macroscopic behavior of ion channels at the synapse. For example, the phosphorylation state of receptors or their association with cytoskeletal elements can affect their kinetics (Greengard *et al.* 1991; Moss *et al.* 1992; Rosenmund and Westbrook 1993; Paoletti *et al.* 1994; Jones and Westbrook 1997; Traynelis and Wahl 1997; Lieberman and Mody 1999) and possibly their single-channel conductance (Clark *et al.* 1997; Benke *et al.* 1998). Furthermore, the number of postsynaptic channels (Silver *et al.* 1996*b*; Nusser *et al.* 1997), the geometry of the synaptic cleft (Barbour and Häusser 1997; Kruk *et al.* 1997), and the spatial distribution of transmitter binding proteins (Diamond and Jahr 1997) can shape the waveform of transmitter in the cleft and set the occupancy of the postsynaptic receptors. Additional complications can ensue if transmitter spills over from neighbouring synapses (Barbour and Häusser 1997; Kullmann and Asztely 1998), since the shape of the transmitter profile and receptor occupancy will then depend on the distance between synapses and the mean release probability (Silver *et al.* 1996*b*)

Understanding the many variables that can influence receptors, and hence synaptic behavior, is important if we wish to fully understand the process of transmission in the CNS. Unfortunately, the tools available for characterizing the functional properties of synaptic receptors are limited in resolution and are rather indirect. In this chapter we review these methods and their limitations. We also discuss what they reveal about functional differences between synaptic and extra-synaptic receptors. The chapter focuses on ionotropic receptors activated by the transmitters glutamate and γ-aminobutyric acid (GABA). For information about metabotropic receptors, such as $GABA_B$ and metabotropic glutamate receptors, we recommend several recent reviews (Kerr and Ong 1995; Conn and Pin 1997; Bettler *et al.* 1998).

Pharmacological identification of synaptic receptors

A variety of receptor/channel properties can be determined by relatively simple pharmacological techniques. At a very basic level, drugs may be used to identify the broad classes of receptor involved in transmission. At glutamatergic synapses, for example, the presence of N-methyl-D-aspartate (NMDA), α-amino-3-hydroxy-5-methyl-4-isoazolepropionic acid (AMPA) or kainate receptors can be determined through the use of specific antagonists or combinations of antagonists, notably D-2-amino-5-phosphonopentanoic acid (AP5), 2,3-benzodiazepine compounds (e.g. GYKI 53655) and 6-cyano-7-nitroquinoxaline-2,3-dione (CNQX). These pharmacological tools isolate different families of receptors produced by genes encoding several different subunits. For example, NMDA receptors are composed of subunits NR1, NR2A-D, and NR3A, AMPA receptors of subunits GluR1–4, and kainate receptors of subunits GluR5–7, KA1 and KA2. Further diversity occurs as a result of alternative splicing and nuclear RNA editing. Although there is some difference in the regional expression of subunits, *in situ* hybridization and PCR studies have shown that many of the mRNAs coding different glutamate receptor subunits are distributed widely throughout the CNS. This heterogeneity at the molecular level results in heterogeneity in behavior of the functional receptors. Receptors composed of different combinations of subunits (within their particular gene family) can display different kinetics, channel conductance and calcium permeability (e.g. Mosbacher *et al.* 1994; Geiger *et al.* 1995; Swanson *et al.* 1997; Fisher and MacDonald 1998; Wyllie *et al.* 1998). Given this potential for heterogeneity in channel function, understanding the precise molecular composition of postsynaptic receptors can be important for predicting the details of transmission at a particular synapse.

The presence of specific subunits at identified synapses can be shown immunohistochemically (see Chapter 4) or, in some cases, deduced pharmacologically. Both approaches, however, are restricted by the availability of appropriate tools (subunit-specific antibodies or specific antagonists) and, in the absence of other data, neither can be used to establish how the identified subunits are assembled to produce receptors of a specific type. Nevertheless, valuable information has come from the use of selective antagonists or modulators. For example, ifenprodil, haloperidol and CP101,606 preferentially block NMDA receptors containing the NR2B subunit (Williams 1993; Ilyin *et al.* 1996; Stocca and Vicini 1998) while N, N, N', N'-tetrakis-(2-pyridylmethyl) ethylenediamine (TPEN), a zinc ion chelator, modulates receptors containing the zinc-sensitive NR2A subunit (Paoletti *et al.* 1997). Similarly, AMPA receptors lacking the edited form of the GluR2 subunit can be identified by their sensitivity to polyamine spider toxins (Tóth and McBain 1998) or internal polyamines such as spermine (Bowie and Mayer 1995; Kamboj *et al.* 1995; Koh *et al.* 1995), while the level of expression of the flip *versus* flop isoforms can be indicated by their sensitivity to the modulator cyclothiazide (Partin *et al.* 1993; Fleck *et al.* 1996)

Pharmacological approaches have also proved valuable for investigating inhibitory synaptic transmission in the CNS. Again, a distinction between the broad classes of inhibitory ionotropic receptors can be made with specific antagonists (such as strychnine for glycine receptors and bicuculline for $GABA_A$ receptors; Farrant and Webster 1988; Becker 1992; see also Jonas *et al.* 1998). As with glutamate receptors, drugs that modulate $GABA_A$ receptors (for review see Barnard *et al.* 1998) can, in theory, be used to identify the presence of specific subunits. Unfortunately, few of the many agents available allow an unequivocal identification. One reasonably clear example, however, is the selective inhibition by furosemide of benzodiazepine-insensitive $GABA_A$ receptors containing α_6 subunits (Korpi *et al.* 1995; Thompson *et al.* 1999).

Biophysical properties of synaptic channels

Understanding the class (or classes) of receptor(s) involved in transmission is a necessary preliminary to establishing a quantitative understanding of the key bio-physical parameters shaping transmission at a particular synapse. These parameters include the kinetics and conductance of the postsynaptic channels present at each contact, the total number of receptors exposed to neurotransmitter, the fraction of receptors that bind transmitter and the mean number of channels open at the peak of the PSC (postsynaptic current). These variables determine both the quantal size and the amount of charge injected into the postsynaptic cell, and therefore govern the effectiveness of information transfer from one neuron to the next. In the next few sections we discuss the difficulties inherent in determining such parameters and the various techniques that have been devised to overcome them.

The time-course of the synaptic conductance

Analysis of synaptic channel properties obviously depends on an ability to obtain an accurate recording of the electrical events occurring at the synapse. Unfortunately, for the majority of central glutamatergic synapses, even such a basic parameter as the time course of the AMPA receptor-mediated conductance change is not known with any accuracy. This is due to difficulties in achieving adequate space-clamp in most neurons (Fig. 5.1). Somatic recordings from neurons with extensive dendritic trees often give EPSC decay times in the 5–20 ms range, while studies on cells with compact electrotonic structures or with synapses close to the soma reveal current decay time constants of ~ 0.3–3 ms, depending on subunit composition of the receptors and the recording temperature (Finkel and Redman 1983; Silver *et al.* 1992, 1996*b*; Forsythe and Barnes-Davies 1993; Geiger *et al.* 1997). Various strategies can be used to optimize the voltage clamp in cells which are not electrically compact and voltage errors arising from the electrode series resistance can be corrected for (Silver *et al.* 1998; Traynelis 1998). However, these approaches do not compensate for errors that arise from dendritic cable filtering (Fig. 5.1). If the cell morphology and the location of active synapses is known, these errors can be estimated using compartmental models (Johnston and Brown 1983; Jonas *et al.* 1993; Major 1993; Spruston *et al.* 1993), with the reliability of the final result being dependent on the accuracy of the model used.

A more direct method for estimating the time course of the synaptic conductance from somatic voltage-clamp recordings is based on measuring charge recovery of the synaptic current from voltage clamp steps taken at different times during the synaptic conductance (Häusser and Roth 1997*a*). This method is, in principle, virtually independent of the series resistance of the recording electrode and the electrical remoteness of the synapse, although in practice it works best for synaptic conductances of intermediate electronic distance and size due to signal-to-noise considerations. In neocortical pyramidal cells the method revealed a fast AMPA-

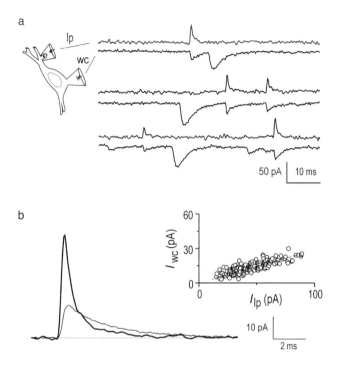

Fig. 5.1   Distortion of synaptic currents by dendritic filtering. Simultaneous synaptic and somatic recordings from a hippocampal pyramidal cell in culture. (a) Schematic diagram of the recording configuration. The upper trace shows currents from a synaptic loose-patch recording (lp) while the lower trace shows the somatic whole-cell (wc) recording from the same cell. mEPSCs originating at the synapse enclosed in the loose-patch pipette appear synchronously in both traces. (b) Comparison of the average synaptic current from 130 paired mEPSCs recorded at the synaptic site (thick trace) and at the soma (thin trace). Note the much smaller amplitude and slower time course of mEPSCs recorded at the soma due to dendritic filtering. Inset: correlation between amplitudes of single-synapse minis measured at the synaptic site (I_{lp}) and at the soma (I_{wc}) within the same experiment. Modified, with permission, from Forti *et al.* (1997).

mediated synaptic conductance with a decay time constant of 1.7 ms, less than half that of somatically recorded EPSCs (3.8 ms; Häusser and Roth 1997*a*). If the reversal potential of the synaptic current is known, measuring the actual reversal potential of the somatic EPSC using voltage jumps also allows an estimation of the attenuation of synaptic charge along the dendrite (Häusser and Roth 1997*a*).

Two other more technically demanding approaches are worth mentioning. The first of these involves whole-cell recording from a dendrite close to the synaptic connection (Häusser 1994; Benke *et al.* 1998). Unlike the charge recovery approach, which involves making an average of many responses, direct dendritic recording can measure PSC variability, which can be used for estimating channel conductance (Benke *et al.* 1998) or quantal parameters. While minimizing space-clamp problems, this method does not overcome the electrode series resistance, which can limit the quality of the voltage clamp. A second approach involves loose-patch recording from individual boutons on the dendrite (Forti *et al.* 1997; Fig. 5.1). This yields data from a single synapse and is, therefore, very powerful. Unfortunately, the technical difficulty of this method limits its application to cell culture preparations.

These methods show that the synaptic conductance change is consistently faster than the PSC recorded at the soma of most central neurons. This is in agreement with modeling studies, which also predict a substantial peak attenuation of somatically recorded EPSCs arising from dendritic synapses (Rall and Segev 1985; Major 1993; Spruston *et al.* 1993; Häusser and Roth 1997*a*). The distortion of the synaptic signal by the electrode-cell circuit must therefore be taken into account when estimating functional synaptic properties from dendritic synapses.

Recordings from dendritic patches

High-resolution recordings of ion-channel behavior can be achieved with the outside-out configuration of the patch-clamp technique. Furthermore, channels in outside-out patches can be activated in a way that mimics the synaptic current using rapid perfusion of transmitter (Fig. 5.2). This approach is potentially very powerful and has been widely used to investigate synaptic mechanisms by comparing the kinetics of receptor deactivation and desensitisation with the time course of the synaptic current (e.g. Lester *et al.* 1990; Colquhoun *et al.* 1992; Hestrin 1992; Jonas *et al.* 1992; Trussell *et al.* 1993; Jones and Westbrook 1995; Silver *et al.* 1996*a*). However, the majority of studies that have used this approach have been carried out using patches excised from the soma. These studies therefore rely on the assumption that the extrasynaptic channels in the patches behave identically to those at the synapse. As discussed elsewhere, there is now direct evidence that this may not always be the case. Two studies have attempted to circumvent this assumption by studying patches excised from the dendrites of central neurons, in the hope that these patches are enriched in synaptic receptors (Fig. 5.2; Spruston *et al.* 1995; Häusser and Roth 1997*b*). In these studies the functional properties of dendritic glutamate receptors were found to be remarkably similar to those in the soma. Unfortunately, from this result it is not possible to conclude that *synaptic* and *extrasynaptic* channels are similar: it remains unclear whether patches excised from the dendrite contain synaptic channels or, as with somatic patches, they simply contain extrasynaptic channels. It is clear, however, that for $GABA_A$ receptors, currents activated in somatic patches consistently show slower deactivation kinetics than synaptic currents (Tia *et al.* 1995; Galarreta and Hestrin 1997; Mellor and Randall 1997; Perrais and Ropert 1999). This may reflect heterogeneity in subunit composition of receptors, changes in their phosphorylation state or interaction with the cytoskeleton (e.g. Jones and Westbrook 1997).

Synaptic channel conductance: direct resolution

To determine the number of channels activated during transmission one requires both an accurate estimate of the synaptic conductance change and knowledge of the single-channel conductance of the channels underlying the PSC. For such

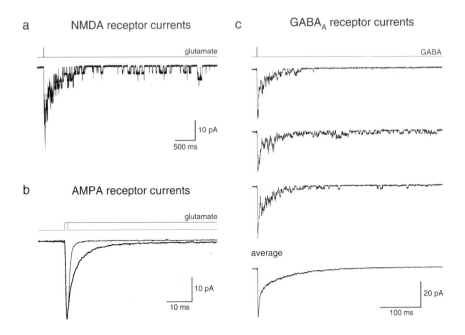

Fig. 5.2   Activation of dendritic transmitter-gated channels in outside-out patches with fast agonist application. (a) Response of an outside-out patch taken from a CA1 pyramidal cell dendrite to a 1ms pulse of 1 mM glutamate in external solution designed to isolate NMDA receptor channels (containing 10 μM glycine, 10 μM CNQX, and no added Mg^{2+}). The holding potential was –80 mV, and the resulting single NMDA receptor channel openings have a mean conductance of 43 pS. Here and in the other panels, the period of transmitter application is represented by the rectangular pulse above the trace. (Modified, with permission, from Sprustion *et al.* 1995). (b) Averaged responses of an outside-out patch taken from a cerebellar Purkinje cell dendrite to brief (1 ms; thin trace) and long (100 ms; thick trace) applications of 1 mM glutamate, which generate an AMPA receptor-mediated current. The deactivation time constant of the current (measured from the response to the 1 ms pulse) was 1.0 ms, and the desensitization time constant (measured from the response to the 100 ms pulse) was 4.5 ms. (Modified, with permission, from Häusser and Roth 1997*b*). (c) Responses of an outside-out patch from a Purkinje cell dendrite to 1 ms applications of 1 mM GABA (holding potential –80 mV). Three individual sweeps are shown, revealing single $GABA_A$ receptor channel openings in the tail of the current. The mean single-channel conductance was 28 pS (cf. Llano *et al.* 1988). The bottom trace shows the average of 40 such sweeps, which was fit with deactivation time constants of 4.5 ms (60%) and 75 ms (40%). (Unpublished data provided by M. Häusser).

calculations most studies have used values of channel conductance determined from somatic recordings. As discussed above, such extrasynaptic receptors may differ from those at the synapse. The most reliable estimates of synaptic channel conductance come from direct resolution of channel transitions in the decay of the PSC. This approach works well at synapses where the channels are of large conductance with long-lived open states, and where the postsynaptic cell is electrically compact with a low background noise level so that high resolution recordings can be made (Fig. 5.3). Although these conditions are rarely met, synaptic channels have been resolved in recordings of glycinergic IPSCs in spinal cord neurons (Takahashi and Momiyama 1991) and cerebellar Golgi cells (Dieudonné 1995); glutamatergic (NMDA) EPSCs in hippocampal neurons (Robinson *et al.* 1991) and cerebellar granule cells (Figs 5.3a,b; Silver *et al.* 1992; Clark *et al.* 1997); GABAergic (GABA$_A$) IPSCs in neurons from the superior colliculus (Kraszewski *et al.* 1992), melanotropes from Xenopus (Borst *et al.* 1994) and cerebellar granule cells (Figs 5.3c,d; Brickley *et al.* 1999). Several of these studies have demonstrated that the single-channel conductance of extrasynaptic channels is indistinguishable from that of synaptic channels under the same experimental conditions (Takahashi and Momiyama 1991; Kraszewski and Grantyn 1992; Dieudonné 1995; Clark *et al.* 1997; but see Brickley *et al.* 1999). Unfortunately, the special conditions required for this approach rule out its application to the majority of synapses in the CNS. This is particularly true for synaptic currents mediated by ligand-gated ion channels with low conductance and/or fast kinetics, such as the AMPA and kainate receptors (Wyllie *et al.* 1993; Swanson *et al.* 1996, 1997).

Estimation of synaptic channel conductance with non-stationary fluctuation analysis

The limited resolution of synaptic recordings acted as a spur to the development of other methods for determining the conductance of postsynaptic channels. Early electrophysiological studies established the utility of noise analysis in extracting information about the biophysical properties of channels from fluctuations in macroscopic currents (Katz and Miledi 1970, 1972; Anderson and Stevens 1973; Conti *et al.* 1975; see also Traynelis and Jaramilo 1998). This approach was extended to non-stationary sodium currents where the number of channels in the population and the channel open probability (at a particular time-point in the decay) remained constant from one trial to the next (Sigworth 1980). The approach involves calculating the variance of current fluctuations about the mean during the current decay. The single channel current, total number of channels and open probability can then be determined by fitting the plot of variance against mean current with a simple binomial model. However, unlike the situation for sodium currents (Sigworth 1980) variations in PSC amplitude at most synaptic connections reflect the activation of different numbers of release sites. As a result, the amplitude of fluctuations around the mean PSC will reflect the quantal size, not the underlying single-channel current. The technical challenge is therefore to isolate current fluctuations arising from the underlying channels from the potentially much larger fluctuations arising from other sources.

Two variants of non-stationary fluctuation analysis were developed for estimating synaptic channel conductance, and both used scaling of the mean current waveform to overcome this problem. In the first method, the mean PSC waveform (or a theoretical function) was fitted to each individual PSC and fluctuations extracted by subtraction (Robinson *et al.* 1991). The main disadvantage of this method (as the authors pointed out) is that the least squares fitting procedure minimizes the variance

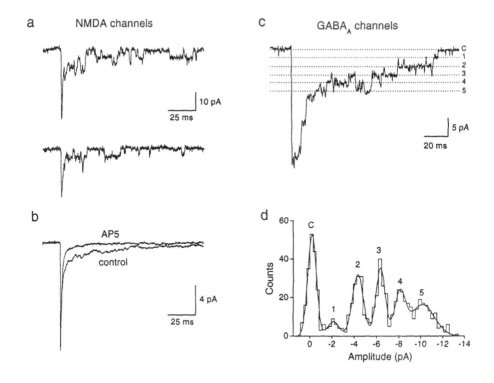

Fig. 5.3 Direct resolution of individual synaptic channels in cerebellar granule cells. (a) Two individual mEPSCs recorded in cerebellar granule cells at –60mV. Synaptic NMDA receptor channel openings can be resolved after the initial rapid non-NMDA component has decayed. In panel (b) 'control' is an average of 115 mEPSCs and 'AP5' is an average of 70 mEPSCs in the presence of 10μM AP5, which abolished the NMDA channel openings. (c) An individual spontaneous IPSC recorded from a cerebellar granule cell at –70mV. GABA$_A$ channel transitions are clearly discernible as the current decays. (d) The same current plotted as an all-point amplitude histogram. The IPSC has five resolvable steps in its decay, seen as equally peaks in its amplitude histogram. The positions of the baseline (C) and the numbered dashed lines (1–5) in panel (c) are taken from the fit of six Gaussian components to the amplitude histogram in panel (d). Modified, with permission, from Silver *et al.* (1992) and Brickley *et al.* (1999).

between the scaled mean waveform and individual PSC, resulting in an underestimate of channel conductance. In the second method the mean PSC waveform was scaled to the peak of each individual PSC and fluctuations around the mean extracted by subtraction (Fig. 5.4a; Traynelis *et al.* 1993; DeKoninck and Mody 1994). The principle behind this method is that variance arising from fluctuations in the quantal content are removed by the peak-scaling procedure leaving current fluctuations arising from channels as they close from the open state at the peak of the current. Several points are worth noting about this approach. By using the method of peak-scaling the mean PSC waveform, information about the total number of channels exposed to transmitter is lost (Traynelis *et al.* 1993; Silver *et al.* 1996*b*). The method can only provide estimates of the weighted mean single-channel current and the mean number of channels *open at the peak* of the PSC. Since the fluctuations arise from channels closing from the open state they depend on the conditional channel open probability and are therefore independent of spatial and temporal non-uniformities in the absolute channel open probability. This feature is important as such non-uniformity can result from variability in vesicle size and dilution of trans-mitter with distance from the release site (Kruk *et al.* 1997).

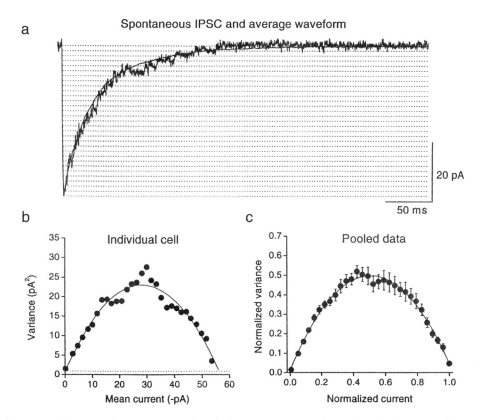

Fig. 5.4 Estimation of synaptic channel conductance with peak-scaled non-stationary fluctuation analysis. (a) The average waveform of 74 spontaneous GABAergic IPSCs (smooth solid trace) scaled to the peak of an individual IPSC (noisy trace). The horizontal dotted lines represent the 30 amplitude bins used to determine values of mean current and variance. (b) Plot of peak-scaled variance (σ_{ps}^2) against mean current ($\bar{I}$) for the cell shown in (a). The plot is fitted with a parabolic relationship $\sigma_{ps}^2 = i\bar{I} - \bar{I}^2/N_p + \sigma_B^2$ to give the weighted-mean single-channel current (i) and the number of channels open at the peak (N_p). The dotted line indicates the baseline variance. (c) Plot of peak-scaled variance normalised by the maximum current against normalised current for data pooled from 10 cells (error bars show s.e.m.). The relationship is well fit by the theoretical parabolic function and gives an estimate of the weighted mean single-channel conductance (27.6 ps) not significantly different from the conductance measured from directly resolved channel closures (26.4 ps) and illustrated in Fig. 5.3. Modified, with permission, from Brickley *et al.* (1999).

Although peak-scaled non-stationary fluctuation analysis is applicable under conditions when conventional non-stationary analysis is not (i.e. when the number of channels activated changes from one PSC to the next or the channel open probability is not uniform) it still relies on a number of assumptions. The main assumptions are that channels are independent and that mean PSC waveform is the same at all synaptic contacts. Contributing synapses must therefore be at the same electrotonic location. Examining whether correlations exist between amplitude, rise and decay time course can test this. Problems also arise if the currents are fast decaying, since asynchrony in release of vesicles can contribute significant variance (Traynelis *et al.* 1993). Ideally, a single release site should be studied (Fig. 5.5c; Silver *et al.* 1996*b*), or a single connection (Silver *et al.* 1996*b*; Momiyama *et al.* 1997; Yoshimura *et al.* 1999). Having said this, the analysis of spontaneous PSCs works well for cells where voltage and space clamp are acceptable (Traynelis *et al.* 1993; DeKoninck and Mody 1994; Nusser *et al.* 1997; Brickley *et al.* 1999). In cerebellar granule cells, for example, GABA$_A$ channel conductance determined by non-stationary fluctuation analysis agrees exactly with that measured by direct resolution of channel closures in the decay of the IPSC (Figs 5.3c,d and 5.4; Brickley *et al.* 1999).

Implicit assumptions in the theory of peak-scaled non-stationary fluctuation analysis are that the postsynaptic channels are identical and have one open state and, that all channels contributing to the decay are open at the peak of the PSC (Traynelis *et al.* 1993). In practice the method is reasonably robust and can be used under many conditions when new channels open after the peak and when channels have multiple conductance levels and/or are heterogeneous. However, some of these conditions, such as the opening of channels for the first time after the peak, distort the shape of the theoretically parabolic relationship between variance and mean current (Figs 5.3b,c and 5.5c). In such cases the channel conductance can be estimated independently from the tail of the PSC (i.e. the low probability end of the mean–variance relationship; Traynelis *et al.* 1993).

Application of peak-scaled non-stationary fluctuation analysis to central synapses has shown that, unlike the situation at the neuromuscular junction, relatively few channels are involved in transmission. At excitatory synapses in the cerebellum the number of non-NMDA channels open at the peak of a uniquantal EPSC ranges from around 15 at the mossy fibre–granule cell synapse (Traynelis *et al.* 1993; Silver *et al.* 1996*b*) to around 70 at the climbing fibre (Momiyama *et al.* 1997). This range of values is similar for GABA$_A$ receptor-mediated currents. The number of channels open at the peak of the synaptic current is around 40–50 for spontaneous IPSCs in cerebellar and hippocampal granule cells (DeKoninck and Mody 1994; Brickley *et al.* 1999), and around 90 for miniature IPSCs (mIPSCs) in cerebellar stellate cells (Nusser *et al.* 1997). Estimating the number of channels open at the peak of the PSC becomes more difficult in large, poorly voltage-clamped neurons. As discussed above, it can be difficult to determine the conductance change at the synapse since distortion of the PSC by dendritic filtering (Fig. 5.1) will lead to underestimation of the peak conductance. This is complicated by the fact that the single-channel conductance is often estimated from the tail of the PSC which is slower, and is thus attenuated less by filtering than the peak of the PSC. If this type of error is not accounted for it will result in an underestimation of the number of channels open at the peak of the PSC.

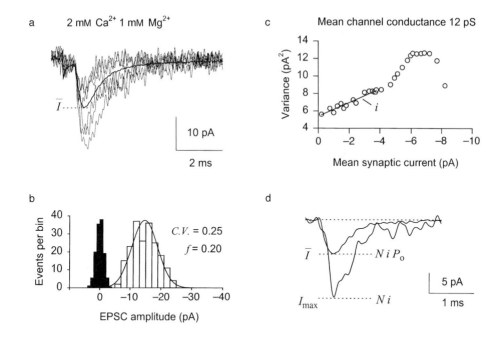

Fig. 5.5 Estimating functional parameters at an excitatory uniquantal synaptic connection. (a) EPSCs from an identified uniquantal mossy fibre–granule cell connection which showed, characteristic, large fluctuations around the mean current (smooth trace). (b) EPSC peak amplitude distribution which was well fit by a single Gaussian function. (c) The single-channel current of non-NMDA receptors underlying the uniquantal connections was estimated from the initial slope of current-variance plots from peak-scaled non-stationary fluctuation analysis. Estimation of the single-channel current (i), mean peak current ($\bar{I}$) and the coefficient of variation of EPSCs allowed a lower limit of $P_o = 0.38$ to be estimated. (d) The mean EPSC and one of the largest EPSCs observed at a uniquantal connection. An upper limit of $P_o = 0.51$ was estimated from the ratio of mean EPSC amplitude and maximum EPSC amplitude (I_{max}) where N is the total number of channels exposed to transmitter at the peak of the EPSC. Modified, with permission, from Silver *et al.* (1996*b*).

Receptor number, receptor occupancy and channel open probability

Thus far, the methods we have discussed allow estimation of the number of channels *opened* by neurotransmitter. For a more detailed understanding of transmission we would like to know how many receptors are *exposed* to transmitter, the fraction of these that bind transmitter (receptor occupancy) and the fraction that subsequently open (open probability, P_o).

Receptor occupancy during transmission is particularly important as it determines 'higher level' properties of the synapse directly. If postsynaptic receptors are not saturated by transmitter the quantal size and the all-or-none behavior observed at uniquantal connections (i.e. those that can generate a maximum of one quantal event; also known as single release site synapses) will be determined presynaptically (Silver 1998). The quantal size will be limited by the amount of transmitter in each vesicle and the all-or-none behavior of the connection will result from the behavior of the release process itself. By contrast, if postsynaptic receptors are saturated, the response to the release of one vesicle, or more than one vesicle, will be the same. In this case the all-or-none behavior of a uniquantal connection is of postsynaptic origin, the quantal size is set by the number of receptor channels in the synaptic membrane. From this it can be seen that level of receptor occupancy not only determines the variability in PSC amplitude at a release site, and thus transmission reliability, but also the possible mechanisms by which a synapse may express plasticity; saturation obviously precludes an increase in synaptic strength *via* an increase in the amount of transmitter per vesicle.

Although receptor occupancy and the total number of channels exposed to transmitter are generally rather difficult to determine, there are several published estimates for these parameters at both excitatory and inhibitory synapses. Pharmacological techniques have been widely used to study the occupancy of $GABA_A$ receptors in particular, albeit with somewhat mixed results. Benzodiazepine agonists increase the affinity of $GABA_A$ receptors, through an increase in the GABA binding rate (Rogers *et al.* 1994; Lavoie and Twyman 1996; Mellor and Randall 1997; Perrais and Ropert 1999), and are thought to increase the amplitude of mIPSCs only if postsynaptic receptors are not saturated following the release of a quantal packet of GABA. While some studies have reported marked increases in mIPSC amplitude in the presence of benzodiazepines (Frerking *et al.* 1995; Mellor and Randall 1997; DeFazio and Hablitz 1998; Perrais and Ropert 1999), and have, therefore, concluded that postsynaptic $GABA_A$ receptors are not fully occupied following the release of a single quantum, others have found little or no change in the peak amplitude of the synaptic current (Otis and Mody 1992; DeKoninck and Mody 1994; Poncer *et al.* 1996). Some, but not all, of this diversity may be accounted for by the recent observation of a confounding temperature-dependent action of benzo-diazepines, such that the amplitude of responses to a sub-saturating concentration of GABA are increased at room temperature but not at physiological temperatures (Perrais and Ropert 1999). Nevertheless, it is likely that there exists a genuine difference in the degree of receptor occupancy among different cell types and at different synapses on the same cell. For example, Nusser *et al.* (1997) have shown for cerebellar stellate cells that the low number of $GABA_A$ receptors present at small synapses are saturated during an mIPSC, while at large synapses, containing more than about 80 receptors, there is incomplete occupancy. In the same cells, $GABA_A$ receptor occupancy, estimated from the interaction of closely spaced quantal events, was also shown to be non-uniform and estimated to be $\sim 75\%$ on average (Auger and Marty 1997). This relatively high average occupancy contrasts with results from retinal amacrine cells in culture where both pre- and postsynaptic receptors sample the same quantum of transmitter. At this somewhat unusual 'dynapse' the large variability in IPSC amplitude and the strong correlation between pre- and post-synaptic responses suggest a low receptor occupancy and a quantal size determined by presynaptic factors (Frerking and Wilson 1995).

Excitatory transmission has also been investigated pharmacologically, both with low affinity competitive antagonists and with agents that interact with transmitter uptake. These studies indicate that transmitter remains in the cleft for a short time (Clements *et al.* 1992; Clements 1996) and that at hippocampal synapses in culture AMPA receptors are not saturated by a vesicle of glutamate (Tong and Jahr 1994*b*; Diamond and Jahr 1997; Liu *et al.* 1999). Additionally, these studies revealed that in hippocampal cells uptake carriers bind glutamate on a submillisecond time scale and can thus influence transmitter profile (Diamond and Jahr 1997). However, other results using glutamate uptake blockers are more complicated, providing evidence both for and against receptor saturation. At 24 °C, block of uptake transporters had no effect on mEPSCs in cultured hippocampal cells or on the decay of evoked EPSCs in cerebellar granule cells (Sarantis *et al.* 1993; Tong and Jahr 1994*a*; but *cf.* Barbour *et al.* 1994). This finding, together with other evidence, suggested that the synaptic AMPA receptors in hippocampal cultures were saturated by a quantum of trans-mitter (Tong and Jahr 1994*a*). However, block of uptake at 34 °C increased the size of mEPSCs, indicating that receptors were not fully occupied, either as a result of a lowering of AMPA receptor affinity (Tong and Jahr 1994*a*) or more rapid binding of glutamate to transporters at higher temperatures (Diamond and Jahr 1997).

A major difficulty in determining such basic synaptic properties as the number of channels, occupancy and open probability is that measurements are usually made from several release sites. Recently, this problem has been addressed by the identification of uniquantal synaptic connections (Gulyas *et al.* 1993; Arancio *et al.* 1994; Bolshakov and Siegelbaum 1995; Stevens and Wang 1995; Silver *et al.* 1996*b*) or by the selective activation of, or measurements from, a single synaptic bouton (Lui and Tsien 1995; Auger and Marty 1997; Forti *et al.* 1997). In many of these studies receptor occupancy was investigated qualitatively by examining the variability of the synaptic response (Fig. 5.5b). If the variability is greater than the maximum expected from the stochastic gating of postsynaptic channels then it is unlikely that the postsynaptic receptors are saturated. This approach can be taken further by analysing fluctuations in the PSC decay using non-stationary fluctuation analysis. This allows estimation of the total number of channels exposed to trans-mitter and the fraction open at the peak of the PSC (Silver *et al.* 1996*b*; Auger and Marty 1997). For example, at the cerebellar mossy fibre–granule cell synapse approximately 40% of the 30–40 non-NMDA channels exposed to glutamate open at the peak of the synaptic current (Fig. 5.5; Silver *et al.* 1996*b*). This corresponded to a receptor occupancy of approximately 50% as calculated from the ratio of the open probability at the peak of the uniquantal EPSC and the maximum open probability at synapses saturated by transmitter (e.g. at multi-quantal connections; $P_{o,max} = 0.84$; Silver *et al.* 1996*b*). The lack of saturation indicated by these techniques is consistent with the large variability in EPSCs observed at single synaptic contacts onto hippocampal neurons (Lui and Tsien 1995; Forti *et al.* 1997). The alternative conclusion, reached following EPSC occlusion experiments at the same hippocampal synapses in culture (Tang *et al.* 1994), can be reconciled by the fact that these recordings were made in the presence of cyclothiazide, a drug that increases the apparent affinity of AMPA receptors (Yamada and Tang 1993).

At synaptic connections with multiple release sites the situation can be more complicated than expected from simple extrapolation of the uniquantal case. Under these conditions, postsynaptic receptors may sense transmitter release from neighboring release sites on the same connection (Trussell *et al.* 1993; Tong and

Jahr 1994*a*; Silver *et al.* 1996*b*) or from different connections (Barbour and Häusser 1997; Kullmann and Asztely 1998; Rossi and Hamann 1998). For example, at multi-site mossy fibre–granule cell synapses in the cerebellum, this 'spillover' of transmitter results in postsynaptic receptor occupancy and quantal size that is dependent on the mean release probability. The effect is so pronounced at some synapses that the postsynaptic non-NMDA receptors become saturated at high release probabilities (Silver *et al.* 1996*b*).

Recently, two-photon confocal microscopy has been used to investigate the occupancy of NMDA receptors during transmission between CA3 and CA1 hippo-campal neurons (Mainen *et al.* 1999). The experimental approach is very simple and is related to that in which occlusion of two closely spaced PSCs is used to estimate occupancy (Tang *et al.* 1994; Auger and Marty 1997). However, the imaging approach is different in that it is postsynaptic calcium that is measured rather than the PSC. Because calcium accumulation within a single spine can be resolved, this method has the advantage that individual synapses can be examined at multi-site con nections. Mainen *et al.* (1999) found that two closely spaced stimuli produced larger calcium changes in the spine than single shocks, suggesting that not all NMDA receptors are occupied following release of transmitter. This elegant approach relies on the assumption that only one release site is present on the spine and that calcium changes arise only from activation of NMDA receptors at the synapse (*cf.* Emptage *et al.* 1999).

Synaptic function and dendritic location

In most of the studies discussed so far, synaptic parameters have been estimated from single synapses, or a homogeneous population of synapses, usually located close to the soma. This necessarily selective approach obviously minimizes compli-cations that might arise from differences in the functional properties of synapses belonging to different classes of presynaptic neuron or of those at different dendritic locations. Synapses onto a single postsynaptic cell can clearly differ in their characteristics, and there is now a growing body of evidence that, for some cells at least, the functional properties of synapses can be related to their position in the dendritic tree. For example, in the early 1970s Iansek and Redman (1973) concluded from electrophysiological studies in cat spinal motoneurons that the size of unitary (single axon) Ia EPSPs recorded at the soma was independent of synapse location. Furthermore, quantal analysis of the same EPSPs revealed that the estimated quantal size was independent of synapse location (Jack *et al.* 1981). Quantal analysis of excitatory synaptic inputs onto hippocampal CA1 neurons also suggests that quantal size at different synapses, when measured at the soma, is independent of their electronic location (Stricker *et al.* 1996). These findings suggested that an adjustment of synaptic weight throughout the dendritic tree could compensate for signal attenuation arising from cable filtering, with the result that the size of the signal recorded at the soma or in the axon, where action potential initiation occurs, would be independent of the physical location of the synaptic input.

A dendritic gradient of synaptic weights has also been suggested for inhibitory connections onto Mauthner neurons, where quantal variance is low (Korn *et al.*

1982). Subsequent studies with combined anatomical and immunohistochemical techniques provided support for this suggestion by demonstrating that the size and complexity of glycine receptor clusters increased with distance from the soma of these neurons (Triller *et al.* 1990). Changes in synaptic properties are not restricted to the postsynaptic membrane; the average number of active zones per terminal and the area of the presynaptic grid also increased with distance from the soma (Sur *et al.* 1995). More recently, similar approaches have shown that clusters of gephyrin, a protein involved in the clustering of glycine receptors, increase in size and complexity with distance from the soma of motoneurons and Ia inhibitory interneurons (Alvarez *et al.* 1997).

At first sight, compensation for dendritic filtering by control of synaptic weight requires that each synapse 'knows' how far it is from the soma. An important finding that sheds light on how this might be achieved is the inverse relationship shown to exist between mEPSC size and the density of active synapses on a cell (Liu and Tsien 1995). Whatever the homeostatic mechanisms involved (e.g. Stewart *et al.* 1996; Davis and Goodman 1998), this relationship, if generally applicable, would mean that changes in synaptic weight with distance from the soma could result simply from a spatial gradient in the density of synaptic innervation. Such a gradient has been shown in goldfish Mauthner cells (Triller *et al.* 1990) and from spine density measurements of hippocampal CA1 cells, which indicate that synaptic innervation tends to be lower on the smaller, more distal, dendrites (Bannister and Larkman 1995). One complicating factor that should be considered when interpreting electrophysiological recordings from the soma is the presence of voltage-gated channels in dendrites (see Chapters 6, 9 and 10). Activation of dendritic voltage-gated channels can, in theory, alter the synaptic signal in such a way as to effectively overcome passive cable filtering, making the size of the somatic response independent of the location of the synapse on the dendritic tree (e.g. De Schutter and Bower 1994; Cook and Johnson 1999). Whether these voltage-dependent properties of dendrites contribute to the weighting of quantal size remains unclear.

Another way in which spatial heterogeneity in synaptic behavior could occur is if synaptic connections arising from different presynaptic cell types have different properties. In the hippocampus, for example, GABAergic synapses at perisomatic and dendritic sites on pyramidal neurons originate from different populations of interneurons and serve different roles in terms of their influence on subthreshold integration, somatic or dendritic electrogenesis and action potential backpropagation (e.g. Miles *et al.* 1996; Tsubokawa and Ross 1996). For CA1 neurons, $GABA_A$ receptor-mediated IPSCs at proximal and distal sites on the dendritic tree also differ significantly in their kinetics and pharmacology, suggesting the presence of distinct receptor types at each location (Pearce 1993; Banks *et al.* 1998). Similar distinctions have been noted for pyramidal cells in the piriform cortex, with $GABA_A$ receptor-mediated IPSCs having both fast and slow components, the latter being expressed to a greater extent in apical dendrites (Kapur *et al.* 1997*b*). Compartmental modeling suggests that separate circuits controlling inhibition in perisomatic regions and in apical dendrites, with synaptic receptors having appropriately tailored kinetic properties, could enable effective dendritic processing to occur independently of the overall control of neuronal excitability (Kapur *et al.* 1997*a*).

Concluding remarks

Due to the technical difficulties of working on central synapses, in part due to their remote dendritic location, many of our concepts in this field derive from the classical work on the neuromuscular junction (Katz 1969). Although the basic principles of quantal transmission elucidated at the periphery appear to be valid for central synapses, it is now apparent that the functional details of transmission are very different. Unlike the rather homogeneous properties found at the neuromuscular junction, central synapses appear sufficiently heterogeneous to make generalization from any specific synapse inadvisable. Heterogeneity is found from the level of the subunits that make up the postsynaptic receptors, to the gross morphology of the connection (Walmsley *et al.* 1998). Indeed, the more that is known about central synapses the clearer it becomes that each is different. Some of this diversity may well reflect the dynamic nature of individual synapses, which are now recognized as capable of undergoing rapid activity-driven changes in structure and receptor content (e.g. Carroll *et al.* 1999; Engbert and Bonhoeffer 1999; Maletic-Savatic *et al.* 1999; Shi *et al.* 1999). Immunohistochemical, pharmacological and electrophysiological data have also shown that postsynaptic receptors cannot be assumed *a priori* to have the same subunit composition as those in the extrasynaptic membrane. Even if they are of the same subtype or exhibit similar properties in certain circumstances (e.g. Takahashi and Momiyama 1991; Clark *et al.* 1997), it is by no means certain that they will exhibit the same functional behavior in an excised membrane patch as seen *in situ* (Clark *et al.* 1997; Mellor and Randall 1997; Perrais and Ropert 1999). These problems substantially lessen the power of using isolated patches to study synaptic function and demand other approaches that allow a more direct analysis of synaptic receptors.

So, what have synaptic measurements told us about postsynaptic receptor function? As we have described, the development of quantitative methods for analysis of synaptic currents and their application to a range of different excitatory and inhibitory central synapses has allowed estimation of a number of key synaptic parameters. These include the profile of transmitter in the synaptic cleft, the precise kinetics and single-channel conductance of postsynaptic receptors, the number of receptors exposed to transmitter, receptor occupancy and channel open probability. While there is certainly a degree of heterogeneity in these parameters among central synapses, one of the consistent observations to emerge from these studies is that rather few channels are activated by a quantum of transmitter. The number of channels that open usually falls in the range of 10–100, and is clearly far less than the number of transmitter molecules thought to be released (2000–5000; Riveros *et al.* 1986; Burger *et al.* 1989; Bruns and Jahn 1995). This excess of transmitter, coupled with the fast rise times of central synaptic currents, has been taken as support for the hypothesis that receptors at central synapses are saturated by transmitter (for review, see Frerking and Wilson 1995). However, detailed modeling studies (Faber *et al.* 1992; Holmes 1995; Kruk *et al.* 1997) have shown that these are not good indicators of receptor occupancy, since the average occupancy depends critically on the rate constants of the channel kinetic scheme and the concentration profile of transmitter in the cleft. The EC_{50} values of AMPA receptors determined from fast-application experiments cover a tenfold range, depending on the particular subtype of receptor

(Jonas and Sakmann 1992; Raman and Trussell 1992; Koh *et al.* 1995; Häusser and Roth 1997*b*). Simply considering this parameter alone it can be seen that receptor occupancies are unlikely to be similar at synapses expressing different receptor subtypes.

Recent estimates of receptor occupancy at central synapses have shown that non-NMDA receptors at some excitatory synapses are not saturated by a packet of glutamate, even though few channels are activated (Silver *et al.* 1996*b*; Forti *et al.* 1997; Liu *et al.* 1999). It is also clear that receptor occupancy is not as simple a synaptic parameter as first assumed. At inhibitory synapses the level of occupancy depends on the size of the contact (and thus the number of channels) with large contacts having a lower occupancy and open probability (Auger *et al.* 1997; Nusser *et al.* 1997). At both excitatory and inhibitory connections, occupancy and channel open probability can also be complicated by transmitter spillover from neighbouring release sites (Barbour and Häusser 1997; Kullmann and Asztely 1998), resulting in saturation of postsynaptic non-NMDA receptors at some synapses. At present it is unclear whether the higher affinity NMDA receptors are saturated by glutamate. Modeling studies suggest that saturation is not inevitable (Holmes 1995) and indeed data obtained from two-photon imaging indicate that NMDA receptors on spines of CA1 synapses may not be fully occupied following the release of a quantum of transmitter (Mainen *et al.* 1999).

While the various biophysical parameters we have described might seem arcane, it is clear that they have important implications for synaptic behavior. Overall, if there is a central theme to emerge from their characterization, it is that the functional behavior of any one central synapse, be it excitatory or inhibitory, cannot necessarily be extrapolated to all synapses. Perhaps unsurprisingly, differences in synaptic behavior are being increasingly recognized as reflecting the different roles played by synapses at different dendritic locations. Accommodating this heterogeneity represents a significant challenge to those trying to establish realistic, yet manageable, models of information processing at the level of single neurons.

Acknowledgements

R.A.S. and M.F. are supported by The Wellcome Trust (R.A.S. holds a Research Career Development Fellowship). We would like to thank Stephen Brickley and Michael Häusser for help with figures.

References

Alvarez, F. J., Dewey, D. E., Harrington, D. A., and Fyffe, R. E. (1997). Cell-type specific organization of glycine receptor clusters in the mammalian spinal cord. *Journal of Comparative Neurology*, **379**, 150–70.

Anderson, C. R. and Stevens, C. F. (1973). Voltage clamp analysis of acetylcholine produced end-plate current fluctuations at frog neuromuscular junction. *Journal of Physiology*, **235**, 655–91.

Arancio, O., Korn, H., Gulyás, A., Freund, T., and Miles, R. (1994). Excitatory synaptic connections onto rat hippocampal inhibitory cells may involve a single transmitter release site. *Journal of Physiology*, **481**, 395–405.

Auger, C. and Marty, A. (1997). Heterogeneity of functional synaptic parameters among single release sites. *Neuron*, **19**, 139–50.

Banks, M. I., Li, T. B., and Pearce, R. A. (1998). The synaptic basis of GABA$_A$ slow. *Journal of Neuroscience*, **18**, 1305–17.

Bannister, N. J. and Larkman, A. U. (1995). Dendritic morphology of CA1 pyramidal neurones from the rat hippocampus: II. Spine distributions. *Journal of Comparative Neurology*, **360**, 161–71.

Barbour, B. and Häusser, M. (1997). Intersynaptic diffusion of neurotransmitter. *Trends in Neurosciences*, **20**, 377–84.

Barbour, B., Keller, B. U., Llano, I., and Marty, A. (1994). Prolonged presence of glutamate during excitatory synaptic transmission to cerebellar Purkinje cells. *Neuron*, **12**, 1331–43.

Barnard, E. A., Skolnick, P., Olsen, R. W., Mohler, H., Sieghart, W., Biggio, G., *et al.* (1998). International Union of Pharmacology. XV. Subtypes of gamma-aminobutyric acidA receptors: classification on the basis of subunit structure and receptor function. *Pharmacological Reviews*, **50**, 291–313.

Becker, C.-M. (1992). In *Handbook of experimental pharmacology*, (ed. H. Herken and F. Hucho), pp. 539–75. Springer, Berlin.

Benke, T. A., Luthi, A., Isaac, J. T., and Collingridge, G. L. (1998). Modulation of AMPA receptor unitary conductance by synaptic activity. *Nature*, **393**, 793–7.

Bettler, B., Kaupmann, K., and Bowery, N. (1998). GABA$_B$ receptors: drugs meet clones. *Current Opinion in Neurobiology*, **8**, 345–50.

Bolshakov, V. Y. and Siegelbaum, S. A. (1995). Regulation of hippocampal transmitter release during development and long-term potentiation. *Science*, **269**, 1730–4.

Borst, J. G , Lodder, J. C., and Kits, K. S. (1994). Large amplitude variability of GABAergic IPSCs in melanotropes from *Xenopus laevis*: evidence that quantal size differs between synapses. *Journal of Neurophysiology*, **71**, 639–55.

Bowie, D. and Mayer, M. (1995). Inward rectification of both AMPA and kainate subtype glutamate receptors generated by polyamine-mediated ion-channel block. *Neuron*, **15**, 453–62.

Brickley, S. G., Cull-Candy, S. G., and Farrant, M. (1999). Single-channel properties of synaptic and extrasynaptic GABA$_A$ receptors suggest differential targeting of receptor subtypes. *Journal of Neuroscience*, **19**, 2960–73

Bruns, D. and Jahn, R. (1995). Real-time measurement of transmitter release from single synaptic vesicles. *Nature*, **377**, 62–5.

Burger, P. M., Mehl, E., Cameron, P. L., Maycox, P. R., Baumert, M., Lottspeich, F., *et al.* (1989). Synaptic vesicles immunoisolated from rat cerebral cortex contain high levels of glutamate. *Neuron*, **3**, 715–20.

Carroll, R. C., Lissin, D. V., von Zastrow, M., Nicoll, R. A., and Malenka, R. C. (1999). Rapid redistribution of glutamate receptors contributes to long-term depression in hippocampal cultures. *Nature Neuroscience*, **2**, 454–60.

Clark, B., Farrant, M., and Cull-Candy, S. G. (1997). A direct comparison of the single-channel properties of synaptic and extrasynaptic NMDA receptors. *Journal of Neuroscience*, **17**, 107–16.

Clements, J. D. (1996). Transmitter timecourse in the synaptic cleft: its role in central synaptic function. *Trends in Neurosciences* **19**, 163–71.

Clements, J. D., Lester, R. A., Tong, G., Jahr, C. E., and Westbrook, G. L. (1992). The time course of glutamate in the synaptic cleft. *Science*, **258**, 1498–501.

Colquhoun, D., Jonas, P., and Sakmann, B. (1992). Action of brief pulses of glutamate on AMPA/kainate receptors in patches from different neurones of rat hippocampal slices. *Journal of Physiology*, **458**, 261–87.

Conn, P. J. and Pin, J.-P. (1997). Pharmacology and functions of metabotropic glutamate receptors. *Annual Review of Pharmacology and Toxicology*, **37**, 205–37.

Conti, F., DeFelice, L. J., and Wanke, E. (1975). Potassium and sodium ion current noise in the membrane of the squid giant axon. *Journal of Physiology*, **248**, 45–82.

Cook, E. P. and Johnston, D. (1999). Voltage-dependent properties of dendrites that eliminate location-dependent variability of synaptic input. *Journal of Neurophysiology*, **81**, 535–43.

Davis, G. W. and Goodman, C. S. (1998). Synapse-specific control of synaptic efficacy at the terminals of a single neuron. *Nature*, **392**, 82–6.

De Schutter, E. and Bower, J. M. (1994). Simulated responses of cerebellar Purkinje cells are independent of the dendritic location of granule cell synaptic inputs. *Proceedings of the National Academy of Sciences USA*, **91**, 4736–40.

DeFazio, T. and Hablitz, J. J. (1998). Zinc and zolpidem modulate mIPSCs in rat neocortical pyramidal neurons. *Journal of Neurophysiology*, **80**, 1670–7.

DeKoninck, Y. and Mody, I. (1994). Noise-analysis of miniature IPSCs in adult rat brain slices: properties and modulation of synaptic GABA$_A$ receptor channels. *Journal of Neurophysiology*, **71**, 1318–35.

Diamond, J. S. and Jahr, C. E. (1997). Transporters buffer synaptically released glutamate on a submillisecond time scale. *Journal of Neuroscience*, **17**, 4672–87.

Dieudonné, S. (1995). Glycinergic synaptic currents in Golgi cells of the rat cerebellum. *Proceedings of the National Academy of Science USA*, **92**, 1441–5.

Edwards, F. A., Konnerth, A., and Sakmann, B. (1990). Quantal analysis of inhibitory synaptic transmission in the dentate gyrus of rat hippocampal. slices: a patch-clamp study. *Journal of Physiology*, **430**, 213–49.

Emptage, N., Bliss, T. V., and Fine, A. (1999). Single synaptic events evoke NMDA receptor-mediated release of calcium from internal stores in hippocampal dendritic spines. *Neuron*, **22**, 115–24.

Engert, F. and Bonhoeffer, T. (1999). Dendritic spine changes associated with hippocampal long-term synaptic plasticity. *Nature*, **399**, 66–70.

Faber, D. S., Young, W. S., Legendre, P., and Korn, H. (1992). Intrinsic quantal variability due to stochastic properties of receptor–transmitter interactions. *Science*, **258**, 1494–8.

Farrant, M. and Webster, R. A. (1989). GABA antagonists: their use and mechanisms of action. In *Neuromethods, Vol. 12. Drugs as tools in neurotransmitter research.* (ed. A. A. Boulton, G. B. Baker, and A. V. Juorio), pp. 161–219. Humana, Clifton, NJ.

Finkel, A. S. and Redman, S. J. (1983). The synaptic current evoked in cat spinal motoneurones by impulses in single group 1a axons. *Journal of Physiology*, **342**, 615–32.

Fisher, J. L. and Macdonald, R. L. (1997). Single channel properties of recombinant GABA$_A$ receptors containing γ_2 or δ subtypes expressed with α_1 and β_3 subtypes in mouse L929 cells. *Journal of Physiology*, **505**, 283–97.

Fleck, M. W., Bahring, R., Patneau, D. K., and Mayer, M. L. (1996). AMPA receptor heterogeneity in rat hippocampal neurons revealed by differential sensitivity to cyclothiazide. *Journal of Neurophysiology*, **75**, 2322–33.

Forsythe, I. D. and Barnes-Davies, M. (1993). The binaural auditory pathway: excitatory amino acid receptors mediate dual timecourse excitatory postsynaptic currents in the rat medial nucleus of the trapezoid body. *Proceedings of the Royal Society London (B)*, **251**, 151–7.

Forti, L., Bossi, M., Bergamaschi, A., Villa, A., and Malgaroli, A. (1997). Loose-patch recordings of single quanta at individual hippocampal synapses. *Nature*, **388**, 874–8.

Frerking, M., Borges, S., and Wilson, M. (1995). Variation in GABA mini amplitude is the consequence of variation in transmitter concentration. *Neuron*, **15**, 885–95.

Galarreta, M. and Hestrin, S. (1997). Properties of GABA$_A$ receptors underlying inhibitory synaptic currents in neocortical pyramidal neurons. *Journal of Neuroscience*, **17**, 7220–7.

Geiger, J. R., Melcher, T., Koh, D. S., Sakmann, B., Seeburg, P. H., Jonas, P., *et al.* (1995). Relative abundance of subunit mRNAs determines gating and Ca^{2+} permeability of AMPA receptors in principal neurons and interneurons in rat CNS. *Neuron*, **15**, 193–204.

Geiger, J. R., Lübke, J., Roth, A., Frotscher, M., and Jonas, P. (1997). Submillisecond AMPA receptor-mediated signaling at a principal neuron-interneuron synapse. *Neuron* **18**, 1009–23.

Greengard, P., Jen, J., Nairn, A. C., and Stevens, C. F. (1991). Enhancement of the glutamate response by cAMP-dependent protein kinase in hippocampal neurons. *Science*, **253**, 1135–8.

Gulyas, A. I., Miles, R., Sik, A., Tóth, K., Tamamaki, N., and Freund, T. F. (1993). Hippocampal pyramidal cells excite inhibitory neurons through a single release site. *Nature*, **366**, 683–7.

Häusser, M. (1994). Kinetics of excitatory synaptic currents in Purkinje cells studied using dendritic patch-clamp recording. *Society for Neuroscience Abstracts*, **20**, 891.

Häusser, M. and Roth, A. (1997a). Estimating the time course of the excitatory synaptic conductance in neocortical pyramidal cells using a novel voltage jump method. *Journal of Neuroscience*, **17**, 7606–25.

Häusser, M. and Roth, A. (1997b). Dendritic and somatic glutamate receptor channels in rat cerebellar Purkinje cells. *Journal of Physiology*, **501**, 77–95.

Hestrin, S. (1992). Activation and desensitization of glutamate-activated channels mediating fast excitatory synaptic currents in the visual cortex. *Neuron*, **11**, 1083–91.

Holmes, W. R. (1995). Modelling the effect of glutamate diffusion and uptake on NMDA and non-NMDA receptor saturation. *Biophysical Journal*, **69**, 1734–47.

Iansek, R. and Redman, S. J. (1973). The amplitude, time course and charge of unitary excitatory post-synaptic potentials evoked in spinal motoneurone dendrites. *Journal of Physiology*, **234**, 665–88.

Ilyin, V. I., Whittemore, E. R., Guastella, J., Weber, E., and Woodward, R. M. (1996). Subtype-selective inhibition of *N*-methyl-D-aspartate receptors by haloperidol. *Molecular Pharmacology*, **50**, 1541–50.

Jack, J. J. B., Redman, S. J., and Wong, K. (1981). The components of synaptic potentials evoked in cat spinal motoneurones by impulses in single group Ia afferents. *Journal of Physiology*, **321**, 65–96.

Jack, J. J. B., Larkman, A. U., Major, G., and Stratford, K. J. (1994). Quantal analysis of synaptic excitation of CA1 hippocampal pyramidal cells. In *Molecular and cellular mechanisms of neurotransmitter release* (ed. L. Stjärne, P. Greengard, S. Grillner, S. Hökfelt, and D. Otterson), pp. 275–299. Raven, New York.

Johnston, D. and Brown, T. H. (1983). Interpretation of voltage-clamp measurements in hippocampal neurons. *Journal of Neurophysiology*, **50**, 464–86.

Jonas, P. and Sakmann, B. (1992). Glutamate receptor channels in isolated patches from CA1 and CA3 pyramidal cells of rat hippocampal slices. *Journal of Physiology*, **455**, 143–71.

Jonas, P., Major, G., and Sakmann, B. (1993). Quantal components of unitary EPSCs at the mossy fibre synapse on CA3 pyramidal cells of rat hippocampus. *Journal of Physiology*, **472**, 615–63.

Jonas, P., Bischofberger, J., and Sandkuhler, J. (1998). Corelease of two fast neurotransmitters at a central synapse. *Science*, **281**, 419–24.

Jones, M. V. and Westbrook, G. L. (1995). Desensitized states prolong GABA$_A$ channel responses to brief agonist pulses. *Neuron*, **15**, 181–91.

Jones, M. V. and Westbrook, G. L. (1997). Shaping of IPSCs by endogenous calcineurin activity. *Journal of Neuroscience*, **17**, 7626–33.

Kamboj, S. K., Swanson, G. T., and Cull-Candy, S. G. (1995). Intracellular spermine confers rectification on rat calcium-permeable AMPA and kainate receptors. *Journal of Physiology*, **486**, 297–303.

Kapur, A., Lytton, W. W., Ketchum, K. L., and Haberly, L. B. (1997a). Regulation of the NMDA component of EPSPs by different components of postsynaptic GABAergic inhibition: computer simulation analysis in piriform cortex. *Journal of Neurophysiology*, **78**, 2546–59.

Kapur, A., Pearce , R. A., Lytton, W. W., and Haberly, L. B. (1997b). GABA$_A$-mediated IPSCs in piriform cortex have fast and slow components with different properties and locations on pyramidal cells. *Journal of Neurophysiology*, **78**, 2531–45.

Katz, B. (1969). *The release of neural transmitter substances*. Liverpool University Press.

Katz, B. and Miledi, R. (1970). Membrane noise produced by acetylcholine. *Nature*, 226, 962–3.

Katz, B. and Miledi, R. (1972). The statistical nature of the acetylcholine potential and its molecular components. *Journal of Physiology*, **224**, 665–99.

Kerr, D. I. and Ong, J. (1995). GABA$_B$ receptors. *Pharmacology and Therapeutics*, **67**, 187–246.

Koh, D.-S., Burnashev, N., and Jonas, P. (1995). Block of native Ca^{2+}-permeable AMPA receptors in rat-brain by intracellular polyamines generates double rectification. *Journal of Physiology*, **486**, 305–12.

Korn, H., Mallet, A., Triller, A., and Faber, D. S. (1982). Transmission at a central inhibitory synapse. II. Quantal description of release, with a physical correlate for binomial n. *Journal of Neurophysiology*, **48**, 679–707.

Korpi, E. R., Kuner, T., Seeburg, P. H., and Luddens, H. (1995). Selective antagonist for the cerebellar granule cell-specific gamma-aminobutyric acid type A receptor. *Molecular Pharmacology*, **47**, 283–9.

Kraszewski, K. and Grantyn, R. (1992). Unitary, quantal and miniature GABA-activated synaptic chloride currents in cultured neurons from the rat superior colliculus. *Neuroscience*, **47**, 555–70.

Kruk, P. J., Korn, H., and Faber, D. S. (1997). The effects of geometrical parameters on synaptic transmission: a Monte Carlo simulation study. *Biophysical Journal*, **73**, 2874–90.

Kullmann, D. M. and Asztely, F. (1998). Extrasynaptic glutamate spillover in the hippocampus: evidence and implications. *Trends in Neurosciences*, **21**, 8–14.

Lavoie, A. M. and Twyman, R. E. (1996). Direct evidence for diazepam modulation of GABA$_A$ receptor microscopic affinity. *Neuropharmacology*, **35**, 1383–92.

Lester, R. A., Clements, J. D., Westbrook, G. L., and Jahr, C. E. (1990). Channel kinetics determine the time course of NMDA receptor-mediated synaptic currents. *Nature*, **346**, 565–7.

Lieberman, D. N. and Mody, I. (1994). Regulation of NMDA channel function by endogenous Ca^{2+}-dependent phosphatase. *Nature*, **369**, 235–9.

Lieberman, D. N. and Mody, I. (1999). Casein kinase-II regulates NMDA channel function in hippocampal neurons. *Nature Neuroscience*, **2**, 125–32.

Liu, G. and Tsien, R. W. (1995a). Properties of synaptic transmission at single hippocampal synaptic boutons. *Nature*, **375**, 404–8.

Liu, G. and Tsien, R. W. (1995b). Synaptic transmission at single visualized hippocampal boutons. *Neuropharmacology*, **34**, 1407–21.

Liu, G., Choi, S., and Tsien, R. W. (1999). Variability of neurotransmitter concentration and nonsaturation of postsynaptic AMPA receptors at synapses in hippocampal cultures and slices. *Neuron*, **22**, 395–409.

Llano, I., Marty, A., Johnson, J. W., Ascher, P., and Gähwiler, B. H. (1988). Patch-clamp recording of amino acid-activated responses in 'organotypic' slice cultures. *Proceedings of the National Academy of Sciences USA*, **85**, 3221–5.

Mainen, Z. F., Malinow, R., and Svoboda, K. (1999). Synaptic [Ca^{2+}] transients in single spines indicate NMDA receptors are not saturated. *Nature*, **13**, 151–5.

Major, G. (1993). Solutions for transients in arbitrarily branching cables: III. voltage clamp problems. *Biophysical Journal*, **65**, 469–91.

Maletic-Savatic, M., Malinow, R., and Svoboda, K. (1999). Rapid dendritic morphogenesis in CA1 hippocampal dendrites induced by synaptic activity. *Science*, **283**, 1923–7.

Mellor, J. R. and Randall, A. D. (1997). Frequency-dependent actions of benzodiazepines on GABA$_A$ receptors in cultured murine cerebellar granule cells. *Journal of Physiology*, **503**, 353–69.

Miles, R., Tóth, K., Gulyás, A. I., Hájos, N., and Freund, T. F. (1996). Differences between somatic and dendritic inhibition in the hippocampus. *Neuron*, **16**, 815–23.

Momiyama, A., Silver, R. A., and Cull-Candy, S. G. (1996). Conductance of glutamate receptor channels at climbing fibre synapses in rat Purkinje cells in thin slices. *Journal of Physiology*, **494P**, 86.

Mosbacher, J., Schoepfer, R., Monyer, H., Burnashev, N., Seeburg, P. H., and Ruppersberg, J. P. (1994). A molecular determinant for submillisecond desensitization in glutamate receptors. *Science*, **266**, 1059–62.

Moss, S. J., Smart, T. G., Blackstone, C. D., and Huganir, R. L. (1992). Functional modulation of GABA$_A$ receptors by cAMP-dependent protein phosphorylation. *Science*, **257**, 661–5.

Nusser, Z., Cull-Candy, S. G., and Farrant, M. (1997). Differences in synaptic GABA$_A$ receptor number underlie variation in GABA miniamplitude. *Neuron*, **19**, 697–709.

Otis, T. S. and Mody, I. (1992). Modulation of decay kinetics and frequency of GABA$_A$ receptor-mediated spontaneous inhibitory postsynaptic currents in hippocampal neurons. *Neuroscience*, **49**, 13–32.

Paoletti, P., Ascher, P., and Neyton, J. (1997). High-affinity zinc inhibition of NMDA NR1-NR-2A receptors. *Journal of Neuroscience*, **17**, 5711–25.

Partin, K. M., Patneau, D. K., and Mayer, M. L. (1994). Cyclothiazide differentially modulates desensitization of alpha-amino-3-hydroxy-5-methyl-4-isoxazolepropionic acid receptor splice variants. *Molecular Pharmacology*, **46**, 129–38.

Pearce, R. A. (1993). Physiological evidence for two distinct GABA$_A$ responses in rat hippocampus. *Neuron*, **10**, 189–200.

Perrais, D. and Ropert, N. (1999). Effect of zolpidem on miniature IPSCs and occupancy of postsynaptic GABA$_A$ receptors in central synapses. *Journal of Neuroscience*, **19**, 578–88.

Pierce, J. P. and Mendell, L. M. (1993). Quantitative ultrastructure of Ia boutons in the ventral horn: scaling and positional relationships. *Journal of Neuroscience*, **13**, 4748–63.

Poncer, J. C., Durr, R., Gahwiler, B. H., and Thompson, S. M. (1996). Modulation of synaptic GABA$_A$ receptor function by benzodiazepines in area CA3 of rat hippocampal slice cultures. *Neuropharmacology*, **35**, 1169–79.

Rall, W. and Segev, I. (1985). Space-clamp problems when voltage clamping branched neurons with intracellular microelectrodes. In *Voltage and patch clamping with intracellular microelectrodes*, (ed. T. G. Smith Jr., H. Lecar, S. J. Redman, and P. Gage), pp. 191–215. American Physiological Society, Bethesda.

Raman, I. M. and Trussell, L. O. (1992). The kinetics of the response to glutamate and kainate in neurons of the avian cochlear nucleus. *Neuron*, **9**, 173–86.

Redman, S. (1990). Quantal analysis of synaptic potentials in neurons of the central nervous system. *Physiological Reviews*, **70**, 165–98.

Riveros, N., Fiedler, J., Lagos, N., Munoz, C., and Orrego, F. (1986). Glutamate in rat brain cortex synaptic vesicles: influence of the vesicle isolation procedure. *Brain Research*, **386**, 405–8.

Robinson, H. P., Sahara, Y., and Kawai, N. (1991). Nonstationary fluctuation analysis and direct resolution of single channel currents at postsynaptic sites. *Biophysical Journal*, **59**, 295–304.

Rogers, C. J., Twyman, R. E., and Macdonald, R. L. (1994). Benzodiazepine and β-carboline regulation of single GABA$_A$ receptor channels of mouse spinal neurones in culture. *Journal of Physiology*, **475**, 69–82.

Rosenmund, C. and Westbrook, G. L. (1993). Calcium-induced actin depolymerization reduces NMDA channel activity. *Neuron*, **10**, 805–14.

Rossi, D. J. and Hamann, M. (1998). Spillover-mediated transmission at inhibitory synapses promoted by high affinity α_6 subunit GABA$_A$ receptors and glomerular geometry. *Neuron*, **20**, 783–95.

Sarantis, M., Ballerini, L., Miller, B., Silver, R. A., Edwards, M., and Attwell, D. (1993). Glutamate uptake from the synaptic cleft does not shape the decay of the non-NMDA component of the synaptic current. *Neuron*, **11**, 541–9.

Shi, S. H., Hayashi, Y., Petralia, R. S., Zaman, S. H., Wenthold, R. J., Svoboda, K., and Malinow, R. (1999). Rapid spine delivery and redistribution of AMPA receptors after synaptic NMDA receptor activation. *Science*, **284**, 1811–16.

Sigworth, F. J. (1980). The variance of sodium current fluctuations at the node of ranvier. *Journal of Physiology*, **307**, 97–129.

Silver, R. A. (1998). Neurotransmission at synapses with single and multiple release sites. In *Central synapses: quantal mechanisms and plasticity*, (ed. D. S. Faber, H. Korn, S. J.

Redman, S. M. Thompson, and J. Altman), pp. 130–9. Human Frontiers Science Programme, Strasbourg.

Silver, R. A., Traynelis, S. F., and Cull-Candy, S. G. (1992). Rapid-time-course miniature and evoked excitatory currents at cerebellar synapses *in situ*. *Nature*, **355**, 163–6.

Silver, R. A., Colquhoun, D., Cull-Candy, S. G., and Edmonds, B. (1996*a*). Deactivation and desensitization of non-NMDA receptors in patches and the time course of EPSCs in rat cerebellar granule cells. *Journal of Physiology*, **493**, 167–73.

Silver, R. A., Cull-Candy, S. G., and Takahashi, T. (1996*b*). Non-NMDA glutamate receptor occupancy and open probability at a rat cerebellar synapse with single and multiple release sites. *Journal of Physiology*, **494**, 231–50.

Silver, R. A., Farrant, M., and Cull-Candy, S. G. (1996*c*). Filtering of synaptic currents estimated from the time course from NMDA channel opening at the rat cerebellar mossy fibre–granule cell synapse. *Journal of Physiology*, **494P**, 85P.

Silver, R. A., Momiyama, A., and Cull-Candy, S. G. (1998). Locus of frequency-dependent depression identified with multiple-probability fluctuation analysis at rat climbing fibre-Purkinje cell synapses. *Journal of Physiology*, **510**, 881–902.

Spruston, N., Jaffe, D. B., Williams, S. H., and Johnston, D. (1993). Voltage- and space-clamp errors associated with the measurement of electrotonically remote synaptic events. *Journal of Neurophysiology*, **70**, 781–802.

Spruston, N., Jonas, P., and Sakmann, B. (1995). Dendritic glutamate receptor channels in rat hippocampal CA3 and CA1 pyramidal neurons. *Journal of Physiology*, **482**, 325–52.

Stevens, C. F. and Wang, Y. (1995). Facilitation and depression at single central synapses. *Neuron*, **14**, 795–802.

Stewart, B. A., Schuster, C. M., Goodman, C. S., and Atwood, H. L. (1996). Homeostasis of synaptic transmission in Drosophila with genetically altered nerve terminal morphology. *Journal of Neuroscience*, **16**, 3877–86.

Stocca, G. and Vicini, S. (1998). Increased contribution of NR2A subunit to synaptic NMDA receptors in developing rat cortical neurons. *Journal of Physiology*, **507**, 13–24.

Stricker, C., Field, A. C., and Redman, S. J. (1996). Statistical analysis of amplitude fluctuations in EPSCs evoked in rat CA1 pyramidal neurones in vitro. *Journal of Physiology*, **490**, 419–41.

Sur, C., Triller, A., and Korn, H. (1995). Morphology of the release site of inhibitory synapses on the soma and dendrite of an identified neuron. *Journal of Comparative Neurology*, **351**, 247–60.

Swanson, G. T., Feldmeyer, D., Kaneda, M., and Cull-Candy, S. G. (1996). Effect of RNA editing and subunit co-assembly single-channel properties of recombinant kainate receptors. *Journal of Physiology*, **492**, 129–42.

Swanson, G. T., Kamboj, S. K., and Cull-Candy, S. G. (1997). Single-channel properties of recombinant AMPA receptors depend on RNA editing, splice variation, and subunit composition *Journal of Neuroscience*, **17**, 58–69.

Takahashi, T. and Momiyama, A. (1991). Single-channel currents underlying glycinergic inhibitory postsynaptic responses in spinal neurons. *Neuron*, **7**, 965–9.

Tang, C.-M., Margulis, M., Shi, Q.-Y., and Fielding, A. (1994). Saturation of postsynaptic glutamate receptors after quantal release of transmitter. *Neuron*, **13**, 1385–93.

Thompson, S. A., Arden, S. A., Marshall, G., Wingrove, P. B., Whiting, P. J., and Wafford, K. A. (1999). Residues in transmembrane domains I and II determine γ-aminobutyric acid type A_A receptor subtype-selective antagonism by furosemide. *Molecular Pharmacology*, **55**, 993–9.

Tia, S., Wang, J. F., Kotchabhakdi, N., and Vicini, S. (1996). Developmental changes of inhibitory synaptic currents in cerebellar granule neurons: role of $GABA_A$ receptor alpha 6 subunit. *Journal of Neuroscience*, **16**, 3630–40.

Tong, G. and Jahr, C. E. (1994*a*). Multivesicular release from excitatory synapses of cultured hippocampal neurons. *Neuron*, **12**, 51–9.

Tong, G. and Jahr, C. E. (1994b). Block of glutamate transporters potentiates postsynaptic excitation. *Neuron*, **13**, 1195–203.

Tóth, K. and McBain, C. J. (1998). Afferent-specific innervation of two distinct AMPA receptor subtypes on single hippocampal interneurons *Nature Neuroscience*, **1**, 572–8.

Traynelis, S. F. (1998). Software-based correction of single compartment series resistance errors. *Journal of Neuroscience Methods*, **86**, 25–34.

Traynelis, S. F. and Jaramillo, F. (1998). Getting the most out of noise in the central nervous system. *Trends in Neurosciences*, **21**, 137–45.

Traynelis, S. F. and Wahl, P. (1997). Control of rat GluR6 glutamate receptor open probability by protein kinase A and calcineurin. *Journal of Physiology*, **503**, 513–31.

Traynelis, S. F., Silver, R. A., and Cull-Candy, S. G. (1993). Estimated conductance of glutamate receptor channels activated during EPSCs at the rat cerebellar mossy fiber-granule cell synapse. *Neuron*, **11**, 279–89.

Triller, A., Seitanidou, T., Franksson, O., and Korn, H. (1990). Size and shape of glycine receptor clusters in a central neuron exhibit a somato-dendritic gradient. *New Biology*, **2**, 637–41.

Trussell, L. O., Zhang, S., and Raman, I. M. (1993). Desensitization of AMPA receptors upon multiquantal neurotransmitter release. *Neuron*, **10**, 1185–96.

Tsubokawa, H. and Ross, W. N. (1996). IPSPs modulate spike backpropagation and associated $[Ca^{2+}]_{(i)}$ changes in the dendrites of hippocampal CA1 pyramidal neurons. *Journal of Neurophysiology*, **76**, 2896–906.

Walmsley, B., Alvarez, F. J., and Fyffe, R. E. (1998). Diversity of structure and function at mammalian central synapses. *Trends in Neurosciences*, **21**, 81–8.

Williams, K. (1993). Ifenprodil discriminates subtypes of the NMDA receptor: selectivity and mechanisms at recombinant heteromeric receptors. *Molecular Pharmacology*, **44**, 851–9.

Wyllie, D. J., Traynelis, S. F., and Cull-Candy, S. G. (1993). Evidence for more than one type of non-NMDA receptor in outside-out patches from cerebellar granule cells of the rat. *Journal of Physiology*, **463**, 193–226.

Wyllie, D. J., Behe, P., and Colquhoun, D. (1998). Single-channel activations and concentration jumps: comparison of recombinant NR1a/NR2A and NR1a/NR2D NMDA receptors. *Journal of Physiology*, **510**, 1–18.

Yamada, K. A. and Tang, C. M. (1993). Benzothiadiazides inhibit rapid glutamate receptor desensitization and enhance glutamatergic synaptic currents. *Journal of Neuroscience*, **13**, 3904–15.

Yoshimura, Y., Kimura, F., and Tsumoto, T. (1999). Estimation of single-channel conductance underlying synaptic transmission between pyramidal cells in the visual cortex. *Neuroscience*, **88**, 347–52.

6

Voltage-gated ion channels in dendrites

Jeffrey C. Magee
Louisiana State University Medical Center

Summary

This chapter focuses on the types and distributions of the main voltage-gated ion channels presently known to exist within the dendrites of CA1 pyramidal neurons, neocortical layer V pyramidal neurons, cerebellar Purkinje cells and olfactory bulb mitral cells. This is a rapidly expanding field so the focus of this chapter has been intentionally limited to these four different neuronal types because of the substantial amount of information available concerning voltage-gated channels in their dendrites, and because of the different forms of dendritic electrogenesis they exhibit. The chapter begins with a short survey of the known dendritic voltage-gated ion channel types and their modulation. A table comparing the physiologically-relevant biophysical properties and some pharmacology of these ion channels is also included. These sections are followed by a look at the distributions of these channels along the dendritic axis of the four cell types. Lastly, some current ideas on how dendritic voltage-gated channels might impact on the physiological functioning of these neurons are introduced.

Introduction

In most central neurons, incoming synaptic inputs are widely distributed across the full extent of complicated dendritic arborizations. The role of dendrites in the integration of such widespread synaptic activity has been the topic of much experimental and theoretical study (reviewed in Johnston *et al.* 1996; Yuste and Denk 1996). The fundamental importance of dendritic integration in the functioning of neurons has insured a continued interest in this issue. Recently, our understanding of the integrative properties of neuronal dendrites has been greatly expanded by the detailed characterizations of many dendritic voltage-gated ion channel populations. This new information has provided an improved appreciation of the factors involved in the coordination and transformation of incoming synaptic input within dendrites.

The voltage-gated ion channels present in dendrites

Na^+ channels

The fast inward current provided by Na^+ channels dramatically increases the excitability of dendrites allowing for the generation and propagation of action potentials as well as shaping of synaptic potentials. Dendritic Na^+ channels have many of the same biophysical and pharmacological characteristics reported for other neuronal TTX-sensitive channels (reviewed in Fozzard and Hanck 1996; Marban et al. 1998). Most of the channels ($\sim 70\%$) are available to be activated at a resting membrane potential (V_{rest}) of -70 mV and significant channel activation begins with depolarizations approximately 20 mV more depolarized than V_{rest}. These channels have rapid activation and inactivation kinetics and an underlying single channel conductance of approximately 15 pS (Huguenard et al. 1989; Stuart and Häusser 1994; Stuart and Sakmann 1994; Magee and Johnston 1995; Bischofberger and Jonas 1997).

Although most channel properties seem fairly uniform along the somato-dendritic axis, there is one key exception in CA1 (and perhaps neocortical) pyramidal neurons. In these cells, Na^+ channels from both the somatic and dendritic membrane possess a separate inactivation state that requires seconds instead of milliseconds for full recovery (Colbert et al. 1997; Jung et al. 1997). Interestingly, the fraction of channels that enter this slow inactivation state is much greater in dendrites compared to the soma, but the time for recovery from this inactivation near V_{rest} is similar in the dendrites and the soma (Colbert et al. 1997; Mickus et al. 1999). As will be discussed further below, the differences between the channel populations in the soma and dendrites appear to be the result of differing levels of phosphorylation (Colbert and Johnston 1998). Alternatively, there may be two separate channel types with different inactivation properties. Whatever the mechanism, this difference in Na^+ channel inactivation underlies the frequency-dependence of action potential back-propagation observed in pyramidal dendrites (Callaway and Ross 1995; Spruston et al. 1995).

The large majority of dendritic, as well as somatic, Na^+ channels are blocked by low concentrations of TTX (high nM range; Stuart and Häusser 1994; Stuart and Sakmann 1994; Magee and Johnston 1995; Bischofberger and Jonas 1997). Thus, in most respects these channels appear to be fairly standard neuronal TTX-sensitive Na^+ channels. There is, on the other hand, quite good evidence of a less standard, persistent Na^+ current in both neocortical pyramidal neurons and Purkinje cells (primarily localized in the somata of Purkinje cells). The evidence from these cells ranges from TTX-sensitive slow depolarizations recorded in somata to sophisticated channel models based on extensive voltage-clamp studies (reviewed in Llinás and Sugimori 1980; Strafstrom et al. 1985; Schwindt and Crill 1995; Crill 1996; Kay et al. 1998). There are less data available confirming the presence of a persistent Na^+ current in CA1 pyramidal neurons or mitral cells. Another type of non-standard Na^+ current is the 'resurgent' Na^+ current, that has been recently described in Purkinje cells (Raman and Bean 1997). Although this current is not likely to be present in the dendrites of Purkinje cells because of the very low density of Na^+ channels in the dendrites of these neurons (see 'Cerebellar Purkinje cells,' below), its presence and distribution in the dendrites of other cell types is not yet known.

Relative to other channel types, less is known about Na^+ channel modulation in general and this also applies to dendritic channels. Detailed studies have been limited to phosphorylation of dendritic Na^+ channels by Ca^{2+}-dependent protein kinase (PKC). While there have been reports of this reducing somatic current amplitude (Numann *et al.* 1991; Cantrell *et al.* 1996), the overwhelming impact of PKC activation on dendritic Na^+ channels is a speeding of the recovery from the prolonged inactivation state (Colbert and Johnston 1998). Increasing PKC activation reduces the drop-off of Na^+ current during 20 Hz trains from 65% to 25%, virtually eliminating the frequency-dependence of action potential backpropagation. Thus, in terms of action potential backpropagation PKC activation increases the overall excitability of dendrites.

A summary of the voltage-dependence and kinetics of activation and inactivation of Na^+ channels, and the major antagonists and modulators, is given in Table 6.1.

Ca^{2+} channels

The relatively slower, more prolonged inward current provided by voltage-gated Ca^{2+} channels further adds to the excitability of dendritic membrane allowing more prolonged single action potentials and bursts of multiple action potentials to occur (reviewed in Dunlap *et al.* 1995; Huguenard 1996). These channels also provide a pathway for Ca^{2+} influx in addition to agonist-gated influx. Ca^{2+} imaging studies and a variety of voltage-clamp recordings have found a mixture of several of the known types of Ca^{2+} channels (i.e., L-, N-, P/Q-, R-, and T-types) to be non-uniformly distributed throughout the dendrites of all neurons thus far tested.

T-type

A Ca^{2+} current and associated Ca^{2+} influx that begins activating at relatively hyperpolarized potentials has been found in several neuronal dendrites (Bindokas *et al.* 1993; Markram and Sakmann 1994; Magee and Johnston 1995; Magee *et al.* 1995; Kavalali *et al.* 1997; Mouginot *et al.* 1997). The corresponding low-voltage-activated (LVA) single channel activity has a small conductance (~ 9 pS) and a higher Ca^{2+}/Ba^{2+} permeability ratio (> 1) than other Ca^{2+} channel types (Magee and Johnston 1995; Kavalali *et al.* 1997; Mouginot *et al.* 1997). In 2 mM Ca^{2+}, the LVA channels begin activating near rest (> -70 mV) with relatively slow activation (~ 5 ms at 0 mV) and rapid inactivation kinetics (~ 30 ms at -60 mV; Kavalali *et al.* 1997; Mouginot *et al.* 1997; Magee, unpublished observations). Only a small fraction of the population is available at rest ($< 20\%$ at -70 mV, 2 mM $CaCl_2$), however, due to a hyperpolarized inactivation range (Kavalali *et al.* 1997; Mouginot *et al.* 1997; Magee, unpublished observations). Compared to other Ca^{2+} channels types, the LVA channels show uniquely slow deactivation kinetics ($\tau_{deact} = \sim 5$ ms at -60 mV; Magee and Johnston 1995; Kavalali *et al.* 1997). Displaying a somewhat distinctive pharmacology they have a high sensitivity to $NiCl_2$ ($IC_{50} \sim 25$ to 250 μM) as well as an nearly complete insensitivity to ω-conotoxin MVIIC and dihydropyridines (Magee and Johnston 1995; Avery and Johnston 1996; Kavalali *et al.* 1997). Together these properties strongly suggest that these are T-type Ca^{2+} channels.

Table 6.1 Channel properties.

Channel	Voltage dependence		Kinetics†			Pharm	Modulate
	Activation*	Inactivation**	Activation	Deactivation	Inactivation		
Na	>-45 mV	$\sim 70\%$	<1 ms	<1 ms	~ 1 ms	TTX	PKC
Ca_T	>-70 mV	$<20\%$	5 ms	~ 5 ms	25 ms	Ni^{2+}	?
Ca_L	>-60 mV	$\sim 100\%$	~ 1 ms	<1 ms	Minimal	Dihydrop.	PKA§
Ca_N	>-20 mV	$>70\%$§	~ 1 ms	<1 ms	50 ms	GVIA	G-protein
Ca_P	>-40 mV	$>90\%$§	~ 1 ms	<1 ms	100s of ms	Aga IVA	G-protein
Ca_R	>-40 mV	$>50\%$§	~ 1 ms	<1 ms	50 ms	Ni^{2+}	?
K_A	>-50 mV	$>70\%$	~ 1 ms	<1 ms	~ 7 ms	4-AP	Kinases
K_D	>-50 mV	$>70\%$	~ 1 ms	<1 ms	~ 20 ms	αDTX	Kinases§
K_S	>-30 mV	$\sim 100\%$	~ 3 ms	<1 ms	Minimal	TEA	Kinases§
H	<-50 mV	$\sim 100\%$	~ 50 ms‡	5 ms‡	None	ZD7288	cAMP, cGMP

*Potentials where channels start activating.
**Percentage of population available at -70 mV.
†Determined at 0, -60 and -20 mV, respectively at $\sim 22°$ C.
§Determined in non-dendritic preparation.
‡Determined at -80 and -45 mV at $35°$ C. See text for references.

L-type

The other more easily identified dendritic channel type is a large conductance, high-voltage activated (HVA) channel ($\sim$25 pS, in 110 Ba^{2+}) that mediates a sustained Ca^{2+} influx in a variety of dendrites (Bindokas *et al.* 1993; Bischofberger and Schild 1995; Christie *et al.* 1995; Magee and Johnston 1995; Markram *et al.* 1995; Magee *et al.* 1996; Kavalali *et al.* 1997). This is a relatively rapid activating ($\sim$1 ms at 0 mV) and deactivating current that due to a lack of voltage-dependent inactivation is quite prolonged. The single channel open time distributions are generally best fit by a double exponential function suggesting that there are two kinetically separable open states, one fast and the other slow ($\sim$0.5 and $\sim$3.0 ms; Magee and Johnston 1995; see also Marrion and Tavalin 1998). These channels are thought to be L-type Ca^{2+} channels because they have high sensitivity to dihydropyridines, a lower sensitivity to Ni^{2+} and are ω-conotoxin MVIIC-insensitive (Magee and Johnston 1995; Kavalali *et al.* 1997). In CA1 pyramidal neurons, the current carried by these channels begins activating near V_{rest} (>-60 mV) in 2 mM Ca^{2+} demonstrating that the HVA distinction applies only when high Ba^{2+} concentrations are used as a charge carrier (Avery and Johnston 1996; Magee *et al.* 1996). It is not clear if this is a unique feature of L-type channels in CA1 dendrites.

N-, P/Q- and R-types

The dendritic Ca^{2+} current that is neither a transient current activated at hyper-polarized potentials or a prolonged dihydropyridine-sensitive current is likely to be some mixture of N-, P/Q- and R-type Ca^{2+} channels (Usowicz *et al.* 1992; Bindokas *et al.* 1993; Bischofberger and Schild 1995; Christie *et al.* 1995; Magee and Johnston 1995; Markram *et al.* 1995; Kavalali *et al.* 1997; Isaacson and Strowbridge 1998). These high-voltage-activated (HVA) currents are mediated by rapidly activating (time to peak $\sim$1 ms at 0 mV) channels with unitary conductances around 15 pS (110 mM $BaCl_2$; Usowicz *et al.* 1992; Magee and Johnston 1995; Kavalali *et al.* 1997). They show a range of inactivation rates, with R-type being the most rapid and P-type showing very slow inactivation kinetics (Usowicz *et al.* 1992; Magee and Johnston 1995; Kavalali *et al.* 1997; see also Randall and Tsien 1997). The voltage ranges of activation for this group of channels are somewhat homogenous (P/Q and R-types start activating >-40 mV) with N-type channels perhaps having a relatively more depolarized activation range (start activating >-20 mV; Randall and Tsien 1997; Liu and Campbell 1998). These channels can be isolated based upon their pharmacology. P-type channels show a unique sensitivity to ω-Agatoxin-IVA, while N-types are highly sensitive to ω-conotoxin GVIA, and both are sensitive to ω-conotoxin MVIIC (Usowicz *et al.* 1992; Magee and Johnston 1995; Kavalali *et al.* 1997). The R-type Ca^{2+} channels do not appear to be sensitive to any of these toxins but do show a high sensitivity to Ni^{2+} (Magee and Johnston 1995; Kavalali *et al.* 1997).

Modulation

Several neuromodulators have been shown to inhibit dendritic Ca^{2+} channels in isolated dendrosomes of hippocampal neurons and action potential-induced Ca^{2+} influx into stratum pyramidale (Chen and Lambert 1997; Kavalali *et al.* 1997). In these studies, metabotropic glutamate, $GABA_B$, somatostatin, serotonin and adenosine receptor activation reduced the HVA Ca^{2+} current and associated Ca^{2+} influx by 12–50% of control. These are all G-protein mediated modulators and they seem to have their largest impact on dendritic N-type Ca^{2+} channels. In cultured mitral cells norepinephrine has been shown to reduce depolarization-induced dendritic Ca^{2+} influx via α_2-adrenoceptor activation while having less of an effect on somatic Ca^{2+} influx (Bischofberger and Schild 1995). This is presumably through the well described α_2 inhibition of N-type channels. T-type channels appear to be uniquely unmodulated, increasing their similarity with Na^+ channels. While there have been no direct studies of adrenoceptor modulation of dendritic L-type channels it would be expected, based on somatic studies, that β-receptor activation would also increase Ca^{2+} influx through these L-type channels (Fisher and Johnston 1990).

A summary of the voltage-dependence and kinetics of activation and inactivation of Ca^{2+} channels, and the major antagonists and modulators, is given in Table 6.1.

K^+ channels

K^+ channels are the main regulators of both dendritic and soma/axonal excitability. The wide variety of electrogenesis observed in central neurons is in large part the result of the wide variety of K^+ channels available (Storm 1990; Jan and Jan 1997; Mathie *et al.* 1998). Most but not necessarily all of the main types of K^+ channels have been found in neuronal dendrites.

Voltage-gated K^+ channels

Dendritic voltage-clamp recordings have revealed substantial outward current densities in several neuronal types. In CA1 and neocortical pyramidal neurons the outward current can be separated into two or three main components while only a single component appears to be present in mitral cells (Bischofberger and Jonas 1997; Hoffman *et al.* 1997; Bekkers and Stuart 1998). The first component is transient, showing rapid activation (~ 1 ms, apparently voltage independent) and inactivation kinetics (~ 5 ms and ~ 20 ms at -30 and $+30$ mV, respectively; Hoffman *et al.* 1997; see also Martina *et al.* 1998). The second is a sustained component that activates more slowly ($\tau_{act} > 2$ ms at -30 mV) and that shows very little if any voltage-dependent inactivation (Hoffman *et al.* 1997; see also Martina *et al.* 1998). Mitral cells do not appear to express the more rapidly activating and inactivating transient component but instead show currents that are more slowly activating and that inactivate over hundreds of milliseconds (Bischofberger and Jonas 1997). Steady-state activation and inactivation curves from CA1 pyramidal neurons indicate that the transient component begins activating with ~ 30 mV depolarizations from rest (-70 mV) while depolarizations of greater than 40 mV are required for activation of the sustained component (Hoffman *et al.* 1997). The outward current in mitral cell dendrites begins activating at about -50 mV (Bischofberger and Jonas 1997). Also, the voltage-range of activation for transient channels located in the distal dendrites of CA1 pyramidal neurons is shifted 10–15 mV hyperpolarized compared to that from the soma/proximal (up to 100 µm) dendrites (Hoffman *et al.* 1997).

In CA1 dendrites, a large fraction of the transient component had voltage-dependent and pharmacological properties (more sensitive to 4-AP than TEA with no H_2O_2 effect) that are most similar to those generally ascribed to a low-voltage activated, A-type K^+ current composed of Kv4 subunits (Hoffman *et al.* 1997; see also Martina *et al.* 1998). The sustained component has voltage-dependent and pharmacological properties (more sensitive to TEA than 4-AP) that are more similar to a delayed-rectifier-type K^+ current perhaps carried by Kv2 subunits. A small fraction of the transient component ($<20\%$) was dendrotoxin-sensitive (and low µM 4-AP sensitive) and thus could perhaps be characterized as a D-type current carried by Kv1 subunits (Hoffman *et al.* 1997; see also Martina *et al.* 1998). Purkinje cell dendrites appear to contain a current that more closely matches the slower inactivation kinetics commonly ascribed to D-type currents (Midtgaard *et al.* 1993). Three distinct types of single K^+ channel activity have been recorded in cell-attached mode from cultured Purkinje cell dendrites but this channel activity is not easily associated with the macroscopic currents described above (Gruol *et al.* 1991).

A summary of the voltage-dependence and kinetics of activation and inactivation of K^+ channels, and the major antagonists and modulators, is given in Table 6.1.

Ca^{2+}-dependent K^+ channels

The Ca^{2+}-dependent K^+ channel types are involved in action potential repolarization, the generation of different duration AHPs and spike frequency adaptation. In comparison to the voltage-gated K^+ channel types, there is relatively little is known about Ca^{2+}-dependent K^+ channels in the dendrites of central neurons (but see Andreasen and Lambert 1995*a*; Sah and Bekkers 1996; Schwindt and Crill 1997). There are, however, at least three different Ca^{2+}-dependent K^+ channel types that have been well characterized in neuronal somata (Storm 1987; reviewed in Sah 1996; Marrion and Tavalin 1998). The first is a large conductance channel (100–400 pS; BK), which has a substantial voltage-dependence along with its relatively low Ca^{2+} sensitivity (0.6–10 µM). A second, smaller conductance channel (5–20 pS; SK) has relatively little voltage-dependence and is more sensitive to Ca^{2+} (100–600 nM). A third channel type (I_{AHP}) apparently has an even smaller single-channel conductance (3–7 pS) and is activated by even lower concentrations of Ca^{2+} (exact sensitivity is undetermined). The time courses of the currents are variable with BK currents appearing most transiently, followed by SK and finally I_{AHP} which can be quite prolonged. BK channels are sensitive to charybdotoxin and low concentrations of TEA, while SK channels are primarily blocked by apamin. I_{AHP} is not blocked by apamin but is inhibited by high concentrations of TEA and a host of neuromodulators like norepinephrine.

Modulation

K^+ channel subunits contain numerous potential phosphorylation sites. Kv4.2; which is the most likely molecular identity of the transient K^+ current component in CA1 pyramidal neurons (Martina *et al.* 1998), has sites for PKA, PKC, CaM Kinase and MAP Kinase phosphorylation (Baldwin *et al.* 1991; Adams *et al.* 1997; Anderson *et al.* 1997). Recent evidence has shown that neuromodulator (β-adrenoceptor, dopamine and muscarinic) activation of PKA and PKC shift the voltage range of activation of the dendritic transient K^+ current component ~ 15 mV depolarized and increase the amplitude of dendritic action potentials (Hoffman and Johnston 1998, 1999). PKA and PKC activation do not significantly affect the sustained component. As with Na^+ channel modulation, kinase activation increases dendritic excitability in CA1 pyramidal neurons. From non-dendritic recordings we know that A-type K^+ channels are modulated or blocked by a wide variety of neurotransmitters and modulators (see Hoffman *et al.* 1998) and the presence of such easily modulated channels provide CA1 pyramidal neurons with a highly trans-formable excitability. Less is known about dendritic K^+ channel modulation in the other cell types.

Inwardly rectifying channels

Inwardly rectifying channels participate in setting the resting membrane potential as well as other basic membrane properties such as input resistance and membrane polarization rates (Holt and Eatock 1995; reviewed in Pape 1996). They also have been shown to have a large impact on the integration of synaptic activity (Magee 1998, 1999; Schwindt and Crill 1998; Stuart and Spruston 1998). In the soma and apical dendrites of hippocampal CA1 pyramidal neurons membrane hyperpolariza-tions evoke inward currents that are slowly activating and deactivating and virtually non-inactivating. Activation curves demonstrate that a significant fraction ($\sim 25\%$) of this hyperpolarization-activated current (I_h) is active near rest and that the voltage range of activation is relatively more hyperpolarized in the distal dendrites (similar to the shift observed for dendritic A-type K^+ channels). As with other I_h types, dendritic I_h demonstrated a mixed Na^+–K^+ conductance that was sensitive to low concentrations of external CsCl and the bradycardic agent ZD7288 (Gasparini and DiFrancesco 1997; Magee 1998). It appears that I_h channels with similar properties are found in the dendrites of both neocortical pyramidal neurons and cerebellar Purkinje cells (Häusser and Clark 1997; Schwindt and Crill 1997; Stuart and Spruston 1998).

While there have not been any direct recordings to date of K_{ir}-type currents from mammalian dendrites there is sufficient indirect evidence to suggest their presence. From somatic recordings we know that these currents are K^+ selective, begin activating around V_{rest} with rapid activation kinetics and show little if any inactivation (Holt and Eatock 1995). These channels are in general sensitive to low concentrations of $BaCl_2$ and many dendritic electrical properties are likewise Ba^{2+}-sensitive (Magee 1999).

Modulation

The I_h activation range is very sensitive to intracellular cAMP and cGMP activities and has been shown in a variety of non-dendritic preparations to be modulated by many neurotransmitters and modulators (Pape 1996). Increases in cAMP or cGMP (such as during β-adrenoceptor activation or application of nitric oxide) shift the activation curve in a depolarized direction increasing the amount of I_h channel activation present at V_{rest}. Decreases in cyclic nucleotides have the opposite effect. An increase in resting I_h activation with increased intracellular cAMP concentrations has been observed in CA1 dendrites (Magee, unpublished observations).

A summary of the voltage-dependence and kinetics of activation and inactivation of I_h channels, and the major antagonists and modulators, is given in Table 6.1.

Subcellular channel distributions

Because voltage-gated ion channels are differentially distributed across the plasma membranes of various neurons, the integrative properties and firing behavior of central neurons vary greatly from cell type to cell type. As examples of this diversity, we examine in detail a few representative neurons which display distinctly different types of electrical signaling and for which there is substantial evidence concerning the dendritic distribution of voltage-gated ion channels. The discussion below is presented in a qualitative manner because methodological differences among the various studies make it difficult to directly compare the specific channel densities.

Hippocampal CA1 pyramidal neurons

Cell-attached patch-clamp recordings from CA1 pyramidal neurons have indicated that Na^+ channel density is maintained at a fairly constant density from the axon initial segment to $\sim 330\ \mu m$ (total dendritic length is about 550 μm) into the dendritic field (Magee and Johnston 1995; Colbert and Johnston 1996; Fig. 6.1a). These data fit well with the recording of TTX-sensitive dendritic action potentials and correlated Ca^{2+} influx (Wong *et al.* 1979; Richardson *et al.* 1987; Herreras 1990; Turner *et al.* 1991; Jaffe *et al.* 1992; Colling and Wheal 1994; Spruston *et al.* 1995; Mackenzie and Murphy 1998). In spite of this uniform Na^+ channel density, the dendritic propagation of action potentials is less robust and the dendritic threshold for action potential initiation is higher than in the axonal regions of the neurons (Magee and Johnston 1997; Golding and Spruston 1998; Mackenzie and Murphy 1998). As discussed further below (see 'Relative Na^+-, K^+-channel densities and action potential backpropagation'), the presence of dendritic K^+ channels is thought to be partly responsible for this situation.

The other main inwardly conducting channel types, Ca^{2+} channels, also seem to be maintained at a fairly constant density (although substantially lower than Na^+ channels) from the soma to 350 μm into the apical dendrites (Magee and Johnston 1995; Fig. 6.1b). While this is true for the total Ca^{2+} current, voltage-clamp recordings and fluorescence imaging studies suggest that the particular sub-types of dendritic Ca^{2+} channels present change with distance from the soma (Christie *et al.* 1995; Magee and Johnston 1995). The Ca^{2+} current of the more proximal regions of the cell appears to be carried predominately by L-type and N-type channels while the Ni^{2+}-sensitive channel types (T- and R-types) appear to play a more dominant role in the more distal regions of the cell (Christie *et al.* 1995; Magee and Johnston 1995; Kavalali *et al.* 1997). A substantial density of N- and P/Q-types has been reported in isolated dendritic segments (Kavalali *et al.* 1997).

While the inward conducting channel types appear to be maintained at a relatively constant density along the dendritic axis, the total outward current density is not. The recorded density of the transient K^+ current component increases linearly with distance from the soma to a density that is more than fivefold higher at $\sim 350\ \mu m$ into the apical dendrites (Hoffman *et al.* 1997; Fig. 6.2a). The current density of the sustained component, however, remains relatively constant (Hoffman *et al.* 1997;

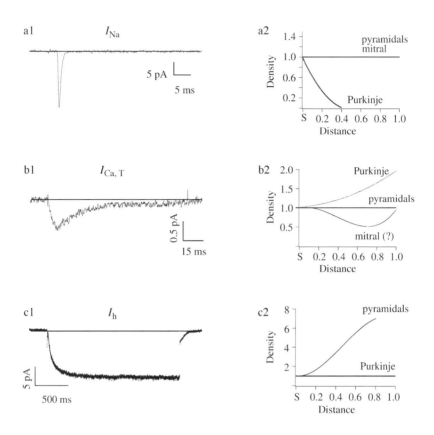

Fig. 6.1   Inward currents in dendrites. (a1–c1) Representative Na$^+$ current (a1), T-type Ca^{2+} current (b1) and hyperpolarization-activated current (c1) recorded in cell-attached patch mode from CA1 pyramidal dendrites. (a2–c2). Schematized plots of approximate channel densities for the four representative cell types. Hypothesized channel density is plotted relative to the somatic density as a function of relative distance from the soma. The maximal distance (1.0) is equal to the maximum length of the dendritic arbor for each cell type. Na$^+$ current (a1) is the average of 10 traces evoked by step depolarizations from –90 to –10 mV. T-type Ca^{2+} current is the average of 30 traces evoked by step depolarizations from –90 to –60 mV in 2.5 mM CaCl$_2$. Ca^{2+} current density plot in b2 is the total composite Ca^{2+} current comprising all channel sub-types. The highly preliminary Ca^{2+} current density in mitral cells is denoted by (?). I_h in (c1) is an average of five traces evoked by step hyperpolarizations from –50 to –110 mV in 110 mM KCl. No data are available for I_h in mitral cells.

Fig. 6.2b). Thus, total outward current density increases dramatically with distance away from the soma.

Ca^{2+}-dependent K$^+$ currents have not been directly recorded from CA1 pyramidal dendrites at this time so it is impossible to be quantitative about their densities. However, we can infer from more indirect data that the density of these channels is very low in more distal regions of the dendrites (Fig. 6.2c). Voltage recordings of more distal dendritic action potentials rarely show any substantial after-hyperpolarizations (AHP), even though a significant Ca^{2+} influx

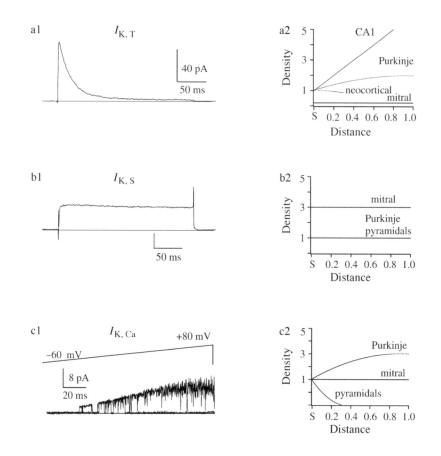

Fig. 6.2 Outward currents in dendrites. (a1–c1). Representative transient K^+ current (a1), sustained K^+ current (b1) and putative Ca^{2+}-dependent K^+ current (c1) recorded in cell-attached patch mode from CA1 pyramidal dendrites. (a2–c2) Schematized plots of approximate channel densities for the four representative cell types. Hypothesized channel density is plotted as in Fig. 6.1. Transient K^+ current (a1) is the average of 30 traces evoked by step depolarizations from –90 to + 50 mV. Available data for neocortical pyramidal neurons is limited to proximal third of arbor (a2). Sustained K^+ current (b1) is the average of 30 traces evoked by step depolarizations from –90 to + 50 mV from the same patch as in (a1) using standard subtraction procedures (Hoffman *et al.* 1997). Available data for neocortical pyramidal neurons is again limited to proximal third of arbor (b2). Putative Ca^{2+}-dependent K^+ current (c1) is two superimposed traces evoked by ramp depolarizations from –60 to + 80 mV. This current was recorded from the proximal dendrite of a two-week-old rat.

can be recorded (Wong and Stewart 1992; Andreasen and Lambert 1995*b*; Spruston *et al.* 1995; Magee and Johnston 1997; Tsubokawa and Ross 1997; Poolos and Johnston 1999; but see Andreasen and Lambert 1995*a*). Furthermore, any AHP that is present in the dendrites is more sensitive to I_h channel blockers than apamin, charybdotoxin or high BAPTA concentrations (Tsubokawa and Ross 1997; Magee 1998; Poolos and Johnston 1999). Again these data suggest that the channels underlying Ca^{2+}-dependent AHPs are in low density in the dendrites compared to the somatic compartment where large AHPs are generated. Finally, BK and SK channels have been shown to co-localize with N- and L-type Ca^{2+} channels, respectively, in CA1 pyramidal neurons and in other neuronal preparations (Sah 1996; Marrion and Tavalin 1998). The relatively lower N- and L-type channel densities present in the more distal dendrites may explain why BK and SK channel activity is hard to find in CA1 pyramidal dendrites.

Like the transient K^+ component, I_h density increases dramatically with distance out the apical dendrites. In CA1 pyramidal neurons I_h density has been observed to increase nearly sevenfold from soma to 350 μm distal (Magee 1998; Fig. 6.1c). This observation is supported by multiple reports of an elevated membrane sag during dendritic hyperpolarizations (a classic hallmark of I_h; Andreasen and Lambert 1995*b*; Tsubokawa and Ross 1996; Magee 1998; Tsubokawa *et al.* 1999). These regional differences can be removed by I_h blockade. Similar indirect data is all that is currently available for inwardly-rectifying K^+ currents. Recently, low concentrations of $BaCl_2$ (100 μM) have been shown to have a larger impact on the input resistance and the membrane kinetics of dendrites compared to that of the soma (Magee, unpublished observations). Although these data are certainly less than conclusive, they suggest that the density of K_{ir} could also increase with distance away from the soma.

Neocortical layer V pyramidal neurons

TTX-sensitive Na^+ currents have been recorded at a fairly constant density from the soma to ∼500 μm (just short of the distal tuft) in neocortical pyramidal neurons (Stuart and Sakmann 1994; Fig. 6.1a). Neocortical neurons also show frequency-dependent backpropagation (Stuart *et al.* 1997) and this phenomenon has been shown to be dependent on the prolonged Na^+ channel inactivation discussed above (Colbert *et al.* 1997; Jung *et al.* 1997). Thus the distribution of dendritic Na^+ channels in neocortical pyramidal neurons appears to be similar to that reported for CA1 pyramidal neurons. Evidence for the presence of Ca^{2+} channels (T, N, P/Q as well as L-type) has also been found along the entire dendritic arbor of neocortical neurons, including the distal tuft and spines (Markram *et al.* 1995; Schiller *et al.* 1998; Fig. 6.1b). While there have been no direct quantitative measures of relative current density, there is enough Ca^{2+} current present in even the most distal regions of neocortical dendrites to generate Ca^{2+}-dependent action potentials (Schiller *et al.* 1997).

In contrast to CA1 pyramidal neurons, there is no evidence of an increasing density of K^+ channels in neocortical pyramidal neurons. At present cell-attached patch recordings have shown that transient and sustained K^+ current components can be recorded from dendrites (recordings have been made out to 300 μm) and that, at this point, the composite density decreases with distance from the soma (Bekkers and Stuart 1998; Figs 6.2a,b). This is a substantial difference in channel complement (compared with CA1 pyramidal neurons) that should greatly influence the backpropagation of action potentials into the arbors of neocortical pyramidal neurons.

Ca^{2+}-dependent K^+ currents have not been directly recorded from dendrites of neocortical pyramidal neurons. Here again though, we can infer from more indirect data that the density of these channels is very low in the more distal regions of the dendrites (but see Schwindt and Crill 1997; Fig. 6.2c). As with CA1 pyramidal neurons dendritic action potentials rarely show AHPs that are anywhere near the amplitude recorded from the soma (Stuart and Sakmann 1994; Schiller *et al.* 1997; Stuart *et al.* 1997). These data suggest that the channels underlying AHPs are lower in density in the dendrites than in the somatic compartment.

Like CA1 pyramidal neurons there is solid evidence that I_h channels are present in the dendritic arbors of neocortical pyramidal neurons (Schwindt and Crill 1997; Stuart and Spruston 1998). In fact, an elevated dendritic I_h density was required for a realistic neuronal model to match whole-cell data recorded from the soma and dendrites (Stuart and Spruston 1998; Fig. 6.1c). Finally a Ba^{2+}-sensitive voltage-dependent inward rectification has been observed in isolated neocortical dendrites (Takigawa and Alzheimer 1998). This rectification is thought to be the result of dendritic inward rectifying K^+ channels. With one major exception the voltage-gated ion channel complements are very similar between the two types of pyramidal neurons. As will be discussed below, however, the differences in K^+ channel density should greatly effect the ability of these channels to regulate action potential backpropagation in these two cell types.

Cerebellar Purkinje cells

Purkinje cells have a substantially different distribution of voltage-gated ion channels than the pyramidal neurons discussed above. The most prominent difference is that the Na^+ channel density has been shown, by a variety of methods, to drop off rapidly with distance from the soma (Lev Ram *et al.* 1992; Stuart and Häusser 1994; Callaway and Ross 1997; Fig. 6.1a). This situation determines that Na^+-dependent action potentials initiated in the soma-axonal region do not actively propagate into the dendrites (Llinás and Sugimori 1979; Llinás and Sugimori 1980; Stuart and Häusser 1994; Callaway *et al.* 1995). This does not, however, mean that Purkinje dendrites are incapable of active electrogenesis. In fact, dendritic recordings and imaging studies have shown Ca^{2+}-dependent action potentials and associated dendritic Ca^{2+} influx that are TTX-insensitive (Llinás and Sugimori 1979; Llinás and Sugimori 1980; Lev Ram *et al.* 1992; Midtgaard *et al.* 1993; Callaway *et al.* 1995). These studies demonstrated that although Purkinje dendrites are relatively devoid of voltage-gated Na^+ channels, they contain a substantial density of voltage-gated Ca^{2+} channels (Fig. 6.1b). Later studies revealed that the Ca^{2+} channels located in the arbor are mainly P- and T-type Ca^{2+} channels (Usowicz *et al.* 1992; Bindokas *et al.* 1993; Mouginot *et al.* 1997; Watanabe *et al.* 1998). The T channels are capable of generating a highly localized Ca^{2+} influx in response to subthreshold synaptic activity, while both channel types (although P-type channels play the predominate role) are involved in the large Ca^{2+} influx associated with dendritic Ca^{2+} action potentials. It has been hypothesized that the dendritic Ca^{2+} channel density may be elevated when compared to that of the soma, especially in localized areas where there may be 'hotspots' of particularly high Ca^{2+} channel density (Llinás and Sugimori 1980; Jaeger *et al.* 1997).

Dendritic Ca^{2+} spiking in these cells is terminated by a prominent AHP that is presumably generated by a high density of Ca^{2+}-dependent K^+ channels located throughout the dendrite (Llinás and Sugimori 1980; Jaeger *et al.* 1997; Fig. 6.2c). The available evidence suggest that delayed rectifier-like K^+ channels (or a sustained voltage-gated component similar to that described above) are primarily located in the somatic and proximal dendritic regions where they are involved in the fast spike repolarization. The more distal dendritic regions appear to contain a high density of a 4-AP sensitive (mM) outward current (perhaps similar to the transient component described above but with slower inactivation kinetics) that plays an important role in the regulation of dendritic Ca^{2+} spiking (Midtgaard *et al.* 1993; Midtgaard 1994; Jaeger *et al.* 1997; Watanabe *et al.* 1998).

From voltage recordings of approximately similar hyperpolarization-induced membrane potential 'sag', there appears to be a uniform density of I_h in the somatic and dendritic compartments (Häusser and Clark 1997; Fig. 6.1c). Little information is available concerning the distribution of inwardly rectifying K^+ currents in the dendrites on Purkinje cells.

In summary, in part because of a low density of dendritic Na^+ channels action potentials do not actively backpropagate into Purkinje cell dendrites. Instead, slowly inactivating Ca^{2+} channel types in the dendrites provide a prolonged inward current that generates Ca^{2+} spikes which are terminated once the intracellular Ca^{2+} concentration becomes sufficiently elevated to activate Ca^{2+}-dependent K^+ channels. The threshold voltages required for the generation of these dendritic Ca^{2+} spikes may be regulated by a transient outward current located in the dendrites themselves. This type of dendritic electrogenesis contrasts sharply with that of the pyramidal cell types discussed above.

Olfactory bulb mitral cells

These cells represent yet another class of dendritic electroresponsivity that is the result of a different voltage-gated ion channel complement and distribution. Like the pyramidal neurons discussed above, mitral cells have a constant Na^+ channel density along the somato-dendritic axis (Bischofberger and Jonas 1997; Fig. 6.1a). Unlike the pyramidal neurons, the K^+ channel density (which is comparatively quite high) is primarily composed of slower activating and inactivating currents (similar to the sustained K^+ component discussed above), that are also maintained at a constant density along the entire recorded dendrite (Bischofberger and Jonas 1997; Fig. 6.2(a,b)). Because of the slow activation kinetics of these currents, action potential amplitude is relatively insensitive to K^+ channel blockade while the duration is prolonged. The voltage-gated Na^+–K^+ channel complement and density of both the somatic and dendritic compartments of mitral cells is similar to that of CA1 pyramidal somata. Although Ca^{2+}-dependent K^+ currents have not been directly recorded, the presence of similarly sized fast AHPs in both the soma and dendritic recordings suggest that the density of these channels is also uniform throughout mitral cells (Bischofberger and Jonas 1997; Chen *et al.* 1997; Isaacson and Strowbridge 1998; Fig. 6.2c). The presence of N-type Ca^{2+} channels in mitral cell dendrites (see below) supports the idea that these channels (BK type) are co-localized.

There appears to be an inhomogeneous distribution of Ca^{2+} channel subtypes in these neurons. Imaging data from cultured mitral cells suggested that the density of L-type channels is restricted to the proximal regions of the cell, while N-type channels are distributed throughout the arborization (Bischofberger and Schild 1995;

Isaacson and Strowbridge 1998). Additional studies have shown that P/Q-types are also found along with N-type Ca^{2+} channels in the dendrites and that these channels play an important role in dendro-dendritic inhibition in the olfactory bulb (Isaacson and Strowbridge 1998). There is no evidence of T-type Ca^{2+} channels in mitral cell dendrites. Finally, action potential-evoked Ca^{2+} signals have been reported to decrease with distance from the soma in the primary and lateral dendrites until the distal tuft region where influx appears to increase back to somatic levels (Isaacson and Strowbridge 1998). This preliminary data suggests that Ca^{2+} channel density may be lower in the non-tuft regions of the dendritic arbor of mitral cells (Fig. 6.1b).

Location-dependent channel modulation

While there is no reason to suspect that specific channel types are differentially modulated depending on their location within the cell, the non-uniformity of channel densities suggest that similar location-dependent differences in receptor types and associated second messenger systems may exist. In fact, Na^+ channels, the transient K^+ component, N-type Ca^{2+} channels and I_h channels all seem to be differentially modulated along the somato-dendritic axis (Bischofberger and Schild 1995; Hoffman *et al.* 1997; Colbert and Johnston 1998; Magee 1998). For dendritic Na^+ and A-type channels there seems to be less PKC-dependent and PKA-dependent phosphorylation, respectively (Colbert and Johnston 1998; Hoffman and Johnston 1998). For dendritic I_h there seems to be less cAMP-dependent channel modulation, through what is thought to be a direct modulation by cAMP (Magee 1998). One cannot, however, rule out less PKA-dependent phosphorylation here also, as the exact mechanism of cAMP modulation of I_h has not been convincingly established (Pape 1996). Therefore, all three of these channel types could be in a relatively less phosphorylated state. This may be indicative of an elevated dendritic phosphatase activity or lower concentrations of other second messengers (e.g. cAMP). Although such a situation may be somewhat of an over-simplification, given the diversity and complexity of modulatory mechanisms, large regional differences in basal channel modulatory state do appear to exist in CA1 pyramidal neurons.

Relative Na$^+$-, K$^+$-channel densities and action potential backpropagation

Most action potential properties, such as threshold, amplitude, duration, and repetitive firing characteristics, are determined by the relative densities of inward (Na^+ and Ca^{2+}) and outward (K^+) currents located within the membrane. As discussed above this important ratio is quite variable among the dendrites of the different neurons (see Fig. 6.3a).

In mitral cells the ratio is relatively high (more Na^+ than fast K^+) and is maintained at a constant level along the entire somato-dendritic axis (Fig. 6.3a). As a result, a large amplitude action potential (peaking near E_{Na}), reminiscent of the traditional 'all-or-none' axonal action potential, is constantly maintained throughout most regions of the cell (Bischofberger and Jonas 1997; Chen *et al.* 1997;

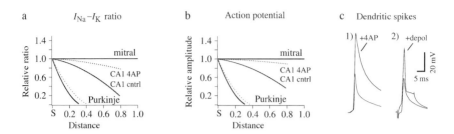

Fig. 6.3   Channel complements shape the pattern of action potential backpropagation. (a1) Schematized Na^+–K^+ (fast activating) current density ratios as a function of distance for the three representative cell types. Plotted as in Figs 6.1 and 6.2. Dashed lines represents the presumed ratios during the blockade of the transient K^+ current (4-AP), with the only significant effect being on the ratio of CA1 cells. (b) Schematized action potential amplitude as a function of distance for four representative cell types. Plotted as in (a). Dashed lines represent the presumed amplitudes during the blockade of the transient K^+ current (4-AP), with the only significant effect again being on the amplitude of CA1 cells. (c1) Dendritic action potentials recorded from CA1 dendrite under control conditions and in the presence of 5 mM 4-AP. (c2). Dendritic action potentials recorded from CA1 dendrite under control conditions and when paired with depolarizing ($\sim$15 mV) current injection. Both manipulations increase action potential amplitude by presumably decreasing dendritic K^+ current density.

Isaacson and Strowbridge 1998; Fig. 6.3b). Because this large amplitude action potential already peaks near E_{Na} and the density of fast K^+ channels is low, these spikes should propagate with a high safety factor and have very little possibility of amplitude modulation.

Purkinje cells lie at the other end of the spectrum. In these cells the Na^+–K^+ current density ratio declines very rapidly with distance from the soma as a result of a rapidly decreasing Na^+ channel density (see Fig. 6.3a). Thus Na^+-dependent action potentials are not capable of actively propagating any significant distance into Purkinje cell dendrites and consequently spike amplitude drops off quickly (Llinás and Sugimori 1979; Llinás and Sugimori 1980; Stuart and Häusser 1994; Callaway *et al.* 1995; see Fig. 6.3b). In this case action potential amplitude is quite small in the more distal regions and because of the lack of Na^+ channels is virtually unchangeable. On the other hand, the Ca^{2+}-dependent action potential plays a prominent role in Purkinje cell dendrites and its generation and propagation is accordingly regulated by dendritic K^+ channels (Midtgaard *et al.* 1993).

Hippocampal CA1 pyramidal neurons lie somewhere in the middle of this spectrum. Like Purkinje neurons, there is a large shift from an inward dominated current ratio in the proximal regions to one that is predominantly fast outward current in the more distal regions (see Fig. 6.3a). Unlike Purkinje neurons, however, the reason for this shift is the large increase in dendritic transient outward current instead of a decrease in dendritic Na^+ channel density. Because of this the inward current required for the generation of large amplitude action potentials is always available and any substances which modulate the transient K^+ component will greatly effect the amplitude of the backpropagating spike (see above; see Fig. 6.3b). Additionally, because A-type K^+ channels exhibit rapid voltage-dependent inactivation at potentials near V_{rest}, moderate depolarization (as could be provided by synaptic activity) can rapidly reduce the available K_A channel population. In this scheme, synaptically active regions of the dendrite will be released from the dampening effect of the high A-channel density and large amplitude action potentials will be generated (Hoffman *et al.* 1997; Kamondi *et al.* 1997; Magee and Johnston 1997; Magee *et al.* 1998; Fig. 6.3c).

These three different types of neuron represent three distinct forms of dendritic action potential backpropagation. Mitral cell dendrites propagate (and initiate) full amplitude, all-or-none action potentials. Purkinje neurons do not generate any form of dendritic Na^+-dependent spikes, but instead generate large amplitude Ca^{2+} spikes. Finally, in neocortical and CA1 pyramidal neurons action potential backpropagation is decremental and readily modulated. These distinct forms of action potential backpropagation are in part the direct result of differences in dendritic voltage-gated ion channel complements and densities.

Concluding remarks

The intent of this chapter is to provide some detailed characteristics of the known voltage-gated ion channels in the dendritic arborizations of a few central neurons. The presence of this wide variety of channels, and their potential for modulation, undoubtably increases the diversity and complexity of dendritic function. The size of this chapter is certain to grow rapidly in the coming years as other channel and neuronal types are investigated. These investigations are sure to produce information that will continue to alter our fundamental understanding of neuronal function.

Acknowledgements

I would like to thank Bill Ross and Dan Johnston for helpful comments on the manuscript.

References

Adams, J. P., Anderson, A. E., Johnston, D., Pfaffinger, P. J., and Sweatt, J. D. (1997). Kv4.2: a novel substrate for MAP kinase phosphorylation. *Society of Neuroscience Abstract*, **23**, 1176.

Andreasen, M. and Lambert, J. D. C. (1995a). The excitability of CA1 pyramidal cell dendrites is modulated by a local Ca^{2+}-dependent K^+-conductance. *Brain Research*, **698**, 193–203.

Andreasen, M. and Lambert, J. D. C. (1995b). Regenerative properties of pyramidal cell dendrites in area CA1 of the rat hippocampus. *Journal of Physiology*, **483**, 421–41.

Anderson, A. E., Adams, J. P., Swann, J. W., Johnston, D., Pfaffinger, P. J., and Sweatt, J. D. (1997). Kv4.2; a fast transient A-type potassium channel is a substrate for PKA and PKC. *Society of Neuroscience Abstract*, **23**, 1394.

Avery, R. B. and Johnston, D. (1996). Multiple channel types contribute to the low-voltage-activated calcium current in hippocampal CA3 pyramidal neurons. *Journal of Neuroscience*, **16**, 5567–82.

Baldwin, T. J., Tsaur, M.-L., Lopez, G. A., and Jan, L. Y. (1991). Characterization of a mammalian cDNA for an inactivating voltage-sensitive K$^+$ channel. *Neuron*, **7**, 471–83.

Bekkers, J. M. and Stuart, G. (1998). Distribution and properties of K$^+$ channels in the soma and apical dendrites of layer 5 cortical pyramidal neurons. *Society of Neuroscience Abstract*, **24**, 2019.

Bindokas, V. P., Brorson, J. R., and Miller, R. J. (1993). Characteristics of voltage sensitive calcium channels in dendrites of cultured rat cerebellar neurons. *Neuropharmacology*, **32**, 1213–20.

Bischofberger, J. and Jonas, P. (1997). Action potential propagation into the presynaptic dendrites of rat mitral cells. *Journal of Physiology*, **504**, 359–65.

Bischofberger, J. and Schild, D. (1995). Different spatial patterns of [Ca^{2+}] increase caused by N- and L-type Ca^{2+} channel activation in frog olfactory bulb neurones. *Journal of Physiology*, **487**, 305–87.

Callaway, J. C. and Ross, W. N. (1995). Frequency-dependent propagation of sodium action potentials in dendrites of hippocampal CA1 pyramidal neurons. *Journal of Neurophysiology*, **74**, 1395–403.

Callaway, J. C. and Ross, W. N. (1997). Spatial distribution of synaptically activated sodium concentration changes in cerebellar Purkinje neurons. *Journal of Neurophysiology*, **77**, 145–52.

Callaway, J. C., Lasser-Ross, N., and Ross, W. N. (1995). IPSPs strongly inhibit climbing fiber-activated [Ca^{2+}]$_i$ increases in the dendrites of cerebellar Purkinje neurons. *Journal of Neuroscience*, **15**, 2777–87.

Cantrell, A. R., Ma, J. Y., Scheuer, T., and Catterall, W. A. (1996). Muscarinic modulation of sodium current by activation of protein kinase C in rat hippocampal neurons. *Neuron*, **16**, 1019-26.

Chen, H. and Lambert, N. A. (1997). Inhibition of dendritic calcium influx by activation of G-protein-coupled receptors in the hippocampus. *Journal of Neurophysiology*, **78**, 3484–8.

Chen, W. R., Midtgaard, J., and Shepherd, G. M. (1997). Forward and backward propagation of dendritic impulses and their synaptic control in mitral cells. *Science*, **278**, 463–7.

Christie, B. R., Eliot, L. S., Ito, K., Miyakawa, H., and Johnston, D. (1995). Different Ca^{2+} channels in soma and dendrites of hippocampal pyramidal neurons mediate spike-induced Ca^{2+} influx. *Journal of Neurophysiology*, **73**, 2553–7.

Colbert, C. M. and Johnston, D. (1996). Axonal action-potential initiation and Na$^+$ channel densities in the soma and axon initial segment of subicular pyramidal neurons. *Journal of Neuroscience*, **16**, 6676–86.

Colbert, C. M. and Johnston, D. (1998). Protein kinase C activation decreases activity-dependent attenuation of dendritic Na$^+$ current in hippocampal CA1 pyramidal neurons. *Journal of Neurophysiology*, **79**, 491–5.

Colbert, C. M., Magee, J. C., Hoffman, D. A., and Johnston, D. (1997). Slow recovery from inactivation of Na$^+$ channels underlies the activity-dependent attenuation of dendritic action potentials in hippocampal CA1 pyramidal neurons. *Journal of Neuroscience*, **17**, 6512–21.

Colling, S. B. and Wheal, H. V. (1994). Fast sodium action potentials are generated in the distal apical dendrites of rat hippocampal CA1 pyramidal cells. *Neuroscience Letters*, **172**, 73–6.

Crill, W. E. (1996). Persistent sodium current in mammalian central neurons. *Annual Review of Physiology*, **58**, 349–62.

Dunlap, K., Luebke, J. I., and Turner, T. J. (1995). Exocytotic Ca^{2+} channels in mammalian central neurons. *Trends in Neurosciences*, **18**, 89–98.

Fisher, R. E. and Johnston, D. (1990). Differential modulation of single voltage-gated calcium channels by cholinergic and adrenergic agonists in adult hippocampal neurons. *Journal of Neurophysiology*, **64**, 1291–302.

Fozzard, H. A. and Hanck, D. A. (1996). Structure and function of voltage-dependent sodium channels: comparison of brain II and cardiac isoforms. *Physiological Reviews*, **76**, 887–926.

Gasparini, S. and DiFrancesco, D. (1997). Action of the hyperpolarization-activated current (I_h) blocker ZD 7288 in hippocampal CA1 neurons. *Pflügers Archive*, **435**, 99–106.

Golding, N. L. and Spruston, N. (1998). Dendritic sodium spikes are variable triggers of axonal action potentials in hippocampal CA1 pyramidal neurons. *Neuron*, **21**, 1189–200.

Gruol, D. L., Jacquin, T., and Yool, A. J. (1991). Single-channel K^+ currents recorded from the somatic and dendritic regions of cerebellar Purkinje neurons in culture. *Journal of Neuroscience*, **11**, 1002–15.

Häusser, M. and Clark, B. A. (1997). Tonic synaptic inhibition modulates neuronal output pattern and spatiotemporal synaptic integration. *Neuron*, **19**, 665–78.

Herreras, O. (1990). Propagating dendritic action potential mediates synaptic transmission in CA1 pyramidal cells in situ. *Journal of Neurophysiology*, **64**, 1429–41.

Hoffman, D. A. and Johnston, D. (1998). Downregulation of transient K^+ channels in dendrites of hippocampal CA1 pyramidal neurons by activation of PKA and PKC. *Journal of Neuroscience*, **18**, 3521–8.

Hoffman, D. A. and Johnston, D. (1999). Neuromodulation of dendritic action potentials. *Journal of Neurophysiology*, **81**, 408–11.

Hoffman, D. A., Magee, J. C., Colbert, C., and Johnston, D. (1997). K^+ channel regulation of signal propagation in dendrites of hippocampal pyramidal neurons. *Nature*, **387**, 869–75.

Holt, J. R. and Eatock, R. A. (1995). Inwardly rectifying currents of saccular hair cells from the leopard frog. *Journal of Neurophysiology*, **73**, 1484–502.

Huguenard, J. R. (1996). Low-threshold calcium currents in central nervous system neurons. *Annual Review of Physiology*, **58**, 329–48.

Huguenard, J. R., Hamill, O. P., and Prince, D. A. (1989). Sodium channels in dendrites of rat cortical pyramidal neurons. *Proceedings of the National Academy of Science USA*, **86**, 2473–7.

Isaacson, J. S. and Strowbridge, B. W. (1998). Olfactory reciprocal synapses: dendritic signaling in the CNS. *Neuron*, **20**, 749–61.

Jaeger, D., De Schutter, E., and Bower, J. M. (1997). The role of synaptic and voltage-gated currents in the control of Purkinje cell spiking: a modeling study. *Journal of Neuroscience*, **17**, 91–106.

Jaffe, D. B., Johnston, D., Lasser-Ross, N., Lisman, J. E., Miyakawa, H., and Ross, W. N. (1992). The spread of Na^+ spikes determines the pattern of dendritic Ca^{2+} entry into hippocampal neurons. *Nature*, **357**, 244–6.

Jan, L. Y. and Jan, Y. N. (1997). Voltage-gated and inwardly rectifying potassium channels. *Journal of Physiology*, **505**, 267–82.

Johnston, D., Magee, J. C., Colbert, C., and Christie, B. R. (1996). Active properties of neuronal dendrites. *Annual Review of Neuroscience*, **19**, 165–86.

Jung, H.-Y., Mickus, T., and Spruston, N. (1997). Prolonged Na^+ channel inactivation contributes to dendritic action potential attenuation in hippocampal pyramidal neurons. *Journal of Neuroscience*, **17**, 6639–46.

Kamondi, A., Acsady, L., and Buzsáki, G. (1998). Dendritic spikes are enhanced by co-operative network activity in the intact hippocampus. *Journal of Neuroscience*, **18**, 3919–28.

Kavalali, E. T., Zhuo, M., Bito, H., and Tsien, R. W. (1997). Dendritic Ca^{2+} channels characterized by recordings from isolated hippocampal dendritic segments. *Neuron*, **18**, 651–63.

Kay, A. R., Sugimori, M., and Llinás, R. (1998). Kinetic and stochastic properties of a persistent sodium current in mature guinea pig cerebellar Purkinje cells. *Journal of Neurophysiology*, **80**, 1167–79.

Lev-Ram, V., Miyakawa, H., Lasser-Ross, N., and Ross, W. N. (1992). Calcium transients in cerebellar Purkinje neurons evoked by intracellular stimulation. *Journal of Neurophysiology*, **68**, 1167–77.

Liu, H. and Campbell, K. P. (1998). Structural determinates of calcium channel beta subunit function. In *Low-voltage-activated T-type calcium channels.* (ed. R. W. Tsien) Adis, Chester, UK.

Llinás, R. and Sugimori, M. (1979). Calcium conductances in Purkinje cell dendrites: their role in development and integration. *Progress in Brain Research,* **51**, 323–34.

Llinás, R. and Sugimori, M. (1980). Electrophysiological properties of *in vitro* Purkinje cell dendrites in mammalian cerebellar slices. *Journal of Physiology,* **305**, 197–213.

Mackenzie, P. J. and Murphy, T. H. (1998). High safety factor for action potential conduction along axons but not dendrites of cultured hippocampal and cortical neurons. *Journal of Neurophysiology,* **80**, 2089–101.

Magee, J. C. (1998). Dendritic hyperpolarization-activated currents modify the integrative properties of hippocampal CA1 pyramidal neurons. *Journal of Neuroscience,* **18**, 1–12.

Magee, J. C. (1999). Dendritic I_h normalizes temporal summation in hippocampel CA1 neurons. *Nature Neuroscience,* **2**, 508–14.

Magee, J. C. and Johnston, D. (1995). Characterization of single voltage-gated Na^+ and Ca^{2+} channels in apical dendrites of rat CA1 pyramidal neurons. *Journal of Physiology,* **487**, 67–90.

Magee, J. C. and Johnston, D. (1997). A synaptically controlled, associative signal for Hebbian plasticity in hippocampal neurons. *Science,* **275**, 209–13.

Magee, J. C., Avery, R. B., Christie, B. R., and Johnston, D. (1996). Dihydropyridine-sensitive, voltage-gated Ca^{2+} channels contribute to the resting intracellular Ca^{2+} concentration of hippocampal CA1 pyramidal neurons. *Journal of Neurophysiology,* **76**, 3460–70.

Magee, J. C., Hoffman, D., Colbert, C., and Johnston, D. (1998). Electrical and calcium signaling in dendrites of hippocampal pyramidal neurons. *Annual Review of Physiology,* **60**, 327–46.

Marban, E., Yamagishi, T., and Tomaselli, G. F. (1998). Structure and function of voltage-gated sodium channels. *Journal of Physiology,* **508**, 647–57.

Markram, H. and Sakmann, B. (1994). Calcium transients in dendrites of neocortical neurons evoked by single subthreshold excitatory postsynaptic potentials via low-voltage-activated calcium channels. *Proceedings of the National Academy of Sciences USA,* **91**, 5207–52011.

Markram, H., Helm, P. J., and Sakmann, B. (1995). Dendritic calcium transients evoked by single backpropagating action potentials in rat neocortical pyramidal neurons. *Journal of Physiology,* **485**, 1–20.

Marrion, N. V. and Tavalin, S. J. (1998). Selective activation of Ca^{2+}-activated K^+ channels by co-localized Ca^{2+} channels in hippocampal neurons. *Nature,* **395**, 823–926.

Martina, M., Schultz, J. H., Ehmke, H., Monyer, H., and Jonas, P. (1998). Functional and molecular differences between voltage-gated K^+ channels of fast-spiking interneurons and pyramidal neurons of rat hippocampus. *Journal of Neuroscience,* **18**, 8111–25.

Martina, M. and Jonas, P. (1997). Functional differences in Na^+ channel gating between fast-spiking interneurons and principal neurons of the rat hippocampus. *Journal of Physiology,* **505**, 593–603.

Mathie, A., Wooltorton, J. R., and Watkins, C. S. (1998). Voltage-activated potassium channels in mammalian neurons and their block by novel pharmacological agents. *General Pharmacology,* **30**, 13–24.

Mickus, T., Jung, H., and Spruston, N. (1999). Properties of slow, cumulative sodium channel inactivation in rat hippocampal CA1 pyramidal cells. *Biophysical Journal,* **76**, 846–60.

Midtgaard, J. (1994). Processing of information from different sources: spatial synaptic integration in the dendrites of vertebrate CNS. *Trends in Neurosciences,* **17**, 166–73.

Midtgaard, J., Lasser-Ross, N., and Ross, W. N. (1993). Spatial distribution of Ca^{2+} influx in turtle Purkinje cell dendrites *in vitro*: role of a transient outward current. *Journal of Neurophysiology,* **70**, 2455–69.

Miyakawa, H., Lev-Ram, V., Lasser-Ross, N., and Ross, W. N. (1992). Calcium transients evoked by climbing fiber and parallel fiber synaptic inputs in guinea pig cerebellar Purkinje neurons. *Journal of Neurophysiology,* **68**, 1178–89.

Mouginot, D., Bossu, J., and Gähwiler, B. H. (1997). Low-threshold Ca^{2+} currents in dendritic recordings from Purkinje cells in rat cerebellar slice cultures. *Journal of Neuroscience*, **17**, 160–70.

Numann, R., Catterall, W. A., and Scheuer, T. (1991). Functional modulation of brain sodium channels by protein kinase C phosphorylation. *Science*, **254**, 115–18.

Pape, H.-C. (1996). Queer current and pacemaker: the hyperpolarization-activated cation current in neurons. *Annual Review of Physiology*, **58**, 299–327.

Poolos, N. P. and Johnston, D. (1999). Calcium-activated potassium conductances contribute to action potential repolarization at the soma but not the dendrites of hippocampal CA1 pyramidal neurons. *Journal of Neuroscience*, **19**, 5205–12.

Raman, I. M. and Bean, B. P. (1997). Resurgent sodium current and action potential formation in dissociated cerebellar Purkinje neurons. *Journal of Neuroscience*, **17**, 4517–26.

Randall, A. D. and Tsien, R. W. (1997). Contrasting biophysical and pharmacological properties of T-type and R-type calcium channels. *Neuropharmacology*, **36**, 879–93.

Richardson, T. L., Turner, R. W., and Miller, J. J. (1987). Action potential discharge in hippocampal CA1 pyramidal neurons: current source-density analysis. *Journal of Neurophysiology*, **58**, 981–6.

Sah, P. (1996). Ca^{2+}-activated K$^+$ currents in neurons: types, physiological roles and modulation. *Trends in Neurosciences*, **19**, 150–4.

Sah, P. and Bekkers, J. M. (1996). Apical dendritic location of slow afterhyperpolarization current in hippocampal pyramidal neurons: implications for the integration of long-term potentiation. *Journal of Neuroscience*, **16**, 4537–42.

Schiller, J., Schiller, Y., Stuart, G., and Sakmann, B. (1997). Calcium action potentials restricted to distal apical dendrites of rat neocortical pyramidal neurons. *Journal of Physiology*, **505**, 605–16.

Schiller, J., Schiller, Y., and Clapham, D. E. (1998). NMDA receptors amplify calcium influx into dendritic spines during associative pre- and postsynaptic activation. *Nature Neuroscience*, **1**, 114–8.

Schwindt, P. C. and Crill, W. E. (1995). Amplification of synaptic current by persistent sodium conductance in apical dendrite of neocortical neurons. *Journal of Neurophysiology*, **74**, 2220–4.

Schwindt, P. C. and Crill, W. E. (1997). Modification of current transmitted from apical dendrite to soma by blockade of voltage- and Ca^{2+}-dependent conductances in rat neocortical pyramidal neurons. *Journal of Neurophysiology*, **78**, 187–98.

Spruston, N., Schiller, Y., Stuart, G., and Sakmann, B. (1995). Activity-dependent action potential invasion and calcium influx into hippocampal CA1 dendrites. *Science*, **268**, 297–300.

Storm, J. F. (1987). Action potential repolarization and a fast after-hyperpolarization in rat hippocampal pyramidal cells. *Journal of Physiology*, **385**, 733–59.

Storm, J. F. (1990). Potassium currents in hippocampal pyramidal cells. *Progress in Brain Research*, **83**, 161–87.

Strafstrom, C. E., Schwindt, P. C., Chubb, M. C., and Crill, W. E. (1985). Properties of persistent sodium conductance and calcium conductance of layer V neurons from cat sensorimotor cortex *in vitro*. *Journal of Neurophysiology*, **53**, 152–70.

Stuart, G. J. and Häusser, M. (1994). Initiation and spread of sodium action potentials in cerebellar Purkinje cells. *Neuron*, **13**, 703–12.

Stuart, G. J. and Sakmann, B. (1994). Active propagation of somatic action potentials into neocortical pyramidal cell dendrites. *Nature*, **367**, 69–72.

Stuart, G. J. and Spruston, N. (1998). Determinants of voltage attenuation in neocortical pyramidal neuron dendrites. *Journal of Neuroscience*, **18**, 3501–10.

Stuart, G. J., Schiller, J., and Sakmann, B. (1997). Action potential initiation and propagation in rat neocortical pyramidal neurons. *Journal of Physiology*, **505**, 617–32.

Takigawa, T and Alzheimer, C. (1998). Electroresponsiveness of acutely isolated dendritic segments of rat neocortical pyramidal cells-evidence for constitutive and transmitter-activated inwardly-rectifying K-currents. *Society for Neuroscience Abstracts*, **24**, 2019.

Tsubokawa, H. and Ross, W. N. (1996). IPSPs modulate spike backpropagation and associated $[Ca^{2+}]_i$ changes in the dendrites of hippocampal CA1 pyramidal neurons. *Journal of Neurophysiology*, **76**, 2896–906.

Tsubokawa, H. and Ross, W. N. (1997). Muscarinic modulation of spike backpropagation in the apical dendrites of hippocampal CA1 pyramidal neurons. *Journal of Neuroscience*, **17**, 5782–5791.

Tsubokawa, H., Miura, M., and Kano, M. (1999). Elevation of intracellular Na^+ induced by hyperpolarization at the dendrites of pyramidal neurones of mouse hippocampus. *Journal of Physiology*, **517**, 135–42.

Turner, R. W., Meyers, D. E. R., Richardson, T. L., and Barker, J. L. (1991). The site for initiation of action potential discharge over the somatodendritic axis of rat hippocampal CA1 pyramidal neurons. *Journal of Neuroscience*, **11**, 2270–80.

Usowicz, M. M., Sugimori, M., Cherksey, B., and Llinás, R. (1992). P-type calcium channels in the somata and dendrites of adult cerebellar Purkinje cells. *Neuron*, **9**, 1185–99.

Watanabe, S., Takagi, H., Miyasho, T., Kirino, Y., Kudo, Y., and Miyakawa, H. (1998). Differential roles of two types of voltage-gated Ca^{2+} channels in the dendrites of Purkinje neurons. *Brain Research*, **79**, 43–55.

Wong, R. K. S. and Stewart, M. (1992). Different firing patterns generated in dendrites and somata of CA1 pyramidal neurons in guinea-pig hippocampus. *Journal of Physiology*, **457**, 675–87.

Wong, R. K., Prince, D. A., and Basbaum, A. I. (1979). Intradendritic recordings from hippocampal neurons. *Proceedings of the National Academy of Sciences USA*, **76**, 986–90.

Yuste, R. and Denk, D. W. (1996). Dendritic integration in mammalian neurons, a century after Cajal. *Neuron*, **16**, 701–16.

7

Dendrites as biochemical compartments

Fritjof Helmchen

Bell Laboratories

Summary

Dendrites have both an electrical and a biochemical character which are closely linked. In this chapter we discuss dendrites as compartments for chemical signals such as concentration changes of ions or other second messengers, which can cause activation of enzymes. In particular, we focus on the question to what extent these signals can be confined to only part of the dendritic tree. This is an important issue because such 'compartmentalization' is considered the basis of local modifications of dendritic properties, for example to achieve input-specific changes of synaptic strength. Following an introduction we first discuss general factors that affect compartmentalization of chemical signals including diffusion, intracellular binding, and removal mechanisms. We then provide examples of dendritic ion and second-messenger signaling, with the main focus on calcium signaling, for which the most detailed information is available from imaging studies. Subsequently, in an attempt to define functional units, we present an overview of the different spatial scales of dendritic compartmentalization spanning a range of three orders of magnitude. Finally, we describe two examples of how chemical signals are used for dendritic information processing.

Introduction

Experience-dependent changes in the nervous system, such as the regulation of synaptic strength of neuronal connections, are induced by specific patterns of electrical activity. They are mediated and expressed, however, through biochemical cellular mechanisms. Dendritic trees, which receive most of the synaptic inputs, display a rich diversity of morphology. The anatomical characteristics of dendrites may be important not only in shaping electrical signals, but also in providing neurons with a means to confine or segregate chemical signals. Electrical and biochemical activity are tightly coupled in neurons (Fig. 7.1a). Synaptic activity can cause electrical excitation of the postsynaptic neuron through ionic current flow as well as second-messenger formation *via* activation of G-protein coupled receptors. These events, in turn, can modulate electrical signaling and neuronal function in a variety of ways. Ion concentration changes can directly affect membrane potential changes by changing the driving forces for ionic current flow or by activating enzymes. Activation of protein kinases or phosphatases, either by calcium or by other second messengers such as inositol 1,4,5-trisphosphate (IP$_3$) or adenosine 3,5-cyclic mono-phosphate (cAMP) (Fig. 7.1b), can cause modifications of the membrane proteins responsible for electrical signaling, namely voltage-gated ion channels and receptor proteins (see Chapters 5 and 6). In addition, a variety of effects including structural changes (see Chapter 14), local protein synthesis (see Chapter 3), and gene expression (Bito *et al.* 1997) may be triggered by the activation of intracellular enzymes. Calcium ions have a special role as second messengers because they can enter the cytosol through several pathways including voltage-dependent calcium channels and release from intracellular stores (Fig. 7.1c), and because they bind to a variety of intracellular proteins, regulating their activity (for reviews see Clapham 1995; Ghosh and Greenberg 1995).

Neurons are highly polarized structures with nerve terminals, axon, soma and dendrites as specialized cellular compartments with different structures and functions. It is obvious that chemical signals such as calcium concentration changes can be spatially confined to these compartments (for a review see Wang and Augustine 1999). More recently it has become clear that subdivisions into functional compartments exist within dendritic trees. Such compartmentalization enables a neuron to spatially segregate signaling cascades and to restrict their effects to certain dendritic regions. In particular, second-messenger signals are involved in the induction of synaptic plasticity. At least some forms of long-term potentiation and depression depend on postsynaptic calcium and can display input specificity according to the Hebbian rule that only those synapses are modified which experience both pre- and postsynaptic activity (for reviews see Bliss and Collingridge 1993; Linden 1994). In addition, synaptic modifications may be associative, meaning that a weak synaptic input is modified when it is paired with a strong neighboring one. Under certain circumstances, synaptic changes can spread to inactive neigh-boring synapses to some extent (Bonhoeffer *et al.* 1989; Schuman and Madison 1994; Engert and Bonhoeffer 1997), indicating that the relevant messenger molecules are diffusible. In view of the various effects of different induction protocols on synaptic plasticity, it seems likely that the exact temporal and spatial pattern of the relevant signaling molecules as well as their interactions are of crucial importance in determining the overall effect. The following questions naturally arise: to what extent are chemical signals localized within dendritic trees? How far do they spread and how long do they persist? What are the cellular mechanisms involved? How are localized chemical signals related to the induction of synaptic plasticity and eventually to animal behavior?

During the last decade new experimental tools to address these questions have been developed and existing ones have been greatly improved. The traditional way of applying effectors or inhibitors to study chemical pathways has been supplemented with high-resolution imaging and photolysis techniques that allow the measurement and the control of the activity of second messengers, respectively. A large number of fluorescent indicators for ions and cAMP (for reviews see Tsien 1989; Adams *et al.* 1993) have been used for imaging of dendritic signaling (for reviews see Regehr and Tank 1994; Denk *et al.* 1996; Eilers and Konnerth 1997). The combination of

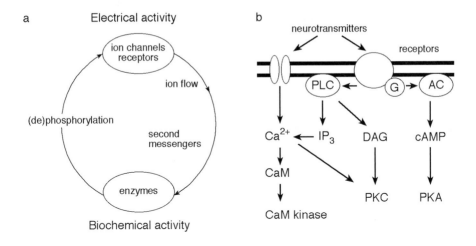

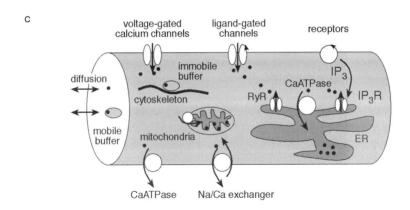

Fig. 7.1 Overview of second-messenger signaling pathways. (a) Coupling of electrical and chemical signaling. Ion fluxes and receptor activation cause ion and second-messenger concentration changes. Activation of cytosolic enzymes in turn leads to modifications of membrane proteins. (b) Main pathways of protein kinase activation *via* G-protein coupled receptors. cAMP production by adenylate cyclase (AC) is controlled by G-proteins and activates cAMP-dependent protein kinase (PKA). Activation of phospholipase C (PLC) leads to generation of diacylglycerol (DAG), which activates protein kinase C, and of inositol 1,4,5-trisphosphate (IP$_3$), which causes calcium release from internal stores *via* the IP$_3$ receptor. Among various other effects Ca^{2+} binds to calmodulin (CaM) and activates CaM kinases. (c) Components of neuronal Ca^{2+} homeostasis. Calcium ions are indicated by black dots. Pathways for Ca^{2+} entry are voltage- and ligand-gated ion channels and release from endoplasmic reticulum (ER) *via* IP$_3$ receptors or ryanodine receptors (RyR). Cytosolic calcium diffuses and binds to mobile or fixed buffers. Clearance mechanisms include extrusion across the plasma membrane *via* a CaATPase and an Na$^+$/Ca^{2+} exchanger, uptake into the ER *via* a CaATPase and uptake into mitochondria *via* a uniporter.

electrophysiology and a camera system or a confocal microscope has proven useful for many applications of imaging dendrites in brain slices (for reviews see Lasser-Ross *et al.* 1991; Eilers *et al.* 1995*b*). For optical measurements from dendrites deep in neuronal tissue, however, two-photon microscopy (Denk *et al.* 1990) is particularly advantageous because of reduced light scattering at the longer excitation wavelengths, reduced photodamage and photobleaching, and the confinement of the excitation to the focal spot, which makes a detection pinhole unnecessary (Denk and Svoboda 1997). Two-photon microscopy enables imaging of dendrites in the intact mammalian brain (Svoboda *et al.* 1997, 1999). Currently, measurements down to about half a millimeter below the brain surface are possible. Fig. 7.2 shows examples of two-photon images of neocortical neurons in the somatosensory cortex of anesthetized rats. Individual dendritic spines are clearly resolved. *In vivo* two-photon microscopy thus opens a whole new field for the investigation of chemical compartmentalization in the intact brain and may allow the study of its behavioral relevance.

Photolytic activation of caged compounds using high-intensity light pulses provided by a flash-lamp or a laser enables the control of the initial localization, the spatial extent and the amplitude of a biochemical signal. Caged compounds have been designed for a variety of molecules, including many nucleotides, neurotransmitters, IP_3, Ca^{2+}, and nitric oxide (for a review see Nerbonne 1996). Focal uncaging allows the generation of highly localized changes of second-messenger or neurotransmitter concentration (Wang and Augustine 1995).

Given the large variety of dendritic morphologies and the differences in expression pattern and subcellular distribution of proteins, the extent and functional importance of compartmentalization varies between different neuronal cell types. We cannot account for this variety here. Rather than listing all different cell types we prefer to focus on general principles of second-messenger signaling in dendrites and use certain cell types as characteristic examples.

Determinants of compartmentalization

The main factors contributing to compartmentalization in dendrites are the pattern of synaptic input, morphological characteristics such as geometrical constraints and distribution of proteins, membrane potential, intracellular diffusion, and messenger binding and removal mechanisms (Fig. 7.3a). The aim of this section is to provide a general introduction that is applicable to any diffusible dendritic messenger. More specific information about different messenger substances is given in the following section.

Spatiotemporal activation pattern

The initial localization of a particular chemical signal depends on the activation pattern of the receptors, membrane conductances, or enzymes that mediate that signal. The dendritic distribution of these proteins is therefore of crucial importance (see Chapters 4 to 6), together with the pattern of afferent innervation. In some cases dendritic trees are innervated in a topographic manner (Borst and Egelhaaf 1994). Dendrites of pyramidal cells in the neocortex are contacted by the different classes of inhibitory cells in characteristic locations (Douglas and Martin 1998), and Purkinje

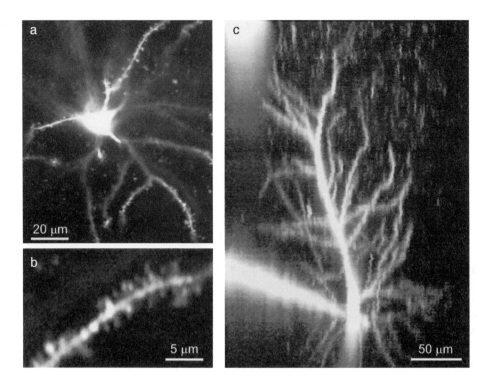

Fig. 7.2 Two-photon microscopy enables the study of dendritic compartmentalization in the intact brain. (a) Two-photon excitation fluorescence image of a pyramidal neuron in the neocortex of an anesthetized rat. The neuron was filled with the calcium indicator Calcium Green-1 *via* an intracellular electrode. The image is a top view from the brain surface showing a cross-section through the soma and basal dendrites 160 μm below the pial surface. (b) Detail of the neuron shown in (a) demonstrating that dendritic spines are clearly resolved. (c) Side-projection of a different layer 2/3 neuron calculated from a stack of images. The electrode is visible on the left side. The soma was 300 μm below the pial surface (reprinted with permission from Svoboda *et al.* 1999).

cell dendrites in the cerebellum receive anatomically segregated excitatory input from parallel fibers and climbing fibers (Palay and Chan-Palay 1974). In other cells this important issue of dendritic innervation patterns is unresolved. Activation of a specific afferent pathway thus may result in a local activation of the postsynaptic dendrites (Fig. 7.3a). The initial production of second messengers by G-protein coupled receptors is mostly confined to the sites of presynaptic transmitter release. The spatial pattern of ion influx depends, in addition, on the postsynaptic membrane potential because of the presence of voltage-dependent ion channels in dendrites (see Chapter 6). For example, excitatory postsynaptic potentials (EPSPs) may locally reach the threshold for activation of calcium channels, causing spatially restricted calcium transients (Miyakawa *et al.* 1992; Eilers *et al.* 1995*a*; Magee *et al.* 1996; Schiller *et al.* 1997). Backpropagating action potentials can lead to a more wide-spread dendritic calcium influx, depending on how far the action potentials invade

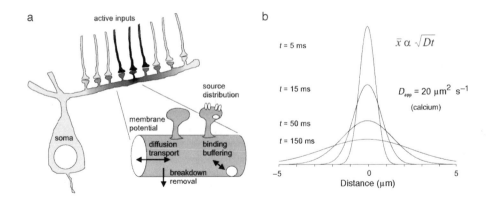

Fig. 7.3 Factors contributing to compartmentalization. (a) Schematic diagram showing the main determinants of compartmentalization using a local increase of ion or second-messenger concentration in a dendritic branch as an example. (b) The square-root-law of diffusion illustrated for the example of buffered calcium diffusion. The theoretical Gaussian distributions of the diffusional spread following a brief calcium injection at the origin are shown at four time points after the injection. Note that for a ten times longer time period the curves broaden by only a factor of $\sqrt{10}$.

the dendrites (Jaffe *et al.* 1992; Schiller *et al.* 1995; Spruston *et al.* 1995; Svoboda *et al.* 1999). The electrical characteristics of the dendritic tree are therefore of vital importance in determining the spread of these signals (see Chapters 9 and 10).

Clearly, not only the distribution of sources but also the spatial organization of the target proteins is of importance. Signaling proteins can be held in place by anchoring proteins and they may be translocated following stimulation (for a review see Mochly-Rosen 1995). A very recent example is the translocation of CaMKII to postsynaptic densities upon NMDA receptor stimulation (Shen and Meyer 1999). In addition, the speed and duration of second-messenger production may be of relevance for the actual activation pattern of the targets. Second-messenger production by enzymes usually is relatively slow, on a time scale of hundreds of milliseconds or longer (Kasai and Petersen 1994). In contrast, calcium influx during an action potential can be as short as a millisecond. It may be important to distinguish between short, pulse-like injections of calcium and slower calcium increases, e.g. during prolonged membrane depolarizations. The reason is that intracellular targets with different binding kinetics can be activated differentially depending on whether calcium ions enter the cytosol rapidly or slowly (Markram *et al.* 1998). Targets with fast binding rates are favored by brief calcium injections because they outcompete slower proteins on a short time scale (see also the section on binding affinities and kinetics below).

Morphology

The anatomical structure of dendrites is the major factor in controlling the diffusional spread of intracellular messengers. The length and the diameter of dendritic branches, the branching pattern, and the density of spines influence the ability of a neuron to spatially confine chemical signals (see Chapter 1). Importantly, excitatory neurons generally bear dendritic spines, whereas inhibitory cells have smooth dendrites (Douglas and Martin 1998). The reason for this difference is unknown, but may reflect different requirements for biochemical compartmentalization.

Partially isolated small cellular volumes such as spines and thin dendritic branches enable a neuron to amplify chemical signals in the sense that the same transmembrane ion flux—or the same amount of enzymatic second-messenger production—causes larger concentration changes if confined to a smaller subcellular volume. In other words, the surface-to-volume ratio is a crucial determinant of the absolute concentrations reached. For dendrites, which are approximately cylindrical, the surface-to-volume ratio depends roughly inversely on the radius. It should be noted that the accessible cytosolic volume is reduced due to the presence of intracellular organelles; the relative degree of volume exclusion in spines and dendritic shafts caused by intracellular organelles remains unknown. Structural changes of dendrites (see Chapter 14) could have a pronounced effect on the local amplitude of chemical signals if they alter the surface-to-volume ratio. Finally, the branching pattern of a dendritic tree defines not only the electronic but also the 'chemical distance' between any two dendritic sites. Analogously to propagation of electrical potentials, the spread of chemical signals in the dendritic tree will depend not only on the density of branching, but also on the relative diameters of parent and daughter dendrites at branch points, with increases in diameter causing further dilution. The degree of chemical isolation between two sites, however, also critically depends on the nature of the messenger substance, as discussed below. In the extreme case, two spines on neighboring branches may be far apart with respect to intracellular diffusion but very close with respect to a freely diffusible substance such as nitric oxide.

Diffusion

We now turn our attention to the mechanisms that affect the spread of chemical signals in dendrites once they have been generated locally. We limit our description to a few fundamental ideas. A more comprehensive treatment of diffusion and buffering can be found in Koch (1998). We do not consider active transport mechanisms in dendrites, which operate on a slower time scale (Sheetz *et al.* 1998). For simplicity we consider the one-dimensional case. Since dendrites typically are long and thin cylindrical structures, such a description often is a useful approximation.

Mobile substances in the cytosol spread by diffusion. Diffusion is a probabilistic process arising from to the thermal agitation of molecules. If we are interested in the temporal change of the concentration $[C(x,t)]$ of a diffusible substance C at a position x along a dendrite, we have to take the difference between the influx and efflux from both sides, both of which depend on the local concentration gradient. The resulting balance equation is the *diffusion equation*:

$$\frac{\partial[C(x,t)]}{\partial t} = D\frac{\partial^2[C(x,t)]}{\partial x^2} \tag{1}$$

where D is the diffusion coefficient. For large molecules (molecular weight $M > 1000$) D depends mainly on their radius and therefore on the cubic root of M. Ions have relatively small diffusion coefficients, partially because of the formation of hydration shells in aqueous solution. Typical aqueous diffusion coefficients for ions, second messengers, and proteins range from 0.1 to 10 μm^2 ms^{-1} (Table 7.1). Cytoplasmic diffusion coefficients are generally two- to threefold smaller because of the higher viscosity and the physical restrictions in the cytosol (Woolf and Greer 1994). In addition, binding to immobile proteins further slows down diffusion of a substance (see the discussion on buffering below). For example, the apparent diffusion coefficient of calcium in the cytosol is only about 0.02 μm^2 ms^{-1} because of intracellular binding (Allbritton *et al.* 1992). For local injection of a substance into an infinite cylinder, the solution of the diffusion equation is a Gaussian distribution of the substance along the dendrite that broadens with time (Fig. 7.3b). An important characteristic of this spreading is that the mean displacement $\bar{x}$ from the point of injection is proportional to the square root of time:

$$\bar{x} \alpha \sqrt{Dt} \qquad (2)$$

Hence, a substance with a diffusion coefficient of 0.1 μm^2 ms^{-1} spreads about 0.3 μm in 1 ms, 1 μm in 10 ms, 3 μm in 100 ms, and 10 μm in 1 s. This illustrates that—given lifetimes of intracellular messengers of less than a second to a few seconds—chemical signals can be quite effectively compartmentalized in long dendrites solely as a result of this square-root-law of diffusional processes. Furthermore, the concentration of a messenger after local elevation increasingly dilutes while spreading, which further limits the spatial range of substrate activation.

Buffering

Second messengers and ions act through binding to target molecules, causing conformational changes and alterations in their activity. At least for H^+ and for

Table 7.1 Aqueous (D_{aqu}) and cytosolic (D_{cyto}) diffusion coefficents for several ions, second messengers and proteins.

Substance	D_{aqu} (μm^2 ms^{-1})	D_{cyto} (μm^2 ms^{-1})
NO	3.8§	
H^+	8‡	0.1–0.2‡ (buffered)
Na^+	1.33§	
K^+	1.96§	
Cl^-	2.03§	
Ca^{2+}	0.6§	0.223* (free)
		0.013—0.065* (buffered)
IP_3	0.72¶	0.28*
cAMP	0.72¶	0.33–0.78†
Calmodulin	0.13¶	0.045¶
CaM kinase II	0.034¶	0.006¶
PKA	0.1¶*	0.032¶

Numbers are from the following references and references cited therein:
*Allbritton *et al.* 1992, †Bacskai *et al.* 1993, ‡Irving *et al.* 1990, §Koch 1998, ¶Woolf *et al.* 1994.

Ca^{2+} the concentration of binding sites can be so large that the majority of ions is bound and only a small fraction remains free. Thus, pH and intracellular free calcium concentration ($[Ca^{2+}]_i$) are buffered effectively. Many Ca^{2+}-binding proteins have reversible binding of calcium as their only known function and are commonly referred to as 'calcium buffers' (Clapham 1995). We now ask how intracellular buffering affects compartmentalization in dendrites. The binding of a substance C to a buffer B can be described by a second-order binding scheme:

$$C + B \Longleftrightarrow CB$$

Binding occurs with an association rate k_{on} and the complex CB dissociates with a rate k_{off}. The affinity of B for binding C is given by the dissociation constant $K_B = k_{off}/k_{on}$. If we include binding to a single buffer species in our description of the spatiotemporal dynamics of [C] (eqn 1) we obtain the *reaction–diffusion equations*:

$$\frac{\partial [C]}{\partial t} = D_C \frac{\partial^2 [C]}{\partial x^2} - k_{on}[C] \cdot [B] + k_{off}[CB]$$

$$\frac{\partial [B]}{\partial t} = D_m \frac{\partial^2 [B]}{\partial x^2} + k_{on}[C] \cdot [B] - k_{off}[CB] \tag{3}$$

$$[B]_T = [B] + [CB]$$

Square brackets denote concentrations, which depend on x and t. We assume that the diffusion coefficient of both the free and the bound buffer is D_m and that the total buffer concentration is $[B]_T$, which in general can be spatially inhomogeneous but in the following is considered constant. eqn 3 is a relatively complex coupled system of partial differential equations, which is difficult to solve analytically. This reflects the enormous increase in complexity of signaling when high concentration levels of intracellular binding sites are present. Useful approximations of eqn 3 can be derived on different spatial scales and with appropriate assumptions.

A frequently used assumption is that the substance and its substrate are in chemical equilibrium at all points in time and in space. Although this assumption is not justified for very brief time periods or on a small spatial scale (< 1 μm; see the section on calcium domains below) it holds reasonably well on a larger scale. In chemical equilibrium the concentration of the bound form of the buffer is given by:

$$[CB] = \frac{[C] \cdot [B]_T}{[C] + K_B} \tag{4}$$

The effectiveness of a buffer to maintain the concentration at a given level (its binding capacity) is given by the ratio of the change in buffer-bound concentration to the change in free concentration of the substance, the so called 'binding ratio' (for a review see Neher 1995)

$$\kappa_B = \frac{\partial [CB]}{\partial [C]} = \frac{[B]_T K_B}{([C] + K_B)^2} \tag{5}$$

which is the first derivative of eqn 4 with respect to [C]. At a given concentration of C, κ_B depends on the total concentration and the dissociation constant of the buffer.

For low concentration levels ($[C] \ll K_B$) the binding ratio simplifies to $[B]_T/K_B$. Later in the chapter we will discuss estimates of dendritic Ca^{2+} binding ratios.

How can we use the concept of binding ratios to describe diffusion in dendrites in the presence of buffering? By adding the two equations in eqn 3 and considering that

$$\partial[CB]/\partial t = \kappa_B \, \partial[C]/\partial t$$

we obtain the following differential equation for the spatiotemporal dynamics of $[C]$:

$$(1 + \kappa_B) \frac{\partial[C]}{\partial t} = D_C \frac{\partial^2[C]}{\partial x^2} + D_m \frac{\partial^2[CB]}{\partial x^2} \tag{6}$$

For immobile buffers ($D_m = 0$) this readily reduces to a simple diffusion equation:

$$\frac{\partial[C]}{\partial t} = D_{app} \frac{\partial^2[C]}{\partial x^2} \tag{7}$$

with an apparent diffusion coefficient:

$$D_{app} = \frac{D_C}{1 + \kappa_B} \tag{8}$$

Thus, on a spatial scale where chemical equilibrium is reached, the diffusion of substances is slowed down in the presence of binding to immobile intracellular proteins. Intuitively this is clear, because fixed buffers hold the substances in place and thus hinder their diffusional spread. When both mobile and fixed buffers are considered, eqn 6 can be simplified to a diffusion equation with an apparent diffusion coefficient given by (Irving *et al.* 1990; Gabso *et al.* 1997):

$$D_{app} = \frac{D_C + \kappa_m D_m}{(1 + \kappa_f + \kappa_m)} \tag{9}$$

where D_m is the diffusion coefficient of the mobile buffer, and κ_m and κ_f denote the binding ratios of the mobile and the fixed buffers, respectively. For a mobile buffer with $D_m > D_C/(1 + \kappa_f)$ the apparent diffusion of a substance is faster than when only a fixed buffer is present. The explanation is that a highly mobile buffer captures the substance near the source and facilitates the diffusional spread by transporting it in 'piggyback' fashion. In summary, intracellular buffers can both slow down or facilitate the diffusional spread of a substance depending on their concentration, affinity, and mobility. This leaves room for speculation that the spatial extent of dendritic calcium compartments might not be stationary but dynamically regulated depending on the expression level of Ca^{2+}-binding proteins.

Binding affinities and kinetics

As we have seen in the previous section, the diffusion of a second-messenger substance is affected by the presence of intracellular binding sites. The actual activation pattern of intracellular targets, however, may depend on the properties of the targets themselves. For example, the activation of a low-affinity binding protein may be more restricted in space compared to a high-affinity protein because it needs higher messenger concentrations for substantial binding. The activation pattern of target molecules can become far more complex if one considers kinetic effects. For example, the rate constants of Ca^{2+}-binding proteins cover several orders of magnitude ($k_{on} \approx 10^6-10^9$ M^{-1} s^{-1}, $k_{off} \approx 1-10^3$ s^{-1}, Falke *et al.* 1994). Markram *et al.* (1998) explored the competition for incoming calcium ions between multiple proteins with different binding kinetics prior to full equilibration. Using numerical simulations they found that proteins with fast kinetics initially outcompete slower proteins, in particular during very brief calcium injections such as those evoked by action potentials. In a subsequent slower phase calcium ions are passed over to slower targets, although these may be bypassed altogether in the presence of calcium removal mechanisms. Another situation where such non-equilibrium effects are significant is calcium binding in the immediate vicinity of open calcium channels (Naraghi and Neher 1997; see the section on calcium domains below). In other words, different proteins may 'see' quite different signals depending on their affinities and their relative kinetic properties. Sequential binding of calcium has been investigated in detail in muscle (Falke *et al.* 1994), but its possible role for dendritic signaling has so far been neglected. For a further exploration of non-equilibrium effects not only the localization and affinity of binding proteins in dendrites need to be known but also their kinetic properties.

Further complexity may arise from multiple binding sites on one protein. The Ca^{2+}-binding protein calmodulin, for example, has four Ca^{2+}-binding sites with different affinities which bind calcium in a cooperative way. The Ca^{2+}-calmodulin complex is a versatile activator of a variety of enzymes (Ghosh and Greenberg 1995). Due to multi-site and cooperative binding the activation of calmodulin depends steeply on the calcium concentration confining it to regions of high concentration (Gamble and Koch 1987; Koch 1998).

Removal mechanisms

Following a period of activity neurons have to reestablish the resting concentrations of ions and second messengers in order to maintain the ability to produce electrical and chemical signals. This is achieved through ion pump mechanisms or enzymatic breakdown. The simplest mathematical description of removal from the cytosol is a non-saturable mechanism which linearly depends on the messenger concentration with a single rate constant γ (in units of s^{-1}). Such a removal mechanism can be considered as the low-concentration limit of a saturable pump or enzyme, e.g. one following Michaelis–Menten kinetics. Although simple, this approximation often provides a reasonable fit to experimental data, for example to calcium transients measured in dendrites or nerve terminals (Helmchen and Tank 1999). The removal rate depends on the surface-to-volume ratio of the cellular compartment, being faster in thinner dendrites. Therefore the structural subdivision of dendrites into many small volumes not only amplifies concentration changes but also facilitates rapid signaling.

How do removal mechanisms affect the diffusional spread of messengers? A dendritic segment in this case resembles a leaky pipe because the messenger substance is either degraded or extruded while diffusing. If we include a linear removal mechanism in eqn 7—with both a mobile and a fixed buffer present—we obtain the *linearized reaction–diffusion equation*:

$$(1 + \kappa_f + \kappa_m) \frac{\partial [C]}{\partial t} = (D_C + \kappa_m D_m) \frac{\partial^2 [C]}{\partial x^2} - \gamma [C] \tag{10}$$

This equation is equivalent to the cable equation (see Chapter 9). Therefore a useful analogy between chemical and electrical signaling can be drawn (Kasai and Petersen 1994; Zador and Koch 1994). The diffusion coefficient relates to the intracellular resistivity, the removal rate corresponds to the inverse of the membrane resistance, and buffers act similar to a capacitance (for more details see Koch 1998). In the idealized case of an infinite cylinder the chemical equivalents of space and time constants can be defined based on cable theory. The 'chemical length constant' or diffusion length is given by:

$$\lambda_{ch} = \sqrt{D_{app} \tau_{ch}} = \sqrt{\frac{D_C + \kappa_m D_m}{\gamma}} \tag{11}$$

where the time constant is defined as:

$$\tau_{ch} = \frac{1 + \kappa_m + \kappa_f}{\gamma} \tag{12}$$

The diffusion length is small for large removal rates γ. Inserting reasonable numbers in eqn 11 yields a wide range of diffusion length for different messengers. For buffered calcium the diffusion length is a few micrometers or less. In contrast, IP_3 as well as cAMP or cGMP have diffusion lengths of tens of micrometers or more (Allbritton *et al.* 1992; Kasai and Petersen 1994). Therefore, calcium can act as a short-range messenger, while IP_3 and cAMP have to be considered more as long-range messengers (Kasai and Petersen 1994). Notably, even the largest diffusion lengths are at least an order of magnitude shorter than typical electrical space constants, indicating that in general dendritic chemical signals are much more confined than electrical signals.

The above considerations assume a localized increase in the concentration of a messenger molecule. If the dendritic concentration rises in concert in large parts of the dendritic tree, for example in the case of calcium transients evoked by back-propagating action potentials, the diffusional term in eqn 10 can be neglected entirely, and the description reduces to a simple single compartment model (Regehr and Tank 1994; Helmchen and Tank 1999). The calcium transients in this model have an exponential decay with a time constant given by eqn 12.

The approximations of the reaction–diffusion equations and of removal mechanisms given in this section may provide a reasonable description of second-messenger dynamics for individual dendritic segments and in the low concentration regime. The underlying assumptions, however, do not hold for real dendritic trees. Deviations from the above equations arise from the complex geometry of dendrites and spines as well as from non-linearities such as saturation of buffers or pumps. For more realistic and detailed models of second-messenger dynamics in dendrites the full differential equations—possibly including saturable removal mechanisms—have to be solved on the basis of morphological reconstructions and using numerical methods. This can be done either for single dendritic branches or spines (Gamble and Koch 1987; Woolf and Greer 1994) or for entire dendritic trees using compartmental models of reconstructed cells (De Schutter and Smolen 1998).

Examples from dendritic ion and second-messenger signaling

In this section we discuss some examples of measurements of the spatiotemporal dynamics of ion or second-messenger concentrations in dendrites. The emphasis will be on what is known—from imaging or uncaging experiments—about diffusion, buffering, and removal mechanisms in dendrites.

Ion concentration changes

Ion concentration changes evoked by neuronal activity may have a variety of effects. They can cause shifts in the reversal potentials by changing the concentration gradients across the plasma membrane, and they may directly affect membrane conductances through binding. Ion concentration changes in small dendrites and dendritic spines can be large and rapid, so that intradendritic diffusion of ions cannot be neglected for the calculation of membrane potential dynamics. The electrical cable model in this case must be generalized by including ion diffusion. For details about such an electro–diffusion model consult Sejnowski and Qian (1992).

pH
Due to the pH sensitivity of most enzymes and ion channels, the intracellular pH needs to be highly regulated in cells. Not surprisingly high values of pH buffering have been reported for muscles and neurons, corresponding to a binding ratio of more than 10 000 (Irving *et al.* 1990; Tombaugh 1998). Diffusion of hydrogen therefore is relatively slow in the cytoplasm (see Table 7.1). It seems likely that localized changes of intracellular pH occur in dendrites during neuronal activity (Chesler and Kaila 1992). A possible function of these pH changes could be a negative feedback effect on dendritic calcium influx since voltage-gated calcium channels are highly pH-sensitive (Tombaugh 1998).

Sodium
The spatial distribution of Na^+ concentration increases in dendrites has been monitored using the Na^+-sensitive dye SBFI. Lasser-Ross and Ross (1992) observed large somatic Na^+ transients in cerebellar Purkinje neurons, but they were not able to detect dendritic $[Na^+]_i$ changes evoked by fast sodium spikes or during calcium action potentials, which is consistent with a low density of Na^+ channels in these dendrites. Dendritic Na^+ influx, however, was observed upon climbing fiber stimulation and—more recently and localized to dendritic branches—upon

parallel fiber stimulation (Callaway and Ross 1997). This influx was attributed to the activation of ligand-gated channels. Also, diffusion of Na^+ from the sites of entry to nearby locations seemed to be quite rapid, which is in contrast to similar experiments on local $[Ca^{2+}]_i$ increases (Eilers *et al.* 1995), and reflects the differences in apparent cytosolic diffusion coefficients between Na^+ and Ca^{2+}. More widespread $[Na^+]_i$ increases have been reported for hippocampal neurons (Jaffe *et al.* 1992) and for neocortical neurons evoked by persistent Na^+ current (Mittmann *et al.* 1997). Most recently, hyperpolarization-induced $[Na^+]_i$ elevations were observed in apical dendrites of mouse hippocampal neurons and were attributed to dendritic hyperpolarization-activated currents (Tsubokawa *et al.* 1999). In most of these studies the Na^+ transients displayed a relatively slow decay of several seconds; however, this may at least partially be caused by buffering of SBFI. Besides affecting $[Na^+]_i$-dependent mechanisms such as the Na^+/Ca^{2+}-exchanger, local $[Na^+]_i$ increases have been implicated in the induction of cerebellar LTD (Linden 1994).

Chloride

Transient chloride influx into neurons is mainly mediated by $GABA_A$ and glycine receptors. Chloride clearance mechanisms include chloride–bicarbonate exchangers, $Na^+/K^+/2Cl^-$ cotransporters, and an ATP-driven chloride pump. An uneven distribution of these removal mechanisms between soma and dendrites of cultured hippocampal neurons has been suggested to generate a gradient of intracellular chloride concentration at rest (Hara *et al.* 1992). Such a standing gradient as well as transient local chloride concentration increases due to receptor activation could shift the reversal potential for chloride in dendritic regions, and thus determine if GABAergic inputs cause hyperpolarizing or depolarizing synaptic potentials (Sejnowski and Qian 1992; Staley *et al.* 1995; Kaila *et al.* 1997). Further investigation of this controversial issue now seems possible by application of fluorescent chloride indicators to single neurons in brain slices (Inglefield and Schwartz-Bloom 1997).

Calcium

The most detailed information is available for the mechanisms involved in dendritic calcium signaling, although little is still known about the molecular identity as well as the spatial distribution of the proteins involved in Ca^{2+} buffering and removal. The pathways of Ca^{2+} entry and their dendritic distribution have been discussed in Chapters 4 to 6. Here we focus on the questions: what happens to calcium ions after they entered the cytosol? What is known about diffusion of calcium ions and of Ca^{2+}-binding proteins in dendrites? How strongly is $[Ca^{2+}]_i$ buffered in dendrites? How rapidly and by what mechanisms is cytosolic Ca^{2+} removed?

Calcium diffusion

The diffusional properties of Ca^{2+} in dendrites have not yet been directly measured. In cytosolic extracts from Xenopus oocytes Allbritton *et al.* (1992) found a low diffusion coefficient of calcium caused by buffering (Table 7.1). An important related question is how mobile the endogenous Ca^{2+}-binding proteins are. If their mobility is low, the usage of highly mobile Ca^{2+} indicators may strongly alter the apparent Ca^{2+} diffusion (eqn 9). Gabso *et al.* (1997) used brief local intracellular injections of calcium into axons of *Aplysia* neurons to address this question. They found an upper limit of 16 μm^2 s^{-1} for the diffusion coefficient of endogenous Ca^{2+} buffers, suggesting that they are either immobilized or of high molecular weight. Similar measurements should be possible on long apical dendrites. A hint that dendritic Ca^{2+} buffers may be rather stationary also comes from calcium measurements on proximal dendrites of neocortical neurons, where no significant wash-out of buffers through the whole-cell pipette could be observed (Helmchen *et al.* 1996). As a consequence of this low mobility of endogenous Ca^{2+} buffers, distortion of Ca^{2+} diffusion by diffusible indicators is probably severe.

Calcium buffering

The endogenous Ca^{2+}-binding capacity (eqn 5) can be determined by systematically measuring the effect of adding an exogenous buffer, for example a Ca^{2+} indicator, on the intracellular $[Ca^{2+}]_i$ changes evoked by a constant calcium influx (for a review see Neher 1995). Depending on the 'baseline buffering' of the endogenous buffers, lower or higher concentrations of added buffer will cause a significant reduction and prolongation of the transients (see eqn 12). Using this approach the Ca^{2+}-binding ratio of the endogenous Ca^{2+} buffers in proximal apical dendrites was estimated to be about 120 in neocortical and 200 in hippocampal pyramidal neurons (Helmchen *et al.* 1996), values comparable to those found for many cell somata (Neher 1995). An extreme case was found in cerebellar Purkinje cell dendrites where the Ca^{2+}-binding ratio ranged from 900 in 6-day-old rats to 2000 in 14-day-old rats (Fierro and Llano 1996). These values also indicate that the expression of Ca^{2+}-binding activity is developmentally regulated. These studies were done on proximal dendrites, and it is likely that the distribution of calcium buffers is non-uniform in dendrites and dendritic spines, in particular since a large fraction of buffers seems to be rather immobile. Possible inhomogeneities of the dendritic Ca^{2+}-binding ratios need further exploration.

Little is known about the identity and nature of the Ca^{2+}-binding proteins that contribute to the measured Ca^{2+}-binding capacities. The relatively high values found for Purkinje neurons are consistent with immunocytochemical studies showing that Ca^{2+}-binding proteins such as parvalbumin, calbindin D28k and calcineurin are abundant in Purkinje cells (Baimbridge *et al.* 1992). It is notable that GABAergic neurons in general seem to have higher expression levels of several types of Ca^{2+}-binding proteins (Baimbridge *et al.* 1992). A promising approach to relate the presence of Ca^{2+}-binding proteins to a specific function is the investigation of mutant mice lacking one or more of these proteins. In a recent study, climbing fiber-evoked dendritic calcium transients in Purkinje neurons of mice lacking calbindin D28k displayed an initial fast decaying component which was absent in wild type mice, indicating that calbindin D28k acts as a fast and high-affinity buffer that shapes the dendritic calcium transient (Airaksinen *et al.* 1997). Since the mutant mice showed deficits in motor coordination tests, this cellular function seems to be of behavioral importance. Further studies are necessary to resolve the nature, distribution and functional role of dendritic Ca^{2+}-binding proteins. Due to the possible importance of non-equilibrium effects (Markram *et al.* 1998) not only the affinities but also the kinetic properties of the Ca^{2+}-binding proteins need to be studied.

Calcium clearance

Calcium removal mechanisms include extrusion *via* plasma membrane Ca-ATPases and Na^+/Ca^{2+} exchangers, uptake into the endoplasmic reticulum (ER) *via* endo-plasmic Ca-ATPases, and uptake into mitochondria *via* a uniporter (Fig. 7.1c; for a review see Blaustein 1988). The linear removal rate γ can be estimated from the decay of calcium transients if the Ca^{2+}-binding ratio is known (eqn 12). The decay time constant of dendritic calcium transients is about 100 ms in neocortical pyramidal neurons (Markram *et al.* 1995; Helmchen *et al.* 1996; Svoboda *et al.* 1997). Assuming a Ca^{2+}-binding ratio of about 100 this implies a dendritic removal rate on the order of $1000\ s^{-1}$.

Only a few studies to date have investigated the mechanisms involved in dendritic calcium clearance. Markram *et al.* (1995) measured the effect of blockers of extru-sion and uptake mechanisms on the decay time of calcium transients in proximal dendrites of neocortical pyramidal neurons. While blockers of the Na^+/Ca^{2+} ex-changer and the plasma membrane Ca-ATPases had only little effect on the decay time, blockers of the ER Ca-ATPases significantly prolonged the transients. In Purkinje cell somata, these three clearance systems contributed about equally at low $[Ca^{2+}]_i$, while uptake into the ER and extrusion *via* the Na^+/Ca^{2+} exchanger were more effective at high calcium concentrations (Fierro *et al.* 1998). Uptake into mitochondria apparently was not effective at the low $[Ca^{2+}]_i$ levels in these studies; however, a possible role of mitochondria in clearing large calcium loads cannot be excluded.

These findings indicate that sequestration of calcium by internal stores is a major sink for cytosolic calcium, consistent with anatomical studies demonstrating the presence of smooth ER in dendrites and spines (see Chapter 1). In addition, ryanodine-sensitive calcium stores were found to be involved in the sequestration of cytosolic calcium in hippocampal pyramidal dendrites (Garaschuk *et al.* 1997). Most notably, these calcium stores were partially filled during the resting state, implying that they not only serve as calcium sinks but—under appropriate conditions—may function as calcium sources by releasing calcium ions from the ER.

Calcium release

The possibility of calcium-induced calcium release from ryanodine-sensitive stores has been demonstrated in cerebellar Purkinje cells (Llano *et al.* 1994; Kano *et al.* 1995) and hippocampal neurons (Garaschuk *et al.* 1997) in brain slices, as well as in dendritic spines of cultured hippocampal neurons (Korkotian and Segal 1998). Calcium release from ryanodine-sensitive as well as from IP_3-operated stores has been suggested to amplify and prolong dendritic calcium rises, in particular in dendritic spines. In fact, several recent studies demonstrated synaptically induced calcium release in dendritic spines. Release was mediated by activation of metabo-tropic glutamate receptors (mGluRs) and subsequent IP_3 production in cerebellar Purkinje cells (Finch and Augustine 1998; Takechi *et al.* 1998), but presumably was induced by calcium influx through NMDA receptors in cultured hippocampal neurons (Emptage *et al.* 1999). In view of a possible involvement of these mechanisms in synaptic plasticity (for review see Bliss and Collingridge 1993; Svoboda and Mainen 1999) further investigations are necessary.

Other messengers

IP₃

Inositol trisphosphate causes calcium release from internal stores and thereby controls a variety of cellular processes (Berridge 1993). IP_3 is produced by phospholipase C, the activity of which is controlled by a large number of G-protein-linked receptors. It is degraded by the IP_3 3-kinase and 5'-phosphomonoesterase and appears to have a lifetime of a few seconds (Allbritton *et al.* 1992; Wang *et al.* 1995). Although IP_3 is not appreciably bound to buffers in cytosolic extracts of Xenopus oocytes (Allbritton *et al.* 1992), it is not clear if high expression levels of IP_3 receptors, for example in cerebellar Purkinje cell dendrites (Berridge 1993), may cause significant buffering of IP_3. IP_3-mediated calcium release following activation of metabotropic glutamate receptors has been implicated in hippocampal and cerebellar synaptic plasticity (Bliss and Collingridge 1993; Linden 1994). For example, photolytic release of IP_3 was shown to induce parallel fiber LTD in cerebellar Purkinje neurons (Khodakhah and Armstrong 1997; Finch and Augustine 1998). This will be further discussed later in the chapter.

cAMP

cAMP is produced by adenylate cyclase, which is regulated by a variety of G-protein coupled receptors, and is degraded by phosphodiesterase. The lifetime of cAMP in cells presumably is in the range of seconds to minutes (Bacskai *et al.* 1993; Kasai and Petersen 1994). Increases in cAMP concentration can have both local and more widespread effects. PKA is known to modulate dendritic ion channels, for example it recently has been shown to downregulate transient K^+ channels in dendrites of hippocampal neurons (Hoffmann and Johnston 1998). Thus, it might be involved in the regulation of local dendritic excitability (Magee *et al.* 1998). On the other hand, cAMP is known to be part of signaling pathways to the nucleus that cause gene activation (Bito *et al.* 1997). It is therefore important to measure the spatiotemporal dynamics of cAMP concentration, which can be achieved by applying an optical probe based on fluorescence resonance energy transfer between labelled subunits of cAMP-dependent protein kinase PKA (Adams *et al.* 1993). Using this probe application of serotonin onto *Aplysia* sensory neurons evoked large cAMP concentration changes which were highest in the fine processes reaching levels of more then 10 µm (Bacskai *et al.* 1993). Subsequently, the cAMP concentration gradients dissipated due to cAMP diffusion with an apparent diffusion coefficient similar to estimates for aqueous solutions. This suggests that buffering of cAMP is negligible in these neurons. In another study, afferent stimulation of the lobster somatogastric ganglion generated local increases of cAMP in fine neurite branches of neurons which eventually spread to the cell body by diffusion (Hempel *et al.* 1996). These studies demonstrate compartmentalization of cAMP signals as well as its ability to act as a long-range messenger. Similar optical measurements of cAMP signals in dendrites of mammalian central neurons have yet to be done.

Degrees of compartmentalization

Depending on the various factors discussed in the last sections chemical signals can be localized in space and time to different degrees (Fig. 7.4). Using mainly calcium as example, we give here an overview of the wide range and functional significance of chemical compartmentalization in dendrites.

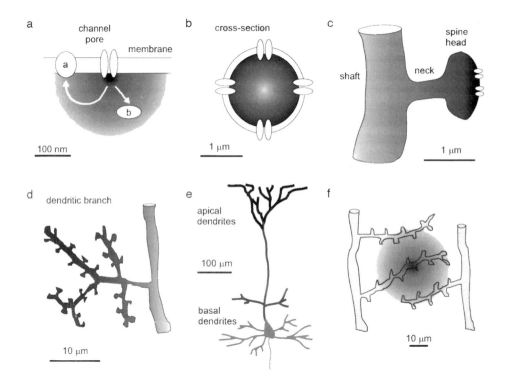

Fig. 7.4 Overview of the degrees of compartmentalization. (a) Domains of high calcium concentrations develop rapidly (<0.1 ms) near the open mouth of a calcium channel. Calcium ions can bind to nearby proteins localized in the membrane (a) or in the cytosol (b). (b) Calcium influx from the extracellular space causes radial concentration gradients which dissipate within milliseconds. (c) Dendritic spines are specialized features which enable the cell to confine concentration increases on the micrometer scale. (d) Calcium elevations can be restricted to dendritic branches. In this case the branches can serve as functional units for 'chemical integration' of incoming synaptic input while the soma remains subthreshold. (e) Calcium accumulation may be relatively widespread but restricted to only parts of the entire dendritic tree, for example the distal dendritic tuft. (f) Compartmentalization differs for freely diffusible messengers such as nitric oxide. In this case a three-dimensional volume—defined by the mobility and lifetime of the messenger—is the affected compartment. The signal can spread to neighboring branches of the same cell or to neighboring cells.

Calcium domains

On the smallest scale, ion flux through an open ion channel causes steep concentration gradients in the immediate vicinity of the channel pore (Fig. 7.4a). In the case of calcium-permeable channels domains of high $[Ca^{2+}]_i$ develop beneath the plasma membrane, reaching peak concentrations of > 100 μM and extending over only a few hundred nanometers (for a review see Neher 1998). Most of the properties of these 'calcium domains' have been inferred from theoretical studies (for example Naraghi and Neher 1997) since they still are challenging to resolve experimentally (but see Llinás *et al.* 1992). Domains develop and collapse extremely rapidly (within a few tens or hundreds of microseconds) following channel opening and closure (Roberts 1994). While immobile buffers have no influence on the steady-state spatial profile of $[Ca^{2+}]_i$, mobile buffers can effectively narrow the spatial extent of domains and prevent binding to nearby targets (Fig. 7.4a). They cause an exponential term in the spatial profile with a length constant λ_D that is given by:

$$\lambda_D = \sqrt{D_{Ca} \tau_D} = \sqrt{D_{Ca}/(k_{on}[B])} \tag{13}$$

where D_{Ca} is the diffusion coefficient of free calcium and $\tau_D = (k_{on}[B])^{-1}$ is the mean time for a calcium ion to be bound by the buffer (note again the square-root relationship). As λ_D depends on the association rate, mobile buffers with either slow (e.g. EGTA) or fast (e.g. BAPTA) kinetics are often used to estimate the distance between intracellular targets and calcium channels.

Besides their importance in controlling neurotransmitter release from presynaptic terminals (Neher 1998) as well as at dendrodendritic synapses (Woolf and Greer 1994; Yuste and Tank 1996), calcium domains have been implicated in various other cellular mechanisms that might be important for dendritic function, such as Ca^{2+}-dependent inactivation of calcium channels (Imredy and Yue 1992) and the activation of $[Ca^{2+}]$-activated potassium channels (Roberts 1994; Marrion and Tavalin 1998). Thus, they may provide a highly localized feedback signal on the electrical membrane properties.

Another interesting possibility is the activation of a third messenger within calcium domains which subsequently is translocated to other parts of the cell. Such a mechanism has been suggested for the phosphorylation of the transcription factor 'cAMP-response element binding protein' (CREB) which promotes nuclear gene expression and has been implicated in the formation of long-term memory (Bito *et al.* 1997). CREB phosphorylation in cultured hippocampal neurons specifically depends on calcium influx during synaptic activation, and calcium was shown to activate calmodulin in a highly localized manner. Calmodulin subsequently is translocated to the nucleus where it activates a CaM kinase which then phosphorylates CREB (Deisseroth *et al.* 1998). The advantage of such an activation cascade is that it combines the specific local initiation of a chemical signal with a widespread effect.

Radial diffusion

Calcium influx from the extracellular space has been shown to cause radial $[Ca^{2+}]_i$ gradients in cell somata (Hernández-Cruz *et al.* 1990). Radial concentration gradients in dendrites (Fig. 7.2b) have not been demonstrated experimentally so far, because these gradients are at the limit of both the spatial and temporal resolution of current imaging techniques (according to eqn 2 diffusional equilibration in a 1 μm thick dendritic segment occurs within a few milliseconds). Therefore, it is not clear if such gradients are of any significance. Numerical simulations of the effect of strategically placing Ca^{2+}-binding proteins within a dendrite, however, indicate that the unequal initial sharing of calcium between competing proteins with different kinetics (see the section on binding affinities and kinetics) can be weakened or enhanced depending on which proteins are placed near the center of the dendrite (Markram *et al.* 1998). Further exploration of such effects awaits more information on the localization and the kinetic properties of target molecules. For many purposes it is justified to neglect radial diffusion and to treat the calcium distribution in dendritic cylinders as a one-dimensional problem (Zador and Koch 1994).

Dendritic spines

Since diffusional equilibration on the micron scale occurs relatively rapidly, one might wonder if cells have developed strategies to localize signals on this scale. Indeed, the structure of dendritic spines appears to be well suited for this purpose (Fig. 7.4c; see also Chapter 1). Dendritic spines are considered as multifunctional compartments with one aspect being chemical compartmentalization (for reviews see Koch and Zador 1993; Harris and Kater 1994; Shepherd 1996). Initially suggested by modeling studies (Gamble and Koch 1987; Wickens 1988), the confinement of calcium signals to individual spines has been demonstrated directly using imaging techniques (for a review see Denk *et al.* 1996). As an example, Fig. 7.5a shows a calcium signal evoked by synaptic activation that is confined to a single dendritic spine in a hippocampal pyramidal neuron. Similar observations were made in spines of hippocampal (Müller and Connor 1991; Yuste and Denk 1995) and neocortical (Koester and Sakmann 1998) pyramidal neurons and of cerebellar Purkinje neurons (Denk *et al.* 1995). Several sources contribute to the calcium influx, including voltage-dependent calcium channels and NMDA receptor channels (Yuste and Denk 1995; Koester and Sakmann 1998; Schiller *et al.* 1998), but possibly also calcium-permeable AMPA or kainate receptors (Denk *et al.* 1995; Yuste *et al.* 1999) as well as calcium release from intracellular stores (Finch and Augustine 1998; Takechi *et al.* 1998; Emptage *et al.* 1999). The relative contribution of these sources depends on the postsynaptic membrane potential and thus could make it possible for a spine to detect coincident pre- and postsynaptic activity as further discussed later in the chapter. Using imaging of calcium in spines, it is possible to detect stochastic failures of synaptic transmission, which may allow optical quantal analysis (Murphy *et al.* 1994; Yuste and Denk 1995; Yuste *et al.* 1999).

The diffusional coupling between spine and shaft has been investigated directly in hippocampal CA1 (Svoboda *et al.* 1996) and cerebellar Purkinje (Häusser *et al.* 1997) neurons by fluorescence recovery from photobleaching or by local uncaging (Fig. 7.5b). Time constants of the diffusional exchange are between 20 and 100 ms for fluorescein dextran (3 kD). Exchange is faster for shorter spines, demonstrating the importance of the spine neck geometry for chemical isolation. For calcium and other second messengers the presence of binding sites and removal mechanisms in

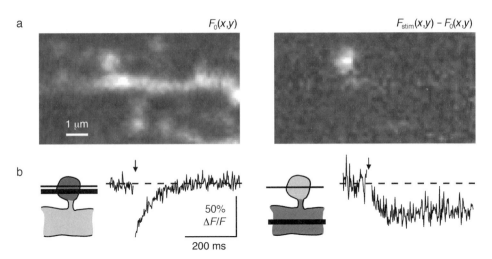

Fig. 7.5 Dendritic spines as biochemical compartments. (a) Two-photon excitation fluorescence image of a dendritic branch and spines of a hippocampal CA1 pyramidal neuron in a brain slice (left). The cell was filled with Calcium Green-1. The difference image of images taken during (F_{stim}) and before (F_0) subthreshold synaptic stimulation (40 Hz, 125 ms) demonstrates that this stimulation produces a calcium accumulation restricted to an individual spine (right). Reprinted with permission from Nature (Yuste and Denk 1995). Copyright (1995) Macmillan Magazines Limited. (b) Measurement of the diffusional coupling between a dendritic spine and the shaft. A hippocampal CA1 pyramidal neuron was filled with fluorescein dextran ($D \approx 0.04 \ \mu m^2 \ ms^{-1}$). Fluorescence was monitored in a dendritic spine head (thin line). Photobleaching was induced with a high-power light exposure for 2 ms (thick line) either in the spine head (left) or in the shaft (right). The time course of the relative fluorescence changes ($\Delta F/F$) reflects the diffusion of unbleached (left) or bleached fluorescein (right) into the spine. Time constants were in the range of 20 to 90 ms. Reprinted with permission from Svoboda *et al.* 1996. Copyright (1996) American Association for the Advancement of Science.

spine necks will further restrict concentration increases to individual spine heads (Woolf and Greer 1994). The confinement of chemical signals to single dendritic spines may be important for the induction of synapse-specific plasticity (Harris and Kater 1994).

Dendritic branches

Calcium elevations may also be restricted to single dendritic branches including several spines and dendritic branchlets (Fig. 7.4d). This degree of compartmentalization has been observed in cerebellar Purkinje cells upon subthreshold parallel fiber activation (Miyakawa *et al.* 1992; Eilers *et al.* 1995; Hartell 1996) as well as in hippocampal CA1 pyramidal neurons upon subthreshold Schaffer collateral stimulation (Magee *et al.* 1995). These localized calcium transients occurred in regions near the synaptic input but were not due to calcium influx through glutamate receptors. Rather, low-voltage activated calcium channels, which were opened by the local synaptic potentials, served as the main entry pathway. Subthreshold activation of dendritic calcium channels was also found in neocortical pyramidal neurons

(Markram and Sakmann 1994). The generation of localized calcium transients by synaptic potentials which remain subthreshold at the soma can be interpreted as a chemical form of synaptic integration (Eilers *et al.* 1995), which could serve to modify synapses locally. In Purkinje cells localized calcium signals indeed are capable of inducing parallel fiber long-term depression (Hartell 1996; Eilers *et al.* 1997). Interestingly, Callaway *et al.* (1995) described local inhibition of widespread calcium increases in Purkinje cell dendrites by IPSPs, which represents the inverse situation compared to localized calcium elevations on a low $[Ca^{2+}]_i$ background. Thus, the spatial pattern of $[Ca^{2+}]_i$ is highly regulated by the spread of membrane potential changes.

Localized calcium transients in Purkinje cell dendrites have also been observed following focal uncaging of IP_3 (Wang and Augustine 1995; Finch and Augustine 1998). In addition, slow onset localized calcium transients due to calcium release were evoked by repetitive parallel fiber stimulation and were restricted to branchlets or even individual spines (Finch and Augustine 1998; Takechi *et al.* 1998). The peak IP_3 concentration produced by such parallel-fiber stimulation was estimated to be on the order of 1 μm. Local increases of IP_3 were shown to be sufficient to induce spatially restricted parallel-fiber long-term depression (Finch and Augustine 1998), demonstrating that IP_3 is capable of defining functional compartments in Purkinje cell dendrites. In contrast to these spatially confined calcium release events in Purkinje cells, waves of calcium release have been observed in soma and dendrites of CA1 hippocampal neurons following local application of mGluR agonists (Jaffe and Brown 1994). It is not clear, however, under what conditions of synaptic stimulation such propagating calcium waves may occur in dendritic trees.

A different example of compartmentalization on the level of dendritic branches has been observed *in vivo* in the visual system of the fly (Borst and Egelhaaf 1994; Single and Borst 1998). In this case calcium accumulations were spatially restricted to those branches that corresponded to the topographic projections of the stimulated part of the visual field.

Dendritic subtrees

Widespread calcium accumulations in dendritic trees or in dendritic subtrees such as basal or distal dendrites (Fig. 7.4e) can be caused by regenerative electrical potentials which involve activation of voltage-gated calcium channels. Backpropagating sodium action potentials (see Chapters 6 and 10) evoke dendritic calcium transients, which may serve as a chemical feedback signal about the output of the cell to parts of the dendritic tree (see also the section on encoding of firing rate below). The spatial extent of the calcium elevations caused by backpropagating action potentials depends on the effectiveness of backpropagation. In Purkinje cells, where backpropagation of the sodium action potential is severely attenuated (Stuart and Häusser 1994), calcium increases during somatic spiking are restricted to the soma and the most proximal dendrites (Lev-Ram *et al.* 1992). In hippocampal and neocortical pyramidal neurons, the calcium transients activated by backpropagating action potentials are typically more extensive, being largest in the proximal dendrite and decreasing further distally (for reviews see Regehr and Tank 1994; Yuste and Tank 1996; Eilers *et al.* 1997). Action potential backpropagation, however, appears to be under the neuromodulatory control of various neurotransmitter systems

(Tsubokawa and Ross 1997; Hoffman and Johnston 1999). *In vivo* calcium imaging using two-photon microscopy has shown that active action potential backpropagation is nearly absent in layer 2/3 pyramidal neurons in anesthetized rats, restricting action potential evoked calcium transients to the proximal dendrites (Svoboda *et al.* 1999). Finally, failure of action potential propagation into subregions of the dendritic tree, for example by frequency-dependent attenuation of backpropagation, can cause corresponding heterogeneity in the calcium signals in different regions (Spruston *et al.* 1995).

While calcium signals evoked by fast action potentials usually are confined to more proximal regions, widespread calcium accumulations can also occur in distal dendrites. One example are the large $[Ca^{2+}]_i$ elevations in Purkinje cell dendrites that are produced by climbing fiber activation (Miyakawa *et al.* 1992). Large calcium transients restricted to the distal dendritic tuft have also been observed in layer V pyramidal neurons (Schiller *et al.* 1997). In this case, the calcium influx depended on the generation of a dendritic calcium action potential which could remain sub-threshold at the soma. The dendritic calcium action potential may serve to amplify distal synaptic input and the distal dendritic $[Ca^{2+}]_i$ elevations may regulate the synaptic efficacy of the distal cortico-cortical afferents to layer V neurons.

Extracellular diffusion

All examples described so far considered cytosolic compartments defined by the dendritic anatomy. A different situation is illustrated in Fig. 7.4f, where the local production of a freely diffusible messenger is considered. For example, nitric oxide (NO) is a gaseous and extremely membrane-permeant messenger which has been implicated in the induction of hippocampal and cerebellar synaptic plasticity (Linden 1994; Schuman and Madison 1994). From its diffusion coefficient (Table 7.1) and a lifetime of 4–5 s one can estimate that NO spreads about 100–200 μm from the site of its production before it degrades. Therefore, it may also affect synapses which have not participated in the induction of synaptic plasticity located either on neighboring dendritic branches of the same neuron or on branches of neighboring cells (Fig. 7.4f). Indeed, non-Hebbian synaptic changes in neighboring neurons within a radius of about 100 μm have been observed in hippocampal slices (Schuman and Madison 1994). More recently, Engert and Bonhoeffer (1997) found in cultured hippocampal slices that LTP spreads 50 to 100 μm along the dendrite of the same neuron. Although they could not conclusively determine whether an intra- or extracellular messenger was responsible for this effect, the dependence on absolute rather than 'cytoplasmic' distance argued in favor of a freely diffusible substance. Similar principles have been suggested to underlie changes in inhibitory transmission mediated by retrograde messengers (reviewed by Alger and Pitler 1995).

Biochemical information processing

In this last section, we address the question of the computational role of biochemical variables in dendritic information processing. Koch (1997) noted that the brain can be thought of as a hybrid computer, operating both in the digital and the analog domain. In a simple view, information is passed digitally from one cell to the other by all-or-none action potentials (see Chapter 10). The spatial and temporal pattern of the digital inputs then is converted into graded biochemical variables such as ion concentrations, membrane protein properties, or enzyme activities, which are further processed in the analog domain and eventually determine the digital output of a postsynaptic neuron. Here we present two examples of how dendritic calcium can encode certain aspects of the digital information transfer between neurons.

Coincidence detection

The first example is the detection of coincidence of a pre- and a postsynaptic action potential which is critical in determining synapse-specific changes of synaptic strength (Markram *et al.* 1997). Several recent studies on pyramidal cells have demonstrated that $[Ca^{2+}]_i$ accumulations in single spines can detect the coincidence of a postsynaptic action potential with the presynaptic neurotransmitter release onto that spine (Yuste and Denk 1995; Koester and Sakmann 1998; Schiller *et al.* 1998; Yuste *et al.* 1999). The basic phenomenon is a supralinear summation of calcium concentration changes caused by pairing of synaptic activation and backpropagating action potentials (Fig. 7.6a). The amplitude of the calcium transient measured when transmitter release is paired with the postsynaptic action potentials is larger than the arithmetic sum of the calcium transients evoked by each stimulus alone. The mechanism underlying this non-linearity could be the relief of the voltage-dependent Mg^{2+}-block of the NMDA-receptor by the backpropagating action potential, which causes additional calcium influx. Evidence consistent with this idea comes from experiments in which focal uncaging of glutamate was used to dissect different pathways for calcium influx in spines of layer V cortical pyramidal neurons (Schiller *et al.* 1998). Although voltage-dependent calcium channels were found to be the main source for calcium rises evoked by glutamate, it was the NMDA-receptor-dependent component which selectively was amplified by pairing protocols. Alternatively or in addition, calcium release from intracellular stores could be involved, e.g. induced by Ca^{2+} influx through NMDA receptors (Emptage *et al.* 1999). At present it is not well understood under which conditions and to what extent these mechanisms contribute to the supralinear spineous $[Ca^{2+}]_i$ accumulations.

Electrophysiological studies have shown that the direction of synaptic changes may be sensitive to the relative timing of pre- and postsynaptic action potentials (Bell *et al.* 1997; Markram *et al.* 1997). If dendritic spines act as coincidence detectors these timing differences should be reflected in the calcium concentrations. Indeed, calcium accumulations in spines critically depend on the relative order of EPSPs and backpropagating action potentials, switching from sublinear summation when EPSPs precede the action potentials to supralinear summation when EPSPs are followed by action potentials (Koester and Sakmann 1998; Yuste *et al.* 1999). At first this might seem consistent with earlier suggestions that the absolute levels of post-synaptic $[Ca^{2+}]_i$ determine whether a synapse is potentiated or depressed (Lisman 1989). However, it is not clear how the average spine calcium concentration—which is measured by imaging techniques—should accomplish this task. For example, it is likely that a burst of postsynaptic action potentials causes similar average calcium concentration changes in the spine head as during pairing of a single action potential

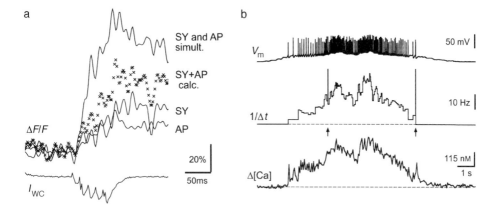

Fig. 7.6 Chemical information processing in dendrites. (a) Dendritic spines as coincidence detectors. The relative fluorescence changes ($\Delta F/F$) of Calcium Green-1 in an individual spine of a hippocampal CA1 pyramidal neuron in a brain slice are shown in response to sub-threshold synaptic stimulation (SY; 5 EPSCs at 75 Hz), postsynaptic spikes (AP) and their simultaneous combination (SY + AP simult.). Pairing of synaptic stimulation and postsynaptic action potentials produces supralinear calcium accumulations in spines, since the response to the combination of the stimuli is larger than the calculated sum of the response to each individual stimulus (SY + AP calc.). Reprinted with permission from Nature (Yuste and Denk 1995). Copyright (1995) Macmillan Magazines Limited. (b) Mean dendritic calcium levels can encode firing rate. Calcium accumulation (Δ[Ca]) in the proximal dendrite of a layer V pyramidal neuron in a brain slice during action potential firing (V_m) with variable frequency evoked by variable somatic current injection. The neuron was filled with Fura-2. The time course of the instantaneous frequency is shown by plotting the inverse of the interspike intervals ($1/\Delta t$). Two bursts with very short interspike intervals occurred at the times indicated by the arrows (peaks are truncated) (reprinted with permission from Helmchen *et al.* 1996).

with an EPSP. Also, recent experiments using photolysis of caged Ca^{2+} question the hypothesis of different $[Ca^{2+}]_i$ thresholds (Neveu and Zucker 1996). This suggests that the average calcium concentration alone is not sufficient to account for the observed differential effects on synaptic changes, but that the exact localization of kinases and phosphatases and the pattern of calcium influx on a submicron scale may be important aspects, as has already been pointed out by Lisman (1989).

Encoding of firing rate

The second example is the encoding of spike frequency by the mean $[Ca^{2+}]_i$ level. As described above, each backpropagating action potential leads to a relatively wide-spread calcium transient in dendrites of hippocampal and neocortical neurons, characterized by a sudden $[Ca^{2+}]_i$ increase due to brief influx through voltage-dependent calcium channels and a roughly exponential decay with a time constant on the order of 100 ms. If action potentials occur with short intervals compared to this decay time, the amplitude of the calcium transient scales with the number of action potentials (Svoboda *et al.* 1997). During slower repetitive firing, however, the dendritic calcium accumulation can be thought of as a 'leaky integrator', which is characterized by a steady-state mean calcium level that linearly depends on the action potential frequency (Helmchen *et al.* 1996; Helmchen and Tank 1999). Indeed, the average calcium concentrations in proximal dendrites of cortical pyramidal neurons reflect the firing frequency well up to a frequency of 30 Hz (Fig. 7.6b). Changes in the firing frequency can be followed on a time scale of 0.1 s, since the time to reach a steady-state level is given by the decay time constant of the individual transients (Helmchen and Tank 1999). The effective time constant to reach a plateau $[Ca^{2+}]_i$ level may even be shorter in the presence of spike adaptation, which would make it possible that the mean $[Ca^{2+}]_i$ level follows frequency fluctuations in the 10–100 ms range (Wang 1998). Given this temporal limitation one can speak of a 'calcium code' for the firing rate (Johnston 1996).

A functional role of these relatively widespread calcium signals could be to provide the dendrites with a feedback signal to control activity-dependent processes. For example, calcium may activate Ca^{2+}-dependent K^+-channels causing hyperpolarization and reducing the cells ability to generate action potentials. The behavioral relevance of intracellular calcium accumulations acting on a calcium-activated K^+-conductance has been demonstrated for the forward masking effect in omega neurons in the cricket auditory pathway where a masking input suppresses the neuronal response to a subsequent test input (Sobel and Tank 1994).

Concluding remarks

In summary, compartmentalization of chemical signals is an important aspect of dendritic signaling. Different messenger substances may have different spatial and temporal ranges of action, and even a single messenger ion such as calcium can exert various functions on different spatial scales. More detailed information about the cellular mechanisms governing the diffusional spread of messenger signals as well as about the ultrastructural organization of dendrites is necessary to elucidate the functional role of these complex signals. Advances in optical imaging techniques should make it possible to further define the relationship between localized dendritic chemical signals and changes in synaptic efficacy. Eventually these techniques may allow one to determine the behavioral relevance of dendritic biochemical compartments.

Acknowledgments

I thank Winfried Denk, Guy Major, David W. Tank, and Samuel S.-H. Wang for their helpful comments on the manuscript.

References

Adams, S. R., Bacskai, B. J., Taylor, S. S., and Tsien, R. Y. (1993). Optical probes for cyclic AMP. In *Fluorescent and luminescent probes for biological activity.* (ed. W. T. Mason) pp. 133–149. Academic Press, London.

Airaksinen, M. S., Eilers, J., Garaschuk, O., Thoenen, H., Konnerth, A., and Meyer, M. (1997). Ataxia and altered dendritic calcium signaling in mice carrying a targeted null mutation of the calbindin D28k gene. *Proceedings of the National Academy of Sciences*, **94**, 1488–93.

Alger, B. E. and Pitler, T. A. (1998). Retrograde signaling at $GABA_A$-receptor synapses in the mammalian CNS. *Trends in Neurosciences*, **18**, 333–40.

Allbritton, N. L., Meyer, T., and Stryer, L. (1992). Range of messenger action of calcium ion and inositol 1,4,5-triphosphate. *Science*, **258**, 1812–15.

Bacskai, B. J., Hochner, B., Mahaut-Smith, M., Adams, S. R., Kaang, B.-K., Kandel, E. R. *et al.* (1993). Spatially resolved dynamics of cAMP and protein kinase A subunits in Aplysia sensory neurons. *Science*, **260**, 222–6.

Baimbridge, K. G., Celio, M. R., and Rogers, J. H. (1992). Calcium-binding proteins in the nervous system. *Trends in Neurosciences*, **15**, 303–8.

Bell, C. C., Han, V. Z., Sugawara, Y., and Grant, K. (1997). Synaptic plasticity in a cerebellum-like structure depends on temporal order. *Nature*, **387**, 278–81.

Berridge, M. J. (1993). Inositol trisphosphate and calcium signalling. *Nature*, **361**, 315–25.

Bito, H., Deisseroth, K., and Tsien, R. W. (1997). Ca^{2+}-dependent regulation in neuronal gene expression. *Current Opinion in Neurobiology*, **7**, 419–29.

Blaustein, M. P. (1988). Calcium transport and buffering in neurons. *Trends in Neuroscience*, **11**, 438–43.

Bliss, T. V. P. and Collingridge, G. L. (1993). A synaptic model of memory: long-term potentiation in the hippocampus. *Nature*, **361**, 31–9.

Bonhoeffer, T., Staiger, V., and Aertsen, A. (1989). Synaptic plasticity in rat hippocampal slice cultures: local 'Hebbian' conjunction of pre- and postsynaptic stimulation leads to distributed synaptic enhancement. *Proceedings of the National Academy of Sciences*, **86**, 8113–7.

Borst, A. and Egelhaaf, M. (1994). Dendritic processing of synaptic information by sensory interneurons. *Trends in Neurosciences*, **17**, 257–63.

Callaway, J. C. and Ross, W. N. (1997). Spatial distribution of synaptically activated sodium concentration changes in cerebellar Purkinje neurons. *Journal of Neurophysiology*, **77**, 145–52.

Callaway, J. C., Lasser-Ross, N., and Ross, W. N. (1995). IPSPs strongly inhibit climbing fiber-activated $[Ca^{2+}]_i$ increases in the dendrites of cerebellar Purkinje neurons. *Journal of Neuroscience*, **15**, 2777–87.

Chesler, M. and Kaila, K. (1992). Modulation of pH by neuronal activity. *Trends in Neurosciences*, **15**, 396–402.

Clapham, D. E. (1995). Calcium signaling. *Cell*, **80**, 259–68.

Deisseroth, K., Heist, E. K., and Tsien, R. W. (1998). Translocation of calmodulin to the nucleus supports CREB phosphorylation in hippocampal neurons. *Nature*, **392**, 198–202.

Denk, W. and Svoboda, K. (1997). Photon upmanship: why multiphoton imaging is more than a gimmick. *Neuron* **18**, 351–7.

Denk, W., Strickler, J. H., and Webb, W. W. (1990). Two-photon laser scanning fluorescence microscopy. *Science*, **248**, 73–6.

Denk, W., Sugimori, M., and Llinás, R. (1995). Two types of calcium response limited to single spines in cerebellar Purkinje cells. *Proceedings of the National Academy of Sciences*, **92**, 8279–82.

Denk, W., Yuste, R., Svoboda, K., and Tank, D. W. (1996). Imaging calcium dynamics in dendritic spines. *Current Opinion in Neurobiology*, **6**, 372–8.

De Schutter, E. and Smolen, P. (1998). Calcium dynamics in large neuronal models. In *Methods in neuronal modeling: from ions to networks*, (2nd edn). (ed. C. Koch and I. Segev), pp. 211–50, MIT Press, Cambridge.

Douglas, R. J. and Martin, K. A. C. (1998). Neocortex. In *The Synaptic organization of the brain*, (4th edn) (ed. G. M. Shepherd), pp. 459–510. Oxford University Press, New York.

Eilers, J. and Konnerth, A. (1997). Dendritic signal integration. *Current Opinion in Neurobiology*, **7**, 385–90.

Eilers, J., Augustine, G. J., and Konnerth, A. (1995*a*). Subthreshold synaptic Ca^{2+} signalling in fine dendrites and spines of cerebellar Purkinje neurons. *Nature*, **373**, 155–8.

Eilers, J., Schneggenburger, R., and Konnerth, A. (1995*b*). Patch clamp and calcium imaging in brain slices. In *Single-channel recording*, (2nd edn) (ed. B. Sakmann and E. Neher), pp. 213–229. Plenum Press, New York.

Eilers, J., Takechi, H., Finch, E. A., Augustine, G. J., and Konnerth, A. (1997). Local dendritic Ca^{2+} signaling induces cerebellar long-term depression. *Learning and Memory*, **3**, 159–68.

Emptage, N., Bliss, T. V. P., and Fine, A. (1999). Single synaptic events evoke NMDA receptor-mediated release of calcium from internal stores in hippocampal dendritic spines. *Neuron*, **22**, 115–24.

Engert, F. and Bonhoeffer, T. (1997). Synapse specificity of long-term potentiation breaks down at short distances. *Nature*, **388**, 279–84.

Falke, J. J., Drake, S. K., Hazard, A. L., and Peersen, O. B. (1994). Molecular tuning of ion binding to calcium signaling proteins. *Quarterly Reviews of Biophysics*, **27**, 219–90.

Fierro, L. and Llano, I. (1996). High endogenous calcium buffering in Purkinje cells from rat cerebellar slices. *Journal of Physiology*, **496**, 617–25.

Fierro, L., DiPolo, R., and Llano, I. (1998). Intracellular calcium clearance in Purkinje cell somata from cerebellar slices. *Journal of Physiology*, **510**, 499–512.

Finch, E. A. and Augustine, G. (1998). Local calcium signalling by inositol 1,4,5-trisphosphate in Purkinje cell dendrites. *Nature*, **396**, 753–6.

Gabso, M., Neher, E., and Spira, M. E. (1997). Low mobility of the Ca^{2+} buffers in axons of cultured Aplysia neurons. *Neuron*, **18**, 473–81.

Gamble, E. and Koch, C. (1987). The dynamics of free calcium in dendritic spines in response to repetitive synaptic input. *Science*, **236**, 1311–15.

Garaschuk, O., Yaari, Y., and Konnerth, A. (1997). Release and sequestration of calcium by ryanodine-sensitive stores in rat hippocampal neurones. *Journal of Physiology*, **502**, 13–30.

Ghosh, A. and Greenberg, M. E. (1995). Calcium signaling in neurons: molecular mechanisms and cellular consequences. *Science*, **268**, 239–47.

Hara, M., Inoue, M., Yasukura, T., Ohnishi, S., Mikami, Y., and Inagaki, C. (1992). Uneven distribution of intracellular Cl^- in rat hippocampal neurons. *Neuroscience Letters*, **143**, 135–8.

Harris, K. M. and Kater, S. B. (1994). Dendritic spines: cellular specializations imparting both stability and flexibility to synaptic function. *Annual Reviews in Neuroscience*, **17**, 341–71.

Hartell, N. (1996). Strong activation of parallel fibers produce localized calcium transients and a form of LTD that spreads to distant synapses. *Neuron*, **16**, 601–10.

Häusser, M., Parésys, G., and Denk, W. (1997). Coupling between dendritic spines and shafts in cerebellar Purkinje cells. *Society for Neuroscience Abstracts*, **23**, 2006.

Helmchen, F. and Tank, D. W. (1999). A single compartment model of calcium dynamics in nerve terminals and dendrites. In *Imaging living cells: a laboratory manual*, (ed. R. Yuste, F. Lanni, and A. Konnerth). Cold Spring Harbor Laboratory Press.

Helmchen, F., Imoto, K., and Sakmann, B. (1996). Ca^{2+} buffering and action potential-evoked Ca^{2+} signaling in dendrites of pyramidal neurons. *Biophysical Journal*, **70**, 1069–81.

Hempel, C. M., Vincent, P., Adams, S. R., Tsien, R. Y., and Selverston, A. I. (1996). Spatio-temporal dynamics of cyclic AMP signals in an intact neural circuit. *Nature*, **384**, 166–9.

Hernández-Cruz, A., Sala, F., and Adams, P. R. (1990). Subcellular calcium transients visualized by confocal microscopy in a voltage-clamped vertebrate neuron. *Science*, **247**, 858–62.

Hoffman, D. A. and Johnston, D. (1998). Downregulation of transient K^+ channels in dendrites of hippocampal CA1 pyramidal neurons by activation of PKA and PKC. *Journal of Neuroscience*, **18**, 3521–8.

Hoffman, D. A. and Johnston, D. (1999). Neuromodulation of dendritic action potentials. *Journal of Neurophysiology*, **81**, 408–11.

Imredy, J. P. and Yue, D. T. (1992). Submicroscopic Ca^{2+} diffusion mediates inhibitory coupling between individual Ca^{2+} channels. *Neuron*, **9**, 197–207.

Inglefield, J. R. and Schwartz-Bloom, R. D. (1997). Confocal imaging of intracellular chloride in living brain slices: measurement of $GABA_A$ receptor activity. *Journal of Neuroscience Methods*, **75**, 127–35.

Irving, M., Maylie, J., Sizto, N. L., and Chandler, W. K. (1990). Intracellular diffusion in the presence of mobile buffers. *Biophysical Journal*, **57**, 717–21.

Jaffe, D. B. and Brown, T. H. (1994). Metabotropic glutamate receptor activation induces calcium waves within hippocampal dendrites. *Journal of Neurophysiology*, **72**, 471–4.

Jaffe, D. B., Johnston, D., Lasser-Ross, N., Lisman, J. E., Miyakawa, H., and Ross, W. N. (1992). The spread of Na^+ spikes determines the pattern of dendritic Ca^{2+} entry into hippocampal neurons. *Nature*, **357**, 244–6.

Johnston, D. (1996). The calcium code. *Biophysical Journal*, **70**, 1095.

Kaila, K., Lamsa, K., Smirnov, S., Taira, T., and Voipio, J. (1997). Long-lasting GABA-mediated depolarization evoked by high-frequency stimulation in pyramidal neurons of rat hippocampal slice is attributable to a network-driven, bicarbonate-dependent K^+ transient. *Journal of Neuroscience*, **17**, 7662–72.

Kano, M., Garaschuk, O., Verkhratsky, A., and Konnerth, A. (1995). Ryanodine receptor-mediated intracellular calcium release in rat cerebellar Purkinje neurones. *Journal of Physiology*, **487**, 1–16.

Kasai, H. and Petersen, O. H. (1994). Spatial dynamics of second messengers: IP_3 and cAMP as long-range and associative messengers. *Trends in Neurosciences*, **17**, 95–101.

Khodakhah, K. and Armstrong, C. M. (1997). Induction of long-term depression and rebound potentiation by inositol trisphosphate in cerebellar Purkinje neurons. *Proceedings of the National Academy of Sciences*, **94**, 14009–14.

Koch, C. (1997). Computation and the single neuron. *Nature*, **385**, 207–10.

Koch, C. (1998). *Biophysics of computation. Information processing in single neurons*, pp. 248–279. Oxford University Press.

Koch, C. and Zador, A. (1993). The function of dendritic spines: devices subserving biochemical rather than electrical compartmentalization. *Journal of Neuroscience*, **13**, 413–22.

Koester, H. and Sakmann, B. (1998). Calcium dynamics in single spines during coincident pre- and postsynaptic activity depend on relative timing of back-propagating action potentials and subthreshold excitatory postsynaptic potentials. *Proceedings of the National Academy of Sciences*, **95**, 9596–601.

Korkotian, E. and Segal, M. (1998). Fast confocal imaging of calcium released from stores in dendritic spines. *European Journal of Neuroscience*, **10**, 2076–84.

Lasser-Ross, N. and Ross, W. N. (1992). Imaging voltage and synaptically activated sodium transients in cerebellar Purkinje cells. *Proceedings of the Royal Society London B*, **247**, 35–9.

Lasser-Ross, N., Miyakawa, H., Lev-Ram, V., Young, S. R., and Ross, W. N. (1991). High time resolution fluorescence imaging with a CCD camera. *Journal of Neuroscience Methods*, **36**, 253–61.

Lev-Ram, V., Miyakawa, H., Lasser-Ross, N., and Ross, W. N. (1992). Calcium transients in cerebellar Purkinje neurons evoked by intracellular stimulation. *Journal of Neurophysiology* **68**, 1167–77.

Linden, D. J. (1994). Long-term depression in the mammalian brain. *Neuron*, **12**, 457–72.

Lisman, J. (1989). A mechanism for the Hebb and the anti-Hebb processes underlying learning and memory. *Proceedings of the National Academy of Sciences*, **86**, 9574–8.

Llano, I., DiPolo, R., and Marty, A. (1994). Calcium-induced calcium release in cerebellar Purkinje cells. *Neuron*, **12**, 663–73.

Llinás, R., Sugimori, M., and Silver, R. B. (1992). Microdomains of high calcium concentration in a presynaptic terminal. *Science*, **256**, 677–9.

Magee, J. C., Christofi, G., Miyakawa, H., Christie, B., Lasser-Ross, N., and Johnston, D. (1995). Subthreshold synaptic activation of voltage-gated Ca^{2+} channels mediates a localized Ca^{2+} influx into dendrites of hippocampal pyramidal neurons. *Journal of Neurophysiology*, **74**, 1335–42.

Magee, J. C., Hoffmann, D., Colbert, C., and Johnston, D. (1998). Electrical and calcium signaling in dendrites of hippocampal neurons. *Annual Reviews in Physiology*, **60**, 327–46.

Markram, H. and Sakmann, B. (1994). Calcium transients in dendrites of neocortical neuron evoked by single sub-threshold excitatory post-synaptic potentials *via* low-voltage-activated calcium channels. *Proceedings of the National Academy of Sciences*, **91**, 5207–11.

Markram, H., Helm, P. J., and Sakmann, B. (1995). Dendritic calcium transients evoked by single back-propagating action potentials in rat neocortical pyramidal neurons. *Journal of Physiology*, **485**, 1–20.

Markram, H., Lübke, J., Frotscher, M., and Sakmann, B. (1997). Regulation of synaptic efficacy by coincidence of postsynaptic APs and EPSPs. *Science*, **275**, 213–15.

Markram, H., Roth, A., and Helmchen, F. (1998). Competitive calcium binding: implications for dendritic calcium signaling. *Journal of Computational Neuroscience*, **5**, 331–48.

Marrion, N. V. and Tavalin, S. J. (1998). Selective activation of Ca^{2+}-activated K^+ channels by co-localized Ca^{2+} channels in hippocampal neurons. *Nature*, **395**, 900–5.

Mittmann, T., Linton, S. M., Schwindt, P., and Crill, W. (1997). Evidence for persistent Na^+ current in apical dendrites of rat neocortical neurons from imaging of Na^+-sensitive dye. *Journal of Neurophysiology*, **78**, 1188–92.

Miyakawa, H., Lev-Ram, V., Lasser-Ross, N., and Ross, W. N. (1992). Calcium transients evoked by climbing fiber and parallel fiber synaptic inputs in guinea pig cerebellar Purkinje neurons. *Journal of Neurophysiology*, **68**, 1178–88.

Mochly-Rosen, D. (1995). Localization of protein kinases by anchoring proteins: a theme in signal transduction. *Science*, **268**, 247–51.

Müller, W. and Connor, J. A. (1991). Dendritic spines as individual neuronal compartments for synaptic Ca^{2+} responses. *Nature*, **354**, 73–6.

Murphy, T. H., Baraban, J. M., Wier, W. G., and Blatter, L. A. (1994). Visualization of quantal synaptic transmission by dendritic calcium imaging. *Science*, **263**, 529–32.

Naraghi, M. and Neher, E. (1997). Linearized buffered Ca^{2+} diffusion in microdomains and its implications for calculation of $[Ca^{2+}]$ at the mouth of a calcium channel. *Journal of Neuroscience*, **17**, 6961–73.

Neher, E. (1995). The use of fura-2 for estimating Ca buffers and Ca fluxes. *Neuropharmacology*, **34**, 1423–42.

Neher, E. (1998). Vesicle pools and Ca^{2+} microdomains: new tools for understanding their roles in neurotransmitter release. *Neuron*, **20**, 389–99.

Nerbonne, J. M. (1996). Caged compounds: tools for illuminating neuronal responses and connections. *Current Opinion in Neurobiology*, **6**, 379–86.

Neveu, D. and Zucker, R. S. (1996). Postsynaptic levels of $[Ca^{2+}]_i$ needed to trigger LTD and LTP. *Neuron*, **16**, 619–29.

Palay, S. and Chan-Palay, V. (1974). *Cerebellar cortex*. Springer, Heidelberg.

Regehr, W. and Tank, D. W. (1994). Dendritic calcium dynamics. *Current Opinion in Neurobiology*, **4**, 373–82.

Roberts, W. M. (1994). Localization of calcium signals by a mobile calcium buffer in frog saccular hair cells. *Journal of Neuroscience*, **14**, 3246–62.

Schiller, J., Helmchen, F., and Sakmann, B. (1995). Spatial profile of dendritic calcium transients evoked by action potentials in rat neocortical pyramidal neurons. *Journal of Physiology*, **487**, 583–600.

Schiller, J., Schiller, Y., Stuart, G., and Sakmann, B. (1997). Calcium action potentials restricted to distal apical dendrites of rat neocortical pyramidal neurons. *Journal of Physiology*, **505**, 605–16.

Schiller, J., Schiller, Y., and Clapham, D. E. (1998). NMDA receptors amplify calcium influx into dendritic spines during associative pre- and postsynaptic activation. *Nature Neuroscience*, **1**, 114–8.

Schuman, E. M. and Madison, D. V. (1994). Locally distributed synaptic potentiation in the hippocampus. *Science*, **263**, 532–6.

Sejnowski, T. J. and Qian, N. (1992). Synaptic integration by electro-diffusion in dendritic spines. In *Single neuron computation*. (ed. T. McKenna, J. Davis, and S. F. Zornetzer), pp. 117–40. Academic Press, London.

Sheetz, M. P., Pfister, K. K., Bulinski, J. C., and Cotman, C. W. (1998). Mechanisms of trafficking in axons and dendrites: implications for development and neurodegeneration. *Progress in Neurobiology*, **55**, 577–94.

Shen, K. and Meyer, T. (1999). Dynamic control of CaMKII translocation and localization in hippocampal neurons by NMDA receptor stimulation. *Science*, **284**, 162–6.

Shepherd, G. M. (1996). The dendritic spine: a multifunctional integrative unit. *Journal of Neurophysiology*, **75**, 2197–210.

Single, S. and Borst, A. (1998). Dendritic integration and its role in computing image velocity. *Science*, **281**, 1848–50.

Sobel, E. C. and Tank, D. W. (1994). *In vivo* Ca^{2+} dynamics in a cricket auditory neuron: an example of chemical computation. *Science*, **263**, 823–6.

Spruston, N., Schiller, Y., Stuart, G., and Sakmann, B. (1995). Activity dependent action potential invasion and calcium influx into hippocampal CA1 dendrites. *Science*, **268**, 297–300.

Staley, K. J., Soldo, B. L., and Proctor, W. R. (1995). Ionic mechanisms of neuronal excitation by inhibitory $GABA_A$ receptors. *Science*, **269**, 977–81.

Stuart, G. and Häusser, M. (1994). Initiation and spread of sodium action potentials in cerebellar Purkinje cells. *Neuron*, **13**, 703–12.

Svoboda, K. and Mainen, Z. F. (1999). Synaptic $[Ca^{2+}]$: intracellular stores spill their guts. *Neuron*, **22**, 427–30.

Svoboda, K., Tank, D. W., and Denk, W. (1996). Direct measurement of coupling between dendritic spines and shafts. *Science*, **272**, 716–19.

Svoboda, K., Denk, W., Kleinfeld, D., and Tank, D. W. (1997). *In vivo* dendritic calcium dynamics in neocortical pyramidal neurons. *Nature*, **385**, 161–5.

Svoboda, K., Helmchen, F., Denk, W., and Tank, D. W. (1999). Spread of dendritic excitation in layer 2/3 pyramidal neurons in rat barrel cortex *in vivo*. *Nature Neuroscience*, **2**, 65–73.

Takechi, H., Eilers, J., Konnerth, A. (1998). A new class of synaptic response involving calcium release in dendritic spines. *Nature*, **396**, 757–60.

Tombaugh, G. C. (1998). Intracellular pH buffering shapes activity-dependent Ca^{2+} dynamics of CA1 interneurons. *Journal of Neurophysiology*, **80**, 1702–12.

Tsien, R. Y. (1989). Fluorescent probes of cell signaling. *Annual Reviews in Neuroscience*, **12**, 227–53.

Tsubokawa, H. and Ross, W. N. (1997). Muscarinic modulation of spike backpropagation in the apical dendrites of hippocampal CA1 pyramidal neurons. *Journal of Neuroscience*, **17**, 5782–91.

Tsubokawa, H., Miura, M., and Kano, M. (1999). Elevation of intracellular Na^+ induced by hyperpolarization at the dendrites of pyramidal neurones of mouse hippocampus. *Journal of Physiology*, **517**, 135–42.

Wang, S. S.-H. and Augustine, G. J. (1995). Confocal imaging and local photolysis of caged compounds: dual probes of synaptic function. *Neuron*, **15**, 755–60.

Wang, S. S.-H. and Augustine, G. J. (1999). Calcium signaling in neurons: a case study in cellular compartmentalization. In *Calcium in biological function*, (ed. E. Carafoli and C. B. Klee). Oxford University Press, New York.

Wang, S. S.-H., Alousi, A. A., and Thompson, S. H. (1995). The lifetime of inositol 1,4,5-trisphosphate in single cells. *Journal of General Physiology*, **105**, 149–71.

Wang, X.-J. (1998). Calcium coding and adaptive temporal computation in cortical pyramidal neurons. *Journal of Neurophysiology*, **79**, 1549–66.

Wickens, J. (1988). Electrically coupled but chemically isolated synapses: dendritic spines and calcium in a rule for synaptic modification. *Progress in Neurobiology*, **31**, 507–28.

Woolf, T. B. and Greer, C. A. (1994). Local communication within dendritic spines: models of second messenger diffusion in granule cell spines of the mammalian olfactory bulb. *Synapse*, **17**, 247–67.

Yuste, R. and Denk, W. (1995). Dendritic spines as basic units of neuronal integration. *Nature*, **375**, 682–4.

Yuste, R. and Tank, D. W. (1996). Dendritic integration in mammalian neurons, a century after Cajal. *Neuron*, **16**, 701–16.

Yuste, R., Majewska, A., Cash, S. S., and Denk, W. (1999). Mechanisms of calcium influx into hippocampal spines: heterogeneity among spines, coincidence detection by NMDA receptors and optical quantal analysis. *Journal of Neuroscience*, **19**, 1976–87.

Zador, A. and Koch, C. (1994). Linearized models of calcium dynamics: formal equivalence to the cable equation. *Journal of Neuroscience*, **14**, 4705–15.

8

An historical perspective on modeling dendrites

Wilfrid Rall

Scientist Emeritus of the National Institutes of Health

Summary

The advent of microelectrode recordings from neurons with branching dendritic trees presented a new problem for neurophysiologists—how to interpret the data obtained from these nonisopotential structures. An important step was the development of mathematical models of dendrites. The theory behind these models is discussed in Chapter 9. Here I provide an historical perspective of the development of such models, paying attention to the progression from passive, linear models to the more complex case of neurons with extensive branching and nonlinear properties. Several other publications provide examples of my perspective, with only partial overlap (Rall 1977, 1992, 1995; Rall and Agmon-Snir 1998; Segev and Rall 1998).

Introduction

The extensiveness of dendritic branching, for most neurons, has been established for 100 years, since the pioneering research of Ramon y Cajal. The need for a mathematical treatment of dendritic cable properties, however, was not recognized until sharp, micropipette electrodes were first used (in the early 1950s) for intracellular recording from motoneurons of cat spinal cord. Successful impalement was usually made in the motoneuron soma, rarely in a large dendritic trunk, and never in a small dendritic branch. The goal was to understand what effect the extensively branched dendritic membrane has on voltage transients recorded in the soma, and it was quickly recognized that modeling was essential for the interpretation of the data. As mathematical modeling has evolved over the years, the key to success has been a recognition of the important interplay between theory and experiment.

Sharp electrodes and membrane time-constant

In the late 1940s, Graham, Ling and Gerard, at the University of Chicago, began to use sharp micropipettes for intracellular recording from single muscle fibers; this application to muscle was extended by Hodgkin and Nastuk, and by Fatt and Katz. Similar electrodes were then applied to motoneurons of cat spinal cord by Woodbury and Patton, by Brock, Coombs and Eccles, and by Frank and Fuortes (early 1950s). It is noteworthy that both Woodbury and Frank learned about these electrodes in the Physiology Laboratories at the University of Chicago; Eccles heard about them from Dexter Easton, who came to Dunedin, New Zealand as a Fulbright Fellow from Seattle, where he had learned about Woodbury's research.

Although I had done extracellular recording with Brock and Eccles, in Dunedin (1949–51), I did not participate in their sharp electrode experiments, because my focus then was on completing my Ph.D. research, aimed at matching experiment and theory for a reflex input/output relation, using monosynaptic responses in spinal cord motoneuron populations. When Eccles moved from Dunedin to Canberra, in the early 1950s, he was succeeded in Dunedin by my good friend, Archie McIntyre, who later moved to Monash University, in Melbourne. In 1956, I moved from Dunedin to Bethesda, where I met Frank and Fuortes; after 17 months at the Naval Medical Research Institute I moved to NIH, where I worked in the Mathematical Research Branch for the next 37 years.

By 1956, two groups (Frank and Fuortes at NIH, and Eccles with collaborators in Canberra) had published membrane time-constant estimates based on their intracellular recordings of voltage transients obtained in response to an electric shock applied across the motoneuron soma membrane by the recording electrode (relative to an extracellular reference electrode). Both groups reported unexpectedly low values for the membrane time-constant; their values, between 1 and 2.5 ms, created a puzzling discrepancy with earlier estimates of approximately 4 or 5 ms, based on synaptic potential decay.

Both groups had analyzed their transient records as if they were composed of a single exponential. Although they did not say so, this meant that they had implicitly assumed a space-clamped neuron, or an isopotential soma, without any dendrites. If one does not postulate an explicit biophysical model that includes such an essential complication as the presence of dendritic cables, then one runs the risk of using overly simple data analysis that yields an incorrect value for the membrane time-constant.

Data analysis needs models that include dendrites

The error was pointed out in a brief note to Science (Rall 1957), followed by a manuscript with a full explanation and discussion submitted to the Journal of General Physiology in 1958. Sadly, this manuscript was rejected, at the urging of a negative referee; however, this manuscript did appear in 1959 as a Research Report of the Naval Medical Research Institute (NMRI) in Bethesda, Maryland. Also, the editors of a new journal, Experimental Neurology, encouraged me to publish this material as two papers; the focus of one (Rall 1959) was on steady-state attenuation and input resistance, that of the other (Rall 1960) was on transients and a method for estimating membrane time-constants.

Frank and Fuortes freely acknowledged their error. Eccles did so only indirectly, by slightly revising his estimates; his postulated residual phase of synaptic current (much illustrated during 1956–8) became reduced in magnitude, and later abandoned. For those readers who might be interested in further details and commentary on the impact of these papers, three references are recommended: pages 27–103 in a book of selected reprints with commentaries (Segev *et al.* 1995); pages 222–225 in a book chapter that describes my research 'path' (Rall 1992); and pages 45–58 in a Handbook chapter (Rall 1977).

From hindsight, we now know that those early transients were also made faster by membrane shunting at the electrode penetration site. In 1959, I did report the interesting clue that large electrode tips tended to yield lower estimates of input resistance, but I did not know the magnitude of the leak until much later, when the patch-clamp method was used for whole-cell recording. The significance of this shunt was discussed in a multiple-authored Physiological Review (Rall *et al.* 1992); also, the mathematical effect of this shunt on the system eigenvalues and time-constants has been solved and discussed (Holmes and Rall 1992; Major *et al.* 1993).

Dendritic synaptic input and EPSP shapes

Once dendritic cable properties had been shown to be important for the interpretation of experimental data, it became clear to me that it was more interesting to investigate the functional implications of synaptic inputs to the dendrites than to pursue refinements in time-constant estimation. This new objective led to two different mathematical models, and to fruitful research collaboration with an NIH experimental group, Burke, Smith, Nelson and Frank, in the Laboratory of Neurophysiology.

For idealized dendritic branching, a dendritic tree was shown to be reducible to an equivalent cylinder of finite length. By making the assumption of passive membrane properties, an analytical solution (Rall 1962a) was used to compute (by slide rule) the first theoretical excitatory synaptic potentials (EPSPs) for nonuniform synaptic input. The synaptic input could be applied to one of two regions (such as soma and proximal dendrites, compared with more distal dendrites). For a brief synaptic input near the soma, the EPSP rises steeply to an early peak, followed by rapid early decay, and then by slower decay. If the same brief synaptic input is delivered to distal dendrites, the EPSP (at the soma) shows a delay, and rises more slowly to a later, more rounded peak, and then decays slowly.

To compare theoretical EPSP shapes with experimentally recorded EPSP shapes, we invented the shape–index plot (Rall *et al.* 1967) in which each shape is a point in a two-dimensional plot of half-width against time-to-peak, or rise-time. It was an exciting time, because many of the data had already been obtained, but had not been plotted in this way. Also, to improve the resolution of theoretical EPSP shapes, I introduced a brief input time-course (now known as an alpha function), and represented the soma plus dendritic trees as a chain of ten compartments. It is noteworthy that compartmental modeling of soma and dendrites was first presented at a 1962 symposium; the published chapter (Rall 1964) has been reprinted in Segev *et al.* (1995) as has the 1967 modeling paper (Rall *et al.* 1967).

This research collaboration culminated in a series of five papers published together in a 1967 issue of the Journal of Neurophysiology. While here avoiding many details, it can be said that this research persuaded the neurophysiological

community that dendritic synaptic input is functional and has predictable characteristics, contrary to what Eccles had maintained. This conclusion was strengthened
by confirmatory experimental studies in Oxford, by Jack, Redman and others, and at
Harvard, by Mendell and Henneman. In all of these studies, we had a population of
EPSP shapes that could be compared with theoretical shape index loci, but we did
not have experimental verification of the presumed proximal and distal dendritic
locations of the synaptic inputs. This deficiency was remedied by the remarkable
experiments of Redman and Walmsley (1983), which provided strong support for the
theoretical relationship between EPSP shape and input location.

Passive *versus* active dendrites and diphasic extracellular voltage transients—theory and experiment

After presenting a seminar in Bern, in 1995, I was asked for a historical perspective
on the question: Why had several early experiments that had been offered as
evidence of active propagation in motoneuron dendrites (Fatt 1957; Terzuolo and
Araki 1961), not been widely accepted as compelling evidence? The answer, I believe,
lies mainly in the demonstration that the key observation, a diphasic extracellular
voltage (V_e) transient, that was recorded in response to antidromic activation of a
single motoneuron soma, was predicted by a computed simulation that assumed
passive properties for the dendritic membrane (Rall 1962*b*). The computed result was
unambiguous, but it was puzzling to many physiologists. Thus, it has been helpful to
provide also the following physical–intuitive explanation.

First phase of diphasic V_e

During the first phase of the somatic action potential, (produced by an antidromic
axonal impulse that fires the soma), the soma membrane is actively depolarized (by
inward flow of sodium ions); there is a passive spread of membrane depolarization
from the soma to the dendrites, but the soma remains the most depolarized during
this first phase. Thus, the flow of intracellular current is from the soma into the
dendrites; the extracellular current flows toward the soma, more or less radially from
the distributed multipolar dendritic membrane. It was shown that such current flow
in the extracellular volume will produce a field of electric potential that is more
negative in the inner extracellular volume (near the soma and proximal dendrites of
that motoneuron), than in the outer extracellular volume (near its distal dendrites
and beyond). This extracellular electric field (generated by activity of this one
motoneuron) is responsible for the initial negative phase of the diphasic (V_e) record,
obtained with an electrode placed in the inner extracellular volume, recording
relative to a reference electrode that is placed near or beyond distal dendritic
branches of this motoneuron.

Second phase of diphasic V_e

During the second phase of this somatic action potential, the soma membrane is
rapidly, actively repolarized (by outward flow of potassium ions); the direction of

current flow is reversed from that in the first phase. During this second phase, the repolarizing soma membrane becomes less depolarized than the dendritic membrane, because the membrane depolarization that had spread passively from soma to dendrites (during the first phase) now decays slowly in the dendrites (because the dendritic membrane is assumed to be passive). The dendritic membrane remains more depolarized than the rapidly repolarizing soma membrane. Thus, the intracellular current flows from dendrites to soma; the extracellular current flows from the soma, more or less radially outward, to the membrane of distal dendritic branches. It was shown that such almost radial flow of current in the extracellular volume will produce a reversed field of electric potential; this field is more positive in the inner extracellular volume (near soma and proximal dendrites), than near or beyond the distal dendritic branches of this motoneuron. The reversed electric field is responsible for the positive (second) phase of the diphasic (V_e) transient obtained with an electrode placed in the inner extracellular volume, recording relative to a distant reference electrode.

The key point, that others had overlooked, is the rapid reversal of current, because of active repolarization of the soma membrane, described above.

Acceptance of V_e **theory and conclusions**

This mathematical modeling result was presented in seminars at NIH and elsewhere (in 1960). It was discussed at length with Frank and Nelson, and others; they all became convinced. This result was then presented at the first International Biophysics Congress, Stockholm, 1961, and was subsequently published in a special issue of the Biophysical Journal (Rall 1962*b*); some of the same figures, with discussion, can be found in pages 228–231 of Rall (1992), or in pages 107–114 of Segev *et al.* (1995).

The conclusion was that these computations do not prove that the dendrites are passive, but they do prove that the observed diphasic extracellular transients can be reproduced theoretically by computations which assume passive dendritic membrane. Consequently, the claim that such experiments provide evidence for active propagation in the dendrites of motoneurons was abandoned; see also discussion by Nelson and Frank (1964).

It is interesting that this issue has not gone away. It still involves careful comparison of theory and experiment. With the greatly improved experimental techniques presented elsewhere in this volume, the new evidence shows that most neuron types do have significant densities of voltage-dependent ion channels in their dendritic membrane. Models suggest that the nonspiny dendrites found in spinal cord motoneurons might also generate action potentials in their dendrites, but this awaits experimental confirmation (Lüscher and Larkum 1998).

Experiment and theoretical modeling of the olfactory bulb

Modeling olfactory bulb field potentials involved several different interactions between theory and experiment. The theory made important use of the insight about diphasic extracellular potentials generated by a single motoneuron (see

'Passive *versus* active dendrites. . .', above), but here we found that it applies also to simultaneous antidromic activation of a cortically arranged population of thousands of mitral cells. Gordon Shepherd had studied such field potentials experimentally at Oxford, with Phillips and Powell. Because they were aware of my modeling of motoneuron V_e transients, they proposed that Gordon should collaborate with me in an effort to understand the highly reproducible spatio-temporal pattern of the field potentials that they had recorded in rabbit olfactory bulb, and had correlated with anatomical depths in the bulb. Thus, my recent modeling and their recent experimental data were brought together at NIH (Rall and Shepherd 1968).

The modeling

We used a compartmental model to simulate antidromic activation of a single mitral cell; we put excitable membrane in the axon and soma compartments; we tried both passive and active membrane in the dendritic compartments. From the V_e transient that had been recorded at the surface of the bulb, we could deduce that the cortical field was an open field (not closed, as it would be for complete spherical symmetry). We called this 'punctured spherical symmetry', and devised a 'potential divider' model to take this into account. With these two models, we could successfully simulate the contribution of the mitral cell population to periods I and II of the field potentials; however, it was clear that mitral cell currents could not generate the depth distribution of the field recorded during the next time interval (period III). This forced the conclusion that the potentials during period III must be generated by currents produced by the very large population of granule cells. We were then led to postulate that the granule cells received their excitatory synaptic input from the secondary dendrites of the mitral cells, and that the depolarized granule cell dendrites do both of the following—they produce the currents that generate the depth distribution of the field potential (during period III), and we postulated that this depolarization might trigger a hypothetical inhibitory synapse back on to the mitral cell dendrites. I had speculated that a single synaptic structure might operate in two modes, first excitatory in one direction and then inhibitory in the other direction. I was proved wrong about the single structure, but I was delighted by what was found.

Dendro-dendritic synapses

Tom Reese and Milton Brightman, who worked independently in electron microscopy at NIH, but who remembered that Gordon had asked about synaptic structures in the external plexiform layer, showed me their new EM images from this layer of olfactory bulb. These images revealed oppositely oriented synaptic contacts between these two kinds of dendrite, and incredible as it might seem, every synaptic contact from a mitral to a granule cell dendrite was of the excitatory type, whereas every synaptic contact from a granule to a mitral dendrite was of the inhibitory type; this was later confirmed by several other laboratories. A four-author manuscript was submitted to Science in 1965; apparently the referee could not believe it, and rejected it; it was published in Experimental Neurology the next year (Rall *et al.* 1966). Here we had dendro-dendritic synapses between two kinds of dendrite—smooth mitral dendrites, and spiny dendrites of granule cells (which have no axon). Each of these dendrites both send and receive synaptically; one sends excitation, the other sends inhibition. Some anatomists could not, at first, accept this; they had thought that dendrites could only receive synaptic input; some suggested that if it sends, it must not be called a dendrite. But time heals wounds, and our theoretical interpretation of this remarkable anatomy and physiology is now generally accepted. I cannot close this paragraph without pointing out that the existence of dendro-dendritic synapses, here and elsewhere in the CNS, opens up a large domain of graded neuronal inter-actions to challenge network modelers; such interactions are completely missing from the usual network models that ignore the existence of dendrites.

Excitable dendritic spines and asymmetric chain reaction

Apart from motoneurons, most neurons have many dendritic spines. The theoretical implications of assuming excitable membrane in dendritic spines were explored by Jack (1975), by Perkel and Perkel (1985), by Miller *et al.* (1985), and by Shepherd *et al.* (1985). Purely hypothetical at first, these studies pointed to synaptic ampli-fication, nonlinear sensitivity to several parameters, and the possibility of chain-reactions, in which several firing spine heads depolarize dendritic membrane; the dendritic membrane could be passive, but under favorable conditions local dendritic depolarization might suffice to bring some adjacent excitable spines to their firing threshold. Would this propagate? If so, how far? Segev and I computed answers to such questions in the context of extensive dendritic branching. We learned that this is more likely to happen in distal branches (because their higher input resistance increases the amount of local depolarization). We also learned that such a chain-reaction tends to propagate more readily into distal dendritic arbors, and less readily toward the soma (in parent branches). Such asymmetry of propagation is related to the asymmetry of passive electrotonic spread in dendritic branches that had been shown in the mid 1970s, in collaboration with Rinzel. It can be understood in terms of contrasting boundary conditions and input resistances—the input resistance into a terminal branch (with a sealed-end) is much higher than the input resistance into a parent branch plus cousin branches.

Functional significance of asymmetric chain-reaction

The importance of such asymmetry in the chain-reaction between excitable spine heads is that it favors nonlinear interactions within subsets of distal branches (i.e. excitable spine clusters in distal arbors); this seems to favor local integration of and discrimination between significantly different synaptic input patterns delivered to the dendrites.

Without this chain-reaction asymmetry, if propagation toward the soma became secure, this would convert the branching system to an all-or-nothing mode, and the neuron would lose the richness inherent in nonlinear local dendritic processing (Rall and Segev 1987; Segev and Rall 1998). Chapters 9 to 11 have more to say about the rich possibilities that are made apparent by such theoretical studies.

Geometric complexity *versus* membrane complexity

An important basic principle of prudent research, both theoretical and experimental, is not to tackle too many complications at once. This was my reason for beginning my modeling with uniform, passive membrane, and with idealized dendritic geometry. Once you solve the reduced problem, you can then begin to deal with some of the complications judged to be functionally important.

Table 8.1, below, has not previously been published, but these ideas did underlie much of my research perspective. Others might find this table useful; it facilitates an overview of interrelated research problems. Thus, Box A3 identifies excitable membrane under space-clamp conditions; by combining space clamp (George Marmont) with voltage clamp (K. S. Cole), and adding the key insight of distinguishing ionic conductances for sodium and potassium ions at different clamped membrane potentials, Hodgkin, Huxley and Katz achieved a major breakthrough in the late 1940s and early 1950s.

Table 8.1 Different combinations of geometric and membrane complications in neuron models.

	1. Passive membrane	2. Synaptic membrane	3. Excitable Membrane
A. Isopotential membrane area	(A.1) Passive soma without dendrites; space-clamped passive membrane	(A.2) Nonlinear effects of synaptic excitation and inhibition; no cable spread	(A.3) Nonlinear ODEs; Hodgkin and Huxley equations; voltage-dependent ionic channel properties
B. Uniform cylinder	(B.1) Cable equation for passive spread of membrane potential; input resistance and spatial decrements	(B.2) Spatial attenuation of EPSP, IPSP and combined; spatio- temporal input patterns contrasted in equivalent cylinder	(B.3) Nonlinear PDEs; propagation of action potential; decrement, block, delay and reflection
C. Dendritic branching	(C.1) Passive cable properties in branched trees; equivalent cylinders; taper and branching	(C.2) Synaptic attenuation in dendritic trees; spatio-temporal input patterns in trees and equivalent cylinders	(C.3) Compartmental models: any specified pattern of branch geometry, of synaptic input, and of membrane nonuniformity
D. Dendritic spines	(D.1) Passive spine properties; spine stem resistance/input resistance ratio; asymmetric decrements	(D.2) Synaptic attenuation; change of relative synaptic weights; extremely local synaptic inhibition	(D.3) Synaptic amplification; non- linear dependence on many spine parameters; asymmetric spread into distal arbors; rich computation potential

Parenthetic note about space, current, and voltage clamp

Some readers may wonder why I entered the names of Cole and Marmont, in the sentence above. The answer is, I was there to witness their contributions. During two summers in Woods Hole (1946–47) I assisted Cole and Marmont in testing the clamping (space, current, voltage) of squid giant axon; indeed, the first long axial intracellular electrode was pulled by me and plated by Marmont in 1947. I was also there when Hodgkin presented a seminar at the University of Chicago in 1948. He reported the research and important new insights achieved with Katz during the previous summer, later published as (Hodgkin and Katz 1949). He also thanked Marmot for discussing his space and current-clamping methods, and thanked Cole for emphasizing the advantages of voltage-clamping. It is noteworthy that Hodgkin (1992, pages 281–3) has described his 1948 visit with Cole and Marmont, including comment about significant observations made in 1947 under voltage-clamp; he acknowledges a visit with Gilbert Ling, during which Ling taught him how to make sharp electrodes. Several earlier relevant references, from 1949, 1968, 1976 and 1985 have been cited in Rall (1992).

I believe that it does not detract from the great achievement of Hodgkin, Huxley, and Katz (experimental, conceptual, and computational), to note the fact that space, current, and voltage clamp of squid axon were first developed by Cole and Marmont. Here we have an interesting example of the interplay between experimental and theoretical innovation; no one, not even Einstein, can advance without building on the work of others.

Geometric complexity

Returning now to Table 8.1, if we wish to explore geometric complexity, we first assume passive membrane; see boxes B.1 and C.1. For these cases, it proved possible to find analytical solutions for uniform cylinders of finite length. It was shown that there is a class of dendritic branching that can be transformed into an equivalent cylinder (Rall 1962*a*); analytical solutions were provided for nonuniform synaptic input (two regions), and the effect on EPSP shape was first demonstrated (Rall 1962*a*).

By using superposition of mathematical solutions (steady state and transient), Rinzel and I provided analytical solutions for input (injected current) to a single branch of a dendritic tree (branches meet constraints for an equivalent cylinder) (Rall and Rinzel 1973) and (Rinzel and Rall 1974). These papers also discuss physiological implications; they are among the reprints collected in Segev *et al.* (1995).

Recently, complicated analytical solutions for dendritic trees with arbitrary branching patterns have been presented and computed (Major *et al.* 1993), a mathematical tour de force. Also, essentially equivalent solutions for a compartmental representation of arbitrary branching (Holmes *et al.* 1992) have been presented and computed. Powerful as these two sets of analytical solutions are, it must be pointed out that they are limited by their dependence on the assumption of passive membrane properties (Boxes B.1 and C.1 in Table 8.1).

Compartmental nonuniformity of inputs and nonlinear membrane

Fortunately, it is now possible to use compartmental models to simulate nonlinear membrane properties (Column 3 in Table 8.1); these nonlinearities can be distributed nonuniformly over the dendritic compartments (C.3 and D.3). Also, the synaptic inputs can be distributed nonuniformly, and the branching need not satisfy the equivalent-cylinder constraints.

Reduced compartmental models

Although modern computers enable one to specify thousands of compartments for one dendritic neuron, my own preference is to avoid using so many, even if the branching data might suggest it. I would rather use fewer compartments, and put my effort into finding the best compartmental assignment of different ion-channel densities and of different synaptic input patterns. An important example is that of Traub *et al.* (1991). For some purposes, such a model can be reduced even further; Pinsky and Rinzel (1994) reduced it to two compartments, where one compartment collected the ion channels and inputs of the soma membrane (including proximal dendrites) and the other compartment collected the ion channels and inputs of most of the dendritic membrane. Such a reduced model can preserve the most essential nonuniformity of channels and inputs (over soma and dendrites), and can facilitate the construction and computational exploration of neural networks that are physiologically more realistic than networks composed of point neurons.

Challenge to test importance of dendrites

With the advent of new methods for obtaining patch-clamp recordings from dendrites, new insight to the functional properties of dendrites is coming at a rapid pace. Some of these advances are discussed in Chapter 10. In Chapter 11, Bartlett Mel takes a look at how some of these properties can impart functional complexity on the dendritic tree. Such analyses present a new frontier in computational neuroscience; understanding the relationship between dendritic physiology and network function.

   To me, it is a useful exercise to look for physiologically interesting network simulations that make use of dendritic compartments with nonlinear membrane properties and inputs that are different from those at the soma (and perhaps also from those at other dendritic compartments), and then to test the importance of these nonuniformities for generating that interesting behavior. The test is simple; begin with a successful model containing nonuniformities, then perform and compare a new computation where the neuronal nonuniformity is removed, either by lumping the dendritic compartments with the soma, or equivalently, by giving all compartments the same nonlinear membrane properties and the same inputs. Good examples of such test computations provide strong support for the essential functional role of dendrites and dendritic synapses.

Concluding remarks

Retired and 77, I am pleased to participate in this book, and to know that such able investigators are carrying forward the adventure of increasing our understanding of dendritic function, using both theory and experiment. My focus has shifted to imagining and making sculptures.

References

Fatt, P. (1957). Electric potentials occurring around a neurone during its antidromic activation. *Journal of Neurophysiology*, **20**, 27–60.

Hodgkin, A. L. (1992). *Chance and Design*. Cambridge University Press.

Hodgkin, A. L. and Katz, B. (1949). The effect of sodium ions on the electrical activity of the giant axon of the squid. *Journal of Physiology*, **108**, 37–77.

Holmes, W. R. and Rall, W. (1992). Electrotonic length estimates in neurons with dendritic tapering or somatic shunt. *Journal of Neurophysiology*, **68**, 1421–37.

Holmes, W. R., Segev, I., and Rall, W. (1992). Interpretation of time-constant and electrotonic length estimates of multi-cylinder or branched neuronal structures. *Journal of Neurophysiology*, **68**, 1401–20.

Jack, J. J. B., Noble, D., and Tsien, R. W. (1975). *Electrical current flow in excitable cells*. Oxford University Press.

Lüscher, H.-R. and Larkum, M. (1998). Modeling action potential initiation and back-propagation in dendrites of cultured rat motoneurons. *Journal of Neurophysiology*, **80**, 715–29.

Major, G., Evans, J. D., and Jack, J. J. B. (1993). Solutions for transients in arbitrarily branching cables: I. Voltage recording with a somatic shunt. *Biophysical Journal*, **65**, 423–49.

Miller, J. P., Rall W., and Rinzel, J. (1985). Synaptic amplification by active membrane in dendritic spines. *Brain Research*, **325**, 325–30.

Nelson, P. G. and Frank, K. (1964). Extracellular potential fields of single spinal motoneurons. *Journal of Neurophysiology*, **27**, 913–27.

Perkel, D. H. and Perkel, D. J. (1985). Dendritic spines: role of active membrane in modulating synaptic efficacy. *Brain Research*, **325**, 331–5.

Pinsky, P. F. and Rinzel, J. (1994). Intrinsic and network rhythmogenesis in a reduced Traub model for CA3 neurons. *Journal of Computational Neuroscience*, **1**, 39–40.

Rall, W. (1957). Membrane time-constant of motoneurons. *Science*, **126**, 454.

Rall, W. (1959). Branching dendritic trees and motoneuron membrane resistivity. *Experimental Neurology*, **1**, 491–527.

Rall, W. (1960). Membrane potential transients and membrane time-constant of motoneurons. *Experimental Neurology*, **2**, 503–32.

Rall, W. (1962a). Theory of physiological properties of dendrites. *Annals of New York Academy of Sciences*, **96**, 1071–92.

Rall, W. (1962b). Electrophysiology of a dendritic neuron model. *Biophysical Journal*, **2** (part 2), 145–167.

Rall, W. (1964). Theoretical significance of dendritic trees for neuronal input–output relations. In *Neural theory and modeling*, (ed. R. F. Reiss), pp. 73–97. Stanford University Press, Palo Alto.

Rall, W. (1977). Core conductor theory and cable properties of neurons. In *Handbook of physiology, the nervous system, Vol. 1, Cellular biology of neurons*, (ed. E. R. Kandel, J. M. Brookhart, and V. B. Mountcastle), pp. 39–97. American Physiological Society, Bethesda.

Rall, W. (1992). Path to biophysical insights about dendrites and synaptic function. In *The neurosciences: paths of discovery II*, (ed. F. Samson and G. Adelman), pp. 215–240. Birkhauser, Boston.

Rall, W. (1995). Perspective on neuron model complexity. In *Handbook of brain theory and neural networks*, (ed. M. A. Arbib), pp. 728–732. MIT Press.

Rall, W. and Agmon-Snir, H. (1998). Cable theory for dendritic neurons. In *Methods in neuronal modeling*, (2nd edn) (ed. C. Koch and I. Segev), pp. 27–92. MIT Press.

Rall, W. and Rinzel, J. (1973). Branch input resistance and steady attenuation for input to one branch of a dendritic neuron model. *Biophysical Journal*, **13**, 648–88.

Rall, W. and Segev, I. (1987). Functional possibilities for synapses on dendrites and dendritic spines. In *Synaptic function*, (ed. G. M. Edelman, W. E. Gall, and W. M. Cowan), pp. 605–36. Wiley, New York.

Rall, W. and Shepherd, G. M. (1968). Theoretical reconstruction of field potentials and dendrodendritic synaptic interactions in olfactory bulb. *Journal of Neurophysiology*, **31**, 884–915.

Rall, W., Shepherd, G. M., Reese, T. S., and Brightman, M. W. (1966). Dendro-dendritic synaptic pathway for inhibition in the olfactory bulb. *Experimental Neurology*, **14**, 44–56.

Rall, W., Burke, R. E., Smith, T. G., Nelson, P. G., and Frank, K. (1967). Dendritic location of synapses and possible mechanisms for the monosynaptic EPSP in motoneurons. *Journal of Neurophysiology*, **30**, 1169–93.

Rall, W., Burke, R. E., Holmes, W. R., Jack, J. J. B., Redman, S. J., and Segev, I. (1992). Matching dendritic neuron models to experimental data. *Physiological Reviews*, **72**, S159-86.

Redman, S. and Walmsley, B. (1983). The time course of synaptic potentials evoked in cat spinal motoneurones at identified group Ia synapses. *Journal of Physiology*, **343**, 117–33.

Rinzel, J. and Rall, W. (1974). Transient response in a dendritic neuron model for current injected at one branch. *Biophysical Journal*, **14**, 759–90.

Segev, I. and Rall, W. (1998). Excitable dendrites and spines: earlier theoretical insights elucidate recent direct observations. *Trends in Neuroscience*, **21**, 453–60.

Segev, I., Rinzel, J., and Shepherd, G. M. (1995). *The theoretical foundation of dendritic function: selected papers of Wilfrid Rall with commentaries*, (ed. I. Segev, J. Rinzel, and G. M. Shepherd) p. 456. MIT Press.

Shepherd, G. M., Brayton, R. K., Miller, J. P., Segev, I., Rinzel, J., and Rall, W. (1985). Signal enhancement in distal cortical dendrites by means of interactions between active dendritic spines. *Proceedings of the National Academy of Science USA*, **82**, 2192–5.

Terzuolo, C. A. and Araki, T. (1961). An analysis of intra- *vs* extracellular potential changes associated with activity of single spinal motoneurons. *Annals of New York Academy of Sciences*, **94**, 547–58.

Traub, R. D., Wong, R. K. S., Miles, R., and Michelson, H. (1991). A model of a CA3 hippocampal pyramidal neuron incorporating voltage clamp data on intrinsic conductances. *Journal of Neurophysiology*, **66**, 635–60.

9

A theoretical view of passive and active dendrites

Idan Segev and Michael London
Hebrew University

Summary

Models of passive-cable structures were tailored in the last 40 years to explore the biophysical principles that govern the interaction between structure, physiology, and input–output function of dendrites. The insights gained from these models are extended here to highlight the effect of nonuniform distribution of passive ion channels in dendrites as well as of excitable dendritic channels. The chapter shows how these models help in interpreting novel experimental data; general principles involved in the manifestation of excitability in dendrites are also provided. The motivation in this work is driven by the conviction that the complexity of the single neuron enriches significantly the computational power of the nervous system, and that models of dendrites are essential for creating the bridge between the single neuron level and the level of the neuronal network.

Introduction: computing with single neurons, computing with neural networks

The main function of the nervous system is to process information—to compute. Incoming sensory information is first represented, or encoded, by the internal 'language' of the nervous system, comprised of its biophysical (electrical and chemical) signals. These signals are then processed in the nervous system before an output—a decision—is made: the movement of the arm, the recognition of a specific face, the identification of a piece of music. Typically, this process leaves some 'memory' traces within the system, and this is often utilized to improve its performance during later processing.

The elementary building blocks of the nervous system are individual neurons with their large, specialized dendritic and axonal trees. Each of these neurons carries part of the computational burden that the whole system implements. But it is yet largely unclear how the properties of the individual neuron (its specific morphology, the distribution of the transmembrane ion channels over its surface, the site and type of its synaptic input) contribute to the information processing function of the whole system. This is, indeed, one of the major enigmas in neuroscience.

A close look at individual neurons, and specifically at their dendrites, reveals clear organizational rules. In cortical pyramids, for example, inhibitory synaptic inputs 'prefer' to contact the dendritic shaft and the soma, whereas the excitatory synapses are typically distributed throughout the whole dendritic tree, and in particular, on the dendritic spines. In many cell types, synaptic input from different input sources is preferentially mapped on to specific regions of the dendritic tree (Shepherd 1998). These inputs often show activity-dependent dynamics; some depress when repeatedly activated, some facilitate and some remain unchanged. Furthermore, the electrical properties of the dendritic membrane are often spatially inhomogeneous. In some cortical pyramids, for example, the fast inactivating voltage-gated Na^+ channels are distributed uniformly (in low density) over the dendritic membrane but voltage-gated A-type K^+ channels, and the I_h channels, seem to be specifically distributed rather densely in distal dendritic locations (see Chapter 6). Such a specific, well organized, morpho-electrical design of dendrites calls for a functional interpretation at both the level of the single neuron and of the whole network.

But one might claim, not without a reason, that this specific design of single neurons is essentially 'washed away' by the overwhelming effect of the network. Indeed, a central neuron in the mammalian CNS receives on the order of 10^4 synapses on its dendritic surface, and each can be activated 1–100 times s^{-1}. Such a bombardment of synapses has a profound effect on the membrane properties of the dendrites (Bernander *et al.* 1991; Rapp *et al.* 1992; Borg-Graham *et al.* 1998). Thus, the alternative view is that the emergent computations of the nervous system are insensitive to the dynamics of the single neuron and it is the connectivity of the network, rather than the properties of its individual neurons, that determines the network dynamics.

We prefer to take the first view whereby the details at the single neuron level do make an important contribution to the performance of the whole system. In this view, one needs to explore the complexity of the single neuron to understand how it might enrich the computational power of the neuronal network to which it belongs. Namely, one should expose the (morphological) 'face' and the (electro-chemical) 'character' of neurons hoping that, with persistent experimental effort, an understanding of the functional consequences of the 'neuron-ware' will emerge. An integral part in this route of investigation is to construct models of neurons that incorporate their physiological and morphological information. This model is then primarily used to achieve the following goals:

(1) to estimate biophysical parameters (such as the value of the specific membrane resistivity, R_m) over the neuron surface from recordings performed at only one, or a few, locations;

(2) to extract the key biophysical parameters that determine the repertoire of electrical/chemical signals that are generated by the neuron;

(3) to obtain insights regarding the computations that such a device *could* perform with its specific biophysical machinery.

This chapter briefly introduces the theoretical framework within which models of dendrites are constructed. It then emphasizes the main biophysical insights that these models have provided during the last 40 years, since Rall developed his cable theory (Rall 1959) and compartmental modeling approach (Rall 1964) for dendritic neurons. A more complete elaboration of this theory can be found in Jack *et al.* (1975), Segev *et al.* (1995), Rall and Agmon-Snir (1998), and Koch (1999). Next, it introduces a theoretical exploration of some recent, interesting experimental findings in cortical pyramids; namely, that the membrane conductance (the density of membrane ion-channels) is distributed nonuniformly over the dendritic surface, such that the membrane is 'leakier' at distal dendritic regions. The implications of such membrane nonuniformity for the interpretation of experimental results, as well as for the input–output function of dendrites, is considered. The chapter ends with theoretical implications of models of excitable dendrites. The next chapter (Chapter 10) analyzes more fully the possible ways synaptic inputs may be integrated by this dendritic hardware.

Models of dendrites—the foundation

Until very recently, most of the stable electrical recordings from neurons were made from the relatively large soma. It is useful to record from the soma because it is electrically close to the axon where, in most mammalian central nervous system (CNS) neurons, the output—a train of action potentials—is produced. However, most of the membrane area of central neurons is in their dendrites and it is there where the synapses contacts the neuron. Can one learn about what happens locally at the synaptic sites in the dendrites from recordings made at the soma?

This question was the motivation for the formulation of the cable theory for dendrites in the late 1950s by Rall (1959) followed by his compartmental modeling approach (Rall 1964). These groundbreaking studies provided the theoretical framework for most of our present insights regarding the connection between the anatomical and physiological properties of dendrites and their input–output functions.

In the one-dimensional cable theory for dendrites, the dendritic tree (Fig. 9.1a) is decomposed into a set of inter-connected cylindrical cables (Fig. 9.1b). Each of these cables represents a small section of the dendritic tree. At any point along this cable, the axial current (which flows along the axial resistance, r_i) can either continue to flow longitudinally or it can flow into the membrane (either charging the membrane capacitance, c_m, or crossing the membrane resistance, r_m). As a first approximation, Rall assumed that the dendrites are *passive*, namely, that all the electrical parameters are constant (time- and voltage-independent). The flow of current in passive cables can then be described mathematically by the one dimensional passive-cable equation:

$$\left(\frac{r_m}{r_i}\right)\frac{\partial^2 V(x,t)}{\partial x^2} - r_m c_m \frac{\partial V(x,t)}{\partial t} - V(x,t) = 0 \qquad (1)$$

where r_i (in Ω cm^{-1}), r_m (in Ω cm), and c_m (in F cm^{-1}) are all per unit length. The general solution of this equation can be expressed as an infinite sum of decaying exponentials (Rall 1969):

$$V(x,t) = \sum_{i=0}^{\infty} C_i e^{-t/\tau_i} \tag{2}$$

where, for a given tree, the coefficients C_i depend on the point of observation (x) and the input current (the initial conditions) but are independent of time (t). In contrast, the values for the 'equalizing' time constants, τ_i, are independent on input location or input current (Rall 1969) (Note that, for passive-cable structures with sealed ends, $\tau_0 = \tau_m$, the membrane time constant). Rall showed that for any passive tree there is an analytic solution of the cable equation (namely, C_i and τ_i can be written explicitly). Thus, it became possible to combine the anatomical and physiological knowledge about a given dendritic tree and (assuming the tree is passive) to describe analytically how the current flows from any input site to any other dendritic location, and specifically the soma (Rall 1959; Segev *et al.* 1995; Rall and Agmon-Snir 1998). Important insights were obtained when these analytic solutions were applied both to synthetic trees and to real dendritic trees (see below). However, when significant nonlinearities exist in the dendritic tree, such as a strong synaptic input (a transient conductance change rather than a current input) or a voltage-dependent membrane conductance, the passive-cable model for dendrites is inappropriate. The problem is then described by the nonlinear cable equation, and numerical (compartmental) methods should typically be used to solve this equation (Rall 1964; Segev and Burke 1998).

In the compartmental method, the continuous cable equation is discretized into a finite set of compartments; each is a lumped representation of a small section of the dendritic tree (Fig. 9.1c). The whole membrane of this dendritic section is lumped into a single *RC* element, where the membrane resistance (R) can depend on time and/or voltage, whereas the membrane capacitance (C) is typically assumed to be constant. The resistance of the dendritic cytoplasm is lumped into a single (typically passive) axial resistance. Thus, in an unbranched neuron, the current flowing in compartment j is:

$$\frac{d}{4\hat{r}_j} \frac{V_{j+1} - 2V_j + V_{j+1}}{\Delta x^2} - \hat{c}_{mj} \frac{dV_j}{dt} - i_{ion_j} = 0 \tag{3}$$

where $\hat{r}_j$ is the axial resistance, $\hat{c}_{m_j}$, is the membrane capacitance of the jth compartment and i_{ion_j} is the total ionic current that flows through the compartment membrane. This current can be voltage and time dependent (nonlinear). For example, i_{ion_j} may be the excitable current that underlies the initiation of the action potential.

It can be shown that, if the length of this dendritic section is sufficiently small, the solution for the compartmental model converges to that of the corresponding cable model (Rall 1964; Segev and Burke 1998). These two complimentary approaches, the cable and compartmental models, were utilized very successfully and have recently become even more popular because of their implementations in user-friendly software packages, mainly in NEURON (Hines and Carnevale 1997) and GENESIS (Bower and Beeman 1994). The primary applications of these modeling tools are:

a. Physiologically and morphologically characterized neuron

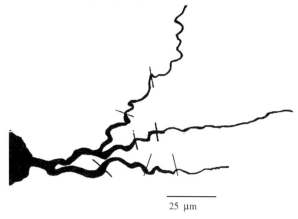

25 μm

b. Cable model

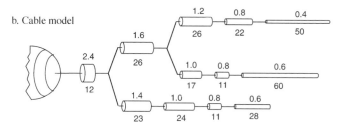

c. Compartmental model

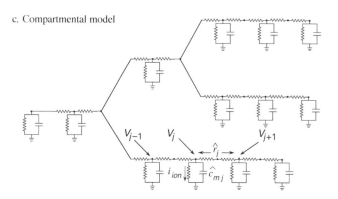

Fig. 9.1 Modeling neuronal dendrites. Dendrites (a) are modeled either as a set of cylindrical membrane cables (b) or as a set of discrete isopotential, RC compartments (c). In the cable representation (b) the voltage at any point in the tree is computed from eqn 9.1 and the appropriate boundary conditions imposed by the tree. In compartmental representation (c) the tree is discretized into a set of interconnected RC compartments; each is a lumped representation of a sufficiently small dendritic segment. Membrane compartments are connected *via* axial cytoplasmic resistances ($\hat{r}_j$). The current at each compartment is described by eqn 9.3; for a tree with N compartments, a set of N ordinary differential equations has to be solved simultaneously. The ion current (i_{ion}) that flows across the membrane resistivity might be a complicated nonlinear function that reflects voltage- and time-dependent properties of the transmembrane ion channels.

1. to estimate, *via* reconciliation between model predictions and experimental results, the electrical properties of remote dendritic arbors and of distal dendritic synapses (including the time-course and the site of the synaptic input) from measurements made at the soma. The models have also suggested further experiments for refining these estimates. Important examples for studies that combine experiments and models of dendrites can be found in Rall *et al.* (1966, 1967, 1992), Redman and Walmsley (1983*a*,*b*), Stratford *et al.* (1989) , Major (1994), Rapp *et al.* (1994), Häusser and Roth (1997), and Stuart and Spruston (1998).

2. to extract the key biophysical parameters that critically determine the input–output capabilities of the dendritic tree. For passive models, these parameters are:

    (1) the specific membrane capacitance (C_m, in F cm^{-2}) and resistivity (R_m, in Ω cm^2);
    (2) the specific axial resistivity (R_i, in Ω cm);
    (3) the input resistance of the neuron (R_N, in Ω);
    (4) the electrotonic length of the dendritic tree ($L = l/\lambda$, in dimensionless units, where *l* is the physical length of the dendrites and $\lambda = (d/4)[(R_m/R_i)]^{1/2}$, in cm, is the space constant and *d* is the diameter of the cylindrical cable); and
    (5) the membrane time constant ($\tau_m = R_m C_m$, in s). For nonlinear models, the properties of the synaptic and excitable channels (type, density, kinetics) at the various dendritic locations have to be specified in addition to the passive properties mentioned above.

3. to gain insights into the principles that underlie the interaction between the morphology and biophysical properties of dendrites (see below).

4. to explore, using the models, the computations that could (in principle) be implemented by the single neuron (see Segev *et al.* 1995; Chapters 10 and 11).

Passive-cable models for dendrites—the seven main insights

The dendritic membrane is endowed with transmitter- and voltage-dependent ion channels which are inherently nonlinear. This can lead to the erroneous (but increasingly popular) notion that passive models of neurons are irrelevant. In the next section this important issue will be fully discussed. Indeed, the insights that were gained from passive models are essential for understanding the behavior of nonlinear signals in dendrites; the passive model should, therefore, be viewed as the skeleton on top of which further (nonlinear) complications are added. Below we summarize the basic insights that were gained from passive models of dendrites.

Dendrites are electrically distributed devices, hence significant voltage attenuation in the dendritic tree is expected

Dendrites tend to ramify and often create large and complicated trees (see Chapter 1). They are thin processes, starting with a diameter of a few microns near the soma; branch diameter typically falls below 1 μm as they successively divide. Many (but not all) types of dendrite are studded with abundant tiny appendages called the dendritic spines (typical area of each spine is 1–1.5 μm^2). When the actual geometry of dendrites is taken into account, together with the specific membrane and axial resistivity (typical values for R_m are between 5000 and 100,000 Ω cm^2 and for R_i between 70 and 250 Ω cm), it is found that neurons are not isopotential units but rather they are electrically distributed. The electrotonic length (L) characterizes the extent of this electrical distribution and in dendrites is on the order of unity (1 space constant from soma to distal dendritic tips). In other words, neurons are not isopotential units, and consequently, a large (tenfold and more) voltage difference (voltage attenuation) can exist between different regions of the dendritic tree (and the soma) after a local synaptic input to the dendrites (Rall and Rinzel 1973).

A significant portion of the synaptic charge reaches the soma even for distal inputs

Because the electrical resistance of the dendritic membrane per unit length is much larger than that of the cytoplasm, the synaptic input current (charge) tends to flow longitudinally along the dendrites rather than being lost *via* the membrane leak to the extracellular space. Consequently, a significant percentage of the synaptic current that is generated at the synaptic input sites reaches the soma. In other words, distal dendritic excitatory synapses do contribute to the depolarization of the soma and axon membrane.

Another consequence of the relatively large R_m value and of the small dimensions of dendrites is that a large input impedance ($\sim 10^3$ MΩ for DC inputs) is expected at distal dendritic arbors. Consequently, even the small amount of current that is produced by a single excitatory synapse can generate locally (e.g. at the spine head membrane) a large excitatory postsynaptic potential (EPSP; 10–20 mV or more). Therefore, nonlinear synaptic saturation is expected at these sites. The same input would produce a much smaller peak depolarization (and less saturation) when placed directly on the soma, where the input resistance could be 10-fold smaller than in the distal location (Rall and Rinzel 1973; Rinzel and Rall 1974; see also Chapter 10).

Voltage attenuation in the dendritic tree is asymmetrical

When current flows from thin distal arbors towards the soma, it encounters a large impedance load ('sink'); the boundary conditions are very different when the current flows in the reverse direction (from soma to dendrites). Because the sink for current is much larger in the dendrite-to-soma direction, the attenuation of voltage in this direction is significantly more severe than in the reverse direction. In other words, the dendritic tree is electrically more compact (voltage is distributed more uniformly) when the input is at (or near) the soma compared with an input given locally at distal dendritic arbors (Rall and Rinzel 1973; Zador *et al.* 1995).

Dendrites are significant time-delay lines for synaptic potentials

As a result of the capacitive properties of the dendritic membrane, a significant delay in peak time is expected when the synaptic potential spreads from distal dendritic locations to the soma (Fig. 9.2a–c). Indeed, the velocity of the synaptic potentials in the dendritic tree (when passive membrane is assumed) is on the order of $2\lambda/\tau_m$ (Jack *et al.*, 1983; Agmon-Snir and Segev, 1993; Zador *et al.*, 1995). With τ_m of approximately 20 ms and λ on the order of 1 mm, the velocity of the EPSP is on the order of 100 μm ms^{-1}, which is rather slow. Thus, the time delay from distal dendritic input sites (located more than 1 mm from the soma) to the soma is expected to be on the order of 10–20 ms (Fig. 9.2c). Indeed, such a range of delays was found experimentally (Nicoll *et al.* 1993; Stuart and Spruston 1998).

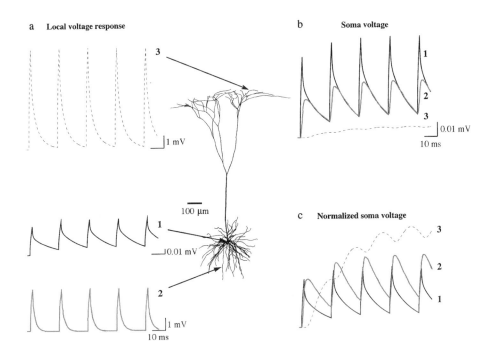

Fig. 9.2 Temporal summation in the dendritic tree depends on input location. Five consecutive current pulses (at 50 Hz) were injected at locations in the dendritic tree of a layer V pyramidal cell depicted at the middle (reconstructed by J. C. Anderson). Point 3 is in the distal apical tuft, point 2 is in a basal arbor and point 1 is at the soma. The local voltage response at the respective input sites is shown in (a). Note that at the two dendritic input locations (2 and 3) there is almost no temporal summation of potential, owing to the small 'effective local time constant' which results from the large 'current sink' imposed on these sites by the dendritic tree. The amplitude of the local voltage response is, however, relatively large because of the large input impedance in these regions. The voltage recorded at the soma in response to these same current injections are shown in (b). Note the very large voltage attenuation of the signal from the dendrites to the soma (compare trace 3 in (a) with that in (b)). In (c), the traces in (b) are normalized to the peak of the first EPSP. This normalization enables one to compare the amounts of temporal summations at the soma as a function of the input location. The summation is larger for the distal apical input. This is because the EPSP arriving from this site becomes significantly broader because of the capacitance that it encounters when spreading towards the soma and consequently, successive EPSPs can summate better with each other. (Model parameters: R_i = 200 Ω cm, R_m = 20,000 Ω cm^2 and C_m = 1 μF cm^{-2}. Current pulse amplitude is 0.01 nA and 2 ms duration).

Another consequence of the membrane capacitance is the increase in the time course of somatic EPSPs when the input originates at distal synapses as compared to the time course arising from proximal inputs (Fig. 9.2c). This difference in time-to-peak and half-width of the somatic EPSP served as the basis for estimating the electrotonic distance of the dendritic synapses from the soma (Rall *et al.* 1967; Redman and Walmsley 1983*a,b*). The 'dendritic delay' and the change in the shape of the EPSP for distal compared with proximal inputs might have important consequences for the information processing capability of neurons (Rall 1964; Segev 1992; Segev *et al.* 1995; and see Chapter 10).

The time-window for the summation of synaptic inputs at the soma is approximately τ_m

For brief synaptic inputs, the duration of the EPSPs *at the soma* is on the order of τ_m. During this time window, synaptic inputs arriving to the soma can temporally summate (integrate) with each other. Indeed, τ_m (which, for cortical pyramids, is on the order of 10–20 ms) sets the upper limit for the temporal resolution (the requirement for input synchronization) in neurons (Agmon-Snir and Segev 1993; Koch *et al.* 1996; Rapp *et al.* 1996).

The temporal resolution at distal dendritic sites (and spines) can be as short as $0.1 \, \tau_m$

Locally, at the dendritic input site, the time-course of the EPSP is determined primarily by the fast flow (loss) of the input current to other regions of the dendritic tree, rather than by τ_m. Namely, the morpho-electrotonic structure of the tree, rather than the membrane properties, determines to a large extent how fast the input current can be lost from the input site. As a result, the local synaptic potential at the input site is briefer than the resultant EPSP at the soma (Fig. 9.2a). Consequently, the effective time window for the summation of synaptic potentials locally at distal dendritic sites can be an order of magnitude shorter than τ_m. A more complete discussion of the functional significance of τ_m is given in Agmon-Snir and Segev (1993), Zador *et al.* (1995), and Koch *et al.* (1996).

Dendritic spines are favorable sites for plastic changes

The special morphology of dendritic spines, that of a small spherical head (volume ranging from 0.005—0.3 μm^3) connected to a thin (0.05–0.2 μm) and often long (1 μm) cylindrical neck, provides favorable conditions for modifying the efficacy of the synaptic input (typically excitatory) that impinges on its head membrane. Rall (1974, 1978) and others (Rinzel 1981; Koch and Poggio 1983; Rall and Segev 1988) have shown in modeling studies that, for an appropriate range of spine parameters, a small change in the spine neck dimensions can result in a large change in the amount of charge that the spiny synapse injects into the dendrite. In addition, the minute volume of the spine head compartment implies a significant change in intracellular ion concentration can occur as a result of the flow of a relatively small number of ions into the spine head (e.g. after the activation of the spiny synapse). This concentration change might trigger a cascade of intracellular processes that might lead to activity-dependent, long-term and very specific changes in the efficacy of spine synapses (see review in Shepherd 1996).

Nonuniform membrane conductance in dendrites

One of the basic assumptions of the classical passive-cable theory is that the specific membrane resistance (or conductance, G_m) is uniform over the dendritic membrane. However, recent experimental evidence shows that both the passive membrane conductance and several types of voltage-dependent ion channels are distributed nonuniformly over the membrane surface (Hoffman *et al.* 1997; Magee 1998; Stuart and Spruston 1998). From these studies it seems that at least in some neuronal types the membrane conductance (G_m) increases with the distance from the soma, such that the membrane at distal locations is leakier than the membrane at regions closer to the soma. As we have already seen above, there is a large attenuation of synaptic potential from the dendrites to the soma. At first glance, it might seem that making the distal membrane leaky would only exaggerate this effect and the synaptic potential will attenuate even more.

In this section we will discuss the effect of such membrane nonuniformity in passive dendritic structure. It is first important to note that when one says 'attenuate more' one must specify what is the reference for the comparison. Indeed, the synaptic potential is greatly affected by the value of G_m *per se* (i.e. both λ and τ_m are functions of this parameter). Thus to separate the effect of the spatial distribution of $G_m(x)$ from that of the average value of G_m, we chose as a reference for comparison the uniform case in which the total amount of conductance remains identical with that of the nonuniform case.

Fig. 9.3a–c, depicts the voltage response at the soma in a simulated hippocampal CA1 pyramidal cell to a current input applied separately at four locations on the dendritic tree. Two cases are shown for each input location. The light line shows the somatic voltage response when the membrane conductance is uniform whereas the solid line is the response when $G_m(x)$ linearly increases with the distance from the soma (see inset in Fig. 9.3d). The total amount of membrane conductance over the whole tree is equal in both cases. Note that, in contrast with the intuitive view, both the amplitude and total area under the voltage response is larger at locations 1–3 in the nonuniform case than in the uniform case (Fig. 9.3b,c). For the most distal input location on the apical tree (point 4), this relation is reversed and the somatic voltage response is larger when the dendritic membrane conductance is uniform.

This general behavior of the uniform case compared with the nonuniform case is depicted in Fig. 9.3d, where the transfer resistance ($R_{x,0}$) between any location in the

(f,h). In (e) and (f) the voltage profile is plotted 2 ms after the stimulus onset, whereas in (g) and (h) it is plotted 60 ms after the end of the stimulus. $R_i = 200\ \Omega$ cm, $R_m = 20\ 000\ \Omega$ cm^2 and $C_m = 1\ \mu F$ cm^{-2} in the uniform case; in the nonuniform case, $G_m(x) = ax$ where $a = 8.6$ 10^{-6} (S cm^{-2}) μm^{-1} and x is the physical distance from the soma.

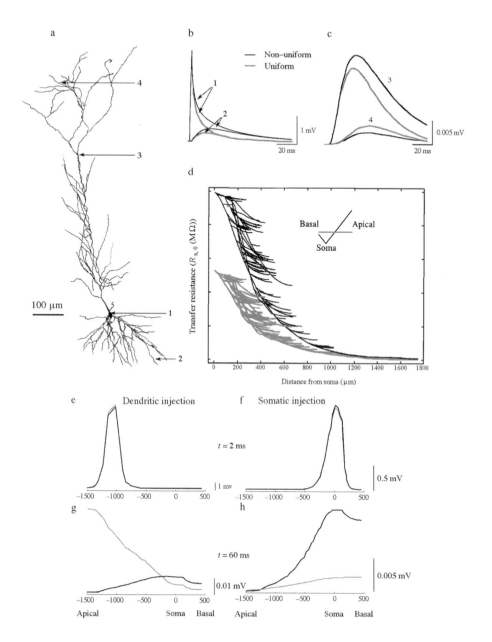

Fig. 9.3 Signal transfer in dendrites with nonuniform membrane conductance. (a) CA1 pyramidal cell (reconstructed by D. Turner). (b,c) Voltage transients recorded at the soma (denoted as point 1) in response to a brief current injection (2 ms, 0.05 nA) at four locations at the dendritic tree. The nonuniform case is depicted by the heavy line whereas the uniform case is depicted by the light line. (d) Transfer resistance, $R_{x,0}$, from any location in the tree to the soma. (e–h) Voltage profile along the path from location 4 ('Apical') to location 2 ('Basal') in response to the same stimulus as in (b) and (c) applied either to location 3 (e,g) or to the soma

modeled tree and the soma is shown. The transfer resistance is the ratio, $V_{\text{soma}}/I_{\text{input}}(x)$, where the input, $I_{\text{input}}(x)$, is a DC current step applied at point x, and V_{soma} is the resultant steady voltage at the soma (point '0' denotes the soma). It can be seen that for almost all input locations, $R_{x,0}$ in the nonuniform case is larger than in the uniform case. This means that for a DC input at almost all input locations, x, the steady-state voltage at the soma will be larger in the nonuniform case. Note that this figure also describes the attenuation of the time integral of the potential (the area under the voltage transient) in the case of transient current injection, because this integral behaves exactly like the voltage under steady-state conditions (Rall and Rinzel 1973; Rinzel and Rall 1974). The difference observed between the uniform and nonuniform cases is quite general. It can be shown analytically that for a cylinder with 'sealed ends' and for a variety of increasing $G_m(x)$ functions (e.g. linear, polynomial, exponential, or sigmoid functions), $R_{x,0}$ is larger for every x in the nonuniform case compared with that of the uniform case. The difference between the two cases becomes larger as the steepness of the $G_m(x)$ increases and when the electrotonic length of the cylinder becomes larger (London *et al.* 1999).

The actual synaptic input is a conductance change with an associated reversal potential (battery) rather than a current input. Thus, for a strong conductance change, the synaptic potential will saturate as it approaches its reversal potential. The larger the local input resistance at the synaptic input site, the larger the voltage saturation at this site for a given synaptic conductance change. This yields an additional difference between the uniform and nonuniform cases. In the nonuniform case, the input resistance at distal locations is smaller because of the leakier membrane at these sites. Thus, less saturation of the synaptic voltage is expected there compared with the corresponding nonuniform case. This reduction in synaptic saturation in the nonuniform case increases the efficacy of most distal synapses in the model shown in Fig. 9.3.

The nonuniformity in the membrane conductance also affects the time-course of voltage transients in a dendritic tree. When a dendritic cable structure has sealed-end boundary conditions (as typically assumed), the final relaxation of voltage is slower in the nonuniform case than in the corresponding uniform case. In other words, for any membrane nonuniformity the slowest (system) time constant, τ_0, is always larger than τ_m, the slowest time constant in the corresponding uniform case (see eqn 9.2). Thus, the final decay (the 'tail') of the excitatory synaptic potentials (e.g. the somatic EPSPs) is expected to be slower when the dendritic membrane conductance is spatially nonuniform. This effect increases with the value of L, the electrotonic length of the structure, and is clearly seen in all the modeled EPSPs shown in Fig. 9.3b,c. This slowing down of the final decay, owing to membrane nonuniformity, increases the effectiveness of temporal summation in nonuniform cable structures.

Another facet of membrane nonuniformity is revealed when considering the spatial relaxation of the voltage with time. In cylinders with uniform membrane and sealed ends, the whole structure becomes isopotential (uniformly polarized) when the voltage reaches a time where it relaxes with the rate governed by τ_m. This is not true for the nonuniform membrane case. Now there is a voltage gradient along the cable structure when the voltage (at any location) relaxes with the final rate, τ_0. The gradient is determined by the spatial profile of the membrane conductance and is independent of the initial conditions (London *et al.* 1999). Such a voltage gradient implies that current flows constantly in the dendritic tree after transient voltage perturbation. This is shown in Fig. 9.3e–h. The same current pulse as in Fig. 9.3b,c was applied either to the soma (f) and (h) or to location 3 on the apical tree (e and g). The voltage profile along the dendritic path from location 4 ('Apical') to location 2 ('Basal') is plotted immediately after the cessation of the current pulse ($t = 2$ ms), and at later times ($t = 60$ ms). Note that the initial response is rather similar in the uniform (light line) and nonuniform (filled line) cases for both input locations. At later times, the voltage in the uniform case is always larger at the injection point. In the nonuniform case, however, the voltage profile is very similar for both input sites and is always larger at proximal (less 'leaky') regions. This voltage profile is very similar to the inverse of the profile of the membrane conductance. Indeed, irrespective of the location of the input after a sufficient time the somatic voltage will be larger than the voltage at any other location in the tree. This result implies that for input injected at distal ('leaky') regions, the local voltage response will initially be larger than the resultant somatic response, but at later times the reverse is true. Thus, voltage 'cross-over' between these two sites is expected (and found experimentally; Stuart and Spruston 1998). Such a cross-over (which is not expected in the uniform case) is a strong indication that the membrane conductance is distributed nonuniformly in the dendritic tree studied (London *et al.* 1999).

With membrane nonuniformity considered above, the membrane conductance near the soma is less leaky than in the corresponding uniform case. This implies that the spike mechanism suffers from a smaller 'sink' in the nonuniform case. In Fig. 9.4a the current–firing (I–f) curves of the neuron modeled in Fig. 9.3 are computed for both the uniform (light line) and nonuniform (heavy line) cases. In both cases, the same excitable axon is attached to the soma. The current required to reach threshold for action-potential initiation is lower in the nonuniform case than in the uniform one. Thus, a smaller number of excitatory synapses is required to fire the axon when the dendrites have a nonuniform conductance distribution. This difference becomes smaller as the stimulus intensity grows and firing frequency increases. Importantly, this figure shows that the firing in the axon depends on the passive properties of the dendritic tree.

To summarize, the above section demonstrates that certain aspects of signal transfer in neurons can be optimized with the re-allocation of passive dendritic ion channels. We have shown that with a fixed number of passive ion channels in the dendritic tree, increasing the channel density at distal dendritic regions (and reducing their density at proximal regions) enhances the efficacy of most of the dendritic synapses as recorded at the soma. Similarly, with re-allocation of the variety of ion channel types available to neurons (both active and passive), a large repertoire of optimization rules could be implemented in the neuron.

Why consider passive models when dendrites have active properties?

The insights summarized above are all based on passive-cable models of dendrites. However, with synaptic inputs (a conductance change) rather than current input and

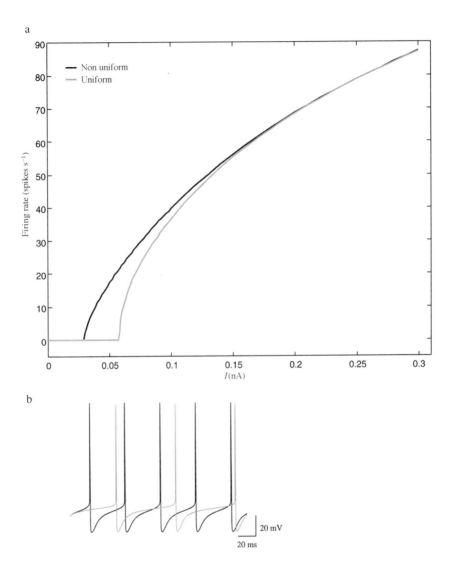

Fig. 9.4 Nonuniformity of membrane conductance changes the load that the dendritic tree imposes on the spike mechanism in the axon. (a) *I–f* curve for the tree shown in Fig. 9.3(a). An excitable axon was attached to the soma (axon parameters are identical to those of Mainen and Sejnowski 1996). Constant current *I* was injected to the soma in both the uniform case (light line) and the nonuniform case (heavy line). In the latter case, the dendritic tree imposes a smaller 'current sink' on the firing mechanism at the axon. Consequently, the *I–f* curve is shifted to the left. (b) Action potentials in the uniform case (light line) and the nonuniform case (heavy line) in a 200 ms time-interval for *I* = 0.065 nA.

with the voltage-dependent ion channels found in dendrites, dendrites are inherently nonlinear devices. In some neuron types, Na^+ or Ca^{2+} spikes can even be generated in the dendritic tree (see Chapter 10). These findings can lead to the erroneous notion that passive models of neurons are essentially irrelevant.

Perhaps the best way to highlight the problem with this erroneous view is to consider the propagation of the action potential in the axon. Axons are highly nonlinear electrical devices, but nevertheless, the propagation of the action potential is strongly affected by their passive properties. Indeed, the propagation velocity of the action potential in unmyelinated axons is directly proportional to the passive space constant, λ (Jack et al. 1975). The intuitive reason is that the 'foot' of the action potential is essentially a passive signal, and so current that spreads 'in front' of the action potential and activates the more distal regions of the axon is strongly affected by the passive properties of the axon.

Similarly, significant spatial averaging takes place in the dendritic tree when input is delivered locally. Because the input current flows rapidly away from the local (synaptic) input site to other dendritic regions, the electrical properties of these not-yet-activated regions have a marked effect on the behavior of the signal at the input site. In other words, the passive properties of the tree shape, to a large extent, the local voltage response at its site of origin even when active channels are involved in the generation of the input signal

Another way to consider the relevance of passive models is by noting that critical electrical parameters, namely, R_i and C_m, are voltage-independent. Because the flow of (both passive and active) electrical signals in cable structures strongly depends on these passive parameters, one cannot ignore passive properties of neurons when analyzing their input–output function.

The passive model should, therefore, be viewed as a skeleton upon which active properties are added. As will be emphasized below when discussing nonlinear cable models, one cannot fully understand active phenomena in neurons without understanding the interplay between the underlying passive and active mechanisms. As shown above, important insights have been gained by careful analysis of the passive case. These insights should then be refined and expanded when the variety of active currents (assuming their properties are known) are incorporated, one-by-one, into the passive model. This is highlighted in the following section that deals with the biophysics of excitable dendrites.

Models of excitable dendrites

As discussed in several chapters in this volume, in the last few years there has been a large leap in our acquaintance with the physiology of dendrites. The advance of new technologies, in particular infrared differential interference contrast video microscopy (Stuart et al. 1993; Dodt and Zieglgänsberger 1994) and two-photon microscopy (Yuste and Denk 1995), have enabled experimenters to measure the electrical properties of the dendritic membrane directly. The fascinating picture that emerges is that dendrites have a large orchestra of voltage-gated channels, which operate with different voltage sensitivity and at different times. Different types of excitable channel are recruited in different regions of the dendritic tree for different input conditions, and their electrical response can range from essentially passive to subthreshold active, to generation of dendritic spikes that spread only locally within the dendritic tree.

Our insights regarding the generation and propagation of electrical signals in *excitable* trees emerged mainly from modeling studies of axonal structures. These models consider highly excitable ('hot') cable structures that, like many real axons, receive depolarizing current at their (somatic) site of origin, and, if generated, the action potential propagates orthodromically to invade the whole (or most) of the axonal tree (e.g. Parnas and Segev 1979; Manor *et al.* 1991).

Compared with axons, the situation with excitable dendritic trees is different in three important ways. First, the synaptic input (both excitatory and inhibitory) may be activated at essentially any location over the dendritic surface. Hence, the active response can start at any region of the dendritic tree. Second, in different instances the input can be spatially distributed or more localized, actively recruiting different regions of the dendritic tree. Third, unlike axons, which have a few hundred to a few thousands excitable ion channels per square micron (Hille 1992), the dendritic tree seems to be less excitable. Consequently, the more confined excitable current that such dendritic channels might generate is expected to be sensitively affected not only by the properties of the excitable channels themselves, but also by the electro-anatomical structure of the tree and the properties (location, strength and distribution) of the synaptic inputs. What are the general principles that underlie the interplay between synaptic inputs, voltage-gated channels and dendritic morphology?

This question is explored below by utilizing carefully chosen simple models of excitable cable structures which receive inputs at different sites. This theoretical investigation provides several general biophysical insights regarding the conditions for the initiation and propagation of electrical signals in excitable dendritic trees (see also Segev and Rall 1998).

Effect of dendritic geometry on the threshold for spike firing

What determines the threshold for spike firing in excitable cable structures such as nerve cells? The intuitive answer is that threshold is set solely by the properties (types, densities, kinetics) of the excitable channels at the site of spike initiation. In this view, the membrane voltage at this site should exceed a critical depolarization, V_{th}, where the net ionic current becomes inward. This inward current will further depolarize the membrane and this will start the regenerative process that underlies the initiation of the action potential.

This view strictly holds only for isopotential structures where the ionic current flows only through the membrane. In real neurons, however, because of their cable properties, a significant portion of the excitable current that is generated at the site of spike initiation flows longitudinally to other regions of the neuron, rather than depolarizing the local membrane. To compensate for this current loss, the voltage threshold in the cable will be larger than the voltage threshold in the corresponding isopotential structure. Indeed, the geometry of the neuron strongly affects the conditions for spike initiation, and as we shall show below, there are cases where excitation can never be realized in cable structures while it could be attained in the corresponding isopotential case (see also Chapter 9 in Jack *et al.* 1975).

In Fig. 9.5, a 1-λ-long excitable cylindrical cable with both ends sealed is modeled. The action potential was initiated separately at two different locations, after a brief depolarizing current pulse. In one case the input current was applied at the end of the cylinder ($X = 0$, where $X = {}^x/\lambda$) and in the other case the current was applied at the middle of the cylinder ($X = 0.5$). In both locations, a minimal current, I_{th} (the *current threshold*), that is required for the initiation of the action potential was applied (lower traces). The *voltage threshold*, V_{th}, is defined as the voltage that was developed at the end of this current pulse (arrows in upper traces).

A few points become immediately evident from this figure. First, although the cylinder is uniformly excitable, V_{th} is larger at the cylinder end than at its midpoint

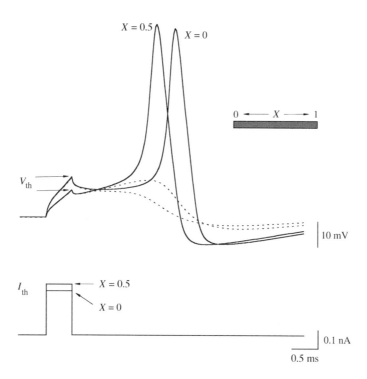

Fig. 9.5 Voltage and current threshold for action-potential initiation in a uniformly excitable cylinder depends on input location. An action potential was initiated with a brief (0.5-ms) threshold current applied at two locations; at one end of the cylinder ($X = 0$) and at the middle of the cylinder ($X = 0.5$). The minimum current, I_{th}, required to initiate an action potential at these sites is shown at the bottom and the two resultant action potentials are superimposed at the top. In each case, a 1% reduction in the amplitude of the applied current resulted with only a local (subthreshold) voltage response (upper trace, dashed lines). The voltage at the end of the current pulse is defined throughout this work as the voltage threshold, V_{th} (arrows in voltage traces). V_{th} is lower at the middle of the cylinder than at its end. In contrast, I_{th} is lower at the end of the cylinder. A cylinder with a cable length of $L = 1$ was modeled, with uniformly excitable membrane described using the standard Hodgkin and Huxley equations at 20° C. Cylinder diameter was 2 μm and the axial resistance was 100 Ω cm (Rapp 1998).

(15 mV and 10 mV, respectively). The opposite is true for I_{th}, which is smaller at the cylinder end (0.24 nA at $X = 0$ compared with 0.28 nA at $X = 0.5$). Another point to note is that the shape of the action potential changes with location; it is somewhat briefer and smaller at $X = 0$ than at $X = 0.5$ (see also Jack *et al.* 1975). Thus, the current and voltage thresholds for action-potential initiation in uniformly excitable cables are a function of both the input site and the electrotonic structure of the cable.

Next, in Fig. 9.6, we consider the case of a branched cable with low excitability (Stuart and Sakmann 1994; Magee and Johnston 1995; Mainen *et al.* 1995; Spruston *et al.* 1995). The parameters used are described in Rapp *et al.* (1996). This excitable cable has a total length of $L = 1$; it branches at its midpoint (at $X = 0.5$) into two daughters such that the $d^{3/2}$ rule of Rall (1959) holds. This structure is electrically equivalent to a single cylinder. Observing V_{th} along the parent branch (Fig. 9.6a), the same qualitative behavior as in the corresponding standard Hodgkin and Huxley case is seen. Now, however, because of the low excitability, V_{th} is much more depolarized at all sites and the minimum point is at $X = 0.3$ rather than at the center of the cable as in highly excitable cylindrical cables.

Moving along the thick daughter ($d = 1.7$ μm), V_{th} looks rather similar to that of the parent branch, with slightly larger values for the corresponding X values. However, near the end of this branch, *spikes could not be initiated at all*; namely V_{th} (and I_{th}, Fig. 9.6b) goes to infinity. At this region, most of the (already reduced) excitable current that is generated locally is lost to the rest of the tree and the remaining inward current is insufficient to initiate the regenerative response that underlies the initiation of the action potential. This failure to initiate an action potential is much more dramatic in the thin ($d = 0.72$ μm) daughter branch where action potential could be initiated only near the branch point.

Because thin dendrites have large input impedance, small currents tend to produce large voltage changes. Accordingly, the current threshold for local regenerative events is relatively low in dendritic branches (Fig. 9.6b; as long as they are not too thin). However, the large impedance load (sink) imposed by the rest of the dendritic tree provide unfavorable conditions for these local regenerative events to actively spread to the other dendritic branches. Experimental observations of such local regenerative events are described in Chapter 10 and their functional significance is considered in Chapter 11.

The situation becomes even more interesting when the stimulus is delivered simultaneously at more than one point. The lower right limb of the graph in Fig. 9.6a represents the case where current was injected simultaneously to the two daughter branches at equal X values (two-point polarization). The input current, I_{stim}, that was applied at each branch was scaled in proportion to the relative input conductance of that branch. The result is striking (although it is directly expected from Rall's 'equivalent cable' conditions in the passive-cable theory). Now the action potential could be initiated in both branches at any input location, X, even at the distal sites of the thin branch. Furthermore, for a given X value, V_{th} at both daughters is identical and is equal to that in the corresponding X value at the parent branch. In other words, this condition is completely identical to the case of a uniform cylinder with $L = 1$. The conclusion is that a distributed input (rather than a spatially localized input) provides more favorable conditions for firing a dendritic action potential.

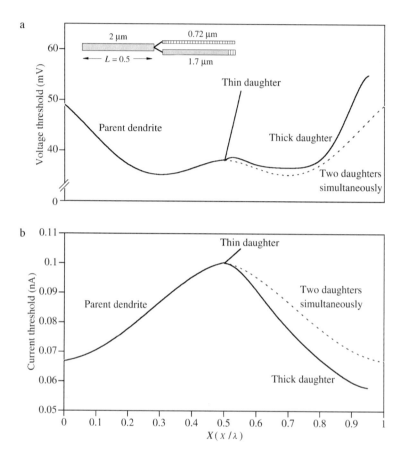

Fig. 9.6 Voltage and current threshold in a weakly excitable branched structure. (a) V_{th} along the dendritic branch. (b) The corresponding I_{th}. In the daughter branches, there are regions in which the weak excitable current cannot overcome the huge conductance load imposed by the parent dendrite and the sister branch, and thus, V_{th} and I_{th} become infinite (striped regions in *inset*). In contrast, a simultaneous input to the two daughters produces an action potential in the daughter branches at all sites (dashed line). Note that although the input impedance in the thin daughter, at $X = 0.55$, is higher than in the parent dendrite, at $X = 0.5$, I_{th} in the thin daughter is higher, rather than lower. In the simultaneously activated case, I_{stim} is injected into each cable is split in proportion to their relative input conductances, that is, the current injected into the branch of diameter d_1 is equal to $I_{stim}d_1^{3/2}/(d_1^{3/2} + d_2^{3/2})$. The current denoted as 'two daughters simultaneously' is the sum of the currents provided to the daughter branches and is equal to I_{th} in the parent dendrite at the same X location. *Inset*: a 0.5-λ-long parent dendrite (2 μm in diameter) is connected to two 0.5-λ-long thick (1.7 μm) and thin (0.72 μm) daughter branches. The model follows Rall's $d^{3/2}$ ratio ('equivalent cylinder' conditions) from Rapp (1998).

The reason for the improved conditions for action-potential initiation with distributed input is that the structure becomes effectively more isopotential compared to the case of a localized input. Relatively less current is lost longitudinally from the input site and more flows to depolarize the local membrane. Consequently, V_{th} is reduced compared to the case of an input to only one branch. (The structure becomes truly isopotential when the current is applied at all locations simultaneously. This then becomes the uniform polarization, or the 'space-clamped' case).

We conclude this section by summarizing its main results. Threshold for spike initiation in dendrites strongly depends both on the cable properties and on input location. The lowest *voltage threshold* is near sites which are effectively most isopotential. This is the case in the middle of highly excitable cylindrical cables with both ends sealed and at (or near) the soma of radial neurons. The lowest *current threshold* is typically obtained at sites with the largest input impedance and in general, these are the favorable sites for action-potential initiation from current (and synaptic) inputs. However, thin dendritic arbors suffer a large impedance load imposed by the tree. Thus, weakly excitable thin arbors are unfavorable sites for spike initiation, although they can have large input impedances. If, however, the thin arbor is highly excitable then the density of the excitable current is sufficiently large to overcome the massive current sink imposed on this arbor. In this case, the increased input impedance in the thin arbor provides favorable conditions (reduced I_{th}) for action-potential initiation. Indeed, it is the interplay between local excitability, amount of current loss, and the input impedance that determines threshold conditions for action-potential initiation at the input site. Finally, an electrically distributed structure becomes effectively more isopotential when the input is spatially distributed rather than spatially localized. Consequently, for a given tree and given location(s), both V_{th} and I_{th} are reduced for a distributed input compared with a more spatially restricted input.

Highly excitable axon and weakly excitable soma and dendrite

What happens when a highly excitable axon is coupled to a weakly excitable soma and dendrites (Moore and Westerfield 1983; Moore *et al.* 1983; Mainen *et al.* 1995; Rapp *et al.* 1996)? Because the soma and dendrites serves as a large sink for the excitable currents generated in the axon, and because the proximal part of the axon might receive a dense inhibitory (symmetrical) synaptic input, the following questions arise in the context of the present study:

1. Where in the axon will the action potential be initiated?
2. What is the effect of inhibition in the proximal part of the axon on the site and timing of action-potential initiation?

A model of a uniformly excitable cylindrical axon, coupled to a weakly excitable isopotential soma and cylindrical dendrite, is schematically depicted in the inset of Fig. 9.7. When a 15-ms current pulse is applied to the model soma, the minimum current (I_{th}) required to generate an action potential in the axon is 0.1 nA. Interestingly, although the current was applied to the soma, the action potential was initiated further down in the axon, approximately 130 μm (0.3 λ) away from the soma, rather than at the proximal end of the axon (Fig. 9.7a). It then propagates

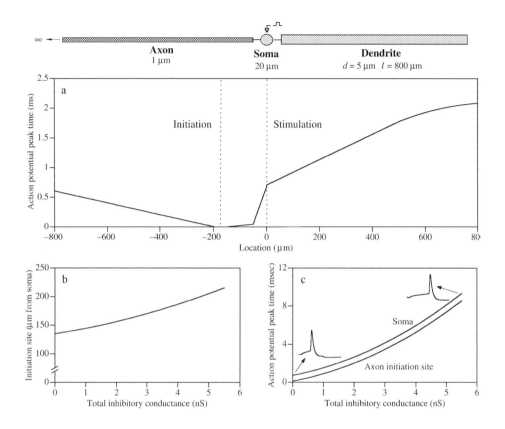

Fig. 9.7 Mixed excitability: A highly excitable axon with weakly excitable soma and dendrite. The model consists of a 20-μm soma, connected to a 800-μm-long, 5-μm dendrite and a long, 1-μm, axon (*Inset* at top). The soma and dendrite are weakly excitable (light gray in *Inset*), whereas the axon is highly excitable (dark gray in *Inset*) Parameters as in Rapp *et al.* (1996). (a) In response to just threshold (0.1-nA, 15-ms) current pulse to the soma, an action potential is initiated in the axon 150 μm away from the soma, rather than in the proximal end of the axon. Then, the action potential propagates forward in the axon (velocity 1.11 m s^{-1}) and backward into the soma and dendrite (0.42 m s^{-1}). (b) A steady-state inhibitory conductance change was uniformly distributed over the first 30 μm of the axon (E_{syn} = –80 mV) and a 0.2-nA current step (twice threshold) was applied to the modeled soma. As a result of the inhibition, the site of action-potential initiation is pushed further away down into the axon; the action potential fails to be initiated with an inhibitory conductance change larger than 6 nS. (c) Synaptic inhibition at the proximal part of the axon delays the time of action-potential initiation in the axon (lower curve), and, consequently, the backpropagating action potential at the soma (upper curve) is also delayed. To demonstrate the effect of inhibition on delaying spike initiation, the *somatic* action potential in the absence of inhibition (left arrow) and with 5.5 nS inhibition (right arrow) are shown (Rapp 1998).

forward along the axon with a velocity of 1.1 m s^{-1}, as well as backward to the soma and the (cylindrical) dendrite with a velocity of 0.42 m s^{-1} (in the linear regime). The initiation of the action potential first in the axon is the result of the increase in channel density in the axon, compared with in the soma and dendrite. The initiation of the action potential down in the axon, rather than near the input site, is the result of a large conductance load imposed on the axon by the (adjacent) soma and dendrites. Because the soma and dendrites are only weakly excitable, they mainly serve as a current sink rather than a current source. Consequently, the voltage threshold for action potential firing in the proximal part of the axon is relatively large. In contrast, the conditions for action-potential initiation are improved at a site located further down in the axon because, at this site, the partial electrical decoupling provided by the axial resistance of the (thin) axon reduces the current sink from this site. In addition, the input impedance at distal axonal sites increases. As a result, the action potential 'prefers' to start somewhere down the axon rather than near the soma (Colbert *et al.* 1996).

Synaptic inhibition in the proximal region of the axon further hinders the condition for action-potential initiation. It shunts the excitable current that is generated at this site even more, and consequently, the action potential is initiated at a greater distance down in the axon (Fig. 9.7b) and with an increased delay (Fig. 9.7c). For the parameters chosen in this model, the site of action-potential initiation is shifted, because of inhibition, to a distance of up to 220 μm away from the soma before it completely fails to fire (when inhibition increases further). The delay in action-potential initiation at this remote initiation zone can be as large as 9 ms compared with the case without inhibition. Clearly, these numbers depend on the kinetics and density of the excitable channels, the morphology and passive properties of the modeled structure, the amount of excitatory current input that reaches the soma, and the properties (time-course, reversal potential, spatial distribution) of the inhibitory synapses in the axon. For example, with increased axonal excitability the site of action-potential initiation will move closer to the soma. In contrast, with an increased conductance load in the dendrites (larger dendritic tree, increased inhibitory conductance in the dendrites) this site will move away from the soma. Still, the general principles that were highlighted here are valid for these different possibilities.

We conclude by stating that the morphology of the relatively thin axon and the large dendritic tree favors the initiation of the action potential down in the axon, perhaps in the first node of Ranvier, rather than near the soma (Colbert *et al.* 1996). Inhibition in the soma and proximal axonal sites could be used to finely modulate both the site and time of action-potential initiation. Similar principles also govern the interaction between dendritic excitability and inhibition, as shown experimentally (Kim *et al.* 1995; see also Miles *et al.* 1996; Chen *et al.* 1997, and Buzsáki and Kandel 1998).

Concluding remarks

In recent years it has become increasingly clear that the complexity of dendrites, in both their morphological faces and physiological character, and in the properties of their synaptic inputs, give rise to a highly nonlinear input–output device. To understand how this device transforms the large number of synaptic inputs it receives into a meaningful output in the axon (which might then also travel back into the dendrites), a modeling framework is required. As shown in this chapter, Rall's cable theory provides a very versatile theoretical framework which enables one to incorporate the rapid increase in morphological and physiological information about dendrites (as demonstrated in this book).

Important insights into the relationship between the structure and function of dendrites were gained using these models. However, very fundamental questions still remain open. What is the functional role of the unique structure of dendrites? Why do some have pyramidal-like structures and others (e.g. cerebellar Purkinje cells) have such different morphological characteristics? Why do some dendrites have excitable Na^+ channels and other cell types do not? But most importantly, what is the functional role of dendrites during the normal operation of the nervous system (e.g. when we write this chapter or when you read it)?

The more we learn about dendrites and neurons the more we realize that they are potentially very powerful, both as computational devices and as plastic devices. But whether *individual* neurons actually enrich the computational capabilities of the *community* of neurons can only be answered in the context of the information-processing task of the network. In other words, the functional meaning of the individual neuron can only be understood within the broader framework of the specific 'language' that the neuronal network uses. We do not yet understand how biological neuronal networks represent and process information. Thus, the biggest challenge for the next century remains to connect the single neuron level to the level of the global operation of the network. It is hoped that this chapter and this book provide a small step in this direction.

Acknowledgments

Special thanks to our colleagues Claude Meunier and Muki Rapp who participated in the research leading to the results presented here. Supported by a grant from the Israeli Academy of Science and the ONR.

References

Agmon-Snir, H. and Segev, I. (1993). Signal delay and propagation velocity in passive dendritic trees. *Journal of Neurophysiology*, **70**, 2066–85.

Bernander, O., Douglas, R. J., Martin, K. A. C., and Koch, C. (1991). Synaptic background activity influences spatiotemporal integration in single pyramidal cells. *Proceedings of the National Academy of Sciences USA*, **88**, 11569–73.

Borg-Graham, L. J., Monier, C., and Fregnac, Y. (1998). Visual input evokes transient and strong shunting inhibition in visual cortical neurons. *Nature*, **393**, 369–73.

Bower, J. M. and Beeman, D. (1994). *The book of GENESIS: exploring realistic neural models with the GEneral NEural SImulation System*. Springer, New York.

Chen, W. R., Midtgaard, J., and Shepherd, G. M. (1997). Forward and backward propagation of dendritic impulses and their synaptic control in mitral cells. *Science*, **278**, 463–7.

Colbert, C. M. and Johnston, D. (1996). Axonal action-potential initiation and Na$^+$ channel densities in the soma and axon initial segment of subicular pyramidal neurons. *Journal of Neuroscience*, **16**, 6676–86.

Dodt, H. U. and Zieglgänsberger, W. (1994). Infrared videomicroscopy: a new look at neuronal structure and function. *Trends in Neurosciences*, **17**, 453–458.

Häusser, M. and Roth, A. (1997). Estimating the time course of the excitatory synaptic conductance in neocortical pyramidal cells using a novel voltage jump method. *Journal of Neuroscience*, **17**, 7606–25.

Hille, B. (1992). *Ionic channels of excitable membranes*. Sinauer, Sunderland, Massachusetts.

Hines, M. and Carnevale, N. T. (1997). The NEURON simulation environment. *Neural Computation*, **9**, 1179–1210.

Hoffman, D. A., Magee, J. C., Colbert, C. M., and Johnston, D. (1997). K$^+$ channel regulation of signal propagation in dendrites of hippocampal pyramidal neurons. *Nature*, **387**, 869–75.

Jack, J. J. B., Noble, D., and Tsien, R. W. (1975). *Electrical current flow in excitable cells.* Oxford University Press.

Kim, H., Breierlein, M., and Connors, B. (1995). Inhibitory control of excitable dendrites in neocortex. *Journal of Neurophysiology*, **74**, 1810–14.

Koch, C. (1999). *Biophysics of computation: information processing in single neurons.* Oxford University Press.

Koch, C. and Poggio, T. (1983). A theoretical analysis of electrical properties of spines. *Proceedings of the Royal Society of London, Series B*, **218**, 455–77.

Koch, C., Rapp, M., and Segev, I. (1996). A brief history of time (constants). *Cerebral Cortex*, **6**, 93–101.

London, M., Meunier, C., and Segev, I. (1999). Signal transfer in passive dendrites with nonuniform membrane conductance. *Journal of Neuroscience*, (in press)

Magee, J. C. (1998). Dendritic hyperpolarization-activated currents modify the integrative properties of hippocampal CA1 pyramidal neurons. *Journal of Neuroscience*, **18**, 7613–24.

Magee, J. and Johnston, D. (1995). Characterization of single voltage-gated Na$^+$ and Ca^{2+} channels in apical dendrites of rat CA1 pyramidal neurons. *Journal of Physiology*, **487**, 67–90.

Mainen, Z., Jeorges, J., Huguenard, J., and Sejnowski, T. (1995). A model of spike initiation in neocortical pyramidal neurons. *Neuron*, **15**, 1427–39.

Major, G. (1994). Detailed passive cable models of whole-cell recorded CA3 pyramidal neurons in rat hippocampal slices. *Journal of Neuroscience*, **14**, 4613–38.

Manor, Y., Koch, C., and Segev, I. (1991). Effect of geometrical irregularities on propagation delay in axonal trees. *Biophysical Journal*, **60**, 1424–37.

Miles, R., Toth, K., Gulyas, A. I., Hajos, N., and Freund, T. F. (1996). Differences between somatic and dendritic inhibition in the hippocampus. *Neuron*, **16**, 815–23.

Moore, J. W. and Westerfield, M. (1983). Action potential propagation and threshold parameters in inhomogeneous regions of squid axons. *Journal of Physiology*, **336**, 285–300.

Moore, J. W., Stockbridge, N., and Westerfield, M. (1983). On the site of impulse initiation in a neurone. *Journal of Physiology*, **336**, 301–11.

Nicoll, A., Larkman, A., and Blakemore, C. (1993). Modulation of EPSP shape and efficacy by intrinsic membrane conductances in rat neocortical pyramidal neurons *in vitro*. *Journal of Physiology*, **468**, 693–710.

Parnas, I. and Segev, I. (1979). A mathematical model for conduction of action potentials along bifurcation axons. *Journal of Physiology*, **295**, 323–43.

Rall, W. (1959). Branching dendritic trees and motoneuron membrane resistivity. *Experimental Neurology*, **1**, 491–527.

Rall, W. (1964). Theoretical significance of dendritic trees for neuronal input-output relations. In *Neural theory and modeling*, (ed. R. Reiss), pp. 73–97. Stanford University Press.

Rall, W. (1969). Time constants and electrotonic length of membrane cylinders and neurons. *Biophysical Journal*, **9**, 1483–508.

Rall, W. (1974). Dendritic spines, synaptic potency and neuronal plasticity. In *Cellular mechanisms subserving changes in neuronal activity*, Brain Information Service Research Report No. 3, (ed. C. D. Woody, K. A. Brown, T. J. Crow, and J. D. Knispel), pp. 13–21. U.C.L.A., Los Angeles.

Rall, W. (1978). Dendritic spines and synaptic potency. *Studies in Neurophysiology*, 203–9.

Rall, W. and Agmon-Snir, H. (1998). Cable theory for dendritic neurons. In *Methods in neuronal modeling: from ions to networks*, (ed. C. Koch and I. Segev), pp. 27–92. MIT Press.

Rall, W. and Rinzel, J. (1973). Branch input resistance and steady attenuation for input to one branch of a dendritic neuron model. *Biophysical Journal*, **13**, 648–88.

Rall, W. and Segev, I. (1988). Dendritic spine synapses, excitable spine clusters and plasticity. In *Cellular mechanisms of conditioning and behavioral plasticity*, (ed. R. Lasek, D. L. Alkon, and N. V. McGaugh), pp. 221–36. Plenum Press.

Rall, W., Shepherd, G. M., Reese, T. S., and Brightman, M. W. (1966). Dendrodendritic synaptic pathway for inhibition in the olfactory bulb. *Experimental Neurology*, **14**, 44–56.

Rall, W., Burke, R. E., Smith, T. G., Nelson, P. G., and Frank, K. (1967). Dendritic location of synapses and possible mechanisms for the monosynaptic EPSP in motoneurons. *Journal of Neurophysiology*, **30**, 1169–93.

Rall, W., Burke, R. E., Holmes, W. R., Jack, J. J. B., Redman, S. J., and Segev, I. (1992). Matching dendritic neuron models to experimental data. *Physiological Reviews*, **72**, 159–86.

Rapp, M. (1998). The computational role of excitable dendrites. Ph.D. thesis, Hebrew University.

Rapp, M., Yarom, Y., and Segev, I. (1992). The impact of parallel fiber background activity on the cable properties of cerebellar Purkinje cells. *Neural Computation*, **4**, 518–33.

Rapp, M., Segev, I., and Yarom, Y. (1994). Physiology, morphology and detailed passive models of cerebellar Purkinje cells. *Journal of Physiology*, **474**, 101–18.

Rapp, M., Yarom, Y., and Segev, I. (1996). Modeling back propagating action potential in weakly excitable dendrites of neocortical pyramidal cells. *Proceedings of the National Academy of Science USA*, **93**, 11985–90.

Redman, S. and Walmsley, B. (1983*a*). Amplitude fluctuations in synaptic potentials evoked in cat spinal motoneurones at identified group Ia synapses. *Journal of Physiology*, **343**, 135–145.

Redman, S. and Walmsley, B. (1983*b*). The time course of synaptic potentials evoked in cat spinal motoneurones at identified group Ia synapses. *Journal of Physiology*, **343**, 117–33.

Rinzel, J. (1981). Models in neurobiology. *Lectures on Applied Mathematics*, **19**, 281–97.

Rinzel, J. and Rall, W. (1974). Transient response in a dendritic neuron model for current injected at one branch. *Biophysical Journal*, **14**, 759–90.

Segev, I. (1992). Single neurone models: oversimple, complex and reduced. *Trends in Neurosciences*, **15**, 414–21.

Segev, I. and Burke, R. E. (1998). Compartmental models of complex neurons. In *Methods in neuronal modeling: from ions to networks*, (ed. C. Koch and I. Segev), pp. 93–136. MIT Press.

Segev, I. and Rall, W. (1998). Excitable dendrites and spines: earlier theoretical insights elucidate recent direct observations. *Trends in Neurosciences*, **21**, 453–460.

Segev, I., Rinzel, J., and Shepherd, G. (1995). *The theoretical foundation of dendritic function*. MIT Press.

Shepherd, G. M. (1996). The dendritic spine: a multifunctional integrative unit. *Journal of Neurophysiology*, **75**, 2197–210.

Shepherd, G. M. (1998). *The synaptic organization of the brain*. Oxford University Press.

Spruston, N., Schiller, Y., Stuart, G., and Sakmann, B. (1995). Activity-dependent action potential invasion and calcium influx into hippocampal CA1 dendrites. *Science*, **268**, 297–300.

Stratford, R. D., Mason, A. J. R., Larkman, A. U., Major, G., and Jack, J. J. B. (1989). The modeling of pyramidal neurons in the visual cortex. In *The computing neuron*, (ed. R. Durbin, C. Miall, and C. Mitchson). Addison–Wesley.

Stuart, G. J. and Sakmann, B. (1994). Active propagation of somatic action potentials into neocortical pyramidal cell dendrites. *Nature*, **367**, 69–72.

Stuart, G. and Spruston, N. (1995). Probing dendritic function with patch pipettes. *Current Opinion in Neurobiology*, **5**, 389–94.

Stuart, G. and Spruston, N. (1998). Determinants of voltage attenuation in neocortical pyramidal neuron dendrites. *Journal of Neuroscience*, **18**, 3501–10.

Stuart, G. J., Dodt, H. U., and Sakmann, B. (1993). Patch-clamp recordings from the soma and dendrites of neurons in brain slices using infrared video microscopy. *Pflügers Archiv*, **423**, 511–18.

Yuste, R. and Denk, W. (1995). Dendritic spines as basic functional units of neuronal integration. *Nature*, **375**, 682–4.

Zador, A., Agmon-Snir, H., and Segev, I. (1995). The morphoelectrotonic transform: a graphical approach to dendritic function. *Journal of Neuroscience*, **15**, 1669–82.

10

Dendritic integration

Nelson Spruston
Northwestern University

Greg Stuart
Australian National University

Michael Häusser
University College London

Summary

The essence of neuronal function is to generate outputs, in the form of action potentials, in response to inputs, in the form of synaptic potentials. The morphology and membrane properties of dendrites are extremely important determinants of this input–output transformation. In this chapter we discuss the many factors affecting the dendritic integration of synaptic potentials, the site of action potential initiation, and dendritic excitability.

Introduction

Dendrites, as illustrated in previous chapters, are morphologically elaborate structures receiving thousands of synaptic inputs. A quick glance at the morphology of various neurons (see Fig. 1 in the Preface) reveals their dramatic structural differences and hints at their functional specialization. Indeed, the functional heterogeneity suggested by morphology is borne out by experimental analysis of different cell types (see Chapter 6). Functionally, dendrites are remarkably complex, with a wide variety of synaptic receptors and voltage-gated channels distributed uniquely in each type of neuron. But what are the functions of dendrites, and how are they enriched by their characteristic mosaic of synapses and channels? With the development of dendritic patch-clamp and imaging methods, significant progress toward answering these questions has been realized in recent years.

Here we review various aspects of dendritic function, including principles that seem to hold for the majority of neurons studied and providing examples of functional specialization in the dendrites of neurons in the mammalian CNS.

The action potential is the final output signal of most neurons

Neurons communicate *via* action potentials—brief, all-or-none reversals of membrane potential polarity mediated by the opening of voltage-gated Na^+ and K^+ channels. Though considerable debate exists regarding the details of information processing in neurons (Shadlen and Newsome 1994, 1995; Ferster and Spruston 1995; Softky 1995), the prevailing view is that action potentials are used to produce a kind of digital code, with the state of the nervous system dictated by a combination of the rate and the precise timing of action potentials across multiple, interconnected neural networks in the brain.

Most cells fire action potentials only when synaptic excitation sufficiently exceeds inhibition[1]. The simplest view of synaptic integration is that excitatory inputs sum, and if the resulting depolarization is large enough to reach threshold, an action potential is generated. In this simple model, inhibition opposes this depolarization, thus increasing the number of active excitatory inputs required to reach threshold. This certainly represents a vast oversimplification of synaptic integration, but serves as a useful starting point.

To influence action potential initiation, postsynaptic potentials (PSPs), both excitatory (EPSPs) and inhibitory (IPSPs), must spread from their site of generation to the action potential initiation zone. This propagation of synaptic potentials is affected by the passive cable properties of dendrites and by the voltage-gated conductances they contain. Furthermore, excitatory and inhibitory potentials sum non-linearly, in a manner determined by the spatial relationship between them. Finally, the process of synaptic integration is potentially complicated by ongoing action potential firing, which can shunt synaptic potentials and change the availability of voltage-gated conductances throughout the neuron. All these factors influence synaptic integration in complicated ways.

Summation and propagation of PSPs depend on dendritic cable properties

The resting potential (V_{rest}) of most neurons is more hyperpolarized than action potential threshold. Furthermore, most unitary PSPs (mediated by one or more contacts between a single presynaptic axon and a postsynaptic dendrite) are too small to bridge the gap between the resting potential and action potential threshold. Multiple synaptic inputs must therefore sum to produce action potential

---

[1] There are some exceptions to this. Some neurons, like Purkinje cells in the cerebellum and dopaminergic cells in the substantia nigra, fire action potentials spontaneously, even when deprived of all synaptic inputs. In such neurons, action potential firing is modulated primarily by inhibition, which reduces the firing rate and may synchronize the firing of many neurons (Yung *et al.* 1991; Häusser and Clark 1997; Gao *et al.* 1996). Other neurons, such as those in the supraoptic nucleus (Bourque and Renaud 1984), fire spontaneously in rhythmic bursts of action potentials. In these neurons, synaptic inputs can modulate these oscillations.

firing in most neurons[2]. This section considers the passive electrical structure of dendrites, and its effects on the integration of PSPs. Later we consider how synaptic integration is further enriched by dendritic voltage-gated channels.

Passive electrical properties and synaptic integration

As discussed in detail later in this chapter, action potentials are initiated in the axon of most neurons. The ability of an EPSP to depolarize the membrane potential (V_m) toward action potential threshold in the axon therefore depends on the size of the PSP and the extent to which it is attenuated as it propagates from the dendrites toward the soma and axon. Chapter 9 summarized several important insights regarding the effects of dendritic cable properties on EPSP amplitude and time-course. Here we build on these insights, by summarizing experimental data on the passive electrical structure of neurons, and illustrating, with examples, how synaptic integration is affected by these properties, the morphology of the cell, the location of a synapse, and the time-course of the synaptic current.

Three passive electrical properties contribute to electrotonic structure of the dendritic tree—the specific membrane resistivity (R_m), the specific membrane capacitance (C_m), and the intracellular resistivity (R_i). High values of R_i and low values of R_m increase the attenuation of synaptic potentials as they propagate passively in dendrites. Attenuation is also greater for brief PSPs compared with more sustained changes in V_m; this arises as a result of the membrane capacitance, which serves to filter transient changes in V_m (Rall 1967; Jack *et al.* 1983; Spruston *et al.* 1994). All these effects are more pronounced for synapses that are located further from the site of action potential initiation.

Fig. 10.1 illustrates the effects of R_m, R_i, and synapse location on synaptic integration. Panels a–c show the responses of a generic pyramidal neuron model to synaptic input in three different locations. In the control case (Fig. 10.1, center column of traces), moving the synapse from the soma (Fig. 10.1a, center) to a proximal dendrite (Fig. 10.1b, center) results in a smaller somatic EPSP because some of the synaptic charge injected onto the dendrite capacitance is lost through the membrane resistance as it propagates toward the soma. This results in a nearly twofold attenuation of the EPSP propagating from the dendrite to the soma in this example. Moving the synapse further out on the dendrite (Fig. 10.1c, center) increases the amplitude of the local synaptic potential in the dendrites, because of the higher input impedance and smaller local capacitance at this dendritic location compared with the soma, and dramatically increases the dendro-somatic EPSP attenuation (nearly tenfold attenuation). These two effects are opposing, resulting in a net reduction of the somatic EPSP amplitude by a factor of three compared with the somatic input shown in A.

---

[2] Exceptions to this include, for example, the spherical bushy cells of the ventral cochlear nucleus (Lieberman 1991), neurons in the magnocellular nucleus of the trapezoid body (Borst *et al.* 1995), and ciliary ganglion neurons (Landmesser and Pilar 1972). In each of these cases a small number of presynaptic axons form a large, calyceal synapse capable of firing the postsynaptic neuron. Another exception is the climbing fiber input to the Purkinje cell, where a single presynaptic fiber reliably generates a stereotyped burst of spikes in the postsynaptic neuron (Llinás and Sugimori 1980*a*).

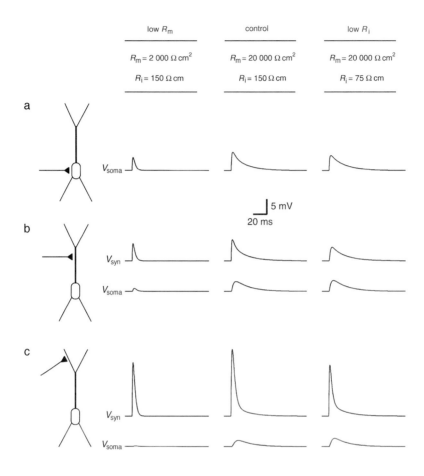

Fig. 10.1 Effects of R_i and R_m on EPSP attenuation. A single excitatory synaptic conductance (g_{syn}) was simulated either at the soma (a), a mid-apical dendrite (b), or a distal apical dendrite (c). Membrane potential at the soma (V_{soma}) and the synapse (V_{syn}) is shown. The center columns are the simulations under control conditions; the left column represents a lower R_m case; the right column represents a lower R_i case. See text for discussion of simulation results. **Simulation methods.** All simulations were performed using NEURON (Hines and Carnevale 1997). The parameters used in the model were: soma, $l = 20$ μm, $d = 20$ μm; main apical dendrite, $l = 350$ μm, $d = 2.94$ μm; distal apical and basal dendrites, $l = 250$ μm, $d = 1.5$ μm; control $R_m = 20\,000$ Ω cm^2; $C_m = 1.0$ μF cm^{-2}; control $R_i = 150$ Ω cm. R_m was halved and C_m doubled to account for spines throughout. Using these parameters, the electrotonic lengths (L) of the apical and basal dendrites are 1.0 and 0.5, respectively. The cell had a resting potential (V_{rest}) of –60 mV. Synapses were placed either at the soma (a), 300 μm from the soma on the main apical dendrite (b, electrotonic distance, X, = 0.43), or 550 μm from the soma on a distal apical dendrite (c, apical, $X = 0.9$). Synapses were modeled as conductance changes ($g_{syn} = 6.38$ nS) with a rising exponential (τ_{rise}) of 0.2 ms and a decaying exponential (τ_{decay}) of 2.0 ms and a reversal potential (E_{rev}) of 0 mV.

Reducing R_m by an order of magnitude has only a modest effect on the amplitude of the local synaptic potential, but has a much bigger effect on the amplitude of the somatic EPSP generated by dendritic synapses (Fig. 10.1, left column). For the most distal synaptic input, the EPSP attenuation for the low R_m value is almost 100-fold (Fig. 10.1c, left), resulting in a somatic EPSP about twenty times smaller than for the same synapse located at the soma. Such large values of dendro-somatic EPSP attenuation have been suggested from modeling of layer V pyramidal neurons (Cauller and Connors 1992; Stuart and Spruston 1998), where a non-uniform distribution of conductances has been shown to result in a leaky apical dendrite (Stuart and Spruston 1998).

The effect of reducing R_i by a factor of two is shown in the right column of Fig. 10.1. For both dendritic synapse locations (Fig. 10.1b,c), this change in R_i results in a reduction of the local dendritic EPSP amplitude that is greater than that produced by the tenfold reduction in R_m. This relatively strong effect of R_i occurs because most of the voltage change during a brief synaptic current results from charging the membrane capacitance; reductions in R_i increase the radial flow of current away from the synapse, thus reducing the amount of charge stored on the local capacitance. Because of this increase in radial current flow along the dendrite, however, the attenuation of the EPSP is reduced. The net effect of a change in R_i therefore is determined by the morphology- and location-dependent effects on the local EPSP amplitude and the dendro-somatic EPSP attenuation. For the intermediate synapse position shown in Fig. 10.1b, these effects are about equal, so the change in R_i has only a small effect on the somatic EPSP amplitude. For the more distal synapse shown in Fig. 10.1c, reducing R_i results in a decrease in the local EPSP but an increase in the amplitude of the somatic EPSP, owing to substantially less EPSP attenuation.

Experimental estimates of passive electrical properties

C_m has been widely regarded as a biological constant with a value of approximately 1 μF cm^{-2}. Recent experimental analysis has provided confirmation of this value for a variety of neurons (Gentet *et al.* 1999). R_m has been measured for a large number of cell types, revealing a wide range of values for different neurons (see below). R_i in mammalian neurons has been estimated using a variety of methods, yielding values ranging from 70–500 Ω cm (Coombs *et al.* 1959; Rall 1959; Lux *et al.* 1970; Barrett and Crill 1974; Cauller and Connors 1992; Fromherz and Muller 1994; Major *et al.* 1994; Rapp *et al.* 1994; Thurbon *et al.* 1994, 1998; Bekkers and Stevens 1996; Meyer *et al.* 1997). Recently, simultaneous somatic and dendritic patch-pipette recordings were used to determine voltage attenuation along the apical dendrites of layer 5 pyramidal neurons (Stuart and Spruston 1998) and the primary dendrites of cerebellar Purkinje neurons (Roth and Häusser 1999). Modeling of these data indicated a value for R_i of 70–140 Ω cm. These experiments provide, arguably, the most reliable estimates of R_i available, because the filtering of transient voltage changes by the dendrites, on which these estimates are based, is very sensitive to R_i.

A particularly critical factor affecting PSP summation is the membrane time-constant (τ_m), which is given by the product of R_m and C_m. For any change in membrane potential, the slowest component of voltage decay is determined by τ_m. Thus, τ_m defines the time window over which synaptic potentials can sum; for presynaptic inputs separated by a few times longer than τ_m, temporal summation becomes diminishingly small.

The membrane time-constant can be estimated directly from the slowest time-constant (τ_0) in a multi-exponential fit of the voltage relaxation following current injection; τ_0 has now been measured for several cell types, revealing a tremendous range in the resting membrane properties of different types of neurons. Given that C_m is likely to be a biological constant, variations in τ_0 are likely to reflect variation in R_m because of differences in the types and densities of ion channels open in the membrane at the resting potential. Hippocampal CA3 pyramidal neurons have among the slowest τ_0 values measured—about 70 ms in brain slices at physiological temperatures (Spruston and Johnston 1992). Even within the hippocampus, τ_0 for other cell types differs from this value; significantly, in CA1 pyramidal neurons τ_0 is less than half this value—about 30 ms in slices (Spruston and Johnston 1992). The fastest τ_0 values recorded so far are from octopus cells in the ventral cochlear nucleus (Golding *et al.* 1999). Patch-pipette recordings from these cells in slices reveal τ_0 values of approximately 0.2 ms. On the basis of τ_0 alone, it can be inferred that CA3 pyramidal neurons will be able to integrate synaptic inputs over a time window about 350-fold longer than in octopus cells. Differences such as these are certain to be functionally important. For example, octopus cells *in vivo* phase lock their firing to clicks of up to 1 kHz (Smith *et al.* 1993). This kind of precise temporal coding would be very difficult to achieve in a neuron with a long membrane time-constant.

Resting membrane properties

Theoretically, τ_m is a purely passive measure, determined only by the membrane capacitance and voltage-independent leak conductances of a neuron. In all cells where this assumption has been tested, however, measured values of τ_0 are voltage-dependent, and influenced by blockers of voltage-dependent conductances. For example, addition of CsCl to the bath (which blocks I_h and inward-rectifying K^+ channels) results in an approximately 50% increase in τ_0 in CA3 and CA1 pyramidal neurons (Spruston and Johnston 1992), a twofold increase in τ_0 in neocortical pyramidal neurons (Stuart and Spruston 1998), and a twentyfold increase in τ_0 in octopus cells (Golding *et al.* 1999). Similarly, even small changes in V_m near V_{rest} have been shown to affect measured values of τ_0 and R_N significantly. These findings suggest that the so-called 'passive' membrane properties of most neurons might be more aptly referred to as 'resting' membrane properties, because they are actually determined in large part by voltage-dependent channels that are open at V_{rest}. The situation is further complicated by the fact that the resting membrane properties of many neurons are unlikely to be uniform. Experimental evidence indicates that many conductances are distributed non-uniformly along dendrites (see Chapter 6). In neocortical and hippocampal pyramidal neurons, conductances that are open at the resting potential, including I_h and others, are present at higher densities in the distal regions of the apical dendrite (Magee 1998; Stuart and Spruston 1998). The net effect of the additional leak in the distal apical dendrites is that distal synapses are even more electrically isolated (from the action potential initiation site in the axon) than they would be in a uniformly passive neuron with the lower, somatic conductance density (Stuart and Spruston 1998). However, as shown by Segev and London (Chapter 9), if a uniformly distributed conductance is redistributed as a non-uniform gradient with progressively leakier dendrites, but with the same total conductance, this redistribution can actually enhance the ability of distal synapses to depolarize the soma (Chapter 9). Another intriguing possibility is that non-uniform channel distributions might equalize temporal summation along the length of the dendrite (Magee 1999). As illustrated in Fig. 10.2, uniform passive membrane properties predict that distal inputs will be summated to a greater extent in the soma because they are broader there than more proximally generated EPSPs (see also Chapter 9). An increased density of I_h in the apical dendrite might, however, compensate for this location-specific dependence of temporal summation (Magee 1999).

Synaptic conductances that are on at rest will also reduce τ_0 by reducing the effective R_m (Bernander *et al.* 1991; Rapp et al 1992). In many brain areas, such as the cerebellar cortex, neurons providing the synaptic input are spontaneously active, thus generating a tonic synaptic conductance that significantly shortens τ_0 (Häusser and Clark 1997). The same is also true in the neocortex, where a reduction of ongoing synaptic activity by local application of TTX has been shown to increase τ_0 and input resistance (R_N) substantially, suggesting that synaptic activity reduces both R_N and τ_0 (Pare *et al.* 1998). Thus, depending on the brain area and the level of background synaptic activity, the time window for temporal summation may be much shorter *in vivo* than *in vitro*.

Dendrites affect spatial and temporal integration

R_m, C_m and R_i are not the only factors that influence summation of synaptic potentials and their propagation to the action potential initiation zone. The structure of the dendritic tree and the position of synapses on the dendrites influences synaptic summation in many ways. To illustrate this, Fig. 10.2a shows a simulation of two synapses on a simple spherical neuron with no dendritic tree. In this isopotential system individual EPSPs decay according to τ_m, and summation is dependent on the timing of the two inputs relative to the membrane time-constant. In the simulation shown in Fig. 10.2a, τ_m is 20 ms, and the EPSPs sum to a peak depolarization 1.37 times the individual EPSP amplitude when the two inputs are separated by 20 ms. The dashed line shows the subtraction of the first response from the paired response. Note that the peak of this subtracted EPSP is slightly smaller than that of the first EPSP (Fig. 10.2a). This occurs because the depolarization associated with the first EPSP produces a slight reduction in driving force for the synaptic current when the second input is activated. Next consider two synapses on a similar soma, but with the addition of apical and basal dendrites (Fig. 10.2b). The synaptic conductances have been scaled up so that the peak of the first EPSP at the soma (6 mV) is the same as in the cell with no dendrites. Note, however, that now the EPSPs rise and decay more quickly, so less summation occurs (Fig. 10.2b; 1.27 times the single EPSP, compared with the simulation with no dendrites—dashed line, from a). This is because only the *final* decay of the EPSP is determined by τ_m; the early decay of the EPSP is accelerated in this case owing to redistribution of charge into

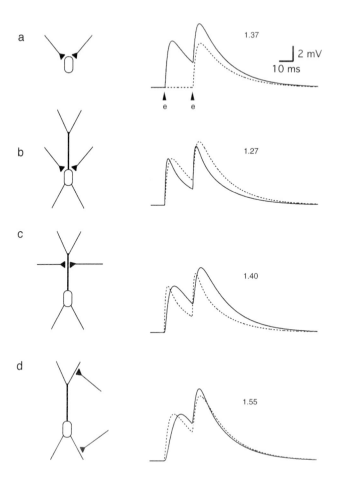

Fig. 10.2 Dendrite structure and synapse location influence EPSP summation. In each panel, the simulation is represented by a schematic diagram with excitatory synapses positioned as shown; the solid line is the simulation of somatic membrane potential following activation of the two excitatory synapses with a 20 ms delay between them. Numbers by each pair of traces represent the peak of the second EPSP relative to the first. (a) Temporal summation in a simple model including only a soma. The dashed line is the subtracted difference between the response to activation of both synapses and just the first (see text). (b) Addition of dendrites to the model accelerates the decay of the somatic EPSPs, reducing temporal summation. (c) Moving the synapses from the soma to the dendrites slows the somatic EPSP, increasing temporal summation. (d) Separating the synapses onto different dendrites maximizes summation (see text). **Simulation methods.** All simulations use the same model described in Fig. 10.1, except for the isolated soma model. In each case two identical synapses were activated, with a delay of 20 ms. Synapses were located at the soma (a,b), 300 μm from the soma on the main apical dendrite (c, $X = 0.43$), 550 μm from the soma on a distal apical dendrite (d, $X = 0.9$), or 200 μm from the soma on a basal dendrite (d, $X = 0.4$). Synaptic conductances were chosen to yield EPSPs of 6 mV in the soma (a, peak $g_{syn} = 1.34$ nS each; b, $g_{syn} = 6.38$ nS each; c, $g_{syn} = 13.25$ nS each; d, apical $g_{syn} = 66.6$ nS, basal $g_{syn} = 16.38$ nS).

the dendrites (see Chapter 9; Rall 1967; Koch *et al.* 1996; Geiger *et al.* 1997; Häusser and Clark 1997). Now consider moving the synapses from the soma to the apical dendrite (Fig. 10.2c). Again the synaptic conductances have been increased in amplitude so that each input produces a 6-mV EPSP at the soma. The time-course of these EPSPs at the soma is slowed, because of the filtering properties of the dendritic membrane between the synapse and the soma (Fig. 10.2c; dashed lines are the simulation from b, for comparison). As a result, more temporal summation occurs (Fig. 10.2c, 1.40 times the single EPSP). Finally, consider the effect of moving the two synapses to different dendrites (Fig. 10.2d). In this case, summation at the soma is maximized (Fig. 10.2d, 1.55 times the single EPSP). This occurs for two reasons— first, the decay of the first EPSP (apical synapse) is slowed because of its greater electrotonic distance from the soma (compared with Fig. 10.2c, dashed line); second, the effect of the first EPSP on the driving force of the second synapse is small, because of the greater electrotonic separation of the two synapses. These simulations illustrate three important points regarding summation in passive neurons:

(1) the presence of dendrites accelerates the EPSP decay near the synapse;

(2) cable filtering of dendritic EPSPs slows their time-course as measured at the soma, thus increasing temporal summation at the soma; and

(3) sublinear summation is expected for synapses located electrotonically close together, but is minimal for electrotonically distant inputs[3].

Excitation–inhibition interactions in dendrites

Dendrites also affect the interaction between excitatory and inhibitory synapses. The principles illustrated in the foregoing discussion of EPSPs apply similarly to IPSPs. The time-course of an IPSP at the soma is slowed if the inhibitory synapse is located on the dendrites. In addition, depolarizations induced by EPSPs, or hyperpolariza-tion by other IPSPs, will affect the driving force for the inhibitory synaptic current more for synapses that are located close together. The latter point is particularly important for IPSPs, because the reversal potential at many inhibitory synapses is close to the resting membrane potential (most notably $GABA_A$ and glycinergic synapses, which activate Cl^- channels). Hence, very small changes in V_m can have relatively large effects on the inhibitory synaptic current. However, the effect of inhibition can be considerable even when IPSPs generate no change in membrane potential themselves. Fig. 10.3a shows the result of activating two excitatory synapses on the soma, either with (solid line) or without (broken line) prior activation of an inhibitory synapse. In these simulations, inhibition is simulated with a reversal potential equal to the resting potential, and hence alone generates no change in membrane potential. Nevertheless, inhibition results in a 35% reduction of the first EPSP, and about a 13% reduction of the second EPSP (Fig. 10.3a). The relative ineffectiveness of the inhibition on the second EPSP occurs because the

---

[3] An elegant example of this is found in the medial superior olive (MSO). In this auditory nucleus, binaural processing is optimized by inputs from each side of the brain contacting separate dendrites of MSO neurons in order to minimize non-linear summation of signals arriving from each ear (Agmon-Snir *et al.* 1998).

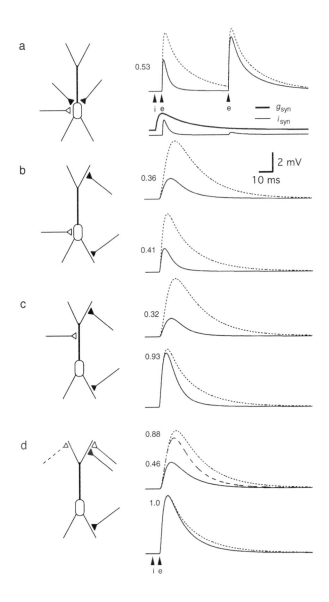

Fig. 10.3 The spatial relationship between inhibition and excitation influences dendritic integration. In each panel, the simulation is represented by a schematic diagram with excitatory (black terminals) and inhibitory (white terminals) synapses positioned as shown. The inhibitory synapse (▲, i) is activated 5 ms before the excitatory synapse (▲, e) and has $E_{rev} = V_{rest}$, meaning that no hyperpolarization is caused by activation of the inhibitory synapse alone. Numbers by each pair of traces represent the peak of the EPSP with inhibition (solid lines) relative to the EPSP without inhibition (dashed lines). (a) Two excitatory synapses on the soma are activated (with a 20-ms delay between them, arrowheads indicate timing) either with inhibition (solid line) or without inhibition (dashed line). The lower traces show the time-course of the inhibitory synaptic conductance (thick line, peak = 50 nS) and current (thin line, peak = 109 pA). (b) Separate responses to activation of the excitatory synapse on the

inhibitory synaptic conductance is largely over by the time the second EPSP arrives. This result demonstrates that inhibition is most effective during the inhibitory synaptic conductance change itself. The special case where inhibition occurs without a change in membrane potential is often referred to as 'shunting inhibition,' because the effect of the inhibitory conductance change is similar to a transient reduction in R_m, which 'shunts' the EPSP without an obvious change in membrane potential. Shunting occurs because the depolarization associated with the EPSP provides an increased driving force for outward current at the inhibitory synapse.

The ability of an inhibitory synapse to shunt current from excitatory synapses depends on the spatial arrangement of the two inputs (Fig. 10.3b–d). Inhibition placed at the soma has a similar effect on EPSPs arriving from all dendritic locations, whereas inhibition located on particular dendrites can be specific for particular inputs. Fig. 10.3b illustrates that somatic inhibition reduces EPSPs originating on different dendrites to similar extents. In fact, somatic inhibition in this case has a slightly more pronounced effect for dendritic excitation than somatic excitation (compare Fig. 10.3a,b). When the inhibitory synapse is moved onto a dendrite, the EPSP generated on the same dendrite is preferentially inhibited, leaving the peak of the other EPSP relatively unaffected (Fig. 10.3c). Dendritic inhibition is most effective at limiting somatic EPSPs if the inhibitory synapse is located 'on path' between the excitatory synapse and the soma. 'Off path' inhibition is only really effective if both the excitatory and inhibitory synapses are located near the end of a dendrite; in this case 'off path' can be almost as effective as the 'on path' inhibition (Fig. 10.3d; this effect is also illustrated nicely in Figure 7.36 of Jack *et al.* 1983). An interesting example where such distal inhibition can be important has been noted in the CA1 region, where inhibitory interneurons with somata in stratum oriens extend axons to stratum lacunosum/moleculare and impinge on the most distal dendrites of CA1 pyramidal neurons (Sik *et al.* 1995). With this arrangement, inhibition would limit the depolarization from the perforant path, which makes excitatory synapses on the distal dendrites of CA1 cells. As shown in Fig. 10.3d, however, distal dendritic inhibition is only effective for excitatory synapses on the same dendritic branch as the inhibitory synapses, and relatively ineffective if located on a different branch.

---

apical dendrite (top traces) or basal dendrite (bottom traces) with and without somatic inhibition. (c) Responses to activation of the same excitatory synapses as in (b) with and without apical dendritic inhibition. (d) Responses to activation of the same excitatory synapses as in (b) and (c) with and without distal apical inhibition. The long-dashed trace indicates simultaneous activation of the excitatory synapse and inhibition on a different branch (peak = 0.88 of control at top and 1.0 at bottom, obscured by the solid line response). Arrowheads indicate the timing of synaptic activation in (b)–(d). **Simulation methods.** All as described in Figs 10.1 and 10.2, including placement and conductance of excitatory synapses for corresponding schematic diagrams. Inhibitory synapses were placed either at the soma (a,b), 300 μm from the soma on the main apical dendrite (c, $X = 0.43$), or at the end of a distal apical dendrite (d, $X = 1.0$). Inhibitory synapses were modeled with the following parameters: $\tau_{rise} = 2$ ms; $\tau_{decay} = 20$ ms; $g_{syn} = 50$ nS; $E_{rev} = V_{rest} = -60$ mV.

Dendritic voltage-gated channels and synaptic integration

On the basis of the above examples it is clear that a postsynaptic neuron can 'count' the presynaptic inputs required to produce an action potential in different ways, depending on the passive membrane properties of dendrites and the location and timing of the inputs. Although some evidence supports the view that synaptic potentials are summated linearly or slightly sublinearly (Burke 1967; Reyes and Sakmann 1996; Cash and Yuste 1998, 1999), dendrites are clearly not passive. Already we have seen that voltage-gated conductances are active at the resting potential, and contribute to the integrative complexity of dendrites. Although theoretical analysis of the electrical properties of dendrites originally focused largely on passive cable properties[4], the importance of active dendrites was considered extensively, and modeled as early as the late 1960s (Rall and Shepherd 1968; Miller *et al.* 1985; Perkel and Perkel 1985; Shepherd *et al.* 1985).

One of the biggest challenges facing neurophysiologists interested in dendritic function is to determine what types of voltage-gated conductance are present in dendrites and how they influence the input–output computations that can be accomplished with synapses on dendrites. Two major obstacles stand in the way of tackling this challenge. First, the small size of dendrites makes them relatively difficult to probe experimentally. Even with the advent of methods for obtaining patch-clamp recordings from dendrites, at present most dendrites are too small to be patched. Advances in our understanding of voltage-gated channels in dendrites will therefore require a combination of approaches including dendritic patch-clamp recording, fluorescent imaging using ion- and voltage-sensitive dyes, and immuno-cytochemical localization of channels.

The second problem is that different types of neurons have different channel distributions, reflecting their distinct functional properties within specialized neural networks. There will be no substitute, therefore, for studying many different cell types using similar methodology and experimental design. Furthermore, these properties are likely to change during development, so each cell type will have to be studied at several development stages (i.e. from neonatal to old age), with special consideration paid to key developmental events affecting the system under study (e.g. eye opening for neurons of the visual system). The distribution and function of voltage-gated channels in dendrites is reviewed in Chapters 4 and 6. Given the burgeoning evidence that dendrites contain voltage-gated channels, it will be important to dissect the contributions of these dendritic channels to synaptic integration. This question is considered below (see 'What are the functions of dendritic excitability?'). First, however, a fundamental question must be resolved— where are action potentials initiated? Our view of synaptic integration depends critically on an accurate answer to this question.

---

[4] The focus of dendritic cable theory on passive behavior was partially based on the fact that passive systems are more easily treated analytically, whereas simulation of active properties such as Hodgkin–Huxley Na^+ and K^+ channels requires numerical approaches. Numerical simulations of active conductances, synaptic conductances, and arbitrary dendritic geometries using compartmental models were introduced later by Rall (1964).

Action potential threshold is lowest in the axon

For many years, experiments have been performed to investigate where action potentials are generated. Early microelectrode recordings from spinal motoneurones revealed that action potentials consisted of two components: an 'initial segment spike' (IS spike) and a 'somatodendritic spike' (SD spike). The IS spike always preceded the SD spike, could be evoked in isolation by antidromic stimulation of the axon, and had a lower threshold than the SD spike (Coombs *et al.* 1957; Fatt 1957; Fuortes *et al.* 1957). These data were interpreted as suggesting that the action potential begins as a low-threshold IS spike in the axon[5], which subsequently triggers the SD spike in the soma and dendrites. This interpretation was later supported by simultaneous intracellular recording from the soma and dendrites of motoneurones *in vivo* (Terzuolo and Araki 1961).

In the years that followed the early experiments on motoneurones, a battery of experiments was performed on other types of neuron. Though some studies offered evidence that spikes can be generated in dendrites (see 'Spikes can be generated in dendrites,' below), a large body of evidence suggested that action potentials are initiated in the axon of most neurons. Field potential recordings in the hippocampus indicated that action potentials were earliest and largest in the somatic and axonal fields (Jefferys 1979; Miyakawa and Kato 1986; Richardson *et al.* 1987), and comparison of somatic and dendritic microelectrode recordings suggested that the fast spikes mediated by Na^+ channels (Na^+ spikes) are generated in the axons of hippocampal and neocortical pyramidal neurons and cerebellar Purkinje cells (Llinás and Sugimori 1980*a,b*; Benardo *et al.* 1982; Amitai *et al.* 1993).

The most direct evidence that action potentials are generated in the axon comes from patch-pipette recordings obtained simultaneously from the soma and a dendrite (or axon) of neurons in brain slices and in culture (Fig. 10.4a). This recording configuration has revealed that Na^+ action potentials usually occur in the soma before those in the dendrites of all cell types studied, including neocortical and hippocampal pyramidal neurons, cerebellar Purkinje cells, spinal motoneurons, mitral cells of the olfactory bulb, and both GABAergic and dopaminergic neurons of the substantia nigra (Stuart and Häusser 1994; Stuart and Sakmann 1994; Häusser *et al.* 1995; Spruston *et al.* 1995*b*; Larkum *et al.* 1996; Bischofberger and Jonas 1997; Chen *et al.* 1997). Furthermore, simultaneous somatic and axonal patch-pipette recordings in a number of neuronal types demonstrated that the action potential always occurred first in the axon and later in the soma (Stuart and Häusser 1994; Stuart and Sakmann 1994; Colbert and Johnston 1996; Stuart *et al.* 1997*a*), directly confirming axonal initiation of the action potential (see Fig. 10.4a). In hippocampal neurons, experiments using local application of TTX suggest that the action potential is generated at the first node of Ranvier (Colbert and Johnston 1996). Nigral dopaminergic cells provide a particularly interesting demonstration of the

---

[5] Ascription of the IS spike to the initial segment was largely posited on the basis of its specialized structural features and proximity to the soma. It is worth noting, however, than no direct evidence contradicts the possibility that the IS spike could be preceded by a spike in a more distal region of the axon, such as the first node of Ranvier.

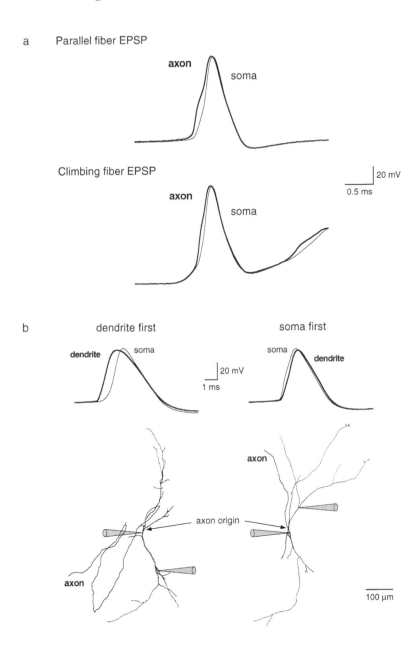

Fig. 10.4 Axonal initiation of action potentials. (a) Simultaneous axonal (7 μm from the soma) and somatic patch-clamp recordings from a cerebellar Purkinje neuron during synaptic stimulation. The top panel shows an action potential resulting from stimulation of the parallel fibers, and the bottom panel shows an action potential activated by stimulation of the climbing fiber. Note that in both cases, the action potential occurs first at the axonal recording site, directly confirming the axonal initiation of the action potential. Adapted from Stuart and Häusser (1994). (b) Simultaneous dendritic (195 μm from the soma) and somatic patch-clamp

axonal site of action potential initiation. In about half of these cells, the action potential occurred first at the dendritic recording site during double somatic-dendritic recording; in those cases, however, staining of the cells revealed that the axon emerged from a dendrite, near the dendritic recording electrode, again indicating an axonal site of action potential initiation (see Fig. 10.4b; Häusser *et al.* 1995).

Theoretical studies suggest that the threshold for action potential initiation might be lowest in the axon because of a 20–1000-fold higher density of Na^+ channels in the axon than is found in the soma and dendrites (Dodge and Cooley 1973; Moore *et al.* 1983; Mainen *et al.* 1995; Rapp *et al.* 1996). Although there is some experimental support for a high density of Na^+ channels in axons (Conti *et al.* 1976; Sigworth 1980; Neumcke and Stampfli 1982; Wollner and Catterall 1986), experimental estimates of Na^+-channel density reveal no differences in the Na^+-channel density of the axon initial segment, soma, or apical dendrites of neocortical and pyramidal neuron dendrites (Colbert and Johnston 1996; G. Stuart, unpublished observations). The finding that action potentials can be generated in the first node of Ranvier, however, indicates that the region of high Na^+-channel density might be in a part of the axon that is still inaccessible to patch-clamp recordings. Other factors also contribute to a low-threshold for action potential initiation in the axon, including the low capacitance of small-diameter axons (Moore *et al.* 1983; Mainen *et al.* 1995) and/or a more hyperpolarized activation voltage for axonal Na^+ channels (Rapp *et al.* 1996). These issues are discussed in more detail in Chapter 9.

Spikes can be generated in dendrites under some conditions

Although action potentials seem to be generated at a low-threshold initiation zone in the axon, there is ample evidence that spikes can be generated in dendrites under some conditions. The first evidence for dendritic spike[6] generation came from field potential recordings in the hippocampus, which indicated an electrogenic response in the apical dendrites of CA1 neurons that preceded the somatic/axonal population spike (Cragg and Hamlyn 1955; Andersen 1960; Fujita and Sakata 1962;

---

recordings from substantia nigra dopamine neurons. The top panels show action potentials at the two recording sites (the dendritic action potential is represented by a thick trace). The bottom panels show the reconstructed biocytin-filled neurons from which the recordings were made. The location of the dendritic and somatic recording sites is indicated by schematic pipettes. Note that in the left-hand neuron the axon originates from a dendrite, 215 μm from the soma, while in the right-hand neuron it originates from the soma. In the left-hand neuron, the action potential was observed first at the dendritic recording site, while in the right-hand neuron the action potential appeared first at the somatic recording site. The reconstructions revealed that the recording site where the action potential appeared first was always the one closest to the site of axon origin, indicating that the action potential is initiated in the axon of these neurons. Adapted from Häusser *et al.* (1995).

Andersen and Lomo 1966; see also Herreras 1990). Around the same time, Eccles and colleagues reported that spikes could be generated in the dendrites of chromatolyzed motoneurones (Eccles *et al.* 1958) and Spencer and Kandel observed small, spike-like events in intracellular recordings from CA1 neurons *in vivo* ('fast prepotentials'), which they inferred were generated in the dendrites (Spencer and Kandel 1961)[7]. Similar events, termed 'dendritic spikes', were observed in recordings from neocortical neurons (Purpura 1967) and cerebellar Purkinje cells (Llinás *et al.* 1968, 1969; Llinás and Nicholson 1971). More recent dendritic recordings from hippocampal and neocortical neurons in slices and *in vivo* support the view that dendrites are capable of generating electrogenic spikes mediated by voltage-gated Na^+ and/or Ca^{2+} channels (Wong *et al.* 1979; Turner *et al.* 1993; Schiller *et al.* 1997; Seamans *et al.* 1997; Stuart *et al.* 1997a; Golding and Spruston 1998; Golding *et al.* 1999b; Kamondi *et al.* 1998). The evidence for dendritic spikes has been reviewed elsewhere (Purpura 1967; Stuart *et al.* 1997b). Here we consider some of the most recent findings.

Recently, simultaneous somatic and dendritic patch-pipette recordings have provided direct demonstration of dendritic spike generation (Fig. 10.5). In both layer 5 and hippocampal pyramidal neurons, dendritic Na^+ and Ca^{2+} spikes have been observed that precede somatic spikes, and the incidence of dendritic spikes is promoted in both cell types by strong synaptic excitation (Golding and Spruston 1998; Golding *et al.* 1999b; Schiller *et al.* 1997; Stuart *et al.* 1997a; see also Turner *et al.* 1989, 1991); dendritic Ca^{2+} spikes preceding or uncoupled from somatic action potentials have also been observed in cerebellar Purkinje cells (Häusser 1996). In neocortex, dendritic spikes in relatively proximal locations are mediated by Na^+ channels, whereas more distal dendritic spikes are mediated largely by voltage-gated Ca^{2+} channels (Schiller *et al.* 1997; Stuart *et al.* 1997a; Larkum *et al.* 1999); in prefrontal cortex the situation is reversed (Seamans *et al.* 1997).

Several observations suggest that dendritic Na^+ and Ca^{2+} spikes propagate poorly to the soma and axon of pyramidal neurons. First, the amplitude of dendritic Na^+ spikes is smaller than the somatically recorded action potential, even when the dendritic spike occurs first. Second, dendritic spikes are sometimes observed in isolation of somatic action potentials in both hippocampal and neocortical pyramidal neurons (Fig. 10.5a). Third, imaging studies show that Ca^{2+} signals associated with distal Ca^{2+} spikes can remain localized to their site of origin in pyramidal cells and Purkinje cells, with little or no calcium signal spreading to the soma (Miyakawa *et al.* 1992; Yuste *et al.* 1994; Eilers *et al.* 1995; Hartell 1996; Schiller *et al.* 1997). Finally, triple recordings from the axon, soma, and apical dendrite of the same neocortical pyramidal neuron indicate that the axonal action potential always precedes the somatic action potential, even when the dendritic spike precedes the somatic action potential (Fig. 10.5a; Stuart *et al.* 1997a). These

---

[6] For convenience, we refer to regenerative events in dendrites as 'dendritic spikes.' Avoiding the term 'action potentials' to refer to these events offers a semantic way of distinguishing dendritic spikes from the all-or-none reliably propagating action potential initiated in the axon.

[7] Whether these events truly represent dendritic spikes is a subject of debate (MacVicar and Dudek 1981; Turner *et al.* 1993; Valiante *et al.* 1995; Nedergaard and Hounsgaard 1996), but more direct evidence now supports the occurrence of dendritic spikes (see below).

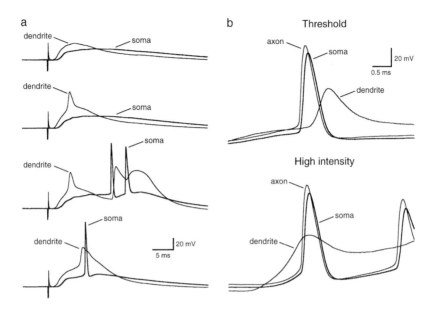

Fig. 10.5   Dendritic spikes and their relation to axonal action-potential initiation. (a) Somatic (thicker traces) and dendritic (440 μm from the soma) recording from a neocortical layer 5 pyramidal neuron during synaptic stimulation in layer 2/3. All recordings from the same cell at similar stimulation intensity. Top: Subthreshold somatic and dendritic EPSPs. Second from the top: Initiation of a dendritic spike in the absence of somatic action potentials. Second from the bottom: Initiation of a dendritic spike in relative isolation from somatic action potentials. Bottom: Initiation of a dendritic spike just prior to a somatic action potential. (b) Somatic (thicker traces), dendritic (300 μm from the soma) and axonal (20 μm from the soma) recording from a neocortical layer 5 pyramidal neuron during synaptic stimulation in layer 2/3. All recordings from the same cell. Top: Synaptic stimulation in layer 2/3 at threshold for axonal action-potential initiation. Bottom: High intensity synaptic stimulation, which initiated a dendritic spike prior to the somatic action potential. Adapted from Stuart *et al.* 1997*a*.

observations suggest that dendritic spikes do not propagate reliably to the soma and axon of neocortical and hippocampal pyramidal neurons. As a consequence, the dendritic spike-mediated depolarization that reaches the soma is small. Usually the somatic depolarization resulting from the EPSP and dendritic spike together are large enough to initiate an axonal action potential, whereas in other cases the EPSP and dendritic spike together produce a subthreshold depolarization in the soma and axon, resulting in an isolated dendritic spike (see Figs 10.5a and 10.7). Dendritic Ca^{2+} spikes are rarely observed in somatic recordings, but can influence action potential initiation through the generation of a burst of action potentials at the soma (Golding *et al.* 1999*b*; Schiller *et al.* 1997; Larkum *et al.* 1999), as originally described in cerebellar Purkinje cells (Llinás and Nicholson 1971; Llinás and Sugimori 1980*b*).
Similar experiments performed in the olfactory bulb reveal that the apical dendrites of mitral cells can generate Na^+ spikes that can, in some circumstances, propagate

to the soma. Though this is a notable difference compared with the behavior of hippocampal or cortical pyramidal cells (see 'Propagation of action potentials and dendritic spikes', below), dendritic Na^+ spikes can also fail to invade the soma and axon of mitral cells, particularly during perisomatic inhibition (Chen *et al.* 1997).

Taken together, the evidence suggests that the local voltage threshold for action potential initiation is lowest in the axon of most neurons. Under some conditions, however, a higher threshold in dendritic regions can be reached first, thus resulting in a dendritic spike. Because the dendrites are relatively weakly excitable compared with the axon, dendritic spikes can only occur if the local synaptic potential in the dendrites is relatively large and fast. If the activated dendrite is sufficiently electrotonically isolated from the axon, the resulting attenuation and delay of the synaptic potential prevent the lower, axonal threshold from being reached before the higher, dendritic threshold. In some cases the attenuation of the EPSP and dendritic spike is large enough that threshold is not reached in the axon, resulting in an isolated dendritic spike (Fig. 10.5a). Electrical isolation of a dendritic spike would be enhanced if it originated on a distal dendrite, had a fast time-course, or occurred during inhibition of the soma and/or axon.

As discussed in the previous chapter by Segev and London, in weakly excitable dendrites, dendritic spikes are most likely to propagate reliably to the soma if the synaptic input occurs on a large-diameter dendrite or is distributed across many dendritic branches. Because of the relatively high input impedance of thin-diameter dendrites, however, the current threshold for locally regenerative events, including dendritic spikes, might be lower in thin dendritic branches, but the propagation of these events to other parts of the dendritic tree will be less reliable. The relative efficacy of inputs on small compared with large dendritic branches, and localized compared with distributed inputs, at evoking dendritic spikes clearly requires further theoretical and experimental study. The data indicate, however, that dendritic spikes in pyramidal neurons only poorly invade the soma, and can fail to trigger an axonal action potential. As such, our view is that these dendritic spikes should be regarded as a form of active synaptic integration and that the final site of synaptic integration is in the axon.

Propagation of action potentials and dendritic spikes

Action potentials propagate through the dendritic tree in a complex way that is influenced by a variety of factors. Here we consider the effects of dendritic morphology, properties of dendritic voltage-gated channels and synaptic inhibition on the propagation of action potentials initiated in the axon and spikes generated in dendrites.

Action-potential backpropagation

After their initiation in the axon, action potentials propagate back into the dendritic tree. The invasion of the dendrites by 'backpropagating action potentials' varies in different cell types. In most neurons where they have been studied, including neocortical and hippocampal pyramidal neurons, dopaminergic and GABAergic neurons in substantia nigra, spinal motoneurons, and mitral cells of the olfactory bulb, action potentials propagate actively back into the dendrites. The amplitude of backpropagating action potentials in these cells types generally diminishes as the action potential propagates away from the soma, but remains well above that expected for passive spread of the action potential (Stuart and Sakmann 1994; Häusser *et al.* 1995; Spruston *et al.* 1995*b*; Larkum *et al.* 1996; Bischofberger and Jonas 1997; Chen *et al.* 1997). This active backpropagation is supported by voltage-gated Na$^+$ channels, which have been shown to be present in the dendrites of several types of neuron (Stuart and Sakmann 1994; Häusser *et al.* 1995; Magee and Johnston 1995; Bischofberger and Jonas 1997). In most neurons, however, back-propagation is decremental, presumably because the density of Na$^+$ channels is too low and K$^+$ channels too high to support non-decremental conduction (Mainen *et al.* 1995; Rapp *et al.* 1996). There is some variation in dendritic Na$^+$ channel densities between cells (see Chapter 6). Pyramidal neurons have a low, but relatively constant, density of Na$^+$ channels along the main apical dendrite (Stuart and Sakmann 1994; Magee and Johnston 1995), whereas mitral cells in the olfactory bulb seem to have a higher density of dendritic Na$^+$ channels and support more reliable backpropagation (Bischofberger and Jonas 1997). Cerebellar Purkinje cells, in contrast, have very low densities of Na$^+$ channels in their dendrites, and do not support active action potential backpropagation (Llinás and Sugimori 1980*a,b*; Lasser-Ross and Ross 1992; Stuart and Häusser 1994). However, the correlation between dendritic sodium channel density and backpropagation is not strict, as substantia nigra dopamine neurons have essentially non-decremental backpropagation, even though they have a lower apparent dendritic Na$^+$-channel density than pyramidal cells (Häusser *et al.* 1995).

Effects of morphology on action potential backpropagation

The morphology of the dendritic tree can affect action potential backpropagation in the same way as has been previously shown for propagation of action potentials in axons. Goldstein and Rall showed that diameter, tapering and branching are important determinants of action potential propagation in axons (Goldstein and Rall 1974). Using simplified analytical solutions of action potential propagation they demonstrated that branch points are particularly sensitive regions where action potentials can fail. Goldstein and Rall quantified branch point geometry using the geometric ratio (GR), defined as:

$$ GR = \sum_j d_j^{3/2} / d_a^{3/2} \tag{1} $$

where d_a is the diameter of the cable along which an action potential is propagating (the 'parent' branch), and d_j are the diameters of the branches the action potential propagates into (the 'daughter' branches; Goldstein and Rall 1974). This geometric ratio defines the impedance mismatch between the parent and daughter dendrites. If one assumes that the membrane properties are uniform and the branch is not near a termination point of a cable, the geometric ratio predicts the behavior of the action potential as it propagates across the branch. If GR = 1 (i.e., if the 3/2 power law is obeyed, and the impedance is 'matched'), propagation is not affected except that the velocity decreases due to the smaller diameter of the distal branches. If GR < 1, a favorable impedance mismatch holds, and action potentials propagate as in cables with a step decrease in diameter. If GR > 1, the impedance mismatch is unfavorable, and action potentials propagate as though they encounter a step increase in diameter, with propagation failing completely for sufficiently high values of GR (the critical value depends on the density and kinetics of the Na^+ and K^+ channels in the different branches, and the passive membrane properties R_m, C_m and R_i). Another way of expressing this is that the safety factor for action potential conduction decreases when an action potential propagates into branches that are just slightly smaller, the same size, or larger than the parent dendrite (Rall 1964).

Similar considerations are expected to hold for action potentials propagating in dendritic trees. Because the safety factor for propagation of action potentials in dendrites is low to begin with (recall that backpropagation is decremental in most neurons), unfavorable impedance mismatches at branch points might result in failure of backpropagating action potentials. Indeed, changes in the shape of backpropagating action potentials in hippocampal dendrites have been observed (Spruston *et al.* 1995*b*), which resemble the shape of action potentials propagating close to failure in axons (Lüscher *et al.* 1994). Furthermore, as discussed earlier in this chapter, different neuronal types show very different degrees of back-propagation (Stuart *et al.* 1997*b*); this might be related to the striking differences in dendritic geometry shown by different cell types. To investigate the contribution of dendritic geometry, a recent study (Häusser *et al.* 1998) performed simulations in which the same complement of active and passive properties was inserted into detailed reconstructions of a large variety of cell types, thus isolating morphology as a variable. Interestingly, the pattern of backpropagation in the different geometries matched the experimental findings, with attenuation being least for substantia nigra dopamine neurons and most for Purkinje cells. Morphological analysis of the dendritic trees revealed that backpropagation was strongly correlated with the way in which membrane area was distributed in the dendritic tree, a function of both the number of branch points and the geometric ratio at individual branch points. This study (Häusser *et al.* 1998) also demonstrated that in very elaborate morphologies, such as Purkinje cells, backpropagation is insensitive to the Na^+-channel density over the physiological range, whereas modulation of Na^+-channel density can produce a wide range of dendritic action potential amplitudes in pyramidal cells. Together, these findings indicate that dendritic morphology, and in particular the branching pattern, is a major determinant of how dendrites will behave functionally, confirming a prediction made by Rall in the mid-1960s (Rall 1964).

Effects of dendritic voltage-gated channels on action potential backpropagation

Non-uniform distributions of channels, and changes in the activation patterns of channels with activity, add a further layer of complexity to our understanding of action potential propagation in dendrites. For example, regional Na^+ channel inactivation or non-uniform distributions of dendritic K^+ channels can have significant effects on propagation. Hoffman and colleagues have shown that the density of A-type K$^+$ channels (K$_A$) in the apical dendrites of CA1 neurons increases as a function of distance from the soma; furthermore, dendritic K$_A$ channels in these cells have a lower activation voltage than do somatic and proximal dendritic K$_A$ channels (Hoffman *et al.* 1997). This channel distribution seems to contribute to a number of physiological features of CA1 neurons, including the relatively high threshold for dendritic spike initiation and the decremental nature of action potential backpropagation (Hoffman *et al.* 1997).

Action potentials backpropagating into CA1 dendrites undergo a marked amplitude attenuation during repetitive activity (Andreasen and Lambert 1995*b*; Callaway and Ross 1995; Spruston *et al.* 1995*b*). A similar form of activity-dependent action potential backpropagation occurs in the distal regions of the apical dendrites of neocortical pyramidal neurons (Stuart *et al.* 1997*a*). This property of action potential backpropagation seem to be largely attributable to the inactivation properties of dendritic Na$^+$ channels (Fig. 10.6a,b). Na$^+$ currents in cell-attached patches from CA1 pyramidal neurons undergo a form of inactivation that develops rapidly but recovers slowly (Colbert *et al.* 1997; Jung *et al.* 1997; Mickus *et al.* 1999). This form of inactivation is particularly pronounced in patches from the apical dendrite. As each action potential invades the dendrites, it leaves a fraction of Na$^+$ channels in a long-lived inactivated state, effectively reducing the density of available Na$^+$ channels to support backpropagation of action potentials arriving even several hundred milliseconds later. Because the safety factor for action potential backpropagation is low, owing to the relatively low Na$^+$-channel density and high K$_A$ channel density in CA1 dendrites, inactivation of even a small number of Na$^+$ channels can significantly affect action potential backpropagation. In this way, slow inactivation of dendritic Na$^+$ channels reduces action potential backpropagation, and induces an activity-dependent decline in action potential amplitude at a single dendritic recording site. This inactivation, together with unfavorable branching geometry, might also contribute to failure of backpropagating action potentials to invade some dendritic branches in CA1 neurons (Spruston *et al.* 1995*b*).

Effects of synaptic inhibition on action potential backpropagation

Synaptic inhibition is another factor that has been shown to influence action potential backpropagation. In CA1 neurons, activation of GABAergic inhibitory conductances limits the invasion of the apical dendrites by backpropagating action potentials (Tsubokawa and Ross 1996). As the time-course of this effect mirrors that of the GABAergic conductance change, the effect seems to be due to a shunting mechanism. Many other details of inhibitory control of backpropagating action potentials are likely to be revealed. For example, it can be predicted that the hyperpolarization associated with inhibition could, if appropriately targeted and timed, increase the recovery of dendritic Na$^+$ channels from the slow inactivated state, thus increasing the amplitude of backpropagating action potentials (Spruston *et al.* 1995*b*; Colbert *et al.* 1997; Jung *et al.* 1997). On the other hand, hyperpolarization could reduce excitability by removing A-current inactivation (Hoffman *et al.* 1997). Thus, the effects of hyperpolarization can be complex, and dependent on the prior firing history of the neuron.

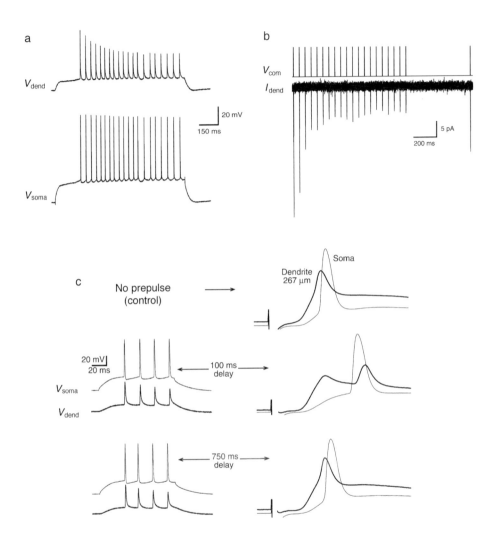

Fig. 10.6 Effects of prolonged Na$^+$ channel inactivation on backpropagating action potentials and dendritic spikes in CA1 pyramidal neurons. (a) A train of action potentials evoked by somatic current injection (300 pA) and recorded simultaneously in the soma and apical dendrite (200 μm from the soma). Repetitive action potential firing results in an activity-dependent decline in the amplitude of backpropagating action potentials (see Spruston *et al.* 1995*b*). (b) Dendritic Na$^+$ currents recorded in a cell-attached patch on an apical dendrite 203 μm from the soma. Brief depolarizations (2 ms, 70 mV) *via* a command potential (V_{com}, relative to V_{rest}) delivered to the patch pipette evoked TTX-sensitive inward currents that accumulated in an inactivated state during the train, due to slow recovery from inactivation. A test pulse 500 ms after the train shows only 38% recovery from inactivation. Adapted from Jung *et al.* 1997. (c) A depolarizing prepulse in a somatic recording (thin traces) evokes four action potentials, which backpropagate into the dendrites, exhibiting activity-dependent amplitude attenuation in a simultaneous dendritic recording (thick traces, 267 μm from the soma). This prepulse of backpropagating action potentials (left) suppressed dendritic spike initiation in response to synaptic stimulation in stratum radiatum when evoked less than 500 ms after the prepulse (right). Adapted from Golding and Spruston 1998.

Dendritic spike propagation

All the factors that influence backpropagating action potentials are likely to have analogous effects on the propagation of dendritic spikes toward the soma and axon. One important feature to consider is the relatively poor forward propagation of dendritic spikes compared with backpropagating action potentials in pyramidal cells (Stuart *et al.* 1997*a*; Golding and Spruston 1998). The morphology of the dendritic tree clearly plays an important role in determining this behavior. Any impedance mismatches that are favorable for action potential backpropagation will be unfavorable for dendritic spikes propagating in the reverse direction, and hence contribute to a reduced safety factor (Goldstein and Rall 1974; Jack *et al.* 1983). Although this might in part explain the observation of the poor forward propagation of dendritic spikes and the occurrence of isolated dendritic spikes (Schiller *et al.* 1997; Stuart *et al.* 1997*a*; Golding and Spruston 1998), other factors are also likely to be important. For example, action potential backpropagation can limit the propagation of dendritic spikes to the soma of CA1 neurons, presumably because of inactivation of dendritic Na^+ channels (Fig. 10.6c; Golding and Spruston 1998). Non-uniform K^+-channel distributions might be another important factor. Although the distribution of dendritic K_A channels (Hoffman *et al.* 1997) probably has the reverse gradient required to explain the poor forward propagation of dendritic spikes, other K^+ channels can also be distributed non-uniformly (e.g. Andreasen and Lambert 1995*a*). The distributions and effects of a variety of K^+ channel subtypes is ripe for further investigation. Interestingly, mitral cells seem to have much better forward propagation than pyramidal cells (Chen *et al.* 1997) under similar experimental conditions. It will be important to determine the mechanisms underlying this difference.

Inhibition has also been shown to influence dendritic Ca^{2+} spikes. In both hippocampal CA3 and neocortical layer 5 pyramidal neurons, inhibition can prevent, delay, or shorten dendritic Ca^{2+} spikes, depending on its timing and strength (Kim *et al.* 1995; Miles *et al.* 1996; Larkum *et al.* 1999). In hippocampal neurons, the effects of inhibition on spike firing depend on the location of the inhibitory input. Dendritic inputs inhibit dendritic Ca^{2+} spikes, whereas perisomatic inhibition suppresses repetitive discharge of somatic action potentials (Miles *et al.* 1996). The effects of inhibition on dendritically generated Na^+ spikes have been explored in mitral cells of the olfactory bulb, where perisomatic inhibition can prevent dendritic Na^+ spikes from invading the soma and axon (Chen *et al.* 1997).

Finally, it should be noted that all of the factors discussed here are subject to modulation and plasticity. Thus, the pattern of action potential backpropagation or dendritic spike propagation may vary according to brain state (McCormick *et al.* 1993). The activity of inhibitory interneurons can be modulated by neurotransmitter systems and activity-dependent and neurotrophin-mediated plasticity (Freund and Buzsáki 1996; Rutherford *et al.* 1998). Muscarinic receptor activation can increase action potential backpropagation in CA1 neurons (Tsubokawa and Ross 1997), perhaps *via* a PKC-mediated modulation of dendritic Na^+ channel inactivation or K^+-channel activation (Colbert and Johnston 1998; Hoffman and Johnston 1998). Even dendritic structure is not static (see Chapter 14), indicating that the effects of morphological changes on action potential and dendritic spike propagation must be considered.

What are the functions of dendritic excitability?

Several possibilities for the function of backpropagating action potentials and dendritic spikes can be envisioned. These include EPSP amplification, triggering transmitter release from dendrites, shunting of EPSPs, generation of action potential burst firing, elevation of dendritic Ca^{2+} concentration, induction of synaptic plasticity.

Dendritic spikes and synaptic integration

The possibility that dendrites might generate spikes has posed a problem; if spikes can be generated in dendrites, the integrative power of the dendritic tree would seem to be minimized, because many of the spatial and temporal interactions involving excitation and inhibition (discussed in the preceding section) would be negated by the generation of a dendritic spike in response to a small number of excitatory inputs. A possible solution to this puzzle was presented as early as 1959, when Lorente de Nó suggested that decremental action potential conduction might play an important role in dendritic integration in the central nervous system (Lorente de Nó and Condouris 1959). In the scenario he envisioned, spikes could be generated in dendrites, but would not propagate reliably to the soma. The effect of dendritic spikes would therefore be to increase the depolarization associated with some synaptic inputs, but would not necessarily trigger an action potential.

A lucid discussion of such conduction failure in dendrites is presented in Chapter 7 of Jack *et al.* (1983). On the basis of theoretical considerations, Jack, Noble and Tsien predicted that dendritic spikes are likely to be generated in active dendrites, but that they might propagate poorly, providing only a limited depolarization of the soma. These authors also pointed out that an obvious possible function of this kind of restricted dendritic spike would be to amplify synaptic potentials, thus increasing the likelihood that a combination of synapses that evoke a dendritic spike will eventually result in an output from the neuron *via* generation of an action potential in the axon. As discussed above, experimental support for this idea has recently been presented (Schiller *et al.* 1997; Seamans *et al.* 1997; Stuart *et al.* 1997*a*; Andreasen and Lambert 1998; Golding and Spruston 1998; Larkum *et al.* 1999). An example of amplification of a somatic EPSP by a dendritic spike is shown in Fig. 10.7. Such amplification might impart computational complexity on dendrites by allowing certain combinations of inputs to summate in the soma and axon, while others could be summated and amplified locally by the generation of a dendritic spike (see Chapter 11).

Subthreshold amplification of EPSPs by Na^+ and Ca^{2+} channels

Amplification of synaptic potentials by dendritic spikes is only one possible scenario. Depending on the types, densities, and distributions of channels in dendrites, PSPs may also be amplified and shaped in more subtle ways by voltage-gated conductances. For example, Na^+ and/or Ca^{2+} channels can amplify EPSPs without generating a spike. One of the first indications that voltage-gated conductances

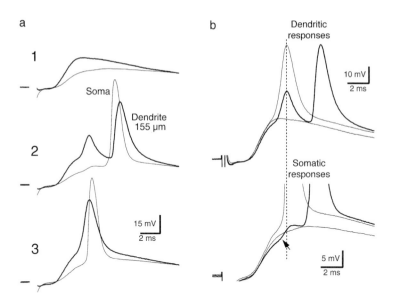

Fig. 10.7 Amplification of EPSPs by dendritic Na$^+$ spikes. (a) Somatic (thin traces) and dendritic (thick traces, 155 μm from the soma) membrane potential recorded simultaneously from a CA1 pyramidal neuron. In the three trials shown, stimulation of stratum radiatum at identical intensity yielded: (1) a subthreshold EPSP, (2) a suprathreshold EPSP with a weak dendritic spike preceding the somatic/backpropagating action potential, and (3) a larger dendritic spike followed by a somatic action potential. (b) Alignment of the dendritic responses (top) and somatic responses (bottom) reveals that in the trace shown in a2 (shown thick here), the occurrence of a dendritic spike triggers an inflection (arrow) on the somatic EPSP, causing the somatic membrane potential to cross threshold for action-potential initiation. Adapted from Golding and Spruston 1998.

might amplify EPSPs in this manner was the observation that a marked increase in the amplitude and integral of EPSPs was observed when pyramidal neurons were held at depolarized potentials (Masukawa and Prince 1984; Stafstrom *et al.* 1985; Deisz *et al.* 1991). A similar voltage-dependent amplification was observed in response to brief somatic current injections used to mimic EPSPs (Deisz *et al.* 1991). Stuart and Sakmann extended this idea by comparing the voltage-dependence of EPSPs and EPSP-like depolarizations evoked by injecting current in the shape of an excitatory postsynaptic current (EPSC) through a dendritic recording electrode (Stuart and Sakmann 1995). They found that the voltage-dependent amplification of both real and 'simulated' EPSPs was blocked by application of TTX. Because the activation of Na$^+$ channels occurred in a voltage range below threshold for action potential initiation, and because the effect of TTX on the EPSP integral was larger than on the peak, the amplification was interpreted as being a result of activation of a non-inactivating, or persistent, Na$^+$ conductance. Furthermore, because the amplification of EPSPs was greatest in the soma, and selectively blocked by local application of TTX to the soma and axon, it seems that this form of amplification occurs primarily because of activation of persistent Na$^+$ current in the soma and axon (Stuart and Sakmann 1995). Schwindt and Crill have reported a TTX-sensitive amplification of currents recorded in the soma in response to prolonged (approximately 1-s) dendritic glutamate iontophoresis (Schwindt and Crill 1995). Because this amplification occurs while the soma (and presumably the axon) are voltage-clamped, this TTX-sensitive current seems to be located in the dendrites. Therefore, it seems that sustained synaptic activation can amplify synaptic currents *via* dendritic persistent Na^+ current, whereas transient EPSPs recruit primarily somatic and axonal current[8].

Inhibitory synaptic potentials (IPSPs) can also be modulated by the persistent Na^+ current, both at the soma and presumably in dendrites (Stuart 1999). At depolarized membrane potentials the hyperpolarization generated by IPSPs turns off the persistent Na^+ current, producing a net outward current, which increases the amplitude and duration of IPSPs. At the soma and axon this increases the ability of inhibition to block action potential generation (Stuart 1999), whereas in the dendrites it is likely to enhance the ability of synaptic inhibition to block dendritic spike generation and propagation.

In the hippocampus, dendritic recordings from CA1 neurons have revealed that Na^+ and Ca^{2+} channels are activated directly by EPSPs (Magee *et al.* 1995). Furthermore, blockers of Na^+ and low-threshold Ca^{2+} channels have been shown to reduce the amplitude and duration of EPSPs measured at the soma in CA1 and CA3 pyramidal neurons (Lipowsky *et al.* 1996; Gillessen and Alzheimer 1997; Urban *et al.* 1998). These experiments provide further support for the idea that Na^+ and Ca^{2+} channels can amplify EPSPs in these neurons.

Subthreshold attenuation by K^+ channels

The effects of K^+-channel activation on EPSPs must also be considered. Dendritic current injection offers the opportunity to perform a controlled examination of the effects of Na^+-channel blockers on the input–output relationship of dendritic EPSPs. In response to varied injections of EPSC-like currents *via* a dendritic patch pipette in CA1 neurons, the resulting simulated EPSPs increase approximately linearly with simulated EPSC amplitude from small to large EPSPs just below action potential threshold; application of TTX reduces the amplitude of the largest simulated EPSPs, such that these events are smaller than expected from linear scaling with the current injection (Spruston *et al.* 1995c). These results suggest that K^+ channels are activated together with Na^+ channels, resulting in no net amplification of the synaptic potential, even when dendritic Na^+ channels are activated by the EPSP. Similar experiments performed in the presence of a high concentration of 4-AP in CA1 neurons reveal that EPSP amplitude is amplified by TTX-sensitive Na^+ channels, but reduced by a 4-AP-sensitive conductance (Hoffman *et al.* 1997). This result suggests that A-type K^+ channels[9], which are present at a high density in CA1 dendrites, counter the amplification produced by dendritic Na^+ channels by dampening subthreshold EPSPs.

---

[8] A component of the amplification in neocortical neurons is blocked by 2 mm Co^{2+}, suggesting the possibility of an additional component mediated by voltage-gated Ca^{2+} channels (Deisz *et al.* 1991).

[9] This high concentration of 4-AP also blocks other types of K^+ channels, including the D-type channel (Rudy 1988).

Further support for activation of voltage-gated K^+ channels in response to subthreshold EPSPs comes from experiments involving iontophoretic application of glutamate to the dendrites of hippocampal pyramidal neurons in culture and in slices. When two separate iontophoretic electrodes are used to mimic excitatory synaptic inputs at two locations, the two simulated EPSPs sum either linearly or sublinearly, depending on the relative locations of the inputs (Cash and Yuste 1998, 1999). The K^+-channel blocker 4-AP either eliminated sublinear summation or revealed a supralinear summation, suggesting that A-type K^+ channels are activated when the two EPSPs summate (Cash and Yuste 1998, 1999). A similar approach using photolysis of caged glutamate to simulate EPSPs at two locations on cultured hippocampal neurons revealed a time-dependence of the effects of voltage-gated channels on summated EPSPs (Margulis and Tang 1998). When the two inputs were activated at an interval of less than 10 ms, the second input was amplified by a TTX-sensitive conductance. At slightly longer intervals (15–100 ms) the second input was depressed by a voltage-gated K^+ conductance. Both the short-latency amplification and longer-latency depression were observed even when the soma was voltage-clamped, suggesting that these effects were mediated by dendritic channels (Margulis and Tang 1998). Experiments using stimulation of perforant path (PP) and mossy fiber (MF) inputs at different time intervals support a similar conclusion regarding K^+-channel activation in CA3 neurons. In these experiments, activation of MF synapses shunted perforant path EPSPs when MF stimulation preceded PP stimulation by less than 20 ms (Urban and Barrionuevo 1998). This effect was voltage-dependent, and blocked by intracellular 4-AP, suggesting that the depolarization by the MF EPSP activates A-type K^+ channels, which then shunts the PP EPSP propagating from the distal dendrites.

The emerging picture in hippocampal pyramidal neurons is that the effects of activation of Na^+ channels by subthreshold EPSPs are dampened by activation of voltage-gated K^+ channels, particularly the A-type channel, which is present at high density in CA1 apical dendrites (Hoffman *et al.* 1997). As discussed previously, however, spikes can be generated in the dendrites of CA1 neurons under some conditions, suggesting that dendritic Na^+ channel activation can tip this balance, particularly during synchronous synaptic excitation (Golding and Spruston 1998). The functional significance of amplification *via* Na^+ and Ca^{2+}-channel activation, both below and above threshold for dendritic spikes remains a matter of speculation, but is likely to receive considerable attention from both experimental and theoretical neurophysiologists.

Dendro-dendritic synapses

Backpropagating action potentials and dendritic spikes may also trigger the release of neurotransmitter from dendrites. Dendrites that act as presynaptic structures have been identified in several areas of the nervous system, including the olfactory bulb, retina, thalamus, substantia nigra, and supraoptic nuclei. In cultured hippocampal neurons, Ca^{2+}-regulated exocytosis of dendritic organelles has been characterized (Maletic-Savatic and Malinow 1998; Maletic-Savatic *et al.* 1998); this could serve as a substrate for dendritic release of transmitters in several cell types.

In the olfactory bulb, mitral cell dendrites form excitatory synapses onto granule cell dendrites, which form reciprocal inhibitory synapses on to mitral cell dendrites

(Rall *et al.* 1966). Action potentials in mitral cells excite adjacent granule cells, resulting in feedback and lateral inhibition of neighboring mitral cells (Jahr and Nicoll 1982). Backpropagating action potentials and dendritically generated spikes in mitral cells are both likely to trigger release at these synapses (Rall and Shepherd 1968; Bischofberger and Jonas 1997; Chen *et al.* 1997, 1998).

Amacrine cells in the retina form dendrodendritic synapses with ganglion cells (Dowling and Boycott 1966). Some amacrine cells have axons capable of generating fast spikes (Stafford and Dacey 1997); most, however, lack axons but are nevertheless capable of generating spikes (Bloomfield 1992). Dendritic spikes recorded in amacrine cells lacking axons have variable amplitudes, suggesting that spikes can be generated at multiple locations and trigger transmitter release from restricted sets of dendrodendritic synapses; in amacrine cells with the largest dendritic trees, dendritic spikes appear to contribute to their relatively large receptive fields (Bloomfield 1996).

In most cases release of excitatory and inhibitory transmitters occurs at specialized synaptic structures. In some neurons, however, neurotransmitters having local modulatory effects can be released from dendrites lacking anatomically identified dendrodendritic synapses. For example, dopamine is released from the dendrites of neurons in the substantia nigra in the absence of specialized presynaptic structures (Cheramy *et al.* 1981; Rice *et al.* 1994). This release is Ca^{2+}- and voltage-dependent and is blocked by TTX (Santiago *et al.* 1992), suggesting that backpropagating action potentials play an important role in the release process (Häusser *et al.* 1995).

The role of backpropagating action potentials and dendritic spikes in triggering neurotransmitter release at dendrodendritic synapses in other cell types is less clear. In the olfactory bulb, dendritic release of GABA from granule cells is likely to occur in the absence of an action potential (Isaacson and Strowbridge 1998; Schoppa *et al.* 1998). At triadic synapses in thalamic relay nuclei, release of GABA from the dendrites of thalamic interneurons is triggered by metabotropic glutamate receptor activation, but occurs even in the absence of somatic spiking (Cox *et al.* 1998). Release of oxytocin and vasopressin from the dendrites of magnocellular neurons in the supraoptic nucleus of the hypothalamus is TTX resistant (Di Scala-Guenot *et al.* 1987; Ludwig and Landgraf 1992; for more on these neurons see Chapter 14). It is possible that backpropagating action potentials or dendritic spikes might be sufficient, but not necessary, to evoke transmitter release from these dendrites.

EPSP shunting by backpropagating action potentials

The backpropagating action potential can also interact with synaptic potentials. The conductances necessary to generate the action potential are large, and therefore generate a substantial drop in apparent membrane resistance, which is localized largely to the axon and soma. This shunt effectively shortens the membrane time-constant in these regions, draining charge from the membrane capacitance. In this way, action potentials can reduce the amplitude of EPSPs and IPSPs, thus providing a mechanism for terminating ongoing synaptic integration. In neocortical pyramidal cells, somatic EPSPs generated by basal synaptic inputs can be attenuated by up to 80% by single action potentials (Stuart and Häusser 1998). The extent to which action potentials shunt synaptic potentials depends not only on the magnitude of the local conductances activated by the action potential, but also on the kinetics of the synaptic conductance. As a consequence, synaptic potentials generated by conductance changes with a slow time-course (e.g. those mediated by NMDA receptors) are least sensitive to shunting, and shunting of dendritic synaptic events locally is small, because of the relatively low density of dendritic conductances activated during action potential backpropagation (Stuart and Häusser 1998).

Action potential bursting and dendritic excitability

Backpropagating action potentials are also important for the generation of action potential burst firing in some neurons. In layer 5 neocortical pyramidal neurons, recruitment of dendritic Ni^{2+}-sensitive Ca^{2+} channels by backpropagating action potentials leads to burst firing (Williams *et al.* 1998). Accordingly, bursting can be prevented by locally applying TTX to the proximal apical dendrite to block action potential backpropagation (Williams *et al.* 1998). Backpropagating action potentials can also facilitate the initiation of distal dendritic Ca^{2+} spikes by synaptic input, resulting in bursts of action potentials detected at the soma (Larkum *et al.* 1999). Activation of dendritic Ca^{2+} conductances is also thought to underlie burst firing in thalamocortical relay cells (Destexhe *et al.* 1998) and cerebellar Purkinje cells (Llinás and Sugimori 1980*b*; Llinás 1988). Consistent with a role of dendritic conductances in burst firing, dendritic depolarization promotes action potential bursts in both CA1 (Wong and Stewart 1992) and neocortical pyramidal neurons (Williams *et al.* 1998). Modeling studies using various dendritic geometries suggest that at least some forms of bursting might be favored in neurons with limited electrical coupling of excitable dendrites to the soma and axon (Pinsky and Rinzel 1994; Mainen and Sejnowski 1996), consistent with the observation of bursting in layer 5 pyramidal neurons in the neocortex (Connors *et al.* 1982; Chagnac-Amitai *et al.* 1990; Larkman and Mason 1990).

Intradendritic calcium elevation by backpropagating action potentials and dendritic spikes

As discussed in Chapter 7, backpropagating action potentials and dendritically generated Na^+ and Ca^{2+} spikes have all been shown to mediate Ca^{2+} entry into dendrites, both *in vitro* (Jaffe *et al.* 1992; Yuste *et al.* 1994; Schiller *et al.* 1995; Yuste and Denk 1995; Schiller *et al.* 1997, 1998) and *in vivo* (Svoboda *et al.* 1997, 1999). Much of this Ca^{2+} elevation is likely to be mediated by voltage-activated Ca^{2+} channels, but other sources of intradendritic Ca^{2+} are also possible. For example, Ca^{2+} entry might also trigger release of Ca^{2+} from intradendritic stores (Ross and Sandler 1998). Receptor activation might also trigger intradendritic Ca^{2+} release (Finch and Augustine 1998; Takechi *et al.* 1998), and some preliminary evidence suggests that concurrent receptor activation and spike backpropagation can act synergistically to release larger amounts of Ca^{2+} in dendrites (Barbara *et al.* 1998). Another important means by which backpropagating action potentials or dendritic spikes could interact with receptor activation is by relieving the voltage-dependent Mg^{2+} block at glutamate-bound NMDA receptors (Spruston *et al.* 1995*a*). This possibility may explain the observation that the Ca^{2+} entry produced by backpropagating action potentials and synaptic activation are larger for an action potential slightly preceded by an EPSP than for the sum of the two Ca^{2+} sources evoked separately (Yuste and Denk 1995; Schiller *et al.* 1998; Yuste *et al.* 1999) or for an EPSP preceded by an action potential (Koester and Sakmann 1998). Another possibility is that synaptic potentials inactivate dendritic A-type K^+ channels, resulting in more effective backpropagation and increased Ca^{2+} influx triggered by the larger action potentials (Hoffman *et al.* 1997; Magee and Johnston 1997).

Synaptic plasticity and dendritic excitability

The possible effects of Ca^{2+} increases in dendrites are numerous. As mentioned above, this is an important step in triggering the release of neurotransmitter from dendrites. During development, Ca^{2+} influx mediated by backpropagating action potentials or dendritic spikes could provide a trigger for activity-dependent dendritic growth. Similarly, such signals could provide the necessary link between presynaptic and postsynaptic activity proposed by Hebb to be required for changes in synaptic strength that underlie learning (see Chapters 13 and 14). Indeed, the relative timing of action potentials and synaptic input are critical in determining changes in synaptic strength (see Chapter 13; reviewed by Linden 1999). In pyramidal neurons, action potentials that precede synaptic activity cause long-term depression of synaptic strength, whereas action potentials that occur during synaptic activation produce long-term potentiation (Gustafsson *et al.* 1987; Debanne *et al.* 1997; Magee and Johnston 1997; Markram *et al.* 1997; Bi and Poo 1998); in other cells the rules are different (Egger *et al.* 1998). Magee and Johnston provided direct support for the idea that action potential backpropagation is a necessary step for these changes to occur by demonstrating that blocking backpropagating action potentials can prevent the induction of long-term potentiation (Magee and Johnston 1997). It seems natural to propose that dendritic spikes could substitute for backpropagating action potentials in this capacity, but this hypothesis has yet to be tested experimentally.

Concluding remarks

Although it has been clear since the turn of the century that dendrites come in all shapes and sizes (see Chapter 1), recent research has shown that this diversity in structure is also associated with a diversity in the active and passive membrane properties of the dendritic membrane. Voltage-gated channels are found in the dendrites of all neurons examined to date, with cell-specific differences in the types, properties and distributions of these channels (Chapter 6). Furthermore, passive membrane properties differ between neuronal types, and even within single neurons. Together, these differences impart a richness to synaptic integration unimaginable in the 1950s, when dendrites were, to some, more a nuisance than an asset to neuronal function (see Chapter 8).

The circumstances under which synaptic activation of dendritic voltage-gated channels causes a departure from the passive behavior of dendrites and thus helps define the input–output relation of neurons remains a matter of intense study.

Generalization across neurons is made difficult by the wide range of behaviors shown by different dendritic trees. Consider, for example, the differences in backpropagation of action potentials observed in different neuronal types (Chapter 6 and above). This diversity reflects the complexity imparted on dendritic processing by the mosaic of active channels and the variety of dendritic morphologies, and undoubtedly is related to the different functional roles of individual neurons in their respective networks. By characterizing this diversity, and searching for the mechanisms underlying it, we will hopefully better understand the way in which individual neurons are tuned to perform their particular computational tasks.

Acknowledgements

We thank Nace Golding, Arnd Roth, and Matthew Larkum for comments on the chapter. We would also like to thank the following organizations for their financial support: the National Institutes of Health (N. S.), the Sloan Foundation (N. S.), the Human Frontiers in Science Program (N. S., G. S., and M. H.), the Klingenstein Foundation (N. S.), the European Commission (M. H.), and the Wellcome Trust (G. S. and M. H.).

References

Agmon-Snir, H., Carr, C. E., and Rinzel, J. (1998). The role of dendrites in auditory coincidence detection. *Nature*, **393**, 268–72.

Amitai, Y., Friedman, A., Connors, B. W., and Gutnick, M. J. (1993). Regenerative activity in apical dendrites of pyramidal cells in neocortex. *Cerebral Cortex*, **3**, 26–8.

Andersen, P. (1960). Interhippocampal impulses. II. Apical dendritic activation of CA1 neurons. *Acta Physiologica Scandanavica*, **48**, 178–208.

Andersen, P. and Lømo, T. (1966). Mode of activation of hippocampal pyramidal cells by excitatory synapses on dendrites. *Experimental Brain Research*, **2**, 247–60.

Andreasen, M. and Lambert, J. D. C. (1995a). The excitability of CA1 pyramidal cell dendrites is modulated by a local Ca^{2+}-dependent K^+-conductance. *Brain Research*, **698**, 193–203.

Andreasen, M. and Lambert, J. D. C. (1995b). Regenerative properties of pyramidal cell dendrites in area CA1 of the rat hippocampus. *Journal of Physiology*, **483**, 421–41.

Andreasen, M. and Lambert, J. D. C. (1998). Factors determining the efficacy of distal excitatory synapses in rat hippocampal CA1 pyramidal neurones. *Journal of Physiology*, **507**, 441–62.

Barbara, J.-G., Sandler, V. M., and Ross, W. N. (1998). A possible involvement of calcium store in action potential evoked calcium transients in CA1 hippocampal pyramidal cells. *Society for Neuroscience Abstracts*, **24**, 80.

Barrett, J. N. and Crill, W. E. (1974). Specific membrane properties of cat motoneurones. *Journal of Physiology*, **239**, 301–24.

Bekkers, J. M. and Stevens, C. F. (1996). Cable properties of cultured hippocampal neurons determined from sucrose-evoked miniature EPSCs. *Journal of Neurophysiology*, **75**, 1250–5.

Benardo, L. S., Masukawa, L. M., and Prince, D. A. (1982). Electrophysiology of isolated hippocampal pyramidal dendrites. *Journal of Neuroscience*, **2**, 1614–22.

Bernander, O., Douglas, R. J., Martin, K. A., and Koch, C. (1991). Synaptic background activity influences spatiotemporal integration in single pyramidal cells. *Proceedings of the National Academy of Science USA*, **88**, 11569–73.

Bi, G. Q. and Poo, M. M. (1998). Synaptic modifications in cultured hippocampal neurons: dependence on spike timing, synaptic strength, and postsynaptic cell type. *Journal of Neuroscience*, **18**, 10464–72.

Bischofberger, J. and Jonas, P. (1997). Action potential propagation into the presynaptic dendrites of rat mitral cells. *Journal of Physiology*, **504**, 359–65.

Bloomfield, S. A. (1992). Relationship between receptive and dendritic field size of amacrine cells in the rabbit retina. *Journal of Neurophysiology*, **68**, 711–25.

Bloomfield, S. A. (1996). Effect of spike blockade on the receptive-field size of amacrine and ganglion cells in the rabbit retina. *Journal of Neurophysiology*, **75**, 1878–93.

Borst, J. G. G., Helmchen, F., and Sakmann, B. (1995). Pre- and postsynaptic whole-cell recordings in the medial nucleus of the trapezoid body of the rat. *Journal of Physiology*, **489**, 825–40.

Bourque, C. W. and Renaud, L. P. (1984). Activity patterns and osmosensitivity of rat supraoptic neurones in perfused hypothalamic explants. *Journal of Physiology*, **349**, 631–42.

Burke, R. E. (1967). Composite nature of the monosynaptic excitatory postsynaptic potential. *Journal of Neurophysiology*, **30**, 1114–37.

Callaway, J. C. and Ross, W. N. (1995). Frequency-dependent propagation of sodium action potentials in dendrites of hippocampal CA1 pyramidal neurons. *Journal of Neurophysiology*, **74**, 1395–403.

Cash, S. and Yuste, R. (1998). Input summation by cultured pyramidal neurons is linear and position-independent. *Journal of Neuroscience*, **18**, 10–15.

Cash, S. and Yuste, R. (1999). Linear summation of excitatory inputs by CA1 pyramidal neurons. *Neuron*, **22**, 383–94.

Cauller, L. J. and Connors, B. W. (1992). Functions of very distal dendrites: experimental and computational studies of layer I synapses on neocortical pyramidal cells. In *Single neuron computation*, (ed. T. McKenna, J. Davis, and S. F. Zornetzer), pp. 199–229. Academic Press, Boston.

Chagnac-Amitai, Y., Luhmann, H. J., and Prince, D. A. (1990). Burst generating and regular spiking layer 5 pyramidal neurons of rat neocortex have different morphological features. *Journal of Comparative Neurology*, **296**, 598–613.

Chen, W. R., Midtgaard, J., and Shepherd, G. M. (1997). Forward and backward propagation of dendritic impulses and their synaptic control in mitral cells. *Science*, **278**, 463–7.

Chen, W. R., Ma, M., Jia, C., and Shepherd, G. M. (1998). Roles of action potential propagation, pre- and postsynaptic NMDA receptors in the activation of olfactory dendrodendritic reciprocal synapses. *Society for Neuroscience Abstracts*, **24**, 321.

Cheramy, A., Leviel, V., and Glowinski, J. (1981). Dendritic release of dopamine in the substantia nigra. *Nature*, **289**, 537–42.

Colbert, C. M. and Johnston, D. (1996). Axonal action potential initiation and Na$^+$ channel densities in the soma and axon initial segment of subicular pyramidal neurons. *Journal of Neuroscience*, **16**, 6676–86.

Colbert, C. M. and Johnston, D. (1998). Protein kinase C activation decreases activity-dependent attenuation of dendritic Na$^+$ current in hippocampal CA1 pyramidal neurons. *Journal of Neurophysiology*, **79**, 491–5.

Colbert, C., Magee, J. C., Hoffman, D. A., and Johnston, D. (1997). Slow recovery from inactivation of Na$^+$ channels underlies the activity-dependent attenuation of dendritic action potentials in hippocampal CA1 pyramidal neurons. *Journal of Neuroscience*, **17**, 6512–21.

Connors, B. W., Gutnick, M. J., and Prince, D. A. (1982). Electrophysiological properties of neocortical neurons *in vitro*. *Journal of Neurophysiology*, **48**, 1302–20.

Conti, F., Hille, B., Neumcke, B., Nonner, W., and Stämpfli, R. (1976). Measurement of the conductance of the sodium channel from current fluctuations at the node of Ranvier. *Journal of Physiology*, **262**, 699–727.

Coombs, J. S., Curtis, D. R., and Eccles, J. C. (1957). The interpretation of spike potentials of motoneurones. *Journal of Physiology*, **139**, 198–231.

Coombs, J. S., Curtis, D. R., and Eccles, J. C. (1959). The electrical constants of the motoneuronal membrane. *Journal of Physiology*, **145**, 505–28.

Cox, C. L., Zhou, Q., and Sherman, S. M. (1998). Glutamate locally activates dendritic outputs of thalamic interneurons. *Nature*, **394**, 478–82.

Cragg, B. G. and Hamlyn, L. H. (1955). Action potentials of the pyramidal neurones in the hippocampus of the rabbit. *Journal of Physiology*, **129**, 608–27.

Debanne, D., Gähwiler, B. H., and Thompson, S. M. (1997). Bidirectional associative plasticity of unitary CA3–CA1 EPSPs in the rat hippocampus *in vitro*. *Journal of Neurophysiology*, **77**, 2851–5.

Deisz, R. A., Fortin, G., and Zieglgänsberger, W. (1991). Voltage-dependence of excitatory postsynaptic potentials of rat neocortical pyramidal neurons. *Journal of Neurophysiology*, **65**, 371–82.

Destexhe, A., Neubig, M., Ulrich, D., and Huguenard, J. (1998). Dendritic low-threshold calcium currents in thalamic relay cells. *Journal of Neuroscience*, **18**, 3574–88.

Di Scala-Guenot, D., Strosser, M. T., and Richard, P. (1987). Electrical stimulations of perifused magnocellular nuclei *in vitro* elicit Ca^{2+}-dependent, tetrodotoxin-insensitive release of oxytocin and vasopressin. *Neuroscience Letters*, **76**, 209–14.

Dodge, F. A. and Cooley, J. W. (1973). Action potential of the motoneuron. *IBM Journal of Research and Development*, **17**, 219–29.

Dowling, J. E. and Boycott, B. B. (1966). Organization of the primate retina: electron microscopy. *Proceedings of the Royal Society of London, Series B, Biological Sciences*, **166**, 80–111.

Eccles, J., Libet, B., and Young, R. R. (1958). The behaviour of chromatolysed motoneurones studied by intracellular recording. *Journal of Physiology*, **143**, 11–40.

Egger, V., Feldmeyer, D., Spergel, D., and Sakmann, B. (1998). Long-lasting modulations of a synapse in the barrel field of rat somatosensory cortex. *Society for Neuroscience Abstracts*, **24**, 157.

Eilers, J., Augustine, G. J., and Konnerth, A. (1995). Subthreshold synaptic Ca^{2+} signalling in fine dendrites and spines of cerebellar Purkinje neurons. *Nature*, **373**, 155–8.

Fatt, P. (1957). Sequence of events in synaptic activation of a motoneurone. *Journal of Neurophysiology*, **20**, 61–80.

Ferster, D. and Spruston, N. (1995). Cracking the neuronal code. *Science*, **270**, 756–7.

Finch, E. A. and Augustine, G. J. (1998). Local calcium signalling by inositol-1,4,5-trisphosphate in Purkinje cell dendrites. *Nature*, **396**, 753–6.

Freund, T. F. and Buzsáki, G. (1996). Interneurons of the hippocampus. *Hippocampus*, **6**, 347–470.

Fromherz, P. and Muller, C. O. (1994). Cable properties of a straight neurite of a leech neuron probed by a voltage-sensitive dye. *Proceedings of the National Academy of Science USA*, **91**, 4604–8.

Fujita, Y. and Sakata, H. (1962). Electrophysiological properties of CA1 and CA2 apical dendrites of rabbit hippocampus. *Journal Neurophysiology*, **25**, 209–22.

Fuortes, M. G. F., Frank, K., and Becker, M. C. (1957). Steps in the production of motoneuron spikes. *Journal of General Physiology*, **40**, 735–52.

Gao, D. M., Hoffman, D., and Benabid, A. L. (1996). Simultaneous recording of spontaneous activities and nociceptive responses from neurons in the pars compacta of substantia nigra and in the lateral habenula. *European Journal of Neuroscience*, **8**, 1474–8.

Geiger, J. R., Lübke, J., Roth, A., Frotscher, M., and Jonas, P. (1997). Submillisecond AMPA receptor-mediated signaling at a principal neuron–interneuron synapse. *Neuron*, **18**, 1009–23.

Gentet, L., Stuart, G., and Clements, J. (1999). Direct measurement of specific membrane capacitance in rat neurons and HEK 923 cells. *Proceedings of the Australian Neuroscience Society*, **10**, 137.

Gillessen, T. and Alzheimer, C. (1997). Amplification of EPSPs by low Ni^{2+}- and amiloride-sensitive Ca^{2+} channels in apical dendrites of rat CA1 pyramidal neurons. *Journal Neurophysiology*, **77**, 1639–43.

Golding, N. L. and Spruston, N. (1998). Dendritic sodium spikes are variable triggers of action potentials in hippocampal CA1 pyramidal neurons. *Neuron*, **21**, 1189–200.

Golding, N. L., Ferragamo, M. J., and Oertel, D. (1999*a*). Role of intrinsic conductances underlying responses to transients in octopus cells of the cochlear nucleus. *Journal of Neuroscience*, **19**, 2897–905.

Golding, N. L., Jung, H., Mickus, T., and Spruston, N. (1999*b*). Dendritic calcium spike initiation and repolarization are controlled by distinct potassium channel subtypes in CA1 pyramidal neurons. *Journal of Neuroscience*. (In press).

Goldstein, S. S. and Rall, W. (1974). Changes of action potential shape and velocity for changing core conductor geometry. *Biophysical Journal*, **14**, 731–57.

Gustafsson, B., Gigström, H., Abraham, W. C., and Huanng, Y.-Y. (1987). Long-term potentiation in the hippocampus using depolarizing current pulses as the conditioning stimulus to single volley synaptic potentials. *Journal of Neuroscience*, **7**, 774–80.

Hartell, N. (1996). Strong activation of parallel fibers produces localized calcium transients and a form of LTD that spreads to distant synapses. *Neuron*, **16**, 601–10.

Häusser, M. (1996). How do active dendrites affect synaptic integration? *European Journal of Neuroscience*, Suppl. 9, 115.

Häusser, M. and Clark, B. A. (1997). Tonic synaptic inhibition modulates neuronal output pattern and spatiotemporal synaptic integration. *Neuron*, **19**, 665–78.

Häusser, M., Stuart, G., Racca, C., and Sakmann, B. (1995). Axonal initiation and active dendritic propagation of action potentials in substantia nigra neurons. *Neuron*, **15**, 637–47.

Häusser, M., Vetter, P., and Roth, A. (1998). Action-potential backpropagation depends on dendritic geometry. *Society for Neuroscience Abstracts*, **24**, 1813.

Herreras, O. (1990). Propagating dendritic action potential mediates synaptic transmission in CA1 pyramidal cells in situ. *Journal of Neurophysiology*, **64**, 1429–41.

Hines, M. L. and Carnevale, N. T. (1997). The NEURON simulation environment. *Neural Computation*, **9**, 1179–209.

Hoffman, D. A. and Johnston, D. (1998). Downregulation of transient K^+ channels in dendrites of hippocampal CA1 pyramidal neurons by activation of PKA and PKC. *Journal Neuroscience*, **18**, 3521–8.

Hoffman, D. A., Magee, J. C., Colbert, C. M., and Johnston, D. (1997). K^+ channel regulation of signal propagation in dendrites of hippocampal pyramidal neurons. *Nature*, **387**, 869–75.

Isaacson, J. S. and Strowbridge, B. W. (1998). Olfactory reciprocal synapses: dendritic signaling in the CNS. *Neuron*, **20**, 749–61.

Jack, J. J. B., Noble, D., and Tsien, R. W. (1983) *Electric current flow in excitable cells*. Oxford University Press.

Jaffe, D. B., Johnston, D., Lasser-Ross, N., Lisman, J. E., Miyakawa, H., and Ross, W. N. (1992). The spread of Na^+ spikes determines the pattern of dendritic Ca^{2+} entry into hippocampal neurons. *Nature*, **357**, 244–6.

Jahr, C. E. and Nicoll, R. A. (1982). An intracellular analysis of dendrodendritic inhibition in the turtle *in vitro* olfactory bulb. *Journal of Physiology*, **326**, 213–34.

Jefferys, J. G. (1979). Initiation and spread of action potentials in granule cells maintained *in vitro* in slices of guinea-pig hippocampus. *Journal of Physiology*, **289**, 375–88.

Jung, H., Mickus, T., and Spruston, N. (1997). Prolonged sodium channel inactivation contributes to dendritic action potential attenuation in hippocampal pyramidal neurons. *Journal of Neuroscience*, **17**, 6639–46.

Kamondi, A., Acsady, L., and Buzsaki, G. (1998). Dendritic spikes are enhanced by co-operative network activity in the intact hippocampus. *Journal of Neuroscience*, **18**, 3919–28.

Kim, H. G., Beierlein, M., and Connors, B. W. (1995). Inhibitory control of excitable dendrites in neocortex. *Journal of Neurophysiology*, **74**, 1810–14.

Koch, C., Rapp, M., and Segev, I. (1996). A brief history of time (constants). *Cerebral Cortex*, **6**, 93–101.

Koester, H. J. and Sakmann, B. (1998). Calcium dynamics in single spines during coincident pre- and postsynaptic activity depend on relative timing of back-propagating action potentials and subthreshold excitatory postsynaptic potentials. *Proceedings of the National Academy of Science USA*, **95**, 9596–601.

Landmesser, L. and Pilar, G. (1972). The onset and development of transmission in the chick ciliary ganglion. *Journal of Physiology*, **222**, 691–713.

Larkman, A. and Mason, A. (1990). Correlations between morphology and electrophysiology of pyramidal neurons in slices of rat visual cortex. II Electrophysiology. *Journal of Neuroscience*, **10**, 1415–28.

Larkum, M. E., Rioult, M. G., and Lüscher, H.-R. (1996). Propagation of action potentials in the dendrites of neurons from rat spinal cord slice cultures. *Journal of Neurophysiology*, **75**, 154–70.

Larkum, M. E., Zhu, J. J., and Sakmann, B. (1999). A novel cellular mechanism for coupling inputs arriving at different cortical layers. *Nature*, **398**, 338–41.

Lasser-Ross, N. and Ross, W. N. (1992). Imaging voltage and synaptically activated sodium transients in cerebellar Purkinje cells. *Proceedings of the Royal Society of London, Series B*, **247**, 35–9.

Lieberman, M. C. (1991). Central projections of auditory-nerve fibers of differing spontaneous rate. I. Anteroventral cochlear nucleus. *Journal of Comparative Neurology*, **313**, 240–58.

Linden, D. (1999). The return of the spike: postsynaptic action potentials and the induction of LTP and LTD. *Neuron*, **22**, 661–6.

Lipowsky, R., Gillessen, T., and Alzheimer, C. (1996). Dendritic Na^+ channels amplify EPSPs in hippocampal CA1 pyramidal cells. *Journal of Neurophysiology*, **76**, 2181–91.

Llinás, R. (1988). The intrinsic electrophysiological properties of mammalian neurons insights into central nervous system function. *Science*, **242**, 1654–64.

Llinás, R., Nicholson, C., Freeman, J. A., and Hillman, D. E. (1968). Dendritic spikes and their inhibition in alligator Purkinje cells. *Science*, **160**, 1132–5.

Llinás, R., Nicholson, C., Precht, W. (1969). Preferred centripetal conduction of dendritic spikes in alligator Purkinje cells. *Science*, **163**, 184–7.

Llinás, R. and Nicholson, C. (1971). Electrophysiological properties of dendrites and somata in alligator Purkinje cells. *Journal of Neurophysiology*, **34**, 532–51.

Llinás, R. and Sugimori, M. (1980*a*). Electrophysiological properties of *in vitro* Purkinje cell somata in mammalian cerebellar slices. *Journal of Physiology*, **305**, 171–95.

Llinás, R. and Sugimori, M. (1980*b*). Electrophysiological properties of *in vitro* Purkinje cell dendrites in mammalian cerebellar slices. *Journal of Physiology*, **305**, 197–213.

Lorente de Nó, R. and Condouris, G. A. (1959). Decremental conduction in peripheral nerve. Integration of stimuli in the neuron. *Proceedings of the National Academy of Science USA*, **45**, 592–617.

Ludwig, M. and Landgraf, R. (1992). Does the release of vasopressin within the supraoptic nucleus of the rat brain depend upon changes in osmolality and Ca^{2+}/K^+? *Brain Research*, **576**, 231–4.

Lüscher, C., Streit, J., Quadroni, R., and Lüscher, H. R. (1994). Action potential propagation through embryonic dorsal root ganglion cells in culture. I. Influence of the cell morphology on propagation properties. *Journal of Neurophysiology*, **72**, 622–33.

Lux, H. D., Schubert, P., and Kreutzberg, G. W. (1970). Direct matching of morphological and electrophysiological data in motoneurons. In *Excitatory synaptic mechanisms*, (ed. P. Andersen and J. K. S. Jansen), pp. 189–98. Universitetsforlaget, Oslo.

MacVicar, B. A. and Dudek, F. E. (1981). Electrotonic coupling between pyramidal cells: a direct demonstration in rat hippocampal slices. *Science*, **213**, 782–5.

Magee, J. C. (1998). Dendritic hyperpolarization-activated currents modify the integrative properties of hippocampal CA1 pyramidal neurons. *Journal of Neuroscience*, **18**, 7613–24.

Magee, J. C. (1999). Dendritic I_h normalizes temporal summation in hippocampal CA1 neurons. *Nature Neuroscience*, **2**, 508–14.

Magee, J. C. and Johnston, D. (1995). Characterization of single voltage-gated Na^+ and Ca^{2+}-channels in apical dendrites of rat CA1 pyramidal neurons. *Journal of Physiology*, **487**, 67–90.

Magee, J. C. and Johnston, D. (1997). A synaptically controlled, associative signal for Hebbian plasticity in hippocampal neurons. *Science*, **275**, 209–13.

Magee, J. C., Christofi, G., Miyakawa, H., Christie, B., Lasser–Ross, N., and Johnston, D. (1995). Subthreshold synaptic activation of voltage-gated Ca^{2+} channels mediates a localized Ca^{2+} influx into the dendrites of hippocampal pyramidal neurons. *Journal of Neurophysiology*, **74**, 1335–42.

Mainen, Z. F. and Sejnowski, T. J. (1996). Influence of dendritic structure on firing pattern in model neocortical neurons. *Nature*, **382**, 363–6.

Mainen, Z. F., Joerges, J., Huguenard, J. R., and Sejnowski, T. J. (1995). A model of spike initiation in neocortical pyramidal neurons. *Neuron*, **15**, 1427–39.

Major, G., Larkman, A. U., Jonas, P., Sakmann, B., and Jack, J. J. (1994). Detailed passive cable models of whole-cell recorded CA3 pyramidal neurons in rat hippocampal slices. *Journal of Neuroscience*, **14**, 4613–38.

Maletic-Savatic, M. and Malinow, R. (1998). Calcium-evoked dendritic exocytosis in cultured hippocampal neurons. Part I: *trans*-Golgi network-derived organelles undergo regulated exocytosis. *Journal of Neuroscience*, **18**, 6803–13.

Maletic-Savatic, M., Koothan, T., and Malinow, R. (1998). Calcium-evoked dendritic exocytosis in cultured hippocampal neurons. Part II: Mediation by calcium/calmodulin-dependent protein kinase II. *Journal of Neuroscience*, **18**, 6814–21.

Margulis, M. and Tang, C. (1998). Temporal integration can readily switch between sublinear and supralinear summation. *Journal of Neurophysiology*, **79**, 2809–13.

Markram, H., Lübke, J., Frotscher, M., and Sakmann, B. (1997). Regulation of synaptic efficacy by coincidence of postsynaptic APs and EPSPs. *Science*, **275**, 213–15.

Masukawa, L. M. and Prince, D. A. (1984). Synaptic control of excitability in isolated dendrites of hippocampal neurons. *Journal of Neuroscience*, **4**, 217–27.

McCormick, D. A., Wang, Z., and Huguenard, J. (1993). Neurotransmitter control of neocortical neuronal activity and excitability. *Cerebral Cortex*, **3**, 387–98.

Meyer, E., Muller, C. O., and Fromherz, P. (1997). Cable properties of dendrites in hippocampal neurons of the rat mapped by a voltage-sensitive dye. *European Journal of Neuroscience*, **9**, 778–85.

Mickus, T., Jung, H., and Spruston, N. (1999). Properties of slow, cumulative sodium channel inactivation in rat hippocampal CA1 pyramidal cells. *Biophysical Journal*, **76**, 846–60.

Miles, R., Toth, K., Gulyas, A. I., Hajos, N., and Freund, T. F. (1996). Differences between somatic and dendritic inhibition in the hippocampus. *Neuron*, **16**, 815–23.

Miller, J. P., Rall, W., and Rinzel, J. (1985). Synaptic amplification by active membrane in dendritic spines. *Brain Research*, **325**, 325–30.

Miyakawa, H. and Kato, H. (1986). Active properties of dendritic membrane examined by current source density analysis in hippocampal CA1 pyramidal neurons. *Brain Research*, **399**, 303–9.

Miyakawa, H., Lev-Ram, V., Lasser-Ross, N., and Ross, W. N. (1992). Calcium transients evoked by climbing fiber and parallel fiber synaptic inputs in guinea pig cerebellar Purkinje neurons. *Journal of Neurophysiology*, **68**, 1178–88.

Moore, J. W., Stockbridge, N., and Westerfield, M. (1983). On the site of impulse initiation in a neurone. *Journal of Physiology*, **336**, 301–11.

Nedergaard, S. and Hounsgaard, J. (1996). Fast Na^+ spike generation in dendrites of guinea-pig substantia nigra pars compacta neurons. *Neuroscience*, **73**, 381–96.

Neumcke, B. and Stampfli, R. (1982). Sodium currents and sodium-current fluctuations in rat myelinated nerve fibres. *Journal of Physiology*, **329**, 163–84.

Pare, D., Shink, E., Gaudreau, H., Destexhe, A., and Lang, E. J. (1998). Impact of spontaneous synaptic activity on the resting properties of cat neocortical pyramidal neurons *in vivo*. *Journal of Neurophysiology*, **79**, 1450–60.

Perkel, D. H. and Perkel, D. J. (1985). Dendritic spines: role of active membrane in modulating synaptic efficacy. *Brain Research*, **325**, 331–5.

Pinsky, P. F. and Rinzel, J. (1994). Intrinsic and network rhythmogenesis in a reduced Traub model for CA3 neurons. *Journal of Computational Neuroscience*, **1**, 39–60.

Purpura, D. P. (1967). Comparative physiology of dendrites. In *The neurosciences: a study program*, (ed. G. C. Quarton, T. Melnechuk, and F. O. Schmitt). Rockefeller University Press, New York.

Rall, W. (1959). Branching dendritic trees and motoneuron membrane resistivity. *Experimental Neurology*, **1**, 491–527.

Rall, W. (1964). Theoretical significance of dendritic trees for neuronal input–output relations. In *Neural theory and modeling*, (ed. R. F. Reiss). Stanford University Press, Palo Alto.

Rall, W. (1967). Distinguishing theoretical synaptic potentials computed for different soma-dendritic distributions of synaptic input. *Journal of Neurophysiology*, **30**, 1138–68.

Rall, W., Shepherd, G. M., Reese, T. S., and Brightman, M. W. (1966). Dendrodendritic synaptic pathway for inhibition in the olfactory bulb. *Experimental Neurology*, **14**, 44–56.

Rall, W. and Shepherd, G. M. (1968). Theoretical reconstruction of field potentials and dendrodendritic synaptic interactions in olfactory bulb. *Journal of Neurophysiology*, **31**, 884–915.

Rapp, M., Yarom, Y., and Segev, I. (1992). The impact of parallel fiber background activity on the cable properties of cerebellar Purkinje cells. *Neural Computation*, **4**, 518–33.

Rapp, M., Segev, I., and Yarom, Y. (1994). Physiology, morphology and detailed passive models of guinea-pig cerebellar Purkinje cells. *Journal of Physiology*, **474**, 101–18.

Rapp, M., Yarom, M., and Segev, I. (1996). Modeling back propagating action potentials in weakly excitable dendrites of neocortical pyramidal cells. *Proceedings of the National Academy of Science USA*, **93**, 11985–90.

Reyes, A. D. and Sakmann, B (1996). Summation of synaptic potentials in layer V pyramidal neurons. *Society for Neuroscience Abstracts*, **22**, 792.

Rice, M. E., Richards, C. D., Nedergaard, S., Hounsgaard, J., Nicholson, C., and Greenfield, S. A. (1994). Direct monitoring of dopamine and 5-HT release in substantia nigra and ventral tegmental area *in vitro*. *Experimental Brain Research*, **100**, 395–406.

Richardson, T. L., Turner, R. W., and Miller, J. J. (1987). Action-potential discharge in hippocampal CA1 pyramidal neurons: current source-density analysis. *Journal of Neurophysiology*, **58**, 981–96.

Ross, W. N. and Sandler, V. M. (1998). Serotonin and spikes synergistically release calcium in dendrites of hippocampal pyramidal cells. *Society for Neuroscience Abstracts*, **24**, 80.

Roth, A. and Häusser, M. (1999). Compartmental models of rat cerebellar Purkinje cells constrained using simultaneous somatic and dendritic patch-clamp recording. *Proceedings of the Physiological Society*, **518**, 142–143P.

Rudy, B. (1988). Diversity and ubiquity of K^+ channels. *Neuroscience*, **25**, 729–49.

Rutherford, L. C., Nelson, S. B., and Turrigiano, G. G. (1998). BDNF has opposite effects on the quantal amplitude of pyramidal neuron and interneuron excitatory synapses. *Neuron*, **21**, 521–30.

Santiago, M., Machado, A., and Cano, J. (1992). Fast sodium-channel dependency of the somatodendritic release of dopamine in the rat's brain. *Neuroscience Letters*, **148**, 145–7.

Schiller, J., Helmchen, F., and Sakmann, B. (1995). Spatial profile of dendritic calcium transients evoked by action potentials in rat neocortical pyramidal neurons. *Journal of Physiology*, **487**, 583–600.

Schiller, J., Schiller, Y., Stuart, G., and Sakmann, B. (1997). Calcium action potentials restricted to distal apical dendrites of rat neocortical pyramidal neurons. *Journal of Physiology*, **505**, 605–16.

Schiller, J., Schiller, Y., and Clapham, D. E. (1998). NMDA receptors amplify calcium influx into dendritic spines during associative pre- and postsynaptic activation. *Nature Neuroscience*, **1**, 114–18.

Schoppa, N. E., Kinzie, J. M., Sahara, Y., Segerson, T. P., and Westbrook, G. L. (1998). Dendrodendritic inhibition in the olfactory bulb is driven by NMDA receptors. *Journal of Neuroscience*, **18**, 6790–802.

Schwindt, P. C. and Crill, W. E. (1995). Amplification of synaptic current by persistent sodium conductance in apical dendrite of neocortical neurons. *Journal of Neurophysiology*, **74**, 2220–4.

Seamans, J. K., Gorelova, N. A., and Yang, C. R. (1997). Contributions of voltage-gated Ca^{2+} channels in the proximal *versus* distal dendrites to synaptic integration in prefrontal cortical neurons. *Journal of Neuroscience*, **17**, 5936–48.

Shadlen, M. N. and Newsome, W. T. (1994). Noise, neural codes and cortical organization. *Current Opinion in Neurobiology*, **4**, 569–79.

Shadlen, M. N. and Newsome, W. T. (1995). Is there a signal in the noise? *Current Opinion in Neurobiology*, **5**, 248–50.

Shepherd, G. M., Brayton, R. K., Miller, J. P., Segev, I., Rinzel, J., and Rall, W. (1985). Signal enhancement in distal cortical dendrites by means of interactions between active dendritic spines. *Proceedings of the National Academy of Science USA*, **82**, 2192–5.

Sigworth, F. J. (1980). The variance of sodium current fluctuations at the node of Ranvier. *Journal of Physiology*, **307**, 97–129.

Sik, A., Penttonen, M., Ylinen, A., and Buzsaki, G. (1995). Hippocampal CA1 interneurons: an *in vivo* intracellular labeling study. *Journal of Neuroscience*, **15**, 6651–65.

Smith, P. H., Joris, P. X., Banks, M. I., and Yin, T. C. T. (1993). Responses of cochlear nucleus cells and projections of their axons. In *The mammalian cochlear nuclei: organization and function*, (ed. M. A. Merchán), pp. 349–60. Plenum Press, New York.

Softky, W. R. (1995). Simple codes versus efficient codes. *Current Opinion in Neurobiology*, **5**, 239–47.

Spencer, W. A. and Kandel, E. R. (1961). Electrophysiology of hippocampal neurons. IV. Fast prepotentials. *Journal of Neurophysiology*, **24**, 272–85.

Spruston, N. and Johnston, D. (1992). Perforated patch-clamp analysis of the passive membrane properties of three classes of hippocampal neurons. *Journal of Neurophysiology*, **67**, 508–29.

Spruston, N., Jaffe, D. B., and Johnston, D. (1994). Dendritic attenuation of synaptic potentials and currents: the role of passive membrane properties. *Trends in Neurosciences*, **17**, 161–6.

Spruston, N., Jonas, P., and Sakmann, B. (1995a). Dendritic glutamate receptor channels in rat hippocampal CA3 and CA1 pyramidal neurons. *Journal of Physiology*, **482**, 325–52.

Spruston, N., Schiller, Y., Stuart, G., and Sakmann, B. (1995b). Activity-dependent action potential invasion and calcium influx into hippocampal CA1 dendrites. *Science*, **268**, 297–300.

Spruston, N., Stuart, G., and Sakmann, B. (1995c). How do voltage-activated channels shape EPSPs in hippocampal CA1 neurons? *Society for Neuroscience Abstracts*, **21**, 584.

Stafford, D. K. and Dacey, D. M. (1997). Physiology of the A1 amacrine: a spiking, axon-bearing interneuron of the macaque monkey retina. *Visual Neuroscience*, **14**, 507–22.

Stafstrom, C. E., Schwindt, P. C., Chubb, M. C., and Crill, W. E. (1985). Properties of persistent sodium conductance and calcium conductance of layer V neurons from cat sensorimotor cortex *in vitro*. *Journal of Neurophysiology*, **53**, 153–70.

Stuart, G. (1999). Voltage-activated sodium channels amplify inhibition in neocortical pyramidal neurons. *Nature Neuroscience*, **2**, 144–50.

Stuart, G. and Häusser, M. (1994). Initiation and spread of sodium action potentials in cerebellar Purkinje cells. *Neuron*, **13**, 703–12.

Stuart, G. and Häusser, M. (1998). Shunting of EPSPs by action potentials. *Society for Neuroscience Abstracts*, **24**, 1810.

Stuart, G. J. and Sakmann, B. (1994). Active propagation of somatic action potentials into neocortical pyramidal cell dendrites. *Nature*, **367**, 69–72.

Stuart, G. and Sakmann, B. (1995). Amplification of EPSPs by axosomatic sodium channels in neocortical pyramidal neurons. *Neuron*, **15**, 1065–77.

Stuart, G. and Spruston, N. (1998). Determinants of voltage attenuation in neocortical pyramidal neuron dendrites. *Journal of Neuroscience*, **18**, 3501–10.

Stuart, G., Schiller, J., and Sakmann, B. (1997a). Action-potential initiation in neocortical pyramidal neurons. *Journal of Physiology*, **505**, 671–632.

Stuart, G., Spruston, N., Sakmann, B., and Häusser, M. (1997b). Action-potential initiation and backpropagation in neurons of the mammalian central nervous system. *Trends in Neurosciences*, **20**, 125–31.

Svoboda, K., Denk, W., Kleinfeld, D., and Tank, D. W. (1997). *In vivo* dendritic calcium dynamics in neocortical pyramidal neurons. *Nature*, **385**, 161–5.

Svoboda, K., Helmchen, F., Denk, W., and Tank, D. W. (1999). Spread of dendritic excitation in layer 2/3 pyramidal neurons in rat barrel cortex *in vivo*. *Nature Neuroscience*, **2**, 65–73.

Takechi, H., Eilers, J., and Konnerth, A. (1998). A new class of synaptic response involving calcium release in dendritic spines. *Nature*, **396**, 757–60.

Terzuolo, C. A. and Araki, T. (1961). An analysis of intra- versus extracellular potential changes associated with activity of single spinal motoneurons. *Annals of the New York Academy of Science*, **94**, 547–58.

Thurbon, D., Field, A., and Redman, S. (1994). Electrotonic profiles of interneurons in stratum pyramidale of the CA1 region of rat hippocampus. *Journal of Neurophysiology*, **71**, 1948–58.

Thurbon, D., Luscher, H. R., Hofstetter, T., and Redman, S. J. (1998). Passive electrical properties of ventral horn neurons in rat spinal cord slices. *Journal of Neurophysiology*, **79**, 2485–502.

Tsubokawa, H. and Ross, W. N. (1996). IPSPs modulate spike backpropagation and associated $[Ca^{2+}]_i$ changes in the dendrites of hippocampal CA1 pyramidal neurons. *Journal of Neurophysiology*, **76**, 2896–906.

Tsubokawa, H. and Ross, W. N. (1997). Muscarinic modulation of spike backpropagation in the apical dendrites of hippocampal CA1 pyramidal neurons. *Journal of Neuroscience*, **17**, 5782–91.

Turner, R. W., Meyers, D. E., and Barker, J. L. (1989). Localization of tetrodotoxin-sensitive field potentials of CA1 pyramidal cells in the rat hippocampus. *Journal of Neurophysiology*, **62**, 1375–87.

Turner, R. W., Meyers, D. E., Richardson, T. L., and Barker, J. L. (1991). The site for initiation of action potential discharge over the somatodendritic axis of rat hippocampal CA1 pyramidal neurons. *Journal of Neuroscience*, **11**, 2270–80.

Turner, R. W., Meyers, D. E., and Barker, J. L. (1993). Fast pre-potential generation in rat hippocampal CA1 pyramidal neurons. *Neuroscience*, **53**, 949–59.

Urban, N. N. and Barrionuevo, G. (1998). Active summation of excitatory postsynaptic potentials in hippocampal CA3 pyramidal neurons. *Proceedings of the National Academy of Science USA*, **95**, 11450–5.

Urban, N. N., Henze, D. A., and Barrionuevo, G. (1998). Amplification of perforant-path EPSPs in CA3 pyramidal cells by LVA calcium and sodium channels. *Journal of Neurophysiology*, **80**, 1558–61.

Valiante, T. A., Velazquez, J. L. P., Jahromi, S. S., and Carlen, P. L. (1995). Coupling potentials in CA1 neurons during calcium-free-induced field burst activity. *Journal of Neuroscience*, **15**, 6946–56.

Williams, S. R., Hendry, I., and Stuart, G. (1998). Mechanism of action potential burst firing in layer 5 neocortical neurones. *Society for Neuroscience Abstracts*, **24**, 2018.

Wollner, D. A. and Catterall, W. A. (1986). Localization of sodium channels in axon hillocks and initial segments of retinal ganglion cells. *Proceedings of the National Academy of Science USA*, **83**, 8424–8.

Wong, R. K. and Stewart, M. (1992). Different firing patterns generated in dendrites and somata of CA1 pyramidal neurones in guinea-pig hippocampus. *Journal of Physiology*, **457**, 675–87.

Wong, R. K. S., Prince, D. A., and Basbaum, A. I. (1979). Intradendritic recordings from hippocampal neurons. *Proceedings of the National Academy of Science USA*, **76**, 986–90.

Yung, W. H., Häusser, M. A., and Jack, J. J. (1991). Electrophysiology of dopaminergic and non-dopaminergic neurones of the guinea-pig substantia nigra pars compacta *in vitro*. *Journal of Physiology*, **436**, 643–67.

Yuste, R. and Denk, W. (1995). Dendritic spines as basic functional units of neuronal integration. *Nature*, **375**, 682–4.

Yuste, R., Gutnick, M. J., Saar, D., Delaney, K. R., and Tank, D., W. (1994). Ca^{2+} accumulations in dendrites of neocortical pyramidal neurons: an apical band and evidence for two functional compartments. *Neuron*, **13**, 23–43.

Yuste, R., Majewska, A., Cash, S. S., and Denk, W. (1999). Mechanisms of calcium influx into hippocampal spines: heterogeneity among spines, coincidence detection by NMDA receptors and optical quantal analysis. *Journal of Neuroscience*, **19**, 1976–87.

11

Why have dendrites? A computational perspective

Bartlett W. Mel
University of Southern California

Summary

In most neurons, dendrites receive the vast bulk of the cell's synaptic input. But why do dendrites exist? What benefits do they confer upon a neuron? What computing operations are carried out in dendritic trees which could not occur within a spatially compact neuron? In this chapter we review evidence from both physiological and computer modeling studies suggesting that dendrites provide space for a large number of compartmentalized nonlinear synaptic interactions. We illustrate the power and generality of this view of dendritic function by enumerating several diverse ways in which intradendritic computations could contribute to classical and extraclassical receptive field properties of neurons in visual cortex.

Introduction

To delimit the scope of our discussion, we begin with the 'null' hypothesis, which holds that dendrites exist strictly to increase the receptive surface area of a neuron, but do not otherwise contribute—or may even detract—from the information processing tasks of the neuron. The essence of this view is that the location of a synapse within the dendritic tree has relatively little importance for postsynaptic integration, a design feature which greatly simplifies the rules needed for the construction and maintenance of a functioning axo-dendritic interface.

As appealing as it may be, the strongest form of this hypothesis faces an immediate challenge. Specifically, passive cable theory makes it clear that spatially extended dendrites, by their nature, create a large disparity among synapses in terms of their ability to influence the final common output signal of neurons—the action potential (Rall and Rinzel 1973; Zador *et al.* 1995). Various authors, however, have proposed a remedy which could salvage a weaker version of the null hypothesis. Specifically, active channels in the dendrites could help to equalize the effects of synapses at the cell body independent of their location in the dendritic tree (Spencer and Kandel 1961; Cauller and Connors 1992; De Schutter and Bower 1994; Cook and Johnston 1999). In this view, a dendritic neuron is made to act more like an idealized 'point' neuron through proper deployment of voltage-dependent channel mechanisms in the dendritic membrane. In the same vein, backpropagating action potentials could help to collapse dendritic space by broadcasting somatic firing activity far afield in the dendrites. Under the null hypothesis, backpropagating action potentials could be interpreted as an adaptation which evolved to allow Hebbian learning mechanisms to be carried out in neurons with distantly scattered synaptic inputs (Magee and Johnston 1997; Markram *et al.* 1997; Koester and Sakmann 1998; Schiller *et al.* 1998)—though the *conditional* penetration of back-propagating action potentials into dendritic subtrees may be cited as evidence against this idea (Spruston *et al.* 1995; Magee and Johnston 1997).

In addition to providing more space for synaptic inputs, there are other potential advantages of a spatially extended axo-dendritic interface which do not relate directly to functional compartmentalization of postsynaptic dendritic processing. For example, a spatially-extended dendritic tree allows an afferent pathway to specifically target a subregion of a dendritic tree, such as the basal versus apical tree, apical tufts *versus* primary trunks, and so on. This type of anatomical segregation is a very common feature of neural organization (Shepherd 1998), but could reflect basic neuroanatomical wiring and targeting constraints. For example, two or more different classes of presynaptic terminals impinging on a neuron may need to be modulated by different signals (Patil *et al.* 1998). In such cases, bulk spatial segregation of the input pathways to distinct dendritic subregions could facilitate the targeting of different modulatory substances to the various classes of presynaptic terminals—again with relatively little significance for postsynaptic integrative processes.

Beyond these wiring-related hypotheses, there exist other possible functions of dendritic trees which involve *bona fide* postsynaptic physiological effects, but which remain outside our present scope. For example, voltage-dependent calcium channels in dendritic compartments have been proposed to contribute to neuronal bursting behavior (Traub 1982; Mainen and Sejnowski 1996), but this type of dendritic function (discussed in Chapter 10) remains largely orthogonal to the main focus of this chapter that is, on dendritic integration involving multiple, compartment-alized nonlinear synaptic interaction domains. Several other recent reviews of dendritic function are available which include a range of different perspectives (Mel 1994; Yuste and Tank 1996; Koch 1998; Segev and Rall 1998).

Compartmentalization of nonlinear processing

For the remainder of this chapter, we consider the ways in which dendritic space impacts on postsynaptic integration. Our main thesis is that:

(1) for some neuron types, spatially extended dendritic trees exist to provide space for a large number of quasi-independent dendritic 'compartments' or 'subunits', where the synaptic input to each compartment is boosted via an accelerating nonlinear input–output relation; and

(2) the integrative function of the dendritic tree as a whole is to compute a sum over the outputs of each of these nonlinear subunits.

We expand upon several aspects of this scenario below.

On expansive local nonlinear operations in dendrites

The term 'expansive' indicates that the response of a dendritic compartment grows faster than linearly with its input over a substantial range of output values—before a compressive (saturating) nonlinearity ultimately sets in. From a physiological point of view, an expansive nonlinearity can arise from any number of mechanisms, singly or in combination, which tend to make weak inputs weaker and/or strong inputs stronger (Fig. 11.1a). For example, several depolarization-gated inward currents exist in dendrites, including NMDA-type synaptic conductances, transient and persistent sodium channels, and several types of voltage-dependent calcium channels—any of which can boost synaptic excitation which is strong enough to enter into the channel's voltage activation range (Thomson *et al.* 1988; Cauller and Connors 1993; Schwindt and Crill 1995, 1996, 1997*a*,*b*, 1998; Lipowsky *et al.* 1996; Gillessen and Alzheimer 1997; Schiller *et al.* 1997; Seamans *et al.* 1997; Stuart *et al.* 1997; Thomson and Deuchars 1997; Golding and Spruston 1998; Margulis and Tang 1998; Urban *et al.* 1998). Less obviously, an outward current which opposes transient depolarizations can nonetheless boost the exponent (i.e. rate of acceleration) of a nonlinear compartmental response; a weakly activated compartment, which spends most of its time far below threshold, is heavily dependent on large transient fluctuations to trigger threshold crossings, and hence to generate action potentials within the compartment. A membrane current which reduces the magnitude of synaptic transients is thus particularly suppressive to the compartment's response under weaker input conditions. We have observed such an effect for the rapidly activating A-type potassium current (Brannon and Mel, unpublished simulations), which exists in high densities in hippocampal CA1 dendrites and acts in part to blunt transient synaptic responses (Hoffman *et al.* 1997)[1]. Thus, a variety of inward and outward currents which are commonly found in dendritic compartments appear designed to suppress weak inputs while boosting stronger inputs—the twin hallmarks of an expansive nonlinear operation.

One of the most common expansive nonlinearities which crops up in models of neural function derives from pairwise multiplication of input signals, such as is embedded in the half-squaring nonlinearity (x^2 for $x > 0$, otherwise zero) at the output stage of many so-called 'energy' models (Pollen and Ronner 1983; Adelson and Bergen 1985; Ohzawa *et al.* 1990; Heeger 1992; Ohzawa *et al.* 1997), along with other models that have been used to describe nonlinear receptive field properties in visual cortex (Peterhaus and von der Heydt 1980). Exponential growth is desirable, in turn, when it is required that one input to a compartment multiplicatively boosts

---

[1] In a compartment driven by a relatively sparse train of excitatory synaptic events, the A-current, which reduces EPSP peak size, can significantly reduce the probability of generating a threshold crossing, and hence of triggering an action potential. However, when the compartment is activated by a more intense barrage of synaptic input (e.g. via multiple synapses, or higher stimulus frequencies), the larger integrated (DC) component of the compartment response holds the compartment much closer to the spike threshold, and thus lessens the need for large transient excursions to cross threshold. The net effect of the A-current is thus to raise the threshold level of synaptic stimulus intensity needed to fire the compartment, without affecting the slope of the response to increasingly potent stimulus conditions. Our simulations used the A-current model as described in Migliore *et al.* (1999).

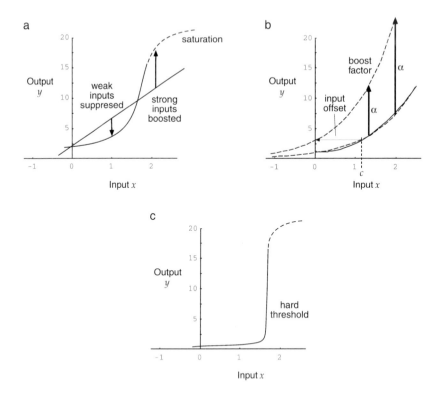

Fig. 11.1 Aspects of boosting nonlinearities. (a) A regime of accelerating growth in a compartment's input–output relation can be generated from an initially linear response curve by 'pushing down' on the low end, and/or by 'pushing up' the high end, possibly using different physiological mechanisms. When the dynamic range of the compartment is exhausted, the response curve saturates, leading to a typical globally sigmoidal structure. (b) An expansive nonlinearity such as a quadratic (solid line) may closely approximate exponential growth over a substantial range of output values (dashed fit). Over this range, any such function has the desirable property that a constant value added to the input x leads to a multiplicative boost in the output y. This holds because $\exp(x+c) = \alpha\exp(x)$, with constant $\alpha = \exp(c)$. (c) When the exponent is 'turned up', an expansive nonlinearity becomes a hard threshold, providing the basis for Boolean operations (e.g. AND and OR gates) and digital computation.

(or suppresses) the effect of the other inputs (Fig. 11.1b). This type of interaction arises, for example, wherever sensory responses are modulated by multiplicative 'gain fields' of one form or another (Zipser and Andersen 1988; Connor *et al.* 1997; McAdams and Maunsell 1999). Despite these different functional roles proposed for quadratic *versus* exponential nonlinearities, it is important to note that these two functional forms can closely approximate each other over an order-of-magnitude range of output values (Fig. 11.1b).

In addition to these continuous forms of accelerating growth, in the limit of a large exponent an expansive nonlinearity behaves like a hard threshold, and can thus underlie the logical AND and OR operations from which conventional digital computations are constructed (Fig. 11.1c).

Expansive nonlinear interactions between synapses have been frequently discussed and/or demonstrated in the biophysical modeling literature (Koch *et al.* 1982; Koch *et al.* 1986; Koch and Poggio 1987, 1992; Rall and Segev 1987; Shepherd and Brayton 1987; Mel 1992*a,b*, 1993; Mel *et al.* 1998*a,b*). Koch *et al.* were among the first to discuss the idea of nonlinear synaptic interactions, during a period in the early 1980s when extensive evidence for dendritic spiking and other active dendritic responses was not yet available. Instead, their focus was on nonlinear multiplicative interactions between depolarizing synaptic excitation and silent inhibition. Synapses with a reversal potential close to the compartment's resting potential, such as a GABA-mediated chloride conductance, were dubbed 'silent' or 'shunting' inhibition, since they act on the input resistance of the compartment rather than on the (resting) membrane potential. Given that the response of a compartment to a DC synaptic current scales with input resistance, the application and/or withdrawal of a silent inhibitory signal could be used to dial up or down the compartment's multiplicative gain in response to slowly varying input signals. Koch *et al.* focused primarily on the divisive 'veto' effect of a large silent inhibitory input, and referred to this pairing of excitation and silent inhibition as an AND–NOT operation.

Dendrites may provide space for multiple nonlinear computations

Reiterating the main thesis of this chapter, dendrites exist primarily to create space for expansive nonlinear synaptic interactions that can be carried out simultaneously in different parts of the tree. An important requirement for this type of dendritic function is that strong nonlinear interactions among synaptic inputs occur only within a compartment, but that compartment outputs combine approximately linearly in terms of their influence on the response of the cell as a whole. As an obvious corollary, the postsynaptic voltage environment in a dendritic neuron which is capable of supporting multiple quasi-independent nonlinear synaptic computations will generally be far from isopotential.

An early discussion of intradendritic physiology involving multiple independent active compartments can be found in Llinas and Nicholson (1971), where it was proposed that synaptically driven local spiking activity could occur independently in different branches of the Purkinje cell dendritic tree. In keeping with this idea, the accumulation of evidence from a large number of experimental studies leads to the conclusion that the dendrites of many neuron types in the mammalian brain support active events which do not reliably propagate throughout the dendritic arbor from their site of origin, whether the site of origin is in the soma or in the dendrites themselves (see Chapter 6 and 10). Several recent *in vitro* and *in vivo* studies illustrate this point, showing that synaptically-generated dendritic spikes do not necessarily propagate to other dendritic branches, or to the soma (Schiller *et al.* 1997; Stuart *et al.* 1997; Golding and Spruston 1998; Kamondi *et al.* 1998). In addition, an *in vitro* study of dendritic integration in CA1 cells using dual iontophoretic glutamate pipettes has recently shown that the main apical trunk of a CA1 cell, which acts as a thick central conduit that gathers current from a large number of oblique branches, typically exhibits sublinear integration—i.e. two inputs to the apical trunk produce a (subthreshold) somatic response which is significantly less than the sum of the individual responses (Cash and Yuste 1999). In contrast, the oblique branches, which emanate from the main apical trunk and are therefore well isolated from each other, show linear summation within a branch *as measured at the cell body*. However, given that an oblique dendrite must drive the somatic response via the apical trunk, which nonlinearly compresses its inputs, a linear response measured at the cell body implies a superlinear—i.e. boosting interaction between the two synaptic inputs to the stimulated oblique branch. This prediction remains unconfirmed, however, given that voltages were not recorded from the stimulated dendritic branches in the course of these experiments.

Given the enormous technical difficulty involved in recording voltage signals simultaneously from multiple locations within the same dendritic tree, and of targeting multiple specific synapses for activation, much of our present understanding of the electrical compartmentalization of spatially-extended dendritic trees derives from computer modeling studies.

An early modeling study by Rall and Rinzel (1973) provided a powerful demonstration of the voltage compartmentalization possible in passive dendritic structures, which derived from the strong attenuation of voltage signals moving from high to low-input-resistance structures—such as in the decay of a distally generated EPSP traveling in the direction of the soma or toward the interface with a main dendritic trunk (for a more recent treatment of passive attenuation issues, see Zador *et al.* 1995). A recent study combining experiments and modeling suggests that some synaptic potentials may attenuate more than 100 fold when propagating from the distal dendrites to the soma of layer V pyramidal neurons (Stuart and Spruston 1998).

In a first detailed look at the compartmentalization of synaptic interactions, Koch *et al.* (1982) took up the case of retinal ganglion cells, and formally defined a dendritic 'subunit' as a region within which the voltage attenuation is small between any pair of synapses within the subunit, but large between every synapse within the subunit and the soma. This definition did not explicitly enforce isolation of subunits from each other, but such isolation was introduced implicitly in the authors' choice of distinct branch tips as subunit seeds. Under reasonable assumptions for the underlying biophysical parameters, Koch *et al.* (1982) found that the relatively large α-type retinal ganglion cell has a considerable capacity for independent voltage processing within its dendritic tree, whereas the physically smaller β-type ganglion cell did not. Woolf *et al.* (1991) carried out a somewhat different analysis of subunit structure in granule cells of the olfactory bulb, which likewise indicated that significant compartmentalization of voltage signals is possible in a passive dendritic tree.

Significantly, the subunit boundaries seen in both of these studies were extremely sensitive to parameters of the analysis, underscoring the fact that voltage communication between any two points in a dendritic tree is in actuality a continuous function of the type of stimulus (small *versus* large, transient *versus* steady-state, etc.), the length of the intervening path, branch geometry, passive cable properties, ongoing synaptic activation, and the numerous voltage-dependent currents found in dendrites. The explicit enumeration of hard-edged subunits within a branched dendritic structure is therefore not feasible.

Without abandoning the basic notion of electrical compartmentalization, however, a more operational approach to the determination of dendritic subunit processing capacity can be sought. Specifically, a dendritic tree can be said to support functional compartmentalization to the extent that nonlinear synaptic interactions can occur simultaneously within multiple dendritic subregions with relatively little crosstalk, i.e. where the local nonlinear response to synaptic input within each subregion is relatively little affected by ongoing activity in other subregions. In lieu of a hard mapping between functional subunits and dendritic subregions, therefore, the capacity of a dendritic tree for compartmentalized nonlinear processing can be quantified by determining empirically the number of distinct sites, perhaps randomly chosen, perhaps optimally chosen, at which quasi-independent nonlinear synaptic interactions can simultaneously occur.

While experimental methods do not currently exist that enable the specific activation of a relatively large, select set (e.g. 10s to 100s) of presynaptic terminals, numerous biophysical modeling studies have shown that dendritic structures are capable of compartmentalizing nonlinear synaptic interactions, in the sense that the response of the neuron differs significantly depending on the relative locations of activated presynaptic terminals distributed across multiple dendritic branches (Koch *et al.* 1986; Rall and Segev 1987; Borg-Graham and Grzywacz 1992; Mel 1992*a,b*, 1993; Zador *et al.* 1992; Mel *et al.* 1998*a,b*). We showed, for example, that dendrites containing active channels in various combinations (NMDA-type synapses, sodium or calcium spiking mechanisms) respond much more strongly when a fixed total amount of excitatory synaptic drive is concentrated within a number of subregions rather than spread diffusely about the dendritic arbor (Mel 1993). This basic phenomenon has been observed for a large range of cell morphologies, channel properties and combinations, with and without spines, from single test pulses to high frequency trains, and for synchronous *versus* asynchronous synaptic input. Intuitively, a small number (e.g. 4) synapses which are activated near to each other, such as on the same dendritic branch, may be sufficient to drive the branch well up into its expansive nonlinear regime, whereas four equally potent synapses activated on separate branches might produce essentially no active response in any branch. Less obvious is the extent to which this scenario can be played out simultaneously at multiple sites throughout the dendritic tree; when some critical density of synaptic excitation is reached, the cell and all of its compartments will be fully activated, regardless of the detailed arrangement of activated synaptic contacts. While the upper limit on this capacity has yet to be worked out for any particular cell morphology and underlying set of biophysical assumptions, for large cells the number of sites at which expansive nonlinear interactions can be carried out with acceptably low levels of crosstalk may be upwards of several dozen (Mel 1993; Mel *et al.* 1998*b*).

This large capacity for a branched dendritic tree to compartmentalize multiple active events can be seen in a model CA1 pyramidal cell with active dendrites, stimulated synaptically with single test pulses (Fig. 11.2). Each pulse activated a randomly distributed population of 70 excitatory synapses confined mostly to the stratum radiatum, and each synapse was modeled with colocalized AMPA and NMDA-type conductances. Dendrites contained voltage-dependent sodium channels and both delayed rectifier and A-type potassium channels, following the CA1 cell model of Migliore *et al.* (1999). Fig. 11.2 shows the local voltage peaks at each of the 70 synapses (black dots) and the soma (open circles) in a series of trials, where in each trial the synapse locations were reassigned at random. The bimodal distribution of peak voltages within a given trial indicates that dendritically initiated spikes, which were typically 40–50 mV in height, were confined within certain subregions, and were only occasionally able to elicit a somatic spike.

Regarding experimental evidence for this type of dendritic integration, several studies have reported nonlinear boosting of synaptic inputs by voltage-dependent channels in the dendrites (Thomson *et al.* 1988; Cauller and Connors 1993; Schwindt and Crill 1995; Lipowsky *et al.* 1996; Schwindt and Crill 1996, 1997*a,b*, 1998; Gillessen and Alzheimer 1997; Schiller *et al.* 1997; Seamans *et al.* 1997; Stuart *et al.* 1997; Thomson and Deuchars 1997; Golding and Spruston 1998; Margulis and Tang 1998; Urban *et al.* 1998). However, a major technical obstacle impedes clarification of this issue—the lack of an available method to stimulate many synapses at known locations. Instead, synaptic activation of a cell is typically achieved by shocking a bundle of fibers which projects into the dendritic field of a target neuron, activating an unknown number of excitatory and inhibitory synapses at unknown locations, through both monosynaptic and polysynaptic pathways. This diffuse, unvisualized spray of synaptic activity is poorly suited to evaluate hypotheses regarding compartmentalization of nonlinear postsynaptic function, since it is impossible to either measure or control the degree of synaptic interaction.

Dendrites could play many computational roles in visual cortex

To this point, we have summarized evidence from physiological and modeling studies which indicates that dendritic neurons are biophysically well suited to support multiple, quasi-independent expansive nonlinear operations, which in some cells may arise from dendritic spiking confined to those subregions receiving concentrated synaptic input. This type of computing device provides a parsimonious account for many kinds of nonlinear processing operations which are known to be carried out in neural tissue (Koch *et al.* 1982*a*, 1986; Koch and Poggio 1987; Mel 1992*a,b*; Mel *et al.* 1998*b*; Poirazi and Mel 1999).

In the remainder of this chapter, we focus on the potential contribution of intradendritic processing to several nonlinear receptive field properties and modulatory influences in the visual cortex, in part to emphasize how the dendrites of a single neuron could participate in several different kinds of processing functions. Some of these ideas have been fleshed out in detail in published studies, while others involve extrapolation and conjecture.

A wide variety of receptive field nonlinearities and modulatory influences seen in visual cortical neurons have been characterized using mathematical or computational models, including position and contrast-invariant orientation tuning (Hubel and Wiesel 1962; Ohzawa *et al.* 1990; Heeger 1992), position-invariant binocular disparity tuning (Ohzawa *et al.* 1997; Livingstone and Tsao 1999), direction selectivity (Adelson and Bergen 1985), motion processing in MT (Nowlan and Sejnowski 1993) and MST (Perrone and Stone 1998), complex shape selectivity coupled with spatial invariance (Fukushima *et al.* 1983; Kobatake and Tanaka

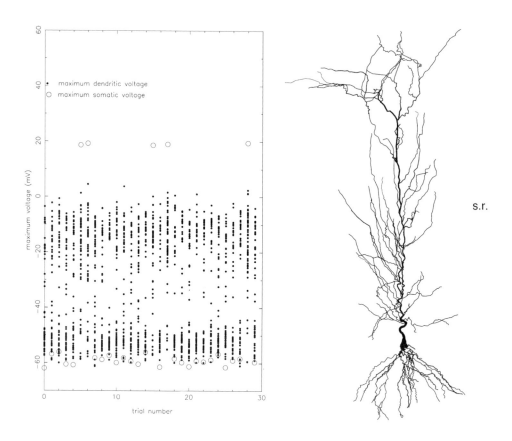

Fig. 11.2 Compartmentalization of synaptically generated dendritic spikes in a model CA1 cell, shown at right (morphology courtesy of D. A. Turner). Dendrites contained an increasing concentration of A-type potassium channels moving from the soma into the dendrites, as first described in (Hoffman *et al.* 1997). Dendrites also contained weak voltage-dependent sodium and potassium currents, which were capable of initiating local dendritic action potentials, but which did not necessarily trigger a somatic spike—and which were not necessarily even recognizable as spikes at a typical slice recording site in the apical trunk. Channel parameters and implementation were courtesy of Michele Migliore, adapted from (Migliore *et al.* 1999). Seventy synapses were distributed at random throughout a restricted portion of the dendritic tree, consisting of any branch falling between 380 and 760 μm from the cell body along the dendritic path length—this corresponded approximately to dendrites falling within the stratum radiatum (s.r.). As in typical slice experiments, the synapses were activated by a single test pulse; the synaptic conductances were modeled as colocalized AMPA and NMDA-type channels. The voltage peak was recorded at each stimulated synapse (black dots) and at the soma (open circles) in a series of 30 trials. Each trial represented a different random distribution of synapse locations. In a typical trial, spiking was in evidence in some, but not all, dendritic compartments, and only in a few cases did dendritic spikes trigger somatic spikes. Biophysical parameters were as follows: $\bar{g}_{AMPA} = 1$ nS, $\bar{g}_{NMDA}/\bar{g}_{AMPA} = 0.6$, $\bar{g}_{Na} = 30$ mS cm^{-2} (soma and dendrites), $\bar{g}_{Na} = 620$ mS cm^{-2} (axon), $\bar{g}_{K_{DR}}/\bar{g}_{Na} = 0.3$ in all cases, and $\bar{g}_{K_A}$ was distributed as an increasing function of distance from the soma. Figure provided by Terrence Brannon.

1994), illusory contour detection (Peterhaus and von der Heydt 1980), contour completion (Kapadia *et al.* 1995), modulation of visual responses by eye-position gain fields (Zipser and Andersen 1988), and stimulus-response modulation via selective attention (Connor *et al.* 1997; McAdams and Maunsell 1999). In each case, the response property in question may be broken down into a set of nonlinear subunit computations of a relatively generic form, i.e. where the input to a subunit—which most often consists of two excitatory synaptic inputs—is summed and then passed through an expansive nonlinearity. The close relation between this type of computation and the biophysical capacities of active dendrites leads to the conjecture that intradendritic processing could contribute in many and varied ways to the response properties of visual cortical neurons.

Fig. 11.3 represents a pictorial conjecture as to how five different nonlinear response properties could arise from dendritic subunit computations within a single layer 2–3 pyramidal cell in visual cortex. The superposition of these several functions within the same neuron is not to be taken too literally, however, since the experimental data relating to these several types of nonlinear receptive field phenomena has been derived from both striate and extrastriate areas in both cats and monkeys.

First, in a recent biophysical modeling study, we demonstrated that the combination of phase invariance and orientation tuning, which are hallmark features of complex cells in visual cortex, could arise in a neuron receiving only monosynaptic, unoriented LGN inputs, as long as:

(1) the LGN inputs are appropriately grouped onto dendritic branches, which act essentially like simple cells; and

(2) the pyramidal cell dendrites contain a sufficient complement of excitatory voltage-dependent channels, including either NMDA-type synaptic conductances, voltage-dependent sodium channels, or both (Mel *et al.* 1998*b*).

In Fig. 11.3, the basic wiring diagram is represented schematically by direct LGN connections (A) to a basal dendrite deep in layer 3, which acts like a single virtual monocular simple cell. Several such groupings with progressively shifted composite receptive fields projected to other dendritic branches. Based only upon these monosynaptic excitatory connections, a modeled cell showed orientation-tuned responses to both light and dark bars over its entire receptive field, which was approximately three times wider than the bar stimulus (Fig. 11.4). In a functionally redundant pathway, two actual simple cells are indicated in Fig. 11.3 with slightly shifted receptive fields are indicated as separate neurons in layer 4 (cells B and B′), both of which drive the overlying complex cell following the tenets of the classical Hubel–Wiesel model (Alonso and Martinez 1998). This notion that complex cells are driven by multiple subunits with shifted spatial phases is one of several neuronal functions which has been compactly encapsulated in the form of an energy model, in which several linear simple-cell-like subunits are each passed through an expansive (half-squaring) nonlinearity before their outputs are combined linearly (Pollen and Ronner 1983; Heeger 1992). In the current context, the key points are that:

(1) an active dendritic branch is biophysically capable of generating the nonlinearity which has traditionally been attributed to the global spiking mechanism of a standalone simple cell; and

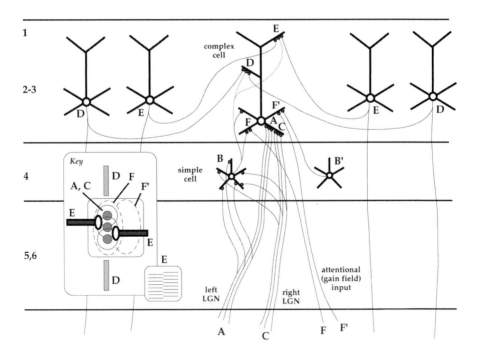

Fig. 11.3 Pictorial conjecture regarding contribution of local expansive nonlinear processing in pyramidal cell dendrites to several visual receptive field properties involving both classical and nonclassical receptive field effects. (A) One simple-cell-like subunits is formed via direct LGN contacts on basal dendrites of a deep layer 2–3 pyramidal cell. (B,B′) Two actual simple cells provide redundant subunit inputs to the overlying complex cell, representing two slightly shifted receptive fields. (C) Direct LGN input contributes to binocular disparity-tuned subunits on complex cell dendrites. (D) Nonlinear boosting of response to stimulus in classical receptive field by colinear stimuli in the extraclassical surround could derive from nonlinear post-synaptic interactions. (E) Pairs of appropriately positioned end-stopped units, consistent with the same illusory contour (see mini-inset), could join in multiplicative conjunctions (as proposed by Peterhaus and von der Heydt 1989) directly within the dendrites of target complex cell. (F,F′) Modulatory inputs, representing gain fields or attentional foci could multiplicatively boost afferents onto target cell via expansive postsynaptic compartment nonlinearity. Boosting can be specific to subregions of the receptive field ((F) vs. (F′)).

(2) the several virtual simple cell subunits needed to compose a phase-invariant complex cell receptive field can be mapped onto several dendritic branches, whose separately thresholded outputs combine linearly to drive the cell's global output.

Second, this monocular scenario can be extended to incorporate binocular disparity tuning. Studies of disparity tuning in cats (Ohzawa *et al.* 1990, 1997) and monkeys (Livingstone and Tsao 1999) indicate that a significant number of complex cells in primarily visual cortex exhibit a sensitivity to horizontal disparity

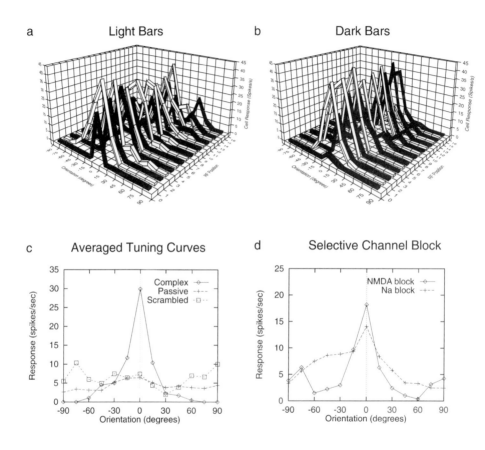

Fig. 11.4 Phase-invariant orientation tuning of a 'complex' cell could derive from simple-cell-like subunits formed within dendritic branches. (a,b) Orientation tuning curves in response to optimal-width light and dark bars over a range of receptive field positions for a single model complex cell. Tuning is roughly invariant to stimulus position and contrast polarity. (c) Average of tuning curves at all positions for light and dark bars is shown in a,b ('Complex'). Tuning is abolished when synapses were spatially scrambled in the dendritic tree ('Scrambled'), or when all voltage-dependent channels (NMDA, dendritic voltage-gated Na^+ and K^+ channels) were blocked leaving an electrically passive cell ('Passive'). (d) Orientation tuning persisted when cells contained either of the two voltage-dependent mechanisms alone. Averaged tuning curves are shown for a cell in which NMDA channels were blocked, leaving only dendritic Na^+ channels to support nonlinear dendritic integration (diamonds). When dendritic voltage-gated Na^+ and K^+ channels were blocked instead, leaving NMDA channels as only source of voltage-dependent dendritic current, the cell remained orientation tuned, though individual tuning curves were broader and noisier; an average tuning curve for 5 complex cells is shown in this case (pluses). Figure reprinted from Mel *et al.* 1998*b*.

much finer than the overall receptive field dimension. This type of nonlinear response has also been described by an energy model (Ohzawa *et al.* 1990, 1997). According to conventional notions, the expansive nonlinearity would again be provided by a separate population of binocular simple cells, in such species where these simple cell precursors exist (Ohzawa *et al.* 1997; they apparently do not in the monkey—see Livingstone and Tsao 1999). However, as indicated in Fig. 11.3, dendritic subunits (A,C) could subserve this function as well (Koch and Poggio 1987; Mel *et al.* 1998*a*).

A third type of nonlinear effect which has been observed in visual cortex involves boosting of the response to an optimally-oriented bar within the classical receptive field of a cell, when it is presented together with a colinear bar in the nonclassical surround—but where the surround stimulus is ineffective on its own (Kapadia *et al.* 1995). Given that the neural signals activated by the surround stimulus are likely carried by horizontal axon collaterals in the superficial layers of cortex (Gilbert 1992), the nonlinear gating interaction between these surround signals and those representing the within-receptive field stimulus could be effected by local post-synaptic boosting within the dendrites of the target neuron (Fig. 11.3D) In the absence of such an account, it is unclear what other intermediary could provide the requisite nonlinearity.

A fourth type of nonlinear effect seen in visual cortex involves a mechanism which could underlie responses to illusory contours. Specifically, some neurons in monkey extrastriate cortex respond to contours which are specified only implicitly by collections of line ends that terminate perpendicularly on the contour in question from both sides (see mini-inset at lower right of Fig. 11.3E)—a visual occurrence which strongly suggests the overlap of two differently textured surfaces (Peterhaus and von der Heydt 1980). These authors proposed a model for the observed neuronal responses in which a set of appropriately-oriented end-stopped neurons (i.e. which are inhibited by a stimulus extending beyond the central receptive field), all consistent with the same physical contour, are grouped in numerous pairwise combinations into AND-like subunits before feeding a conventional oriented contour-sensitive neuron. In a possible dendritic substrate for the needed pairwise conjunctions, a representative pair of end-stopped cells which give rise to excitatory horizontal connections are shown to terminate within the same locally thresholded (i.e. expansively boosted) dendritic subunit (Fig. 11.3E).

A fifth example of a nonlinear visual receptive field interaction involves the multiplicative boosting seen where gain fields modulate neuronal responses (Zipser and Andersen 1988) and in some forms of selective visual attention (Connor *et al.* 1997; McAdams and Maunsell 1999). For example, when a monkey attends a stimulus within the receptive field of a V4 neuron, the orientation tuning curve for the cell is boosted such that the responses at all orientations are scaled up by approximately the same multiplicative factor (1.3). While the biophysical origin of this nonlinear boosting factor is not known, its compatibility with postsynaptic biophysics invites the conjecture that the effect results from an attentionally-modulated synaptic input, properly targeted to the dendritic subunit(s) representing the attended stimulus (Fig. 11.3F). Note that an attentional input representing a slightly shifted locus within the receptive field modulates a different dendritic subunit (Fig. 11.3F′).

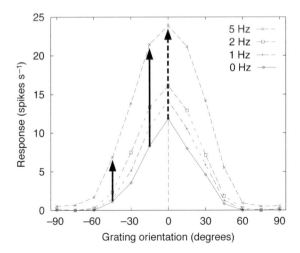

Fig. 11.5   Nonlinear boosting of tuning curves was seen in a detailed biophysical model, as a result of incrementing a weak constant background input to four dendritic branches involved in the computation. Multiplicative boosting of curves (compare tuning curves for 0 Hz and 5 Hz modulatory inputs) is similar to that seen for attended stimuli by McAdams and Maunsell (1999). Figure provided by Kevin Archie.

We tested the feasibility of this dendritic account for response scaling using a pre-existing compartmental model for orientation and disparity tuning which employed a highly reduced morphology, but was otherwise conceptually similar to that described in (Mel *et al.* 1998*a*). A series of orientation tuning curves was generated for the cell under increasing levels of attentional focus, which was modeled by delivering a modulatory input to each compartment, that progressively incremented the background firing rate of every synapse. As shown in Fig. 11.5, the tuning curves exhibit an expansive nonlinear scaling, where strong responses are boosted more than weak responses (compare two solid arrows), though the boost is seen to saturate for the strongest input conditions (dashed arrow).

Concluding remarks

In this chapter we have adopted the view, rooted in numerous experimental and modeling studies, that dendrites provide space for a large number of functionally independent nonlinear synaptic interactions, which can occur simultaneously across the dendritic tree. Thus, unlike the view of dendritic function embodied in the null hypothesis, which emphasizes the effect of each synapse at the cell body, the present perspective emphasizes instead the effect of a synapse *on the effectiveness of other synapses* in its vicinity. In particular, activation of localized groups of synapses may lead to dendritic spikes; multiple spikes arising in different dendritic branches may then sum to drive the cell's output via action potentials traveling down the axon. We have argued that the most important type of compartmentalized synaptic interaction is an expansive nonlinear one, based on:

(1) the properties of channels known to exist in nearly all types of dendrites that have been studied;

(2) experimental studies that indicate synaptic inputs can be amplified by dendritic spikes and/or membrane conductances operating in the subthreshold range;

(3) biophysical modeling studies that confirm the robustness of this type of interaction; and

(4) the repeated appearance of essentially this same nonlinear functional form in diverse models of neural responses.

Viewed in this way, a dendritic neuron is akin to a two-layer artificial neural network with a single output unit, and a set of sigmoidal hidden units driven by partially overlapping sets of input variables. This type of connection has been discussed at length elsewhere (Mel 1992*b*; Poirazi and Mel 1999).

Given that a dendritic branch or other subregion may exhibit the same kind of input–output nonlinearity which is normally attributed to a standalone neuron—whether biological or artificial—it is useful to consider some of the advantages that the brain may accrue by 'loading up' its dendrites with nonlinear subunit processing capacity. First, and most obviously, the power of computer hardware is most often quantified by counting nonlinear subunits of one form or another. For example, the power of a microprocessor is often quantified by the number of transistors it contains, the power of a Boolean logic network is quantified by the number of gates it contains, and the representational power of a neural network is often quantified by the number of hidden units or fixed nonlinear basis functions it contains. Thus, given the opportunity to increase the number of functioning nonlinear elements in a computer by one or two orders of magnitude, while maintaining the same general architecture, the designer is obviously well advised to do so. In the brain, an accidental confluence of spatially-extended neuronal morphologies and voltage-dependent ionic channels may have provided just such an opportunity. Additionally, dendrites retain the capacity for significant growth into adulthood in response to demands of the environment (Greenough and Bailey 1988; Chapter 14), which may allow a neuron to adaptively boost its own nonlinear processing capacity, as needed. In contrast, the option to grow more neurons does not exist in most parts of most nervous systems.

Fig. 11.3 illustrates a diversity of roles that could be played by a single multicompartment neuron, and buttresses the notion that individual dendrites may participate in numerous functions of cortical tissue which have normally been ascribed to whole neurons, or to cortical circuits. However, the choice of examples given here does not necessarily imply that the functions of compartmentalized active dendrites are limited to sensory processing operations. We have in other work, for example, found that compartmentalized dendritic nonlinearities could significantly boost the memory capacity of neural tissue, and that this capacity can be directly exploited using Hebb-like learning rules to establish the mapping of afferent connections onto the dendritic tree (Mel 1992*a,b*; Poirazi and Mel 1999). Possible contributions of active dendritic integration to nonlinear processing operations in many other neural contexts remain to be considered.

Two main avenues for experimental validation of the ideas discussed in this chapter involve:

(1) demonstrating that intracellular blockade of dendritic channels either reduces or eliminates some key form of nonlinear response—for example orientation or disparity tuning in LGN-recipient complex cells; or

(2) demonstrating using either anatomical or live imaging techniques that afferent axons target postsynaptic cells in spatially appropriate ways, i.e. as predicted by the type and degree of nonlinear interactions required among them.

Such experiments are important, in that they could help to establish dendrites as major contributors to the brain's computing capacity—which has to this point largely escaped detection.

Acknowledgements

Thanks to Kevin Archie, Terrence Brannon, Gary Holt, and Nelson Spruston for many useful discussions and help with figures. This work was funded by the National Science Foundation and the Office of Naval Research.

References

Adelson, E. and Bergen, J. (1985). Spatiotemporal energy models for the perception of motion. *Journal of the Optical Society of America*, **A2**, 284–99.

Alonso, J.-M. and Martinez, L. M. (1998). Functional connectivity between simple cells and complex cells in cat striate cortex. *Nature Neuroscience*, **1**, 395–403.

Borg-Graham, L. and Grzywacz, N. (1992). A model of the direction selectivity circuit in retina: transformations by neurons singly and in concert. In *Single neuron computation*. (ed. T. McKenna, J. Davis, and S. Zornetzer), pp. 347–375. Academic Press, Cambridge, MA.

Cash, S. and Yuste, R. (1999). Linear summation of excitatory inputs by CA1 pyramidal neurons. *Neuron*, **22**, 383–94.

Cauller, L. J. and Connors, B. W. (1992). Functions of very distal dendrites: experimental and computational studies of layer I synapses on neocortical pyramidal cells. In *Single neuron computation*, (ed. T. McKenna, J. Davis, and S. Zornetzer), pp. 199–229. Academic Press, Boston.

Cauller, L. J. and Connors, B. W. (1993). Synaptic physiology of horizontal afferents to layer I in slices of rat SI neocortex. *Journal of Neuroscience*, **18**, 751–62.

Connor, C. E., Preddie, D. C., Gallant, J. L., and Van Essen, D. C. (1997). Spatial attention effects in macaque area V4. *Journal of Neuroscience*, **17**, 3201–14.

Cook, E. P. and Johnston, D. (1999). Voltage-dependent properties of dendrites that eliminate location-dependent variability of synaptic input. *Journal of Neurophysiology*, **81**, 535–43.

De Schutter, E. and Bower, J. M. (1994). Simulated responses of cerebellar Purkinje cells are independent of the dendritic location of granule cell synaptic inputs. *Proceedings of the National Academy of Science USA*, **91**, 4736–40.

Fukushima, K., Miyake, S., and Ito, T. (1983). Neocognitron: a neural network model for a mechanism of visual pattern recognition. *IEEE Transactions on Systems, Man and Cybernetics*, **SMC-13**, 826–34.

Gilbert, C. D. (1992). Horizontal integration and cortical dynamics. *Neuron*, **9**, 1–13.

Gillessen, T. and Alzheimer, C. (1997). Amplification of EPSPs by low Ni^{2+}- and amiloride-sensitive Ca^{2+} channels in apical dendrites of rat CA1 pyramidal neurons. *Journal of Neurophysiology*, **77**, 1639–43.

Golding, N. L. and Spruston, N. (1998). Dendritic sodium spikes are variable triggers of action potentials in hippocampal CA1 pyramidal neurons. *Neuron*, **21**, 1189–200.

Greenough, W. and Bailey, C. (1988). The anatomy of memory: convergence of results across a diversity of tests. *Trends in Neurosciences*, **11**, 142–7.

Heeger, D. (1992). Normalization of cell responses in cat striate cortex. *Visual Neuroscience*, **9**, 181–97.

Hoffman, D. A., Magee, J. C., Colbert, C. M., and Johnston, D. (1997). K^+ channel regulation of signal propagation in dendrites of hippocampal pyramidal neurons. *Nature*, **387**, 869–75.

Hubel, D. and Wiesel, T. (1962). Receptive fields, binocular interaction and functional architecture in the cat's visual cortex. *Journal of Physiology*, **160**, 106–54.

Kamondi, A., Acsady, L., and Buzsaki, G. (1998). Dendritic spikes are enhanced by co-operative network activity in the intact hippocampus. *Journal of Neuroscience*, **18**, 3919–28.

Kapadia, M. K., Ito, M., Gilbert, C. D., and Westheimer, G. (1995). Improvement in visual sensitivity by changes in local context: parallel studies in human observers and in V1 of alert monkeys. *Neuron*, **15**, 843–56.

Kobatake, E. and Tanaka, K. (1994). Neuronal selectivities to complex object features in the ventral visual pathway of the macaque cerebral cortex. *Journal of Neurophysiology*, **71**, 856–67.

Koch, C. (1998). *Biophysics of computation*. Oxford University Press, New York.

Koch, C. and Poggio, T. (1987). Biophysics of computation: neurons, synapses, and membranes. In *Synaptic Function*, (ed. G. Edelman, W. Gall, and W. Cowan), pp. 637–697. Wiley, New York.

Koch, C. and Poggio, T. (1992). Multiplying with synapses and neurons. In *Single neuron computation*, (ed. T. McKenna, J. Davis, and S. Zornetzer), pp. 315–45. Academic Press, Cambridge, MA.

Koch, C., Poggio, T., and Torre, V. (1982). Retinal ganglion cells: a functional interpretation of dendritic morphology. *Philosophical Transactions of the Royal Society of London, Series B*, **298**, 227–63.

Koch, C., Poggio, T., and Terra, V. (1986). Computations in the vertebrate retina: gain enhancement, differentiation and motion discrimination. *Trends in Neurosciences*, **9**, 204–11.

Koester, H. J. and Sakmann, B. (1998). Calcium dynamics in single spines during coincident pre- and postsynaptic activity depend on relative timing of back-propagating action potentials and subthreshold excitatory postsynaptic potentials. *Proceedings of the National Academy of Science USA*, **95**, 9596–601.

Lipowsky, R., Gillessen, T., and Alzheimer, C. (1996). Dendritic Na^+ channels amplify EPSPs in hippocampal CA1 pyramidal cells. *Journal of Neurophysiology*, **76**, 2181–91.

Livingstone, M. S. and Tsao, D. (1999). Two-bar interactions in space and time: evidence for common mechanisms for stereopsis and direction selectivity. (Submitted for publication.)

Llinas, R. and Nicholson, C. (1971). Electrophysiological properties of dendrites and somata in alligator Purkinje cells. *Journal of Neurophysiology*, **34**, 534–51.

Magee, J. C. and Johnston, D. (1997). A synaptically controlled, associative signal for Hebbian plasticity in hippocampal neurons. *Science*, **275**, 209–13.

Mainen, Z. F. and Sejnowski, T. J. (1996). Influence of dendritic structure on firing pattern in model neocortical neurons. *Nature*, **382**, 363–6.

Margulis, M. and Tang, C. (1998). Temporal integration can readily switch between sublinear and supralinear summation. *Journal of Neurophysiology*, **79**, 2809–13.

Markram, H., Lübke, J., Frotscher, M., and Sakmann, B. (1997). Regulation of synaptic efficacy by coincidence of postsynaptic APs and EPSPs. *Science*, **275**, 213–15.

McAdams, C. J. and Maunsell, J. H. R. (1999). Effects of attention on orientation-tuning functions of single neurons in macaque cortical area V4. *Journal of Neuroscience*, **19**, 431–41.

Mel, B. W. (1992a). The clusteron: Toward a simple abstraction for a complex neuron. In *Advances in neural information processing systems*, (ed. J. Moody, S. Hanson, and R. Lippmann), pp. 35–42. Morgan Kaufmann, San Mateo.

Mel, B. W. (1992*b*). NMDA-based pattern discrimination in a modeled cortical neuron. *Neural Computation*, **4**, 502–16.

Mel, B. W. (1993). Synaptic integration in an excitable dendritic tree. *Journal of Neurophysiology*, **70**, 1086–101.

Mel, B. W. (1994). Information processing in dendritic trees. *Neural Computation*, **6**, 1031–5.

Mel, B. W., Ruderman, D. L., and Archie, K. A. (1998*a*). Toward a single cell account of binocular disparity tuning: an energy model may be hiding in your dendrites. In *Advances in neural information processing systems*, (ed. M. I. Jordan, M. J. Kearns, and S. A. Solla), pp. 208–14. MIT Press, Cambridge, MA.

Mel, B. W., Ruderman, D. L., and Archie, K. A. (1998*b*). Translation-invariant orientation tuning in visual 'complex' cells could derive from intradendritic computations. *Journal of Neuroscience*, **18**, 4325–34.

Migliore, M., Hoffman, D., Magee, J., and Johnston, D. (1999). Role of an A-type K^+ conductance in the back-propagation of action potentials in the dendrites of hippocampal pyramidal neurons. *Journal of Computational Neuroscience*. (Submitted for publication.)

Nowlan, S. and Sejnowski, T. (1993). Filter selection model for generating visual motion signals. In *Advances in neural information processing systems*, (ed. S. Hanson, J. Cowan, and L. Giles), pp. 369–376. Morgan Kaufmann, San Mateo.

Ohzawa, I., DeAngelis, G. C., and Freeman, R. D. (1990). Stereoscopic depth discrimination in the visual cortex: neurons ideally suited as disparity detectors. *Science*, **249**, 1037–41.

Ohzawa, I., DeAngelis, G. C., and Freeman, R. D. (1997). Encoding of binocular disparity by complex cells in the cat's visual cortex. *Journal of Neurophysiology*, **77**, 2879–909.

Patil, M. M., Linster, C., Lubenov, E., and Hasselmo, M. E. (1998). Cholinergic agonist carbachol enables associative long-term potentiation in piriform cortex slices. *Journal of Neurophysiology*, **80**, 2467–74.

Perrone, J. A. and Stone, L. S. (1998). Emulating the visual receptive-field properties of MST neurons with a template model of heading estimation. *Journal of Neuroscience*, **18**, 5958–75.

Peterhaus, E. and von der Heydt, R. (1980). Mechanisms of contour perception in monkey visual cortex. II. Contours bridging gaps. *Journal of Neuroscience*, **9**, 1749–63.

Poirazi, Y. and Mel, B. W. (1999). The memory capacity of subsampled quadratic classifiers: why active dendrites may remember more. *Neural Computation* (In press).

Pollen, D. and Ronner, S. (1983). Visual cortical neurons as localized spatial frequency filters. *IEEE Transactions on Systems, Man and Cybernetics*, **13**, 907–16.

Rall, W. and Rinzel, J. (1973). Branch input resistance and steady attenuation for input to one branch of a dendritic neuron model. *Biophysical Journal*, **13**, 648–87.

Rall, W. and Segev, I. (1987). Functional possibilities for synapses on dendrites and dendritic spines. In *Synaptic function*, (ed. G. M. Adelman, W. E. Gall, and W. M. Cowan), pp. 605–36. Wiley, NY.

Schiller, J., Schiller, Y., Stuart, G., and Sakmann, B. (1997). Calcium action potentials restricted to distal apical dendrites of rat neocortical pyramidal neurons. *Journal of Physiology*, **505**, 605–16.

Schiller, J., Schiller, Y., and Clapham, D. E. (1998). NMDA receptors amplify calcium influx into dendritic spines during associative pre- and postsynaptic activation. *Nature Neuroscience*, **1**, 114–18.

Schwindt, P. C. and Crill, W. E. (1995). Amplification of synaptic current by persistent sodium conductance in apical dendrite of neocortical neurons. *Journal of Neurophysiology*, **74**, 2220–4.

Schwindt, P. and Crill, W. (1996). Equivalence of amplified current flowing from dendrite to soma measured by alteration of repetitive firing and by voltage clamp in layer 5 pyramidal neurons. *Journal of Neurophysiology*, **76**, 3731–9.

Schwindt, P. C. and Crill, W. E. (1997*a*). Local and propagated dendritic action potentials evoked by glutamate iontophoresis on rat neocortical pyramidal neurons. *Journal of Neurophysiology*, **77**, 2466–83.

Schwindt, P. C. and Crill, W. E. (1997*b*). Modification of current transmitted from apical dendrite to soma by blockade of voltage- and Ca^{2+}-dependent conductances in rat neocortical pyramidal neurons. *Journal of Neurophysiology*, **78**, 187–98.

Schwindt, P. C. and Crill, W. E. (1998). Synaptically evoked dendritic action potentials in rat neocortical pyramidal neurons. *Journal of Neurophysiology*, **79**, 2432–46.

Seamans, J. K., Gorelova, N. A., and Yang, C. R. (1997). Contributions of voltage-gated Ca^{2+} channels in the proximal *versus* distal dendrites to synaptic integration in prefrontal cortical neurons. *Journal of Neuroscience*, **17**, 5936–48.

Segev, I. and Rall, W. (1998). Excitable dendrites and spines: earlier theoretical insights elucidate recent direct observations. *Trends in Neurosciences*, **21**, 453–60.

Shepherd, G. (1998). *The synaptic organization of the brain.* Oxford University Press.

Shepherd, G. M. and Brayton, R. K. (1987). Logic operations are properties of computer-simulated interactions between excitable dendritic spines. *Neuroscience*, **21**, 151–65.

Spencer, W. A. and Kandel, E. R. (1961). Electrophysiology of hippocampal neurons. IV. Fast prepotentials. *Journal of Neurophysiology*, **24**, 272–85.

Spruston, N., Schiller, Y., Stuart, G., and Sakmann, B. (1995). Activity-dependent action potential invasion and calcium influx into hippocampal CA1 dendrites. *Science*, **268**, 297–300.

Stuart, G. and Spruston, N. (1998). Determinants of voltage attenuation in neocortical pyramidal neuron dendrites. *Journal of Neuroscience*, **18**, 3501–10.

Stuart, G., Schiller, J., and Sakmann, B. (1997). Action potential initiation in neocortical pyramidal neurons. *Journal of Physiology*, **505**, 617–32.

Thomson, A. M. and Deuchars, J. (1997). Synaptic interactions in neocortical local circuits: dual intracellular recordings in vitro. *Cerebral Cortex*, **7**, 510–22.

Thomson, A. M., Girdlestone, D., and West, D. C. (1988). Voltage-dependent currents prolong single-axon postsynaptic potentials in layer III pyramidal neurons in rat neocortical slices. *Journal of Neurophysiology*, **60**, 1896–907.

Traub, R. D. (1982). Simulation of intrinsic bursting in CA3 hippocampal neurons. *Neuroscience*, **7**, 1233–42.

Urban, N. N., Henze, D. A., and Barrionuevo, G. (1998). Amplification of perforant-path EPSPs in CA3 pyramidal cells by LVA calcium and sodium channels. *Journal of Neurophysiology*, **80**, 1558–61.

Woolf, T. B., Shepherd, G. M., and Greer, C. A. (1991). Local information processing in dendritic trees: subsets of spines in granule cells of the mammalian olfactory bulb. *Journal of Neuroscience*, **11**, 1837–54.

Yuste, R. and Tank, D. W. (1996). Dendritic integration in mammalian neurons, a century after Cajal. *Neuron*, **16**, 701–16.

Zador, A., Claiborne, B., and Brown, T. (1992). Nonlinear pattern separation in single hippocampal neurons with active dendritic membrane. In *Advances in neural information processing systems*, (ed. J. Moody, S. Hanson, and R. Lippmann), pp. 51–58. Morgan Kaufmann, San Mateo.

Zador, A. M., Agmon-Snir, H., and Segev, I. (1995). The morphoelectrotonic transform: a graphical approach to dendritic function. *Journal of Neuroscience*, **15**, 1669–82.

Zipser, D. and Andersen, R. A. (1988). A back-propagation programmed network that simulates response properties of a subset of posterior parietal neurons. *Nature*, **331**, 679–84.

12

Dendritic processing in invertebrates: a link to function

Gilles Laurent

California Institute of Technology

Summary

While the properties of dendritic voltage-gated currents in vertebrate neurons have recently received considerable (and renewed) attention, their potential functions for circuit integration and behavior remain largely speculative. This chapter summarizes results obtained in neurons within the smaller brains of invertebrates. In such systems, the functional link between neural/dendritic properties and circuit/systems-level activity can often be made, providing an important explanatory bridge between levels of analysis. This chapter also attempts to debunk some of the often-encountered misconceptions about neurons in invertebrate systems, and emphasizes the functional principles common to dendritic processing in both invertebrate and vertebrate networks.

Introduction

Writing about invertebrate neurons (i.e. the neurons of metazoans that are not vertebrates) is a bit like writing about wheels, *except* those of Chevrolets. Clearly, the vast majority of neuron types are found in invertebrates. Just as one finds wheels on space shuttles, scooters, and push-chairs, one finds neurons (and their dendrites) in deep-sea cephalopods, dragonflies, shrimps, mites, jelly-fish and duodenum-dwelling flatworms. Consequently, it is challenging to give a coherent—or even representative—description of neurons in the invertebrate world, a space far more diverse, with about 30 phyla and 97% of the animal species, than that of animals with backbones (and a few other usually forgotten chordates). Neurons are clearly tailored to function within their own, specialized network, yet just as the wheels of all rolling vehicles share a common purpose, neurons in octopuses, ticks, beetles, rats, and presumably cheetahs and pangolins, all serve the same basic function. Virtually all neurons, vertebrate and invertebrate alike, function as information-processing devices that interface with the world and with each other using transmembrane ionic currents and signaling pathways with, for the most part, common evolutionary origins. Thus, there is much to learn about neuronal function by studying invertebrates, and in many cases invertebrate nervous systems are experimentally advantageous. But are insights obtained from studying invertebrate nervous systems valuable for those interested primarily in vertebrate, or mammalian, nervous system function? I believe so, for the following reasons.

At the molecular level, we know for example that many of the signaling devices and pathways found in the nervous system of a simple metazoan, the nematode *Caenorhabditis elegans,* are highly conserved in mammalian neurons (Bargmann 1998). This has been established in *C. elegans* for ion channels (of which 80 are selective for potassium and 90 are ligand-gated), neurotransmitter receptors, neurotransmitter synthesis and exocytosis pathways, PDZ domain proteins and G-protein coupled second messenger pathways. Even the NMDA glutamate receptor, a vertebrate ligand-gated channel with important roles in rhythm generation (Grillner *et al.* 1987; Scrymgeour-Wedderburn *et al.* 1987) and 'Hebbian' synaptic plasticity (Hawkins *et al.* 1993; see Chapter 13), can be found in the brains of marine mollusks (Dale and Kandel 1993; Murphy and Glanzman 1997), indicating common ancestry. Mouse genes involved in mouse eye specification and development can replace their homolog in flies and produce an intact fly eye (Quiring *et al.* 1994), indicating shared developmental instruction pathways. The common ancestors of mice, flies, mollusks and nematodes lived 0.6 to 1.2 billion years ago (Allman 1998). Many of the fundamental molecular building blocks involved in the function and development of contemporary brains thus appear to be highly conserved across the main metazoan phyla. Should we expect greater differences at the supramolecular level?

At the cellular and biophysical levels, classical work by Cole, Hodgkin, Huxley, Katz, Keynes, Armstrong, Bezanilla and their colleagues on squid axon action potential conductances established fundamental facts on spike generation and propagation which, as we now know, apply also to vertebrate neurons (Hodgkin and Huxley 1952; Johnston and Wu 1995). The first non-Hodgkin–Huxley membrane currents were later identified in mollusks, opening the way for the characterization of axonal and dendritic voltage- and ion-gated channels (Johnston and Wu 1995; see Chapters 6 and 10). At the synaptic level, work on the squid giant synapse contributed (and continues to contribute) to our understanding of chemical neurotransmitter release mechanisms. Work by Ratliff and Hartline on lateral inhibition in the *Limulus* retina established the basic principles of organization for early sensory circuits (Ratliff 1965). Wilson (1961) first established the existence of central pattern generating circuits in motor systems (i.e. provided the first experimental support for the idea that sensory feedback is not necessary for the production of a motor pattern) using locust flight behavior, and thus opened the way for a cellular and system's understanding of premotor networks in the vertebrate spinal cord as well as countless other invertebrate preparations (McClelland and Grillner 1983; Grillner *et al.* 1987; Getting 1989). Kandel, Carew, Selverston, Marder, Moulins, Harris-Warrick and their colleagues provided some of the best descriptions of the molecular, cellular and circuit underpinnings of synaptic plasticity and circuit rearrangement in mollusks and crustaceans (Miller and Selverston 1982; Harris-Warrick *et al.* 1992; Hawkins *et al.* 1993; Marder 1998). This partial list illustrates that many functional principles, whether molecular, biophysical, synaptic or related to circuit dynamics, are far more similar across phyla than body plans and gross morphology might suggest. Of course cats are not jellyfish. Differences do exist between taxonomic groups. But emphasizing common principles is, I think, a useful endeavor.

This chapter therefore focuses on recent studies of dendritic integration which share a common scientific thread. This thread is the link between mechanisms and function. Neurons guide and underlie sensation, perception and behavior, phenomena which depend to a great degree on the animal's ecosystem—the nature and statistics of its sensory world, the nature and behaviors of its predators, mates and offspring. Their functions and the signals which they channel can therefore only be ultimately understood within the context in which they evolved to be used.

The invertebrate neuron myths

Before delving into specifics, I would like to dispel some structural and functional myths about the so-called 'invertebrate neurons' and through this, deconstruct the mystique of the pyramidal cell (no offense to neighboring chapters). These myths exist because we tend to forget that invertebrates are diverse and that their brains are complex and heterogeneous (Ramón y Cajal 1909; Strausfeld 1976). The brain of *Aplysia* is no more a ball of interconnected R15 and L3 neurons than a fish brain is composed of *Mauthner* cells. Small brains, like big ones, contain many neuronal types (see Fig. 12.1) and those types that we happen to know typically represent a small minority of the total.

Myth number 1: 'Invertebrate nervous systems are simple'

Invertebrate nervous systems are likely to be simpler than many vertebrate systems. It is partly for this reason (or belief) that some physiologists chose to study them. The brain of an 'average' insect such as a housefly or a honeybee contains between 0.5 and 1 million neurons. An insect's brain is therefore undoubtedly smaller than that of most mammals. At the same time, it is difficult to substantiate the claim that invertebrate brains are simpler (Koch and Laurent 1999). Indeed, if we have learned anything from studying invertebrate brains, it is that even the smallest among them express hard-to-predict properties. Take the stomatogastric ganglion, a network of about 30 neurons whose collective actions control gut motility and food ingestion and grinding in crabs, lobsters and other crustaceans (Harris-Warrick *et al.* 1992). One of many discoveries made about this system is that knowing its *full* synaptic connectivity was not sufficient to allow any useful or realistic prediction about its dynamics or function (Getting 1989; Marder and Meyrand 1989; Marder and Calabrese 1996; Marder 1998). A similar revelation came when the entire nervous system of the *Caenorhabditis elegans* hermaphrodite nematode (which contains 302 neurons *in toto*) was painstakingly mapped by serial electron microscopy, revealing a few hundred gap junctions and a few thousand chemical synapses (White *et al.* 1986). Because so little is known about the physiological properties of its neurons (Goodman *et al.* 1998), the function and internal logic of this network remain largely unknown, in spite of its available connectivity map. Finally, numerical simulations

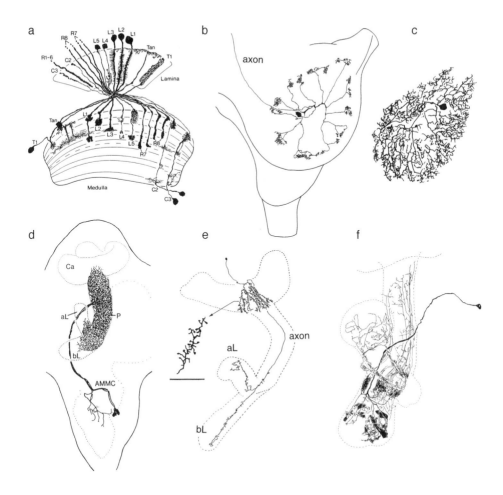

Fig. 12.1 Camera Lucida drawings of selected insect brain neurons. (a) Main neuron types in the *Drosophila* lamina (top) and medulla (bottom) of the optic lobes (portions of the insect brain just proximal to the retina). The R1–8 segments are photoreceptor axon terminals. L1–5 are lamina monopolar interneurons. From K. F. Fischbach, in Stavenga and Hardie (1989), p.196. (b) Locust antennal lobe projection neuron, the insect analog of a vertebrate mitral cell. Note the 20 dendritic tufts, each arborizing in one of the 1000 olfactory glomeruli. Adapted from Laurent and Naraghi (1994). (c) Locust antennal lobe local neuron, analogous to granule cells in the vertebrate olfactory bulb. Same scale as in (b). Note the extensive arborizations, instrumental in the global coordination of projection neuron activity. Adapted from MacLeod and Laurent (1996). (d) Dopaminergic neurons in the locust protocerebrum, with arborizations within the mushroom body pedunculus (P). Ca: calyx of the mushroom body; a-bL: alpha-beta lobes. AMMC: cluster of somata. Adapted from Wendt and Homberg (1992). (e) Locust Kenyon cell, intrinsic neuron of the mushroom body (stippled outline). Note the spiny dendrites (inset). Adapted from Laurent and Naraghi (1994). (f) Locust beta lobe neuron, target of thousands of Kenyon cells as in (e). Note the dense dendritic tufts in the beta lobe and the looser axonal neurites in the alpha lobe and pedunculus. Adapted from MacLeod *et al.* (1998). Note the diversity of shapes, sizes and arbor complexity across these many neurons.

of neural circuit dynamics have, in the last ten years, also made it clear that the many nonlinearities characterizing the function of dendritic trees, synapses, ion channels and receptors make it tremendously difficult to predict accurately the behavior of even the simplest networks, in the absence of precise knowledge and understanding of the many key state variables (Wang and Buszaki 1996; Getting 1989; Marder 1998).

Many invertebrates and vertebrates must solve the same basic problems, simply because they share the same natural world. They must, for example, learn and/or recognize complex patterns (shapes, colors, motions, sound motifs, calls, odors) crucial for feeding, mating, egg-laying, homing and predator avoidance. They must move, often using appendages that require precise coordination. The more closely we look, the more we discover that common problems often find similar neural, computational and integrative solutions in vertebrates and invertebrates, even if the detailed components used (e.g. neurotransmitters, receptors, etc.) often are not precisely identical. One such example is the early olfactory system, whose basic functional architecture and population dynamics are strikingly similar in mammals, fish, reptiles, amphibians, crustaceans, insects and mollusks (Hildebrand and Shepherd 1997). Another example is a common computational solution to the problem of looming object detection in vision by insects and birds (Wang and Frost 1992; Hatsopoulos *et al.* 1995; Sun and Frost 1998; Gabbiani *et al.* 1999). In conclusion, despite being small—with notable exceptions such as the octopus brain (Young 1964)—many invertebrate brains have much of the complexity and richness (Fiorito and Scotto 1992) of the larger vertebrate brains. Geneticists first revealed and then exploited the fact that many genes have been remarkably conserved during the last billion years of animal evolution. This observation has facilitated their studies of—to name but a few—intra- and intercellular signalling pathways, cell trafficking and organismal development in all the major phyla. The same broad-minded view should also illuminate neuroscience.

Myth number 2: 'Invertebrate neurons are large'

One of the great advantages of invertebrate systems is that some of their neurons are very large. In the early days of electrophysiology, voltage-clamp measurements could only be achieved in a few neurons big enough to permit multiple electrode impalement. While techniques and needs have changed, the idea that invertebrate neurons are invariably large remains. First, note that invertebrate bodies can be very small. As J. Z. Young reportedly said, 'there is enough room inside a squid giant axon for two *Drosophila* to walk hand in hand'. Two *Drosophila*, of course, each contain several hundred thousand neurons in their respective brains. But *Drosophila* is not even among the smallest multicellular invertebrates endowed with a brain! The *Circocylliba* mite, for example, is an arthropod that lives lodged on the inner surface of the mandibles of worker ants of the species *Eciton* (Hölldobler and Wilson 1994). How do minuscule neurons work? How are the potentially severe consequences of ion channel noise controlled and counteracted? Are transmembrane ionic gradients subject to massive fluctuations during activity? These problems have received rather little attention (Bekkers and Stevens 1990), except for a recent experimental study in *C. elegans* neurons (Goodman *et al.* 1998). Second, just like the brain of rats contains large Purkinje neurons and small granule cells, the brains of invertebrates contain heterogeneous populations of neurons, of which some are big and others are small. In locusts for example, cell body sizes range from about 100 μm (two metathoracic fast tibial extensor motoneurons; Burrows 1996) to about 6 μm (100 000 Kenyon cells, intrinsic neurons of the mushroom bodies, a brain structure involved in olfaction, multimodal processing and memory; see Fig. 12.1e). Dendritic diameters range between *ca.* 10 and 0.1 μm, allowing routine intradendritic impalements with sharp electrodes in processes 1 μm thick or larger (Burrows 1979*a,b*; Laurent 1993). Similar size ranges can be found in many other arthropod and molluscan brains.

Myth number 3: 'Invertebrate neurons are highly specialized'

This argument is often advanced by people who contrast invertebrate neurons with pyramidal cells, the often-described 'Lego' blocks of the mammalian cortex. This is a false impression caused by comparing things that are not comparable. Pyramidal cells in mammalian cortices should be compared not with gill motoneurons in mollusks or wind-sensitive interneurons in insects, but with invertebrate neurons in a structure whose role is similar to that of the mammalian cortex. A more acceptable comparison is with insect mushroom bodies, whose intrinsic neurons, the Kenyon cells, are both numerous (over 300 000 in the cockroach brain), morphologically homogeneous and functionally versatile. While mushroom bodies are subdivided into several sensory compartments (Mobbs 1982; Yang *et al.* 1995), the Kenyon cells found in each one of these compartments cannot (yet) be identified on morphological criteria or electrophysiological properties alone (Laurent and Naraghi 1994). Conversely, many neuronal types in the brain of vertebrates (take looming-sensitive neurons in *Nucleus Rotundus* of pigeons for example), possess functional and anatomical features which make them remarkably similar to their insect analogs (Sun and Frost 1998; Gabbiani *et al.* 1999). In both phyla, these neurons appear equally 'specialized'.

The concept of the 'identified neuron' is also a hallmark of invertebrate nervous systems. One can reliably identify an R15 neuron in an *Aplysia* abdominal ganglion, a DCMD (descending contralateral motion detector) neuron in a locust brain (Palka 1967; O'Shea *et al.* 1974; O'Shea and Rowell 1976; Rind and Simmons 1992), a PD (pyloric dilator) neuron in a lobster stomatogastric ganglion (Harris-Warrick *et al.* 1992) or an Omega neuron in a cricket prothoracic ganglion (Selverston *et al.* 1985). This feature of reliable identifiability has been one of the most powerful arguments *for* the use of such systems. But one should not forget that, here also, such identifiable features are restricted to a few, well-studied, and usually small subsystems of neurons. No such description could be applied to the tens of thousands of olfactory projection neurons in the crustacean antennal lobe (Wachowiak and Ache 1994). Similarly, one can foresee the not-too-distant day when the molecular identity of individual neurons or groups of neurons in the vertebrate brain will be routinely assessed using molecular probes. In other words, identifiability/nonidentifiability is only a function of our present limited knowledge. Identifiability is an operational description and not, in my opinion at least, an intrinsically profound characteristic of invertebrate neurons.

Myth number 4: 'Invertebrate neurons have a different dynamic polarization'

The somata of arthropod or molluscan neurons are generally located at the periphery of the central nervous system, and thus surround the regions of the neuropil in which most synaptic interactions take place (Burrows 1996). Because individual somata and their neurites (which often include both dendritic and axonal processes) are usually joined by a single process, the soma of these 'monopolar' neurons cannot be considered as the global 'integrator' of dendritic inputs and is also not the point of origin of the axon. Action potentials are generated along a neuritic process, which thereby defines dendrites on one side and axon on the other. The spike initiation zone, a region of membrane with presumed high density of voltage-gated ion channels involved in spike initiation, is therefore located away from the soma. Does this constitute a fundamental functional difference with vertebrate neurons? First, while this description applies to many known and well-studied invertebrate neurons, it also applies to several vertebrate neuronal types, such as striatal and thalamic neurons in the tiger salamander (Herrick 1939), tectal neurons in fish (Meek and Schellart 1978) and reptiles (Ramón y Cajal 1909), and many dopamine neurons in rat substantia nigra (Häusser *et al.* 1995). Similarly, action potential generation also occurs remotely from the soma of dorsal root sensory neurons in the mammalian spinal cord. It is thus not a hallmark of invertebrate neurons. Second, while the soma does not constitute the border between input and output zones, a functional polarization usually remains. This was best demonstrated by Burrows and collaborators in locust local spiking neurons. These local neurons are found in thoracic segments and integrate mechanosensory information from leg receptors. All neurites are confined to a single ganglion, but they can nevertheless be divided clearly into axonal and dendritic compartments by gross morphological features (dendrites appear fine, dense and nonvaricose, while axonal segments are sparse and varicose) and, more importantly, by synaptic ultrastructure (Watson and Burrows 1985). Dendritic and axonal subfields are linked by a single and soma-less dorso–ventral process. Finally, note that this simplistic description of functional polarization of neurons applies, in vertebrates as in invertebrates, to a fraction only (albeit large) of all neural populations. Locust nonspiking local interneurons, for example, possess intermingled input and output synapses (and thus lack any gross functional polarization; Watson and Burrows 1988), just as seen in certain retinal amacrine cells, olfactory bulb neurons or thalamic neurons in mammals (Cox *et al.* 1998).

In conclusion, it is important to note the numerous features that unite invertebrate and vertebrate neurons. I have tried to emphasize that the heterogeneity and complexity of invertebrate neurons and of the circuits they form are probably as high as those of vertebrate neurons and brains. Invertebrate neurons found in small circuits do not appear any simpler or any more linear than the most complex pyramidal cells in rat somatosensory cortex (Koch and Laurent 1999). I also believe that comparisons between phyla are useful and informative *only* when drawn appropriately. Comparing two functionally unrelated neuron types in cats and lobsters is as unsound as comparing spinal and olivary neurons in the same species. It follows that, if one wants to compare the computational and biophysical properties of invertebrate and vertebrate neurons, one should be guided first by function (e.g. wide-field visual motion detection). Once circuits with similar functions have been identified—which may not always be possible—neurons within those circuits can be selected and compared across species and phyla (e.g. wide-field neurons in *Nucleus Rotundus* in birds *versus* wide-field neurons in the *lobula* or *lobula plate* of the optic lobes of insects). Only then can comparisons become meaningful, and useful insights about dendritic biophysics and computations be gained.

The link between biophysics, computation and function

A good reason why one might choose to study invertebrate neurons is that their individual contributions to computation, coding and behavior can be tested more easily than with analogous vertebrate nervous systems. I have selected five examples to illustrate this point. All examples originate from studies of insect nervous systems, simply because I know these best. Similarly good (or possibly better) examples could have been taken from other animal model systems.

Dendritic Ca^{2+} dynamics and selective attention in hearing

Crickets display elaborate acoustic behavior whereby the males attract and court females using specific calling and mating songs while they express bellicosity to competing males through yet another set of song patterns (Pollack 1988; Schildberger and Homer 1988). Crickets' ears are located on the tibiae of their front legs and their primary auditory neuropil is found on each side of the corresponding, prothoracic ganglion. Within this neuropil, are (among many others) two bilateral sensory interneurons (one for each side of the midline) called omega neurons (Selverston *et al.* 1985). They are so called because of their characteristic Ω-shaped neuritic morphology. Each omega neuron receives inputs from one ear through one tip of its Ω-shaped field (thus termed the dendritic field) and contacts its contralateral partner via the other tip (the axonal field). These neurons, which can be readily impaled *in vivo* in walking and orienting animals (Schildberger and Homer 1988), respond to sound chirps in the frequency range corresponding to the males' calling song (*ca.* 5 kHz) by producing bursts of action potentials. The intensity of these responses, however, depends on the context in which the songs are being heard. For example, the response to chirps of 60 dB-SPL, 4.8 kHz syllable triplets is greatly attenuated (and even abolished) if each 60 dB chirp is preceded by a louder (90 dB) but otherwise identical one (Sobel and Tank 1994). This effect, called forward masking, can be considered as a sort of gain control whereby omega neuron sensitivity is lowered so as to allow selective responses only to the louder sound in that frequency range (Pollack 1988). Erik Sobel and David Tank (1994) identified a biophysical dendritic phenomenon likely to be responsible for this response suppression.

Intracellular recordings from the omega neuron show that each chirp-evoked burst of action potentials is followed by a membrane potential hyperpolarization. These hyperpolarizations are larger for sounds of larger intensity and decay upon sound offset with a time constant of 4.3 ± 1.0 s. Using fluorescence imaging of fura-2-filled omega neuron dendrites, Sobel and Tank showed that each chirp leads to a large increase of intracellular calcium, with slow return to resting level ($\tau = 4.5 \pm 1.4$ s) after sound offset, similar to what can be observed electrophysiologically. To test the hypothesis that these phenomena are causally related—i.e. that the sound-evoked hyperpolarization results from intradendritic calcium entry and subsequent activation of a calcium-activated potassium current, they performed two manipulations. In the first, they used the fast and high-affinity calcium-buffering property of fura-2 to prevent the putative activation of calcium-activated K^+ channels. This experiment showed that, in such circumstances, the omega neuron's post-chirp hyperpolarization was suppressed, and even replaced by prolonged firing. In the second experiment, they used a caged calcium compound, DM-Nitrophen, to raise intradendritic calcium concentration transiently upon flash photolysis. This manipulation caused a direct membrane hyperpolarization which, if delivered during a sound-evoked burst of action potentials, mimicked the naturally evoked post-burst hyperpolarization and decreased the omega neuron's sensitivity to sound. In conclusion, forward masking, a cellular property leading to selective responsiveness to the loudest sounds in a background of overlapping sounds, can be explained by a control of cellular excitability brought about by dendritic calcium entry. While the detailed mechanisms underlying this calcium flux and subsequent $I_{K,Ca}$ activation remain unknown in omega neurons, their functional relevance for acoustic behavior has been established.

Voltage-gated potassium channels and visual ecology

This part of the chapter describes some biophysical properties of insect photoreceptors and their relationship with behavior. Although photoreceptors do not possess proper and elaborate dendritic trees, their input (phototransductive) and output (synaptic) domains are usually physically separated by a neurite of variable length. This interposed membrane is not passive but rather expresses (in insects as in vertebrates) complex nonlinear properties due to the presence of numerous voltage-gated ion channel types (Fulpius and Baumann 1969; Hardie 1985, 1989; Hamdorf *et al.* 1988; Jansonius 1990; Weckström *et al.* 1992, 1993; Laughlin and Weckström 1993; Juusola *et al.* 1994; Weckström 1994; Laughlin 1996). The reasons why specific channels with precise intrinsic properties are expressed in a particular photoreceptor of a particular species necessitates a biological understanding of the animal's behavior and ecology. Nowhere is this better illustrated than in insect vision.

Let us first describe the role of K^+ channels in blowfly photoreceptors. Arthropod photoreceptors depolarize in response to light. A dark-adapted blowfly photoreceptor has a sensitivity comparable to that of a vertebrate rod, generating 1–2 mV single-photon bumps from a resting potential of about –65 mV. Once light-adapted, the same photoreceptor has its sensitivity reduced a thousandfold and yet expresses a signal-to-noise ratio and frequency response that match—or even surpass—those of vertebrate cones. This is made possible in part by a very high phototransduction rate (10^6 photons s^{-1}), which itself requires a large area of photoreceptive membrane. The resulting capacitive load causes a long membrane time constant—4 ms in a passive photoreceptor in darkness. While this long time constant is tolerable in the dark, where transduction is slow, it would be severely constraining in daylight, when the animal needs very fast updates of its environment for flight maneuvers. This problem is solved by the activation of several species of voltage-sensitive K^+ channels (some inactivating, some noninactivating) upon light-induced depolarization. A 100-fold increase in membrane conductance brought about by K^+ channel opening in daylight (at steady-state) decreases both response time and sensitivity, thus also preventing saturation and enabling operation in the midrange of the photoreceptor potential, where it is most sensitive to changes in light intensity. Potassium channel activation, therefore, acts as an adaptive and precisely matched gain control device with consequences for both receptor sensitivity and speed (Laughlin and Weckström 1993; Laughlin 1996).

Let us now turn to the adaptation (in an evolutionary sense) of potassium channel kinetics to the animal's ecology. Because the blowfly photoreceptor delayed rectifier (DR) conductance activates relatively slowly, fast depolarizing transients caused by brisk changes in brightness are spared from attenuation, a feature essential for appropriate visual control of fast flight. By comparing photoreceptor K^+ channel kinetics across 20 species of dipteran insects (flies, crane flies, etc.), Matti Weckström and Simon Laughlin established that prominent noninactivating DR conductances are always found in the fast photoreceptors of diurnal species, but never in the dusk- or night-flying ones. By contrast, the photoreceptors of night fliers (which are slow fliers), are slow and express rapidly inactivating K^+ channels, whose activation prevents large voltage transients in highly sensitive receptors. Even more astonishing is the observation that locust photoreceptors switch from a low sensitivity and high acuity state during daytime to a high sensitivity, low acuity state during night time (when they usually migrate). This switch is caused by a circadian regulation of the ratio of sustained to inactivating K^+ currents, possibly mediated by 5HT levels (Hevers and Hardie 1993; Cuttle *et al.* 1995).

While I have limited this description to K^+ currents, other voltage-gated conductances (Na^+, Ca^{2+}) have also been described in insect photoreceptors (Weckström *et al.* 1992), and likely play additional roles in matching the properties of these neurons to the ecology of the animal whose behaviors they guide. In conclusion, an explanation for the varied and adaptive roles of K^+ channel properties in insect photoreceptors has resulted from an understanding of these animals' biology.

Dendritic geometry and computation of visual motion

The third optic lobe of insects (lobula or, in some species such as flies, the lobula plate) contains many complex wide-field motion-sensitive visual neurons. Some respond to translational horizontal or vertical motion (Stavenga and Hardie 1989), others to more complex rotatory visual flow-fields (Krapp and Hengstenberg 1996; Krapp *et al.* 1998) induced by the animal's own motion through space; yet others respond to object motion relative to the animal and are specifically inhibited by flow-fields induced by the animal's own motion (O'Shea and Rowell 1976). A recent study by Sandra Single and Axel Borst (1998) investigates the role played by the complex, fan-shaped dendritic trees of some of these blowfly lobula plate neurons (lobula plate tangential cells or LPTCs) in computing image velocity. Motion detection is assumed to be accomplished first by small field neurons in the neuropil immediately upstream from the lobula, the so-called medulla (Reichardt 1987). Specific retinotopic arrays of medulla elementary motion detectors feed their direction-selective signals (each thought to be calculated by correlation of luminance levels from adjacent photo-receptors, according to the model proposed by Reichardt (1987) to the large dendritic trees of specific LPTCs, thus conferring, through global summation and integration, specific wide-field motion sensitivity onto them.

If a large moving grating is projected onto a fly's retina, a subset of the LPTCs will be activated depending on the direction and orientation of the moving pattern. Because motion computation by medulla neurons is primarily local, the signals received by any activated wide-field LPTC should contain temporally modulated components phase-locked to the local modulations of the luminance pattern. One predicts that such temporal fluctuations of dendritic potential should be local (i.e. detectable from each dendritic compartment whose motion-detecting inputs are being periodically stimulated by the moving grating), and that many such out-of-phase modulated signals (arising from different locations on the retinotopic array) would cancel out by spatial averaging within, or downstream from, the dendritic fan, resulting in a smooth, unmodulated neuronal output. This is precisely what was shown, using *in vivo* Ca^{2+} imaging of LPTC dendrites during motion stimulation (Single and Borst 1998). Many of the LPTCs, such as the VS1 neuron, possess large, roughly planar dendritic fans that spread over many hundreds of μm. By simul-taneously imaging calcium dynamics within the separate dendrites of individual LPTCs (filled by intracellular injection of the calcium indicator Calcium Green), Single and Borst showed that, while local dendritic fluctuations of intracellular Ca^{2+} undergo large periodic fluctuations locked to the grating's motion, each dendritic signal is phase-shifted relative to the others according to their relative spacing within the retinotopic array. The axonal Ca^{2+} signal (indicative of the voltage output of the entire neuron), however, is smooth (i.e. contains a DC component only). To ascertain that the Ca^{2+} signals are caused by membrane potential fluctuations (i.e. are caused by Ca^{2+} entry through voltage-gated rather than ligand-gated channels), they combined hyperpolarizing current injections and visual stimuli. This simple manip-ulation leads to a suppression of the periodic modulation of the visually-evoked Ca^{2+} signal, indicating that Ca^{2+} entry is voltage-dependent and only secondary to synaptically-induced depolarization (NMDA-like currents with mixed ligand and voltage gating are not known to exist in these circuits). This spatial averaging of out-of-phase signals, of course, can only occur if the stimulus motion vector is parallel to the physical plane of the dendrites. If it were normal to the plane of the dendritic tree, all dendrites would undergo voltage modulations in phase, resulting in a periodic global output locked to the moving grating stimulus. One can see, therefore, how the precisely defined geometry of these large dendritic trees is used to optimize the computation of visual motion by averaging out undesirable local fluctuations.

Voltage-dependent modulation of dendritic impedance and linearization of synaptic transfer

We now turn to a class of local, axonless and nonspiking neurons in the locust thoracic nervous system. Nonspiking neurons have been described in many invertebrate and vertebrate nervous systems (Burrows and Siegler 1978; Graubard 1978; Burrows 1979*a,b*, 1980; Hayashi *et al.* 1985; Burrows 1987; Angstadt and

Calabrese 1991; Burrows 1996; Marder and Calabrese 1996; Olsen and Calabrese 1996; Manor *et al.* 1997; Cox *et al.* 1998). The roles, morphology, ultrastructure and modes of action of nonspiking local interneurons in locust sensory-motor circuits and motor control have been thoroughly studied over the last twenty years by Malcolm Burrows and colleagues (reviewed in Burrows 1996). I will focus here on dendro-dendritic processing and on the potential advantages that such a mode of synaptic transmitter release confers. While nonspiking neurons fail to produce Na^+ action potentials upon depolarization, their dendrites (which, as stated earlier contain intermingled pre- and postsynaptic specializations; Watson and Burrows (1988) and are thus mixed dendritic and axonal neurites) are not passive. Indeed, they express several voltage-gated K^+ and Ca^{2+} channel types, with specific activation ranges and kinetics, which have been characterized by intradendritic single-electrode voltage- and current-clamp *in vivo* as well as patch-clamp studies in dissociated cell culture (Laurent 1990, 1991, 1993; Laurent *et al.* 1993). Because they express these channels, nonspiking neuron dendrites behave nonlinearly when their membrane potential is altered by intradendritic current injection, with dramatic consequences for temporal synaptic integration (Laurent 1990, 1993). The basic phenomena are as follows. The normal dynamic range of nonspiking neuron voltage (as recorded in intact and moving animals) is between –65 and –40mV. At the most negative potentials, the membrane behaves passively, with a relatively high input resistance and long time constant (between 20 and 30 ms; Laurent 1990, 1991, 1993). At potentials more positive than –60 mV, DR and A-type K^+ currents activate, causing a drop (tenfold over the –60 to –40 mV range) in input resistance and membrane time constant. Such reduction in dendritic input resistance leads to a drastic reduction in the amplitude and duration of synaptic potentials (Laurent 1990), with important consequences for synaptic transfer (see below). At yet more positive potentials ($\geqslant$ –40 mV), a dendritic Ca^{2+} current is activated which amplifies any local depolarizations, such as those caused by EPSPs (Laurent 1993; Laurent *et al.* 1993). Consequently, the electrical behavior of a nonspiking dendrite, and its response to synaptic inputs, depend critically upon the membrane potential at the time of the input. If this potential is more negative than –60 mV, input resistance and time constant are high, leading to large and long-lasting voltage deviations (e.g. large EPSPs). If the dendritic membrane potential is between –60 and –45 mV, input resistance and time constant are reduced, leading to smaller and shorter PSPs. Finally, if the dendritic membrane potential is more positive than –40 mV, EPSPs are amplified by the action of voltage-gated Ca^{2+} conductances.

The functional significance of these observations emerges once the synaptic properties of the nonspiking neurons are considered. Nonspiking neurons release neurotransmitter tonically in such a way that single EPSPs in a nonspiking neuron can directly affect a postsynaptic neuron (Burrows 1979*a*). By using single-electrode voltage-clamping of nonspiking dendrites and simultaneous dendritic voltage recording of postsynaptic motoneurons, it became possible to describe quantitatively the gain and range of synaptic transfer (at steady-state) at this nonspiking synapse (Laurent 1993). The transfer curve is sigmoidal, with a foot at –65 mV, mid-point around –50 mV and saturation around –40 mV (Laurent 1993). The dynamic gain of synaptic transfer (i.e. the amount of postsynaptic voltage change produced by a given presynaptic voltage change) is given by the slope of the sigmoidal transfer curve, and is thus maximum at the midpoint (–50 mV) and least at both foot (around –65mV) and shoulder (around –40 mV). Hence, when synaptic transfer is most efficient (at around –50 mV), the nonspiking dendrite is itself least responsive to an injected current (e.g. an EPSC). By contrast, at voltages where the dynamic gain of the synapse drops (the two rectifying regions of the sigmoid), the dendrite is more responsive, either because its input resistance is higher (negative potentials) or because boosting Ca^{2+} currents are activated. The nonlinearities of the membrane's electrical behavior and those of the nonspiking synapse therefore appear to be precisely matched to counteract each other, and could thereby potentially linearize transfer through the nonspiking dendrite.

That this is the case was shown directly by the following experiment. A nonspiking dendrite and a postsynaptic motoneuron were simultaneously impaled. A single leg hair afferent was then identified that made a monosynaptic excitatory connection onto the impaled nonspiking neuron (see Laurent and Burrows (1988) for a demonstration of connectivity), providing a chain of three synaptically connected neurons. Each imposed movement of this hair caused an EPSP in the nonspiking neuron, which in turn caused an IPSP in the postsynaptic motoneuron (Fig. 3 in Laurent 1993). The experiment then consisted in measuring the amplitude of the motoneuron IPSP as the membrane potential of the nonspiking dendrite was varied between –95 and –44 mV by direct current injection. Although the amplitude and time integral of the nonspiking neuron EPSP both varied dramatically as functions of the holding potential, the response of the motoneuron to these afferent-evoked EPSPs did not change significantly (Laurent 1993). The amplitude and shape of the disynaptically evoked motoneuron IPSPs therefore appeared to be independent of the state of the interposed nonspiking interneuron. This constitutes, therefore, a dendritic adaptive gain control mechanism where voltage-gated currents linearize the nonlinearities of graded and spike-less chemical synaptic transmission. Because nonspiking transfer is common in many sensory local circuits (e.g. the retina or the olfactory bulb), such complex adaptive mechanisms may have widespread use in providing constancy of processing over wide operating ranges.

Coincidence detection and odor-encoding by synchronized cell assemblies

Recent work in the insect olfactory nervous system indicates that odors are represented by dynamical assemblies of synchronized neurons (Laurent and Davidowitz 1994; Laurent *et al.* 1996; Wehr and Laurent 1996, 1999). These neuronal assemblies are found first in the antennal lobe, a glomerular neuropil analogous to the vertebrate olfactory bulb. This neuropil contains two main neuronal populations: excitatory projection neurons (PNs), whose function is analogous to vertebrate mitral and tufted cells, and inhibitory local neurons (LNs), similar to granule and periglomerular cells in the olfactory bulb. One function played by LNs is to synchronize sets of PNs by widespread distribution of fast and periodic inhibitory inputs (MacLeod and Laurent 1996). By selectively blocking one class of GABA receptors in the antennal lobe, it was possible to show that PN synchronization could be abolished, without other consequences for PN respon-siveness, response patterning or odor tuning (MacLeod and Laurent 1996). This observation was then used to test for the potential functional importance of PN synchronization. A first series of experiments used behavioral tests for odor learning, memorization and discrimination. These tests indicated that PN synchronization is relevant for neither odor learning nor memorization, but rather for *fine* odor discrimination (coarse odor discrimination between chemically distant odors was normal in animals whose PN assemblies had been desynchronized; Stopfer *et al.* 1997). A second series of experiments tested whether the odor tuning of high order olfactory neurons found two synapses downstream from the synchronized PN assemblies could be modified by selective PN desynchronization. These experiments showed that this is indeed the case, even though the desynchronized PNs themselves showed no modification, broadening or loss of specificity of their responses (MacLeod *et al.* 1998). These results showed that PN synchronization is indeed relevant for odor perception and decoding by high order neurons, and that infor-mation about odor stimuli must be contained in, and decoded from, the *relational* aspects of PN activity (i.e. from the relative timing of PN spikes, and not solely from collective firing rates; MacLeod *et al.* 1998). If synchronized PN spikes carry additional information, as the above results indicate, nonlinear biophysical mechanisms should exist that selectively 'sense' groups of coincident PN spikes.

PNs send axons to two main regions of the insect brain: the lateral protocerebral lobe, a region just proximal to the third optic lobes, and the calyx of the mushroom body (MB), a prominent pedunculated structure involved in olfactory, multimodal and memory processes (Erber and Menzel 1980; Mobbs 1982; Heisenberg *et al.* 1985; Heisenberg 1989; Davis 1993). In the MB, PN axon collaterals make direct excita-tory contacts with the spiny dendrites of the MB intrinsic neurons, called Kenyon cells (KCs; Laurent and Naraghi 1994). These KCs are small (6 μm soma diameter, 100–200 nm dendrite and axon diameter) and numerous (5000 in *Drosophila melanogaster*; 100 000 in locusts; over 300 000 in cockroaches), but can nevertheless be recorded intracellularly in intact animals (Laurent and Naraghi 1994). KCs respond to odor presentation with bursts of 20–30 Hz membrane potential oscillations, locked to the MB local field potential and to the collective PN inflow from the antennal lobe. In response to a given odor stimulus, some of the membrane potential oscillatory cycles in a particular KC will cross firing threshold and produce one action potential per oscillatory cycle, phase-locked to the local field potential (Laurent and Naraghi 1994). If an odor stimulus is replaced by electrical stimulation of PNs, the following observations can be made from an intracellularly recorded KC: First, progressive increases in the strength of the PN stimulation lead to incremental steps in the size of the monosynaptic KC EPSP, indicating a large degree of convergence between PNs and KCs. Second, if PN stimulation is increased beyond a certain intensity, the KC EPSP displays an active (voltage-dependent) response with very sharp rising and falling phases (Laurent and Naraghi 1994). That this response is voltage-dependent can be shown by simple manipulation of the postsynaptic holding voltage at the time of stimulation. This response hence constitutes a subthreshold, but nonlinear amplification of the PN-evoked EPSP, bringing membrane voltage closer to spike threshold. It is, therefore, a coincidence detecting mechanism that will selectively raise firing probability if, during a given oscillation cycle, the timings of co-occurring presynaptic spikes show little dispersion. In conclusion, the function of some of the dendritic voltage-gated conductances expressed by KCs is to allow the detection of synchronized input from oscillatory assemblies of projection neurons, and thus participate in the extraction of correlational information encoded across neuronal populations (Laurent and Naraghi 1994; MacLeod *et al.* 1998).

Concluding remarks

These examples hopefully illustrate how the study of dendritic processing in invertebrate neurons can contribute to our understanding of neuronal and brain function. While the biophysical and mechanistic details (channel pharmacology, density, kinetics, precise distribution etc.) of these dendritic phenomena remain generally less well explored in invertebrates than in mammalian cortical or hippo-campal preparations, their functional implications are often much easier to under-stand and establish. What is so promising is the fact that most of the phenomena explored in these small preparations have obvious analogs in the larger brains and circuits of vertebrates. Neural synchronization, for example, is an established phenomenon in many mammalian neural circuits, for which function has as yet been impossible to prove directly (Freeman 1975; Gray and Singer 1989; Singer 1999). Other examples promise very useful discoveries. The LGMD (lobula giant motion detector) neuron in the locust brain, for example, is a large visual neuron specialized for the detection of looming objects (Rind and Simmons 1992; Gabbiani *et al.* 1999). Recent work indicates that its firing rate during object approach can be described mathematically by the multiplication of two terms, respectively functions of the angular size and angular velocity of the moving object (Hatsopoulos *et al.* 1995; Gabbiani *et al.* 1999). Because this computation cannot be carried out by the motion detecting elements presynaptic to LGMD, it must be done by the dendritic tree of LGMD. Biophysical studies of nonlinear processing in this neuron may thus provide an understanding of the mechanisms underlying neuronal multiplication, a compu-tation fundamental in many neural processes such as the computation of gain fields in primate cerebral cortex (Andersen *et al.* 1985). In summary, at a time when the molecular and biophysical processes underlying neuronal function are starting to be well described, the time is ripe to place these smart cellular and sub-cellular devices back into the context in which they evolved to serve. A good starting point is the brain of animals whose behavior can be studied in detail.

References

Allman, J. M. (1998). *Evolving brains*. Freeman, New York.
Andersen, R. A., Essick, G., and Siegel, R. (1985). Encoding of spatial location by posterior parietal neurons, *Science*, **230**, 456–8.
Angstadt, J. D. and Calabrese, R. L. (1991). Calcium currents and graded synaptic transmission between heart interneurons of the leech. *Journal of Neuroscience*, **11**, 746–59.
Bargmann, C. I. (1998). Neurobiology of the *Caenorhabditis elegans* genome. *Science*, **282**, 2028–33.

Bekkers, J. M. and Stevens, C. F. (1990). Two different ways evolution makes neurons larger. *Progress in Brain Research*, **83**, 37–45.

Burrows, M. (1979*a*). Synaptic potentials effect the release of transmitter from locust nonspiking interneurons. *Science*, **204**, 81–3.

Burrows, M. (1979*b*). Graded synaptic transmission between local pre-motor interneurons of the locust. *Journal of Neurophysiology*, **42**, 1108–23.

Burrows, M. (1980). The control of sets of motoneurones by local interneurones in the locust. *Journal of Physiology*, **298**, 213–33.

Burrows, M. (1987). Inhibitory interactions between spiking and nonspiking local interneurones in the locust. *Journal of Neuroscience*, **7**, 3282–92.

Burrows, M. (1996). *The neurobiology of an insect brain*. Oxford University Press.

Burrows, M. and Siegler, M. V. S. (1978). Graded synaptic transmission between local interneurones and motoneurones in the metathoracic ganglion of the locust. *Journal of Physiology*, **285**, 231–55.

Cox, C. L., Zhou, Q., and Sherman, S. M. (1998). Glutamate locally activates dendritic outputs of thalamic interneurons. *Nature*, **394**, 478–82.

Cuttle, M. F., Hevers, W., Laughlin, S. B., and Hardie, R. C. (1995). Diurnal modulation of photoreceptor potassium conductance in the locust. *Journal of Comparative Physiology*, **176**, 307–16.

Dale, N. and Kandel, E. R. (1993). l-Glutamate may be the fast excitatory transmitter of Aplysia sensory neurons. *Proceedings of the National Academy of Sciences USA*, **90**, 7163–7.

Davis, R. L. (1993). Mushroom bodies and *Drosophila* learning. *Neuron*, **11**, 1–14.

Erber, J. and Menzel, R. (1980). Localization of short-term memory in the brain of the bee, *Apis mellifera*. *Physiological Entomology*, **5**, 343–58.

Fiorito, G. and Scotto, P. (1992). Observational learning in *Octopus vulgaris*. *Science*, **256**, 545–7.

Freeman, W. J. (1975). *Mass action in the nervous system*. Academic Press, New York.

Fulpius, B. and Baumann, F. (1969). Effects of sodium, potassium, and calcium ions on slow and spike potentials in single photoreceptor cells. *Journal of General Physiology*, **53**, 541–61.

Gabbiani, F., Krapp, H. G., and Laurent, G. (1999). Computation of object approach by a wide-field, motion-sensitive neuron. *Journal of Neuroscience*. (In press.)

Getting, P. A. (1989). Emerging principles governing the operation of neural networks. *Annual Review of Neuroscience*, **12**, 185–204.

Goodman, M. B., Hall, D. H., Avery, L., and Lockery, S. R. (1998). Active currents regulate sensitivity and dynamic range in *C. elegans* neurons. *Neuron*, **20**, 763–72.

Graubard, K. (1978). Synaptic transmission without action potentials: input–output properties of a non-spiking presynaptic neuron. *Journal of Neurophysiology*, **41**, 1014–25.

Gray, C. M. and Singer, W. (1989). Stimulus-specific neuronal oscillations in orientation columns of cat visual cortex. *Proceedings of the National Academy of Science USA*, **86**, 1698–702.

Grillner, S., Wallén, P., Dale, N., Brodin, L., Buchanan, J., and Hill, R. (1987). Transmitters, membrane properties and network circuitry in the control of locomotion in lamprey. *Trends in Neuroscience*, **10**, 34–41.

Hamdorf, K., Hochstrate, P., Hoglund, G., Burbach, B., and Wiegund, U. (1988). Light activation of the sodium-pump in blowfly photoreceptors. *Journal of Comparative Physiology A*, **162**, 285–300.

Hardie, R. C. (1985). Functional organization of the fly retina. *Progress in Sensory Physiology*, **5**, 1–79.

Hardie, R. C. (1989). A histamine-activated chloride channel involved in neurotransmission at a photoreceptor synapse. *Nature*, **339**, 704–6.

Harris-Warrick, R., Marder, E., Selverston, A. I., and Moulins, M. (ed.) (1992). *Dynamic biological networks: the stomatogastric nervous system*. MIT Press, Cambridge, MA.

Hatsopoulos, N., Gabbiani, F., and Laurent, G. (1995). Elementary computation of object approach by a wide-field visual neuron. *Science*, **270**, 1000–3.

Häusser, M., Stuart, G., Racca, C., and Sakmann, B. (1995). Axonal initiation and active dendritic propagation of action potentials in substantia nigra neurons. *Neuron*, **15**, 637–47.

Hawkins, R. D., Kandel, E. R., and Siegelbaum, S. A. (1993). Learning to modulate transmitter release: themes and variations in synaptic plasticity. *Annual Review of Neuroscience*, **16**, 625–65.

Hayashi, J. H., Moore, J. W., and Stuart, A. E. (1985). Adaptation in the input–output relation of the synapse made by the barnacles photoreceptor. *Journal of Physiology*, **368**, 179–95.

Heisenberg, M. (1989). Genetic approach to learning and memory (mnemogenetics) in *Drosophila melanogaster*. In *Fundamentals of memory formation: neuronal plasticity and brain function*, (ed. B. Rahmann), pp. 3–45. Fischer, New York.

Heisenberg, M., Borst, A., Wagner, S., and Byers, D. (1985). *Drosophila* mushroom body mutants are deficient in olfactory learning. *Journal of Neurogenetics*, **2**, 1–30.

Herrick, C. J. (1939). Cerebral fiber tracts of *Amblystoma tigrinum* in midlarval stages. *Journal of Comparative Neurology*, **71**, 511–612.

Hevers, W. and Hardie, R. C. (1993). Serotonin modulated *Shaker* potassium channels in *Drosophila* photoreceptors. In *Gene-brain-behaviour*, (ed. N. Elsner and M. Heisenberg), p. 631. Thieme, Stuttgart.

Hildebrand, J. G. and Shepherd, G. M. (1997). Mechanisms of olfactory discrimination: converging evidence for common principles across phyla. *Annual Review of Neuroscience*, **20**, 595–631.

Hodgkin, A. L. and Huxley, A. F. (1952). A quantitative description of membrane current and its application to conduction and excitation in nerve. *Journal of Physiology*, **117**, 500–44.

Hölldobler, B. and Wilson, E. O. (1994). *Journey to the ants: a story of scientific exploration.* Belknap Press of Harvard University Press, Cambridge, MA.

Jansonius, N. M. (1990). Properties of the sodium-pump in the blowfly photoreceptor cell. *Journal of Comparative Physiology A*, **167**, 461–7.

Johnston, D. and Wu, S. M.-S. (1995). *Foundations of cellular neurophysiology.* MIT Press, Cambridge, MA.

Juusola, M., Kouvalainen, E., Jarvilehto, M., and Weckström, M. (1994). Contrast gain, signal-to-noise ratio, and linearity in light-adapted blowfly photoreceptors. *Journal of General Physiology*, **104**, 593–621.

Koch, C. and Laurent, G. (1999). Complexity in the nervous system. *Science*. (In press).

Krapp, H. G. and Hengstenberg, R. (1996). Estimation of self-motion by optic flow processing in single visual interneurons. *Nature*, **384**, 463–6.

Krapp, H. G., Hengstenberg, B., and Hengstenberg, R. (1998). Dendritic structure and receptive-field organization of optic flow processing interneurons in the fly. *Journal of Neurophysiology*, **79**, 1902–17.

Laughlin, S. B. (1996). Matched filtering by a photoreceptor membrane. *Vision Research*, **36**, 1529–41.

Laughlin, S. B. and Weckström, M. (1993). Fast and slow photoreceptors—a comparative-study of the functional diversity of coding and conductances in the diptera. *Journal of Comparative Physiology A*, **172**, 593–609.

Laurent, G. (1990). Voltage-dependent non-linearities in the membrane of locust nonspiking local interneurones, and their significance for synaptic integration. *Journal of Neuroscience*, **10**, 2268–80.

Laurent, G. (1991). Evidence for voltage-activated outward currents in the neuropilar membrane of locust nonspiking local interneurones. *Journal of Neuroscience*, **11**, 1713–26.

Laurent, G. (1993). Adaptive gain control by nonlinear properties of local circuit neuron dendrites. *Journal of Physiology (Lond.)* **470**, 45–54.

Laurent, G. and Burrows, M. (1988). Direct excitation of nonspiking local interneurones by exteroceptors underlies tactile reflexes in the locust. *Journal of Comparative Physiology*, **162A**, 563–72.

Laurent, G. and Davidowitz, H. (1994). Encoding of olfactory information with oscillating neural assemblies. *Science*, **265**, 1872–5.

Laurent, G. and Naraghi, M. (1994). Odorant-induced oscillations in the mushroom bodies of the locust. *Journal of Neuroscience*, **14**, 2993–3004.

Laurent, G., Seymour-Laurent, K., and Johnson, K. (1993). Dendritic excitability and a voltage-gated calcium current in locust nonspiking interneurons. *Journal of Neurophysiology*, **69**, 1484–98.

Laurent, G., Wehr, M., and Davidowitz, H. (1996). Odour encoding by temporal sequences of firing in oscillating neural assemblies. *Journal of Neuroscience*, **16**, 3837–47.

MacLeod, K. and Laurent, G. (1996). Distinct mechanisms for synchronization and temporal patterning of odor-encoding neural assemblies. *Science*, **274**, 976–9.

MacLeod, K., Backer, A., and Laurent, G. (1998). Who reads temporal information contained across synchronized and oscillatory spike trains? *Nature*, **395**, 693–8.

Manor, Y., Nadim, F., Abbott, L. F., and Marder, E. (1997). Temporal dynamics of graded synaptic transmission in the lobster stomatogastric ganglion. *Journal of Neuroscience*, **17**, 5610–21.

Marder, E. (1998). From biophysics to models of network function. *Annual Review of Neuroscience*, **21**, 25–45.

Marder, E. and Calabrese, R. L. (1996). Principles of rhythmic motor pattern generation. *Physiological Review*, **76**, 687–717.

Marder, E. and Meyrand, P. (1989). Chemical modulation of an oscillatory neural circuit. In *Neuronal and cellular oscillators*, (ed. J. W. Jacklet), pp.317–38. Marcel Dekker, New York.

McClelland, A. D. and Grillner, S. (1983). Initiation and sensory gating of 'fictive' swimming and withdrawal responses in an *in vitro* preparation of the lamprey spinal cord. *Brain Research*, **269**, 237–50.

Meek, J. and Schellart, N. A. M. (1978). A Golgi study of goldfish optic tectum. *Journal of Comparative Neurology*, **182**, 89–122.

Miller, J. P. and Selverston, A. I. (1982). Mechanisms underlying pattern generation in lobster stomatogastric ganglion as determined by selective inactivation of identified neurons IV. Network properties of pyloric system. *Journal of Neurophysiology*, **48**, 1416–32.

Mobbs, P. G. (1982). The brain of the honeybee *Apis mellifera* I. The connections and spatial organization of the mushroom bodies. *Philosophical Transactions of the Royal Society of London. Series B: Biological Sciences*, **298**, 309–54.

Murphy, G. G. and Glanzman, D. L. (1997). Mediation of classical conditioning in *Aplysia californica* by long-term potentiation of sensorimotor synapses. *Science*, **278**, 467–71.

Olsen, Ø. H. and Calabrese, R. L. (1996). Activation of intrinsic and synaptic currents in leech heart interneurons by realistic waveforms. *Journal of Neuroscience*, **16**, 4958–70.

O'Shea, M. and Rowell, C. H. F. (1976). The neuronal basis of a sensory analyzer, the acridid movement detector system. II. Response decrement, convergence, and the nature of the excitatory afferents to the fan-like dendrites of the LGMD. *Journal of Experimental Biology*, **65**, 289–308.

O'Shea, M., Rowell, C. H. F., and Williams, J. L. D. (1974). The anatomy of a locust visual interneurone; the descending contralateral movement detector. *Journal of Experimental Biology*, **60**, 1–12.

Palka, J. (1967). An inhibitory process influencing visual responses in a fibre of the ventral nerve cord of locusts. *Journal of Insect Physiology*, **13**, 235–48.

Pollack, G. S. (1988). Selective attention in an insect auditory neuron. *Journal of Neuroscience*, **8**, 2635–9.

Quiring, R., Walldorf, U., Kloter, U., and Gehring, W. J. (1994). Homology of the *Eyeless gene of Drosophila* to the *small eye* gene in mice and *aniridia* in humans. *Science*, **265**, 785–9.

Ramón y Cajal, S. (1909). *Histologie du système nerveux de l'homme et des vertébrés*. Tome 1. Instituto Ramón y Cajal, Madrid.

Ratliff, F. (1965). *Mach bands: quantitative studies on natural networks in the retina*. Holden-Day, San Francisco.

Reichardt, W. (1987). Evaluation of optical motion information by movement detectors. *Journal of Comparative Physiology. A, Sensory, Neural, and Behavioral Physiology*, **161**, 313–5.

Rind, F. C. and Simmons, P. J. (1992). Orthopteran DCMD neuron: a reevaluation of responses to moving objectives. I. Selective responses to approaching objects. *Journal of Neurophysiology*, **68**, 1654–66.

Schildberger, K. and Homer, M. (1988). The function of auditory neurons in cricket phonotaxis. 1. Influence of hyperpolarization of identified neurons on sound localization. *Journal of Comparative Physiology A*, **163**, 621–31.

Scrymgeour-Wedderburn, J. F., Reith, C. A., and Sillar, K. T. (1997). Voltage oscillations in *Xenopus* spinal cord neurons: developmental onset and dependence on coactivation of NMDA and 5HT receptors. *European Journal of Neuroscience*, **9**, 1473–82.

Selverston, A. I., Kleindienst, H.-U., and Huber, F. J. (1985). Synaptic connectivity between cricket auditory interneurons as studied by selective photoinactivation. *Journal of Neuroscience*, **5**, 1283–92.

Singer, W. (1999). Striving for coherence. *Science* **397**, 391–3.

Single, S. and Borst, A. (1998). Dendritic integration and its role in computing image velocity. *Science*, **281**, 1848–50.

Sobel, E. C. and Tank, D. W. (1994). *In vivo* Ca^{2+} dynamics in a cricket auditory neuron: an example of chemical computation. *Science*, **263**, 823–6.

Stavenga, D. G. and Hardie, R. C. (1989). *Facets of vision*. Springer, Berlin.

Stopfer, M., Bhagavan, S., Smith, B., and Laurent, G. (1997). Impaired odor discrimination on desynchronization of odor-encoding neural assemblies. *Nature*, **390**, 70–4.

Strausfeld, N. J. (1976). *Atlas of an insect brain*. Springer, Berlin.

Sun, H. and Frost, B. J. F. (1998). Computation of different optical variables of looming objects in pigeon nucleus rotundus neurons. *Nature Neuroscience*, **1**, 296–303.

Wachowiak, M. and Ache, B. W. (1994). Morphology and physiology of multiglomerular olfactory projection neurons in the spiny lobster. *Journal of Comparative Physiology A*, **175**, 35–48.

Wang, X.-J. and Buzsaki, G. (1996). Gamma oscillation by synaptic inhibition in a hippocampal interneuronal network model. *Journal of Neuroscience*, **16**, 6402–13.

Wang, Y. and Frost, B. J. (1992). Time to collision signalled by neurons in the nucleus rotundus of pigeons. *Nature*, **356**, 236–8.

Watson, A. H. D. and Burrows, M. (1985). The distribution of synapses on the two fields of neurites of spiking local interneurones in the locust. *Journal of Comparative Neurology*, **240**, 219–32.

Watson, A. H. D. and Burrows, M. (1988). The distribution and morphology of synapses on nonspiking local interneurones in the thoracic nervous system of the locust. *Journal of Comparative Neurology*, **272**, 605–16.

Weckström, M. (1994). Voltage-activated outward currents in adult and nymphal locust photoreceptors. *Journal of Comparative Physiology A*, **174**, 795–801.

Weckström, M., Juusola, M., and Laughlin, S. B. (1992). Presynaptic enhancement of signal transients in photoreceptor terminals in the compound eye. *Proceedings of the Royal Society London, Series B*, **250**, 83–9.

Weckström, M., Järvilehto, M., and Heimonen, K. (1993). Spike-like potentials in the axons of nonspiking photoreceptors. *Journal of Neurophysiology*, **69**, 293–6.

Wehr, M. and Laurent, G. (1996). Odour encoding by temporal sequences of firing in oscillating neural assemblies. *Nature*, **384**, 162–6.

Wehr, M. and Laurent, G. (1999). Relationship between afferent and central temporal patterns in the locust olfactory system. *Journal of Neuroscience*, **19**: 381–390.

Wendt, B. and Homberg, U. (1992). Immunocytochemistry of dopamine in the brain of the locust *Schistocerca gregaria. Journal of Comparative Neurology*, **321**, 387–403.

White, J. G., Southgate, E., Thomson, J. N., and Brenner, S. (1986). The structure of the nervous system of the nematode *Caenorhabditis elegans. Philosophical Transactions of the Royal Society of London, Series B*, **314**, 1–340.

Wilson, D. M. (1961). The central nervous control of flight in a locust. *Journal of Experimental Biology*, **38**, 471–90.

Yang, M. Y., Armstrong, J. D., Vilinsky, I., Strausfeld, N. J., and Kaiser, K. (1995). Subdivision of the Drosophila mushroom bodies by enhancer trap expression patterns *Neuron*, **15**, 45–54.

Young, J. Z. (1964). *A model of the brain.* Oxford University Press.

13

Functional plasticity at dendritic synapses

Zachary F. Mainen

Cold Spring Harbor Laboratory

Summary

Most synapses are made onto dendrites, and most excitatory connections are made onto dendritic spines. Synaptic plasticity is thus an intrinsically dendritic phenomenon, but the functional significance of the structural, electrical and molecular properties of dendrites for synaptic plasticity is still very poorly understood. Do dendrites have a computational or cell biological role in the modification of synaptic strength that is more than circumstantial? The aim of this chapter is to summarize experimental data and theoretical considerations that may be relevant to the role of dendrites in synaptic plasticity. The focus is on associative Hebbian synaptic plasticity mediated by NMDA receptor activation.

Introduction

Synapses channel information between neurons in the brain, and are dynamically strengthened and weakened by the patterns of neuronal activity flowing through them. Activity-dependent synaptic plasticity is thought to be fundamental to many brain functions, including refinement of connections during development (reviewed in Katz and Shatz 1996 and Cline 1998; see Chapter 2), learning and memory and other forms of information storage (reviewed in Martinez and Derrick 1996 and Stevens 1998), and by extension many higher cognitive functions.

In this chapter, we first discuss the idea of Hebbian synaptic plasticity and the key biophysical characteristics of the NMDA receptor relevant to its role in Hebbian or associative long-term potentiation. The NMDA receptor is sensitive to the conjunction of neurotransmitter release and membrane depolarization and can therefore detect the conjunction of presynaptic and postsynaptic neuronal activity. The location of the receptors on dendritic spines may allow Ca^{2+} signals resulting from NMDA receptor activation to be localized to spines, permitting synapse-specific plasticity. In addition to this primary model, issues concerning other sources of spine Ca^{2+} (e.g. voltage-sensitive Ca^{2+} channels, VSCCs) and other possible coincidence detectors are also raised.

We next discuss how the Hebbian plasticity involving NMDA receptors on spines depends on two roles of dendrites: *integration* of the electrical activity that is detected by the receptor, permitting cooperativity and associativity of synaptic inputs, and *compartmentalization* of chemical messengers or signal transduction cascades, permitting synapse specificity. While the basic aspects of these functions are well understood, the impact of the detailed aspects of the integration and compartmentalization provided by dendrites is just beginning to be explored. We focus in particular on recent experiments concerning the role of dendritic action potentials in plasticity.

We argue that the major role of dendrites in synaptic plasticity may be in modifying the strength of interactions between particular subsets of synapses by virtue of their relative locations within the dendritic tree. This could occur either due to inhomogeneities of electrical signaling across the dendrites or breakdown of chemical compartmentalization between synapses. The complex architecture of dendritic arbors would facilitate the formation of associations between synapses on the same dendritic branches or subparts of the dendritic tree while suppressing associations between synapses located on different dendritic branches.

Dendritic spine NMDA receptors as Hebbian coincidence detectors

Hebb's postulate

Donald Hebb postulated the following synaptic strengthening rule:

When the axon of cell A is near enough to excite cell B or repeatedly or persistently takes part in firing it, some growth process or metabolic change takes place in one or both cells such that A's efficiency, as one of the cells firing B, is increased.

(Hebb 1949).

As a candidate mechanism for information storage in the brain, Hebb's postulate has withstood experimental and theoretical scrutiny like very few other principles of brain function (reviewed in Brown *et al.* 1990). Nevertheless, as a computational or mechanistic description, Hebb's rule clearly demands much further interpretation and fleshing out. How does a synapse 'know' when it has taken part in firing a cell? How are presynaptic and postsynaptic firing encoded in molecular events at the synapse? What molecules detect the conjunction of these events? How are the pre- and postsynaptic signals corresponding to one synapse kept separate from those belonging to other synapses?

Discovery of NMDA receptor-dependent LTP has led to a theory of synaptic plasticity that describes how neurons, dendrites and synapses implement Hebbian plasticity. This theory, which we will refer to as the 'spine-NMDA receptor theory' of LTP, will guide most of the discussion of synaptic plasticity in this chapter. Although the theory is still unproven and is lacking in many details, it is by far the most widely accepted and thoroughly documented account of the mechanisms by which synaptic connections between neurons are strengthened.

The primary omission from Hebb's rule is often considered to be the lack of a provision for decreases in synaptic efficacy. Without a mechanism for depression to complement synaptic potentiation, the brain would eventually face saturation of synaptic efficacy and consequent loss of stored information. What conditions allow for the undoing of synaptic strengthening or the weakening of connections? A number of different generalizations of the Hebb rule have been proposed on theoretical grounds (reviewed in Brown *et al.* 1990). Two forms of synaptic depression have received particular experimental attention: homosynaptic long-term depression (LTD) at hippocampal and neocortical synapses (reviewed in Bear and Malenka 1994), and associative LTD at cerebellar parallel fiber to Purkinje cell synapses (reviewed in Linden 1994). Of particular interest with respect to the role of dendrites is depression that is triggered by pairing of action potentials and EPSPs (discussed below).

Long-term potentiation

Long-term potentiation (LTP) is a particular form of synaptic strengthening (reviewed in Bliss and Collingridge 1993) that has been recognized as displaying the essential elements of Hebb's rule (Kelso *et al.* 1986; Malinow and Miller 1986; Gustafsson *et al.* 1987; Brown *et al.* 1990). LTP was originally described at synapses made between neurons in the entorhinal cortex and the granule cells in the dentate gyrus of the hippocampus (Bliss and Lømo 1973). When this pathway was activated with a brief, high-frequency stimulus train, a rapid and sustained increase in the strength of subsequent test stimuli was observed. Subsequent studies revealed similar forms of long-lasting, activity-dependent synaptic enhancement in all three of the major synapses of the hippocampal formation, as well as in numerous neocortical regions (reviewed in Bear and Kirkwood 1993 and Kirkwood and Bear 1995), amygdala (Chapman *et al.* 1990; Rogan and LeDoux 1995; Huang and Kandel 1998), striatum (Kombian and Malenka 1994; Calabresi *et al.* 1996), and other central as well as peripheral synapses (e.g. Brown and McAfee 1982).

The best-studied form of LTP is that which occurs at synapses of Schaffer commissural-collateral axons from CA3 to CA1 neurons in the hippocampus. The nature of LTP at other synapses, such as in the dentate gyrus or different neocortical synapses, may differ in various details that have not been thoroughly characterized. In general, neocortical LTP appears to have many similarities to CA1 LTP (Bear and Kirkwood 1993). Pyramidal cells in many brain regions appear similarly equipped in terms of plasticity machinery: NMDA receptors, spines, key protein kinases, etc. Nevertheless, it is worth keeping in mind the example of LTP at the mossy-fiber to CA3 synapse, which is mechanistically quite dissimilar to CA1 LTP (reviewed in Johnston *et al.* 1992 and Nicoll and Malenka 1995), but may display many of the same essential features (Derrick and Martinez 1996). Unless indicated otherwise, when speaking of LTP we refer to CA1 LTP, or in some cases neocortical LTP, throughout this chapter.

In contrast to the general agreement about how LTP is triggered or induced, there is much more controversy over the nature of the changes underlying synaptic strengthening, generally referred to as the 'expression mechanism'. Whether expression involves presynaptic or postsynaptic changes, or changes on both sides of the synapse, has significant consequences for information processing (Otmakhov *et al.* 1993), but is somewhat more removed from the function of dendrites than are the mechanisms of induction. This chapter focuses primarily on induction mechanisms and conditions under which LTP is triggered.

NMDA receptor properties

A Hebbian synaptic modification requires the detection of coincident presynaptic and postsynaptic activation (Hebb 1949). The response of a coincidence detector in the presence of both signals should be qualitatively different than the response to either signal alone. Some form of coincidence detection can be accomplished relatively simply by a response element with a supralinear response function such as a threshold. A number of examples of molecules capable of functioning in this way are discussed in Bourne and Nicoll (1993).

The NMDA receptor is a remarkable macromolecular complex with a strong claim to be the Hebbian detector underlying LTP. Sensitivity to specific NMDA receptor antagonists (e.g. 2-amino-5-phosphopentanoic acid, AP5) is usually considered the *sine qua non* of the main form of LTP (Bliss and Collingridge 1993), although NMDA receptor-independent dependent forms of LTP have also been described (reviewed in Johnston *et al.* 1992 and Nicoll and Malenka 1995). By virtue of an unusual set of biophysical characteristics, the NMDA receptor opens only when both the presynaptic and postsynaptic neurons are activated. Specifically, receptor opening requires both a presynaptic chemical signal (neurotransmitter) and a postsynaptic electrical signal (local membrane depolarization). When both occur together, the opening of the receptor allows Ca^{2+} ions to enter the postsynaptic neuron and activate Ca^{2+}-sensitive enzymes that eventually lead to synaptic potentiation or depression.

The excitatory neurotransmitter glutamate activates two primary ion channel-coupled (ionotropic) receptors, the AMPA and NMDA receptors (so named for their artificial agonists, α-amino-3-hydroxy-5-methyl-4-isoxazolepropionate and *N*-methyl-D-aspartate, respectively; reviewed in Edmonds *et al.* 1995). The AMPA receptors are generally seen as providing the primary depolarization associated with synaptic activation, while the NMDA receptors are viewed as a secondary source of depolarization, being primarily involved in plasticity.

The sensitivity of the NMDA receptor for glutamate is high (EC50 in the 1 μM range, Patneau and Mayer 1990) making the receptor more sensitive to lower concentrations of transmitter than the AMPA receptor (EC50 >100 μM; Patneau and Mayer 1990). The high affinity of the NMDA receptor is also associated with a very slow deactivation rate following brief applications of glutamate (100 to >500 ms); meaning that once presynaptically-released glutamate binds to the receptor, it remains bound for a fairly lengthy time period. Therefore the NMDA receptor acts as a long-lasting indicator of presynaptic activity.

A crucial and unusual biophysical characteristic of the NMDA receptor is that it remains 'silent' at normal resting potentials and does not pass current unless the membrane is depolarized. When the receptor is bound by glutamate, the pore of the receptor opens but conduction of the channel is blocked by extracellular Mg^{2+} ions (Mayer *et al.* 1984; Nowak *et al.* 1984). Depolarization of the postsynaptic membrane expels Mg^{2+} from the channel, allowing it to conduct a mixture of Na^+, K^+ and Ca^{2+}. Thus, due to the voltage-sensitivity of the Mg^{2+} block, the conductance of the NMDA receptor is a supralinear function of postsynaptic voltage over the range of potentials from rest to around –20 mV. The kinetics of the Mg^{2+} block are rapid (Nowak *et al.* 1984), so in contrast to the slow deactivation of the receptor, the coupling of depolarization to channel block is nearly instantaneous (on a sub-millisecond time-scale; Spruston *et al.* 1995). It should also be noted that in addition to activation by glutamate and modulation by Mg^{2+}, the NMDA receptor is sensitive to a large and diverse array of molecular signals, including glycine, zinc, polyamines, histamine, pH, redox agents, neurosteroids, calmodulin, kinases, and phosphatases (reviewed in McBain and Mayer 1994).

NMDA receptors display considerable molecular diversity. Functional receptors are composed of NR1 subunits in combination with members of the NR2 gene family. Different NR2 subunits confer different physiological and pharmacological properties on the receptor (reviewed in Feldmeyer and Cull-Candy 1996). In addition, the NR1 subunit also exists in a variety of different splice variants that confer different properties to the receptor (reviewed in Zukin and Bennett 1995). Developmental and cell-type specific regulation of subunit composition and splicing give rise to diversity in the functional properties of NMDA receptors across different neuronal populations. Of particular interest with respect to NMDA receptor plasticity are subunit-specific differences in deactivation and Mg^{2+} sensitivity (Monyer *et al.* 1994). Cells expressing NMDA receptors with different subunit composition may exhibit shorter or longer integration times or sensitivity to post-synaptic depolarization. Diversity of subunit composition within single neurons may also be important, perhaps depending on the class of presynaptic afferent (cf. Maccaferri *et al.* 1998).

The second crucial property of the NMDA receptor is its permeability to Ca^{2+} ions (MacDermott *et al.* 1986; Ascher and Nowak 1988). It is through this second messenger that the receptor couples its activation to downstream enzymes. For example, intracellular postsynaptic application of Ca^{2+} chelators blocks LTP (Lynch *et al.* 1983; Malenka *et al.* 1988). The location of the synaptic NMDA receptors on dendritic spines is thought to restrict the increase in intracellular $[Ca^{2+}]$ to the vicinity of the activated synapse (reviewed in Koch and Zador 1993). The basic structural feature of a head separated from the parent dendrite by a thin neck has been shown by computer simulations (Holmes and Levy 1990; Zador *et al.* 1990) and direct experimental measurement (Svoboda *et al.* 1996; Häusser *et al.* 1997) to hinder diffusion of molecules between the spine head and the dendritic shaft (and *vice versa*). Theoretical and experimental issues regarding the role of dendritic spines and other dendritic compartments in compartmentalizing Ca^{2+} and other (bio)chemicals are the subject of Chapter 7.

Electrical integration and compartmentalization by dendrites

The requirement for both glutamate and postsynaptic depolarization for NMDA receptor activation, and the location of these receptors on dendritic spines, form the basis for the spine-NMDA receptor theory of Hebbian plasticity. This model can

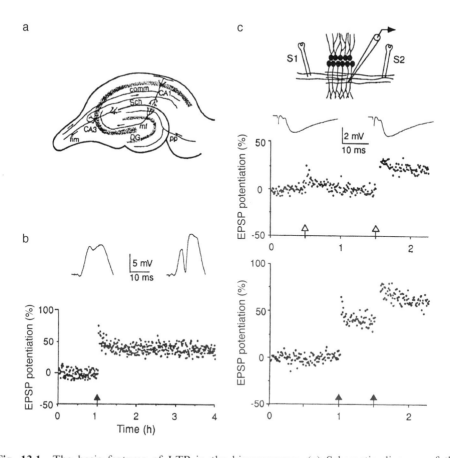

Fig. 13.1 The basic features of LTP in the hippocampus. (a) Schematic diagram of the hippocampus, showing the principal regions (CA1, CA3, and dentate gyrus (DG)) and excitatory pathways (perforant path, pp; mossy fibers, mf; fimbria, fim; Schaffer collaterals, Sch; and commissural fibers, comm). (b) Field potential recordings in the somatic region of the dentate gyrus *in vivo* in response to perforant path stimulation recorded before (left) and 3 h after (right) LTP induction using a 250 Hz, 200 ms tetanus. Note the increase in slope of the population EPSP and in the size of the population spike (downward deflection). The graph plots the slope of the rising phase of the population EPSP following LTP induction (at the time of the arrow). (c) Demonstration of cooperativity, associativity and synapse-specificity of LTP. The top diagram shows a schematic diagram of the arrangement of recording and stimulation electrodes in the CA1 region of a hippocampal slice. Two independent inputs (S1 and S2) are activated by stimulation electrodes placed on either side of the extracellular recording electrode in the dendritic field. The stimulus intensities are adjusted so that S1 provides a weak input, and S2 a strong input. The slopes of the population EPSPs for the two pathways are plotted as a function of time in the lower panels. Tetanic stimulation of S1 (first open arrow) produced no long-lasting increase in synaptic efficacy, since the synaptic drive was below the cooperativity threshold for LTP. A tetanus to S2 (first closed arrow) produced robust LTP in this pathway, but no change in S1, demonstrating synapse-specificity of the potentiation. When both pathways were tetanized together (second open and closed arrows), this coincident activation produced associative LTP in the weak pathway, S1. Representative field EPSPs following S1 stimulation, taken before and after potentiation, are shown above the graphs. Taken, with permission, from Bliss and Collingridge (1993).

explain three central aspects of the phenomenology of LTP induction: *cooperativity*, *associativity* and *synapse-specificity* (see Fig. 13.1). We will discuss these properties in some detail, as they are essential to the role of dendrites in synaptic plasticity. Two other primary characteristics of NMDA receptor-dependent LTP, its rapid induction and persistent expression, while critical to the possible function of LTP in memory storage, are relatively less important with regard to dendritic function.

Cooperative interactions mediated by dendrites

Cooperativity refers to the requirement for the near-simultaneous activation of a threshold level of synaptic input necessary in order to induce LTP. In practice, cooperativity has been seen as sensitivity to either the frequency of stimulation delivered during a tetanization protocol (Bliss and Lømo 1973; Colino *et al.* 1992) or to the intensity of the extracellular stimulus used to activate presynaptic axons during a tetanus (Bliss and Gardner-Medwin 1973; McNaughton *et al.* 1978; Barrionuevo and Brown 1983).

Consistent with the spine-NMDA receptor theory, LTP induction does not appear to require a certain density of activated synapses or frequency of synaptic activation other than what is necessary to produce the requisite NMDA receptor activation. Direct experiments demonstrate that depolarization (applied by a postsynaptic recording electrode) combined with low-frequency stimulation of presynaptic afferents is sufficient to induce LTP (Kelso *et al.* 1986; Wigstrom *et al.* 1986; Colino *et al.* 1992). Conversely, membrane hyperpolarization is sufficient to prevent LTP from taking place during high frequency stimulation that would normally elicit LTP (Kelso *et al.* 1986; Malinow and Miller 1986). These findings provide key support for the idea that the role of synaptic activation in cooperativity is mediated solely through synaptic depolarization (and possible subsequent electrogenesis) and the consequent relief of the NMDA receptor Mg^{2+} block. Conversely, cooperativity does not appear to be related to a threshold for some other signal (e.g. glutamate, presynaptic Ca^{2+}).

Dendrites mediate the *spatial* and *temporal* integration of depolarization produced by active synapses, and therefore dendritic integration shapes the cooperativity property of LTP induction. Without dendritic electrical integration, multiple synapses within a pathway would not sense each other's activity. The simplest form of cooperativity just requires that dendrites sum their synaptic inputs. But what exactly are the detailed spatial and temporal properties of the integrative process? How do spatial or temporal proximity affect the summation (or other interactions) of active inputs? In order to understand the full nature of cooperativity and the rules for when LTP will be generated, a better understanding of dendritic integration is necessary.

If the dendritic arbor were effectively isopotential (i.e. voltage uniformity in all dendritic branches), then the spatial aspect of dendritic integration would be negligible. All synapses, regardless of location, would experience the same postsynaptic depolarization. As discussed in Chapters 9 and 10, dendrites are seldom isopotential. As passive electrical compartments, dendrites low-pass filter signals temporally and attenuate their spread spatially (see Chapters 9 and 10). When the active (voltage-dependent) electrical properties of dendrites are also considered, the rules become potentially much more complex (see Chapters 10 and 11). The initiation of action potentials and the extent of their propagation into the dendritic tree may make an important contribution to the depolarization seen by a synapse. The upshot of these considerations is that the location of a synapse within the dendritic tree may determine to some degree how that synapse will interact with other active synapses (see Chapter 11). Computer simulations suggest that active dendritic conductances (e.g. voltage-gated Na^+ channels or NMDA receptors) increase cooperativity (depolarization) among 'clustered' compared to 'diffuse' synaptic inputs (Mel 1993), and that this may lead to selective strengthening of synapses whose activity is both correlated and dendritically clustered (see below).

The limits of cooperativity requirements have been tested in a variety of experiments. Frequency of presynaptic activation is certainly an important parameter of LTP induction under most circumstances. This is expected for a number of different reasons, including the frequency-dependence of presynaptic release probability, the integration time constant of the postsynaptic membrane, and the sensitivity of Ca^{2+} dependent enzymes such as CaMKII (De Koninck and Schulman 1998). Nevertheless, it has been shown that single very strong afferent stimuli (Abraham *et al.* 1986) as well as weak stimuli paired with maintained intracellular depolarization (Colino *et al.* 1992) can induce LTP even when these stimuli are separated by as much as 1 min. The low success rate of such protocols would be expected from the low probability of transmitter release occurring on a given stimulus. With respect to the role of the number of activated synapses required for the induction process, it has been shown that activation of even a single presynaptic neuron is sufficient to induce LTP if postsynaptic depolarization is applied *via* a recording pipette (Malinow 1991). Together, these findings form an extremely important foundation for the spine-NMDA receptor theory, as they appear to exclude quite convincingly the necessity of activating other coincidence detectors that could mediate cooperativity and associative synaptic interactions by sensing the number of activated synapses through some signal other than depolarization.

Associative interactions mediated by dendrites

In the context of LTP experiments, associativity refers to the ability of a 'test' pathway to be potentiated when activated together with a separate 'conditioning' pathway (e.g. Barrionuevo and Brown 1983). The test pathway is stimulated weakly so that LTP is not induced by this stimulus alone. The conditioning pathway is given strong stimulation, providing sufficient depolarization to induce LTP. The 'associative interaction' describes the ability of the strong pathway to provide the postsynaptic signal needed by the weak pathway so that it too undergoes LTP during co-activation. In general, then, associative interaction refers to cooperation (*via* postsynaptic depolarization) between different sets of synapses. Associativity can also refer to the ability of some other source of postsynaptic depolarization (e.g. by an electrode or by postsynaptic action potentials) to provide the postsynaptic depolarization needed to trigger LTP. Cooperativity between synapses, as discussed above, is essentially the same process.

The associative properties of LTP were first described in the dentate gyrus *in vivo* by pairing weak input from contralateral entorhinal cortex with a strong ipsilateral input (McNaughton *et al.* 1978; Levy and Steward 1979, 1983). Concurrent activation of both pathways achieved potentiation where stimulation of either pathway alone failed to potentiate the weak input. These experiments naturally also demonstrated the synapse specificity of LTP (see below). Later, associativity was also demonstrated in the CA1 region of the hippocampal slice (Barrionuevo and Brown 1983), a preparation in which the effects of inhibition and potential circuit complexities were minimized.

Mechanistically, the properties of the NMDA receptor explain in a simple manner the ability to form associative interactions through the summation of postsynaptic depolarization. Stimulation of the test input provides the release of glutamate required for binding to NMDA receptors. Concurrent stimulation of the conditioning input provides the postsynaptic depolarization, which is also experienced by the test input, necessary to activate the glutamate-bound NMDA receptors by relieving Mg^{2+} block.

Spatial limits on associativity

As with cooperativity, dendritic electrical integration mediates the associative interactions between sets of synapses. Assuming perfect spatial integration (i.e. an isopotential dendritic tree), the relationship of synapses in the test and conditioning inputs (other than shared identity of synapses) is irrelevant—all associations between different synapses or pathways onto a cell are equivalent. But if neurons are not isopotential, then the spatial relationship of synapses in the two pathways will modify the associative interaction. Electrically proximal synapses would be more likely to share depolarization than electrically remote synapses. The contribution of non-isopotential postsynaptic compartments to a Hebbian plasticity rule has been simulated (Mainen *et al.* 1990) and analyzed mathematically (Pearlmutter 1995). Although these studies suggest that electrotonic attenuation will affect patterns of synaptic strengthening, empirical verification of this possibility is very interesting but technically challenging.

Very few experimental data are available on the spatial parameters of associative LTP. One difficulty with this class of experiment is that the locations of active synapses are not well known with most electrophysiological techniques. In a structure with laminated afferents, such as the hippocampus or cerebellar cortex, the position of an extracellular stimulating electrode can be used to try to localize activated afferents (e.g. Andersen *et al.* 1980), but the spatial specificity is nevertheless limited and the precise dendritic locations of synapses are unknown. It is also unclear how results obtained with synchronous activation of relatively large numbers of synapses will resemble physiological (*in vivo*) patterns of activity.

A notable set of studies by Levy and colleagues (White *et al.* 1988, 1990) demonstrated a spatial specificity of associative LTP in the dentate gyrus *in vivo*. Using current source density analysis to map the location of active synapses along the proximo-distal axis of the granule cells, the authors determined the degree of overlap between various pairs of stimulated pathways from the entorhinal cortex. The ability of a strong ipsilateral conditioning input to potentiate a weak contralateral test input depended on the amount of overlap between the two sets of inputs, with an overlap of $> 50\%$ needed for significant potentiation (White *et al.* 1990).

Although it might have been surmised that this spatial specificity arose simply from voltage attenuation between synaptic populations, further studies actually pointed to a critical role for inhibition in the spatial specificity. Blockade of inhibition enhanced associative interactions between non-overlapping synapses (Tomasulo *et al.* 1993). These results were supported by computer simulations which showed that massive local shunting inhibition, but not voltage attenuation alone, would be required to decouple different groups of synapses in these electrotonically compact cells (Holmes and Levy 1997). The role of action potentials in dentate associative LTP remains somewhat unclear (Holmes and Levy 1997; see below). In disinhibited CA1 slices, associative LTP can be produced between basal and apical dendritic inputs separated by hundreds of microns (Gustafsson and Wigstrom 1986).

Modification of associativity by inhibition
These results stress that inhibition may critically regulate the induction of dendritic synaptic plasticity. Feed-forward and feedback inhibitory circuits are often recruited in experimental induction paradigms (unless inhibition is pharmacologically blocked) and are certainly also critical in the physiological activation of local circuits in the hippocampus, neocortex and other brain regions. Blockade of inhibition changes considerably the stimulus conditions necessary for LTP induction and raises the probability of LTP induction in a slice preparation. For example, 'primed burst' (Larson and Lynch 1986) or 'theta burst' stimulation (brief bursts delivered at 200 ms inter-stimulus interval, corresponding to the endogenous theta frequency) is particularly effective in inducing LTP because it results in effective disinhibition of the slice (Pacelli *et al.* 1989) through presynaptic $GABA_B$ autoreceptors on GABAergic terminals (Davies and Collingridge 1996). These studies strongly suggest that dynamic changes in inhibitory circuitry due to activity patterns or neuromodulation provides an important influence on dendritic integration mediating synaptic plasticity *in vivo*.

Inhibition may severely alter the integrative properties of dendritic trees (Häusser and Clark 1997; Holmes and Levy 1997; Paré *et al.* 1998). At a gross level, inhibition interacts with excitatory synaptic drive by summation (hyperpolarizing the membrane) or multiplication (shunting inhibition), lowering the voltage levels reached postsynaptically or preventing the initiation of action potentials. More complex roles of inhibition depend on the precise location of inhibitory synapses within the dendritic tree and temporal relationship of their activation to the activation of excitatory synapses (Raastad *et al.* 1998). Tonic synaptic activity (both inhibition and excitation) can substantially alter the cable properties of dendrites, reducing the effective membrane resistance and thereby increasing electrotonic attenuation (Bernander *et al.* 1991; Häusser and Clark 1997; Paré *et al.* 1998; but see Raastad *et al.* 1998).

The results of Levy and colleagues make a fairly strong case that at least under some conditions, excitatory and inhibitory EPSPs effectively carve out multiple semi-independent units within the dendritic tree. It will be interesting to test whether these results can be extended to other synapses and to finer dendritic sub-regions. Computer simulations suggest that semi-independent synapse 'clusters' may form across individual dendritic branches (Mainen *et al.* 1990). These effects can be expected due to passive electrotonic structure (Korogod *et al.* 1994) or the amplification of local postsynaptic depolarization by dendritic non-linearities (regenerative currents, Mel 1993; Mel *et al.* 1998). The prediction of these models is that statistical properties (i.e. the correlation structure) of the set of inputs to the neuron are represented in the spatial location of the synapses (see Chapter 11). Means for local stimulation and optical monitoring of synaptic activity may be useful in testing these possibilities.

Temporal limits on associativity

xThe temporal requirements of associative LTP are relatively easy to characterize compared to its spatial requirements, and are also quite important. The biophysical properties of the NMDA receptor provide an important prediction regarding the temporal asymmetry of its detection of synaptic conjunctions. Recall that the effect of presynaptic glutamate is long-lasting (the channel deactivates slowly), while the postsynaptic depolarization affects the channel essentially instantaneously through a rapidly flickering Mg^{2+} block. Therefore, one would predict that temporal order of pre- and postsynaptic signals is quite critical. The presynaptic signal may precede the postsynaptic signal by a time window corresponding to the decay time of the NMDA current, but the reverse order would not produce receptor activation. Temporal asymmetry is also found implicitly in Hebb's rule: the requirement that the presynaptic cell 'takes part in firing' the postsynaptic cell (Hebb 1949) suggests a causal relationship which in turn entails that presynaptic activity precedes postsynaptic activity.

Experiments confirm the expectation of Hebb's rule and the spine NMDA receptor theory. Backward conditioning between weak and strong pathways fails to generate LTP (Levy and Steward 1983; Gustafsson and Wigstrom 1986; Kelso and Brown 1986). Recent studies pairing postsynaptic action potentials (APs) with EPSPs have mapped the temporal sensitivity of associative interactions even more precisely. The role of backpropagating action potentials in plasticity is examined in more detail below.

Associativity has been seen as an important property of LTP in relation to its presumptive role in learning and memory. Simple forms of learning such as classical conditioning involve associative interactions which appear somewhat analogous to associative LTP paradigms (reviewed in Quinn 1998). The weak input would correspond to or in some way represent the conditioned stimulus (CS) while the strong input would correspond to the unconditioned stimulus (US). Following pairing of CS and US, the CS response becomes potentiated and can now evoke the response previously exclusive to the US. The temporal requirements of these learning paradigms (CS must predict or precede US) appears to have a direct mapping to the temporal requirements of associative LTP, although this may be coincidental. For instance, it is not clear whether depolarization rather than, for instance, a neuromodulatory signal carries information in the US. Several recent studies have provided remarkable evidence that just such an associative LTP-like phenomenon in the lateral amygdala mediates the acquisition of fear conditioning (Rogan and LeDoux 1995; McKernan and Shinnick-Gallagher 1997; Rogan *et al.* 1997). More complex forms of learning have less clear relationships with the cellular properties of LTP induction and may call for entirely new mechanisms, such as the provision of a global reinforcement signal which is not computed locally by the cell (reviewed by Schultz *et al.* 1997).

Backpropagating action potentials and synaptic plasticity

The presence of voltage-gated Na^+, K^+ and Ca^{2+} channels in the dendritic arbor may profoundly change the function of the dendrites in synaptic integration (see Chapters 9–11). It follows directly that the integrative function of the dendrites in synaptic plasticity will also be critically shaped by these active channels. The function of active dendritic processing may have as much impact on signaling between synapses as on conveying synaptic signals to the soma.

Action potentials are usually initiated in the axon (reviewed by Stuart *et al.* 1997*b*), but the presence of voltage-gated Na^+ channels throughout the dendritic arbor of hippocampal and neocortical pyramidal cells (along with favorable electrical load considerations) promotes the propagation of regenerative currents 'backward' into the dendritic arbor (see Chapters 6, 9 and 10). Thus, a back-propagating action potential may serve to notify synapses throughout the dendritic tree when a spike has been emitted from the axon. The role of backpropagating action potentials in synaptic plasticity has recently become a topic of considerable interest. Under physiological conditions, do these action potentials mediate the postsynaptic depolarization necessary for NMDA receptor opening? If so, this finding would bring the physiology even closer to Hebb's principle requiring firing of both presynaptic and postsynaptic neurons (Hebb 1949).

Are backpropagating action potentials necessary?

It has been demonstrated that action potentials are not strictly necessary for the induction of CA1 LTP (McNaughton *et al.* 1978; Kelso *et al.* 1986; Gustafsson *et al.* 1987). The depolarization necessary for NMDA receptor opening can be directly supplied by current injected through a recording pipette under conditions where spikes are absent postsynaptically. Indeed, a common procedure for inducing LTP in whole-cell recordings is to voltage clamp the neuron at around 0 mV while stimulating presynaptic afferents at low frequency (Malinow and Tsien 1990). The fact that LTP can be readily induced in the absence of postsynaptic firing suggests the simple explanation that the main influence of backpropagating action potentials on LTP is their depolarization of the NMDA receptor and the consequent amplification of NMDA-receptor-mediated Ca^{2+} influx (Koch and Zador 1993; Yuste and Denk 1995; Koester and Sakmann 1998; Schiller *et al.* 1998; Yuste *et al.* 1999), rather than a secondary mechanism such as activation of voltage-gated Ca^{2+} channels (see below).

While postsynaptic action potentials may not be strictly necessary, it is an important and difficult problem to determine under what conditions postsynaptic action potentials are in fact involved in the normal (*in vivo*) induction of LTP. Blockade of postsynaptic action potentials (Scharfman and Sarvey 1985) or specific blockade of their dendritic backpropagation (Magee and Johnston 1997) can prevent LTP induction under some conditions. In some preparations, AP–EPSP pairing can induce LTP where pairing EPSPs and prolonged depolarization or high-frequency stimulation fails (Markram *et al.* 1997; Zhang *et al.* 1998). A *requirement* for action potentials, in the context of the spine-NMDA receptor theory, implies that sub-threshold summation of EPSPs cannot produce enough depolarization to activate NMDA receptors sufficiently to generate potentiation. Thus, synaptic cooperativity under physiological conditions could reflect the necessity for sufficient synaptic depolarization to elicit spikes (Zhang *et al.* 1998). Likewise, associative interactions would depend not on direct sharing of depolarization between synapses, but on the ability of one input to generate the postsynaptic action potentials necessary to bring about NMDA receptor depolarization. Understanding these phenomena will ultimately demand monitoring *in vivo* patterns of pre- and post-synaptic activity and their consequences for the strength of synaptic connections (e.g. Thomas *et al.* 1998).

Relatively few studies have yet tested pairing of presynaptic EPSPs and postsynaptic action potentials to induce LTP. The results of recent experiments in a range of preparations, including neocortical slices (Markram *et al.* 1997); acute hippocampal slices (Magee and Johnston 1997), cultured hippocampal slices (Debanne *et al.* 1998) and dissociated cultures (Bi and Poo 1998); and frog tectal neurons *in vivo* (Zhang *et al.* 1998), are mostly consistent. LTP induced by pairing EPSPs and postsynaptic action potentials is usually (Markram *et al.* 1997; Bi and Poo 1998; Debanne *et al.* 1998; Zhang *et al.* 1998), but not always (Magee and Johnston 1997, see below) blocked by NMDA receptor antagonists. Synapse specificity of EPSP–AP pairing was demonstrated in tectal neurons (Zhang *et al.* 1998). Given that the vast majority of our knowledge of LTP mechanisms stems from experiments using tetanic stimuli (and to a lesser extent from low-frequency pairing with prolonged depolarization), it will be very important to determine whether mechanisms of EPSP–AP-induced LTP are indeed similar. Experiments such as verifying synapse specificity of induction, establishment of the duration of potentiation, and occlusion of tetanically-induced LTP and action potential pairing-induced potentiation would be useful in this regard.

Extracellular monitoring of EPSP–AP pairing-induced LTP would provide a simple experimental protocol that could facilitate the study of issues such as the temporal coincidence windows and sensitivity to pharmacological agents. In whole-cell pairing experiments, postsynaptic action potentials are generated by intracellular current pulses, but they can also be elicited by antidromic activation of postsynaptic cell axons. Perhaps surprisingly, such a protocol has not been successfully used. In one study examining orthodromic-antidromic pairing (Jester *et al.* 1995), conventional NMDA receptor-dependent LTP was not induced, but a form of potentiation known as 'EPSP-spike' (E-S) potentiation (Bliss and Lømo 1973) was seen. This type of potentiation is expressed as an increase in the size of an extracellular population spike relative to the size of the extracellular field EPSP and is neither dependent on NMDA receptor activation nor restricted to active synapses. Although the mechanisms of E-S potentiation are still somewhat obscure, there is evidence for changes in inhibitory circuitry (Chavez-Noriega *et al.* 1990). One modeling study proposed that an increase in dendritic excitability could produce a general increase in the coupling of EPSPs to spike initiation (Wathey *et al.* 1992), but there is no experimental evidence to support this possibility.

Temporal sensitivity of EPSP–AP pairing

As with two-pathway experiments (Levy and Steward 1983; Gustafsson and Wigstrom 1986; Kelso *et al.* 1986), an asymmetrical window of coincidence is seen in EPSP–AP pairing studies: the EPSP must precede the postsynaptic action potential in order to induce LTP (Markram *et al.* 1997; Bi and Poo 1998; Debanne *et al.* 1998). As discussed above, this result can be understood in the context of NMDA receptor properties: the action of presynaptic glutamate decays slowly, but the action of depolarization on the Mg^{2+} block is very rapid.

How close in time must the postsynaptic action potential follow the EPSP in order to trigger plasticity? In layer 5 neocortical pyramidal neurons, a 100 ms interval produced no plasticity regardless of order, while a 10 ms interval produced potentiation when EPSPs preceded action potentials (Markram *et al.* 1997). In cultured hippocampal neurons, a similar protocol also produced LTP with forward pairing and LTD with backward pairing, but with an even more refined temporal requirement—a conjunction window of ~20 ms (see Fig. 13.2; Bi and Poo 1998). This time window is much shorter than can easily be explained by NMDA receptor kinetics, which raises the possibility that the efficacy of EPSP–AP pairing may depend on some other time-dependent effect of the EPSP arrival, e.g. the inactivation of dendritic K^+ channels by the EPSP (Hoffman *et al.* 1997; Magee and Johnston 1997). Interestingly, exactly synchronous pairing may not be effective in inducing potentiation (Debanne *et al.* 1998). This could perhaps be caused by the time needed for NMDA receptors to begin opening (rise time is around 10 ms) or a consequence of the EPSP facilitating backpropagation of a subsequent action potential (see below). The delay due to conduction of the action potential (velocity ~500 μm ms^{-1} along the main apical trunk; Stuart *et al.* 1997*a*) would seem to be relatively short even for distal synapses.

If the order of action potential and EPSP is reversed, so that the action potential precedes synaptic stimulation, LTP does not occur. However, where reverse pairing typically produces no changes in two-pathway associative LTP (Levy and Steward 1983; Gustafsson and Wigstrom 1986; Kelso *et al.* 1986), reverse AP–EPSP pairing produces depression of the paired synapses (Markram *et al.* 1997; Bi and Poo 1998; Debanne *et al.* 1998; Zhang *et al.* 1998). A similar result was originally observed with asynchronous pairing of EPSPs and depolarizing pulses in CA1 neurons of cultured hippocampal slices (Debanne *et al.* 1994, 1997). Remarkably, the switch from maximal potentiation to maximal depression may occur with a time shift of <5 ms (Bi and Poo 1998). The observation of bi-directional plasticity might be explained by findings that potentiation follows from a large increase in $[Ca^{2+}]$ while LTD follows from a smaller sustained increase (Yang *et al.* 1999). Ca^{2+} imaging suggests that the spine $[Ca^{2+}]$ achieved is greater during forward than backward pairing (Koester and Sakmann 1998; Yuste *et al.* 1999). Whether such differences could account for a radical change in the effect on synaptic transmission is unclear; this would be an obvious candidate for simulation studies. It seems apparent that various combinations of stimuli (for example postsynaptic action potentials of varying number) could lead to similar amplitudes of spine $[Ca^{2+}]$ increase. How then could peak spine $[Ca^{2+}]$ alone reliably distinguish a particular AP–EPSP sequence? Activation of downstream enzymes, particularly CaMKII, may sense not only

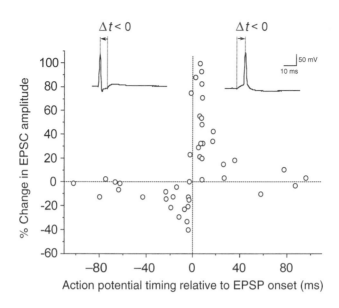

Fig. 13.2 Temporal window for the induction of synaptic potentiation and depression in hippocampal neurons. Persistent potentiation and depression of glutamatergic synapses were induced by correlated spiking of presynaptic and postsynaptic neurons in paired recordings from pyramidal neurons in dissociated hippocampal cultures. The graph shows the percentage change in the postsynaptic EPSC amplitude 20–30 min after repetitive correlated spiking (60 pulses at 1 Hz) plotted against the relative timing of pre- and postsynaptic activity. Action potential timing was defined by the time interval (Δt) between the onset of the EPSP and the peak of the presynaptic action potential during each cycle of repetitive stimulation, as illustrated by the traces above the graph. Only synapses with initial EPSC amplitude of < 500 pA were included, and all EPSPs were subthreshold for data associated with negatively correlated action potential timing. Taken, with permission, from Bi and Poo (1998).

amplitude but also temporal properties of $[Ca^{2+}]$ transients (De Koninck and Shulman 1998). Issues regarding Ca^{2+} signaling are discussed in more detail below (Synapse specificity section).

Regulation of backpropagating action potentials

Various mechanisms have been shown to be capable of modulating the spatial extent of dendritic action potential invasion in pyramidal neurons (see Chapters 6, 9 and 10). Differential invasion of backpropagating action potentials is a mechanism that might limit or reinforce the associations between particular synapses on the basis of their dendritic location. Generally speaking, synapses on a particular dendritic branch are likely to experience identical action potential signals, while synapses on different branches may experience distinct action potential signals. For example, under resting conditions in pyramidal neurons, action potentials typically do not fully invade the dendritic tree (Spruston *et al.* 1995; Stuart *et al.* 1997*a*); only synapses within the proximal regions of the dendritic tree would thus be subject to action potential depolarization and experience potentiation. These proximal synapses would therefore form associations with each other, but not with more distal (uninvaded) synapses. It is possible that invasion of action potentials may be controlled on a much more local level by up- or down-regulation of the activity of voltage-dependent Na^+ and K^+ channels. Thus, similar considerations might apply to individual sub-trees of secondary or even tertiary branches rather than simply to large-scale proximo-distal specificity. Candidate mechanisms for branch-specific regulation of backpropagating action potentials include branch-point failures (Jaffe *et al.* 1992; Regehr and Tank 1992; Spruston *et al.* 1995; Magee and Johnston 1997), excitatory (Hoffman *et al.* 1997; Magee and Johnston 1997; Magee *et al.* 1998) or inhibitory (Buzsaki *et al.* 1996; Tsubokawa and Ross 1996) synaptic input, phosphorylation (Hoffman and Johnston 1998; Magee *et al.* 1998), neuromodulatory transmitters (Tsubokawa and Ross 1997; Hoffman and Johnston 1999; Sandler and Ross 1999), and action potential-dependent inactivation (Colbert *et al.* 1997; Jung *et al.* 1997; Mickus *et al.* 1999).

Whether selective amplification and suppression of the invasion of different regions of the dendritic tree plays an important role in dendritic plasticity remains an intriguing conjecture. However, one very exciting set of studies (Hoffman *et al.* 1997; Magee and Johnston 1997; Magee *et al.* 1998) has gone some way toward demonstrating the possibility of branch-specific EPSP–AP pairing in CA1 pyramidal neurons. First, sub-threshold EPSPs boost the amplitude of backpropagating action potentials (Magee and Johnston 1997) by inactivating transient A-type K^+ channels, that are present at high density in CA1 pyramidal cell dendrites and can control backpropagating action potential amplitude there (Hoffman *et al.* 1997). Second, dendritic hyperpolarizing current injections can prevent induction of LTP by EPSP–AP pairing (Magee and Johnston 1997), perhaps by the fact that such injections can prevent action potential boosting by EPSPs (Magee and Johnston 1997). Third, at the fork of the primary apical dendrite of CA1 neurons, branch-specific boosting of action potentials can be produced by direct depolarizing pulses applied to one branch (see Fig. 13.3; Magee and Johnston 1997; Magee *et al.* 1998). It appears to follow logically, but remains to be demonstrated experimentally, that branch-specific associative LTP can be induced in this way. This might be accomplished by monitoring two weak (sub-threshold and non-EPSP-boosting) test pathways applied to separate branches and inducing potentiation by pairing with a strong (supra-threshold and EPSP-boosting) pathway confined to a single branch (or alternatively direct dendritic depolarization could substitute for the strong pathway). In the context of these action potential boosting experiments, it is interesting to note that the amplitude of Ca^{2+} transients in dendritic spines of neocortical neurons were only affected by AP–EPSP order under conditions in which NMDA receptors were not blocked (Koester and Sakmann 1998). This result could imply that either A-channel inactivation is particularly sensitive to NMDA receptor (*versus* AMPA receptor) EPSPs, or that such mechanisms present in CA1 neurons are absent or working differently in neocortical neurons. The latter suggestion is supported by the low apparent density of A-type K^+ channels in the dendrites of neocortical pyramidal neurons (Bekkers and Stuart 1998; Korngreen *et al.* 1999).

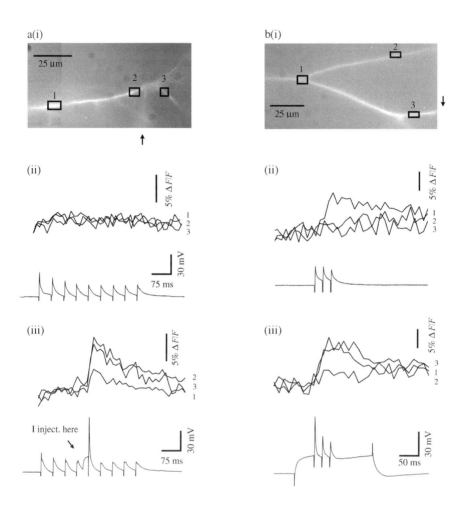

Fig. 13.3 Branch-specific boosting of action potentials in dendrites. (a) (i) CA1 pyramidal cell filled with Fura-2 *via* a dendritic patch pipette (arrow), located ∼290 μm from the soma. The image is oriented so that the more proximal regions of the neuron are located toward the left. (ii) Optical recordings (average $\Delta F/F$) from regions of the neuron delimited by the numbered boxes in (i), with dendritic voltage trace shown below. A train of nine antidromic action potentials (*bottom line*) triggers a very small Ca^{2+} signal in the distal dendrites. (iii) A 40 ms, 0.3 nA current injection causes an increase in dendritic action potential amplitude and associated Ca^{2+} signal. The largest Ca^{2+} signal is located nearest the dendritic pipette suggesting that the largest increase in action potential amplitude is near the point of current injection. A trace with only the current injection was used to correct for bleaching and for any small Ca^{2+} signals ($<1\%$ $\Delta F/F$) caused by the current injection. (b) (i) In a different pyramidal cell, a dendrite was filled with Fura-2 *via* a patch pipette located ∼280 μm from the soma on the lower branch (*arrow*), ∼50 μm distal to the site shown. The major branch point is ∼150 μm away from the soma. (ii) Optical recordings (average $\Delta F/F$) from regions of the neuron delimited by the numbered boxes in (i), with the dendritic voltage shown below. A train of three antidromic action potentials (*bottom line*) induces a Ca^{2+} signal primarily localized to regions of the dendrite proximal to the branch point. (iii) Current injection (0.2 nA) into the lower branch (*arrow*) causes an increase in the amplitude of the first dendritic

Chemical compartmentalization and integration by dendrites

Synapse specificity

Synapse specificity refers to the requirement for an individual synapse to be pre-synaptically activated in order for it to undergo potentiation during a conditioning protocol. Lack of synapse specificity implies a process that is not truly sensitive to the conjunction of pre- and postsynaptic activity. Although mechanisms for regulating the overall amount of synaptic input to a cell may play an important role (Turrigiano and Nelson 1998; Turrigiano *et al.* 1998), synapse specificity is often seen as a prerequisite for a cellular memory mechanism. The issue is basically one of computational or storage capacity. Roughly speaking, if each synapse stores one or a few bits of independent information, the storage capacity of a neuron is multiplied by the number of its synapses, typically 10^4 or more. A catastrophic breakdown of synapse specificity would clearly degrade capacity, but it has been argued that the effects of semi-local potentiation may be beneficial (e.g. Montague *et al.* 1991; Montague 1996).

In the hippocampus, synapse specificity of LTP was deduced from early studies (Andersen *et al.* 1977; Levy and Steward 1979). However, the experimental evidence demonstrating *strict* synapse specificity during LTP induction is perhaps weaker than the documentation of associative and cooperative phenomena. Numerous studies have been conducted with dual pathways of stimulated afferents. Typically, in the hippocampus, these are stimulated using large extracellular electrodes placed some distance (around 0.5–1 mm) apart from one another, either on opposite sides of the recording site or at separate locations along the proximo-distal axis of the cell. Thus, the precise spatial location of activated synapses is not known, but could generally involve either partially interdigitated or mostly segregated populations of synapses. Not knowing the location of active synapses, it remains possible that specificity breaks down on a spatial scale which is small relative to these distances (e.g. between neighboring spines on a small dendritic branch). Notably, in one of the most careful examinations of this issue, the authors found a *lack* of synapse specificity at distances < 150 μm (Engert and Bonhoeffer 1997). This study used local perfusion to pharmacologically isolate groups of nearby synapses in cultured hippocampal slices. Because there was no obvious dependence of the amount of cross-potentiation on the relationship of the groups of synapses to dendritic branching, these results could be interpreted as supporting an extracellularly-diffusing messenger rather than intradendritic diffusion. Similar conclusions were

---

action potential and a large increase in the Ca^{2+} signal in the dendritic branch that received the current injection, whereas only a very small signal is evident in the other branch. This profile suggests that coincident synaptic input can influence back-propagating action potentials to preferentially invade synaptically active regions of the dendrite. The current injection by itself did not produce a Ca^{2+} signal in the displayed regions. Taken, with permission, from Magee *et al.* (1998).

328 Functional plasticity at dendritic synapses

drawn from studies describing intercellular spread of potentiation between synapses on nearby neurons (Kossel *et al.* 1990; Schuman and Madison 1994).

According to the spine-NMDA receptor model, synapse specificity begins with the requirement for the presynaptic terminal to release glutamate directly onto NMDA receptors in order to bind and open them. Non-activated synapses may receive strong postsynaptic depolarization, but without glutamate binding to NMDA receptors, will not receive the necessary NMDA receptor-mediated Ca^{2+} influx. From this point, synapse specificity is believed to first rely on the ability of the postsynaptic dendrites to localize this $[Ca^{2+}]$ signal, and some portion of the signal transduction cascade that it activates, to the region of the synapse. Ultimately, the plasticity is expressed as a change in one or several local synaptic properties (e.g. number of functional postsynaptic receptors in the postsynaptic density). This theory also relies implicitly on an inability of other sources of spine Ca^{2+} (particularly VSCCs) to provide an adequate $[Ca^{2+}]$ signal for potentiation (discussed below).

Achieving synapse specificity may be most problematic with respect to those synaptic modifications that require *de novo* synthesis of plasticity-related proteins. It is believed that the initial maintenance of synaptic potentiation is provided by covalent modifications or translocation of synaptic proteins, but that maintenance of the potentiation beyond a period of some hours requires the recruitment of newly synthesized proteins (reviewed in Bliss and Collingridge 1993). Given that protein synthesis begins with transcription in the nucleus followed by ribosomal translation (either in the cell body or in the dendrites—see Chapter 3), the machinery cannot be contained entirely within a given spine synapse. Therefore, some provision must be made for targeting the newly synthesized proteins preferentially or exclusively to potentiated synapses. A number of hypotheses of how this might be achieved have been proposed (for example through a synaptic 'tag'; reviewed in Frey and Morris 1998). Quasi synapse-specific protein delivery might be achieved by up-regulating translation in a branch-specific manner. True synapse specificity would still require spine-specific markers or tags, such as a particular phosphorylated protein.

Dendritic spine [Ca^{2+}]

NMDA receptors have an unusually high permeability to Ca^{2+} ions (Mayer and Westbrook 1987; Ascher and Nowak 1988). The only well-recognized 'output' of the NMDA receptor is the flux of Ca^{2+} ions into the dendritic spine on which the receptors are located. Insofar as the NMDA receptor is the principal pathway for rises in spine $[Ca^{2+}]$, NMDA receptor activation and spine $[Ca^{2+}]$ activation could be considered equivalent coincidence detectors (but see below). The chemical compartmentalization provided by the spine (see Chapter 7) would provide a means for restricting the rise in $[Ca^{2+}]$ and subsequent activation of Ca^{2+}-sensitive enzymes that would catalyze the enhancement of synaptic strength.

A simple and popular hypothesis concerning the transduction of Ca^{2+} signals into different forms of synaptic plasticity is that the amplitude and duration of local spine $[Ca^{2+}]$ rises determine whether potentiation or depression (or nothing) will occur (Lisman 1989; Bear and Malenka 1994). A rise in postsynaptic $[Ca^{2+}]$ is necessary for LTP and LTD induction, as chelation of Ca^{2+} by intracellular buffers prevents the induction of LTP (Lynch *et al.* 1983; Malenka *et al.* 1988). Following reduction of Ca^{2+} entry through NMDA receptors (by pharmacological block using AP5 or hyperpolarization), a normally LTP-inducing tetanus can induce LTD (Cummings *et al.* 1996). Evidence for the sufficiency of spine $[Ca^{2+}]$ to induce potentiation or depression has been somewhat more difficult to obtain. Many stimuli that increase spine $[Ca^{2+}]$, such as action potentials or depolarizing voltage pulses, typically do not produce LTP, but may produce a transient potentiation (e.g. Kullmann *et al.* 1992). A difficulty in interpreting experiments of this type is that the $[Ca^{2+}]$ actually achieved at test synapses is not known. Protocols for inducing LTP by raising intracellular Ca^{2+} with photolysis of caged-Ca^{2+} compounds have yielded mixed results (Malenka *et al.* 1988; Neveu and Zucker 1996*a,b*). However, it appears that some of the variability observed in these studies may be avoided with a new caged-Ca^{2+} compound (Yang *et al.* 1999). As predicted, raising Ca^{2+} briefly to high levels consistently produced LTP, while raising Ca^{2+} to lower levels for a sustained period produced LTD (Yang *et al.* 1999). In these conditions, presynaptic activity and glutamate release are not necessary for potentiation to occur (but see Kullmann *et al.* 1992; Neveu and Zucker 1996*b*). The exact parameters of the required $[Ca^{2+}]$ rise may also depend on the history of the synapse (i.e. 'meta-plasticity', reviewed in Abraham and Bear 1996).

It is widely held that the main function of postsynaptic spines is to compartmentalize diffusible molecules at a single spine synapse and to prevent them from otherwise diffusing between synapses (Wickens 1988; Holmes and Levy 1990; Koch and Zador 1993; Svoboda *et al.* 1996; Häusser *et al.* 1997). Compartmentalization of synaptic Ca^{2+} transients by spines has been demonstrated with imaging techniques (Muller and Connor 1991; Denk *et al.* 1995; Yuste and Denk 1995; Koester and Sakmann 1998; Mainen *et al.* 1999; Yuste *et al.* 1999). However, it is not clear from these studies to what extent compartmentalization would hold under various stimulation conditions. It is worth noting that there is little evidence for synapse specific plasticity at synapses lacking spines (e.g. synapses onto aspiny inhibitory neurons, Cowan *et al.* 1998), as predicted by this theory of spine function. On the other hand, it is also possible that compartmentalization is achieved on a much smaller spatial scale than even the spine. There is evidence, for example in the process of vesicular release, that Ca^{2+} signaling molecules are located within a microdomain (<100 nm; reviewed by Neher 1998) near the mouth of a Ca^{2+} channel. The role of dendrites in compartmentalizing chemical signals is treated at length in Chapter 7.

Role of voltage-sensitive Ca^{2+} channels

Although the NMDA receptor is clearly a main source of spine Ca^{2+} entry, other sources of Ca^{2+} entry into dendritic spines clearly exist, in particular voltage-gated Ca^{2+} channels and intracellular Ca^{2+} stores. Local uncaging of neurotransmitter produces increases in spine $[Ca^{2+}]$ that are sensitive to various Ca^{2+} channel blockers (Schiller *et al.* 1998). Blockers of Ca^{2+} release from stores can dramatically reduce spine Ca^{2+} transients under some conditions (Emptage *et al.* 1999; but see Mainen *et al.* 1999). Backpropagating action potentials admit Ca^{2+} through voltage-sensitive Ca^{2+} channels (VSCCs) on dendrites and dendritic spines (Yuste and Denk

1995; Koester and Sakmann 1998; Magee *et al.* 1998; Yuste *et al.* 1999). The amount of Ca^{2+} entering the spine *via* NMDA receptor activation and *via* VSCC activation is of comparable magnitude (e.g. Koester and Sakmann 1998), although the NMDA receptor activation may be greatly increased during sustained depolarization. These observations raise the possibility that backpropagating APs or even local depolarization could mediate a plasticity signal independent of NMDA receptor gating.

The actual contribution of VSCCs to associative LTP is still controversial. Ca^{2+} influx through VSCCs is not strictly necessary for LTP, as voltage clamping the neuron at the synaptic reversal potential inactivates VSCCs and prevents then from being opened by EPSPs, but LTP can still be induced simply by paired EPSPs under these conditions (Perkel *et al.* 1993). Furthermore, LTP can be produced in the presence of L-type and T-type VSCC blockers (e.g. Huang and Malenka 1993; Hanse and Gustafsson 1994; Bi and Poo 1998). Blockers of other VSCC types (e.g. N, P, Q/R) affect presynaptic Ca^{2+} channels and block transmitter release, making pharmacological dissection of their roles more difficult to discern. Nevertheless, the possibility of cooperativity between NMDA receptor and VSCC mediated Ca^{2+} entry under particular stimulus conditions is not excluded by these experiments. Assuming that VSCCs are activated primarily during action potential invasion and not by sub-threshold stimulation (i.e. primarily high-threshold VSCCs are involved), the participation of VSCCs in LTP induction would depend on the extent to which action potentials are elicited and backpropagated during a particular induction protocol (Markram *et al.* 1997). When these variables are not measured and depend on the precise stimulation delivered, inconsistent results would be expected. In EPSP–AP pairing experiments, blockade of L-type VSCCs has been shown to partially prevent potentiation (Magee and Johnston 1997; Bi and Poo 1998) and can block depression (Bi and Poo 1998). Other forms of NMDA receptor-independent (and VSCC-dependent) potentiation have been described in neurons that also show NMDA receptor-dependent potentiation. Some of these, such as TEA-induced potentiation (e.g. Hanse and Gustafsson 1994), are heterosynaptic, but an associative form that requires synaptic stimulation (but not NMDA receptor activation) has also been reported (Kullmann *et al.* 1992). The latter study points to the possibility of a secondary coincidence detector (outside the spine-NMDA receptor theory).

How would the enzymes in a spine distinguish between Ca^{2+} arising from NMDA receptor influx and that arising from other Ca^{2+} sources? Is it possible that Ca^{2+} entering through the NMDA receptor has privileged access to a key enzyme by virtue of extreme proximity? The ability of EGTA to prevent LTP induction (Lynch *et al.* 1983) would suggest otherwise, as this chelator does not bind fast enough to prevent Ca^{2+} signaling on the scale of channel 'microdomains'. Furthermore, photolytic activation of fast Ca^{2+} buffers can prevent LTP induction up to 1 s after a tetanus (Malenka *et al.* 1992), indicating that Ca^{2+} must remain elevated for enough time to equilibrate over much larger spatial domains (see Chapter 7 for a discussion of diffusion issues).

The conundrum of how a synapse could distinguish the presynaptically gated NMDA receptor Ca^{2+} from purely postsynaptic sources of Ca^{2+} raises the question as to whether a second pathway parallel to the NMDA receptor might detect presynaptic activity. The main candidates for such a detector are the metabotropic glutamate receptors (mGluRs), which are not permeable to ions but directly activate second messenger pathways. The evidence for the involvement of mGluRs in LTP induction remains controversial (Selig *et al.* 1995). mGluRs might contribute additional Ca^{2+} into the spine *via* activation of Ca^{2+} release from stores (e.g. Emptage *et al.* 1999). In this case, spine $[Ca^{2+}]$ remains the coincidence detector and the problem remains unsolved. Alternatively, a downstream enzyme might integrate the Ca^{2+} signal with the mGluR-activated second messenger, thereby acting as a more precise, second order detector of pre- and postsynaptic activity. Further downstream coincidence detectors are also called upon for mechanisms of LTP expression involving presynaptic changes.

Concluding remarks

Our understanding of the physiology of LTP has been formalized by a theory based on spine NMDA receptors as coincidence detectors. The spine-NMDA receptor theory proposes two main functions for dendrites in explaining the phenomenology of LTP:

Electrical integration. Synapses interact by supplying depolarization (or hyper-polarization) that is sensed eventually by the NMDA receptor. Thus, the integrative function of the dendritic tree is seen as mainly electrical. Most experimental data is consistent with cell-wide summation of synaptic activity, with little exploration to date of how the active and passive propagation of electrical signals within dendrites may give rise to more complex synaptic relationships. The contributions of voltage-sensitive Ca^{2+} channels and coincidence detectors other than the NMDA receptor are still not well understood.

Chemical compartmentalization. Once activated, the NMDA receptor mediates a highly local (spine-specific) biochemical cascade with no interaction occurring between synapses. The dendritic tree, particularly through the dendritic spines on which excitatory synapses are formed, isolates synapses from one another to provide synapse specificity. Thus, the dendrites are seen as achieving chemical compartmentalization. Determination of the net effect of synaptic plasticity by the time course and amplitude of bulk spine $[Ca^{2+}]$ is an attractive, but still unproven hypothesis.

Recent work has indicated that these two concepts represent oversimplifications. Our view of the contribution of the dendritic arbor must take into account the following possibilities, which both imply that, under some circumstances, groups of neighboring synapses can form functional units:

Electrical compartmentalization. The dendritic arbor will promote not only electrical integration but inevitably some degree of compartmentalization or localization of passive and active electrical signaling. Synaptic integration and action potential backpropagation may be subject to dynamic control by a large number of modulatory influences. Associative interactions between synapses within the dendritic tree will therefore have a spatial or topological component, reinforcing synapses with nearby dendritic location and correlated activity. These possibilities remain largely in the realm of conjecture, and will require experimental means to measure and control the location of patterned synaptic activity.

Chemical integration. Dendrites and spines may not fully compartmentalize the signal transduction events downstream of NMDA receptor activation. Ca^{2+} signals may leave spines and travel between adjacent synapses under some conditions. While subsequently activated enzymes may be immobilized in spines, it is still not clear how the delivery of newly synthesized synaptic proteins is achieved in synapse-specific manner. Control of protein translation or protein trafficking may occur on a semi-local (e.g. branch-specific) scale.

References

Abraham, W. C. and Bear, M. F. (1996). Metaplasticity: the plasticity of synaptic plasticity. *Trends in Neurosciences*, **19**, 126–30.

Andersen, P., Sundberg, S. H., Sveen, O., and Wigstrom, H. (1977). Specific long-lasting potentiation of synaptic transmission in hippocampal slices. *Nature*, **266**, 736–7.

Andersen, P., Sundberg, S. H., Sveen, O., Swann, J. W., and Wigstrom, H. (1980). Possible mechanisms for long-lasting potentiation of synaptic transmission in hippocampal slices from guinea-pigs. *Journal of Physiology*, **302**, 463–82.

Ascher, P. and Nowak, L. (1988). The role of divalent cations in the *N*-methyl-D-aspartate responses of mouse central neurones in culture. *Journal of Physiology*, **399**, 247–66.

Barrionuevo, G. and Brown, T. H. (1983). Associative long-term potentiation in hippocampal slices. *Proceedings of the National Academy of Sciences USA*, **80**, 7347–51.

Bear, M. F. and Kirkwood, A. (1993). Neocortical long-term potentiation. *Current Opinion in Neurobiology*, **3**, 197–202.

Bear, M. F. and Malenka, R. C. (1994). Synaptic plasticity: LTP and LTD. *Current Opinion in Neurobiology*, **4**, 389–99.

Bekkers, J. M. and Stuart, G. (1998). Distribution and properties of potassium channels in the soma and apical dendrites of Layer 5 cortical pyramidal neurons. *Society for Neuroscience Abstracts*, **24**, 2019.

Bernander, O., Douglas, R. J., Martin, K. A., and Koch, C. (1991). Synaptic background activity influences spatiotemporal integration in single pyramidal cells. *Proceedings of the National Academy of Sciences USA*, 88, 11569–73.

Bi, G. Q. and Poo, M. M. (1998). Synaptic modifications in cultured hippocampal neurons: dependence on spike timing, synaptic strength, and postsynaptic cell type. *Journal of Neuroscience*, **18**, 10464–72.

Bliss, T. V. P. and Collingridge, G. L. (1993). A synaptic model of memory: long-term potentiation in the hippocampus. *Nature*, **361**, 31–9.

Bliss, T. V. and Gardner-Medwin, A. R. (1973). Long-lasting potentiation of synaptic transmission in the dentate area of the unanaesthetized rabbit following stimulation of the perforant path. *Journal of Physiology*, **232**, 357–74.

Bliss, T. V. and Lømo, T. (1973). Long-lasting potentiation of synaptic transmission in the dentate area of the anaesthetized rabbit following stimulation of the perforant path. *Journal of Physiology*, **232**, 331–56.

Bourne, H. R. and Nicoll, R. (1993). Molecular machines integrate coincident synaptic signals. *Cell*, **72** Suppl, 65–75.

Brown, T. H. and McAfee, D. A. (1982). Long-term synaptic potentiation in the superior cervical ganglion. *Science*, **215**, 1411–13.

Brown, T. H., Kairiss, E. W., and Keenan, C. L. (1990). Hebbian synapses: biophysical mechanisms and algorithms. *Annual Review of Neuroscience*, **13**, 475–511.

Buzsaki, G., Penttonen, M., Nadasdy, Z., and Bragin, A. (1996). Pattern and inhibition-dependent invasion of pyramidal cell dendrites by fast spikes in the hippocampus *in vivo*. *Proceedings of the National Academy of Sciences USA*, **93**, 9921–5.

Calabresi, P., Pisani, A., Mercuri, N. B., and Bernardi, G. (1996). The corticostriatal projection: from synaptic plasticity to dysfunctions of the basal ganglia. *Trends in Neurosciences*, **19**, 19–24.

Chapman, P. F., Kairiss, E. W., Keenan, C. L., and Brown, T. H. (1990). Long-term synaptic potentiation in the amygdala. *Synapse*, **6**, 271–8.

Chavez-Noriega, L. E., Halliwell, J. V., and Bliss, T. V. (1990). A decrease in firing threshold observed after induction of the EPSP–spike (E–S) component of long-term potentiation in rat hippocampal slices. *Experimental Brain Research*, **79**, 633–4.

Cline, H. T. (1998). Topographic maps: developing roles of synaptic plasticity. *Current Biology*, **8**, 836–9.

Colbert, C. M., Magee, J. C., Hoffman, D. A., and Johnston, D. (1997). Slow recovery from inactivation of Na^+ channels underlies the activity-dependent attenuation of dendritic action potentials in hippocampal CA1 pyramidal neurons. *Journal of Neuroscience*, **17**, 6512–21.

Colino, A., Huang, Y. Y., and Malenka, R. C. (1992). Characterization of the integration time for the stabilization of long- term potentiation in area CA1 of the hippocampus. *Journal of Neuroscience*, **12**, 180–7.

Cowan, A. I., Stricker, C., Reece, L. J., and Redman, S. J. (1998). Long-term plasticity at excitatory synapses on aspinous interneurons in area CA1 lacks synaptic specificity. *Journal of Neurophysiology*, **79**, 13–20.

Cummings, J. A., Mulkey, R. M., Nicoll, R. A., and Malenka, R. C. (1996). Ca^{2+} signaling requirements for long-term depression in the hippocampus. *Neuron*, **16**, 825–33.

Davies, C. H. and Collingridge, G. L. (1996). Regulation of EPSPs by the synaptic activation of $GABA_B$ autoreceptors in rat hippocampus. *Journal of Physiology*, **496**, 451–70.

De Koninck, P. and Schulman, H. (1998). Sensitivity of CaM kinase II to the frequency of Ca^{2+} oscillations. *Science*, **279**, 227–30.

Debanne, D., Gähwiler, B. H., and Thompson, S. M. (1994). Asynchronous pre- and postsynaptic activity induces associative long- term depression in area CA1 of the rat hippocampus *in vitro*. *Proceedings of the National Academy of Sciences USA*, **91**, 1148–52.

Debanne, D., Gähwiler, B. H., and Thompson, S. M. (1997). Bidirectional associative plasticity of unitary CA3–CA1 EPSPs in the rat hippocampus *in vitro*. *Journal of Neurophysiology*, **77**, 2851–5.

Debanne, D., Gähwiler, B. H., and Thompson, S. M. (1998). Long-term synaptic plasticity between pairs of individual CA3 pyramidal cells in rat hippocampal slice cultures. *Journal of Physiology*, **507**, 237–47.

Denk, W., Sugimori, M., and Llinas, R. (1995). Two types of calcium response limited to single spines in cerebellar Purkinje cells. *Proceedings of the National Academy of Sciences USA*, **92**, 8279–82.

Derrick, B. E. and Martinez, J. L., Jr. (1996). Associative, bidirectional modifications at the hippocampal mossy fibre-CA3 synapse. *Nature*, **381**, 429–34.

Edmonds, B., Gibb, A. J., and Colquhoun, D. (1995). Mechanisms of activation of glutamate receptors and the time course of excitatory synaptic currents. *Annual Review of Physiology*, **57**, 495–519.

Emptage, N., Bliss, T. V., and Fine, A. (1999). Single synaptic events evoke NMDA receptor-mediated release of calcium from internal stores in hippocampal dendritic spines. *Neuron*, **22**, 115–24.

Engert, F. and Bonhoeffer, T. (1997). Synapse specificity of long-term potentiation breaks down at short distances. *Nature*, **388**, 279–84.

Feldmeyer, D. and Cull-Candy, S. (1996). Functional consequences of changes in NMDA receptor subunit expression during development. *Journal of Neurocytology*, **25**, 857–67.

Frey, U. and Morris, R. G. (1998). Synaptic tagging: implications for late maintenance of hippocampal long- term potentiation. *Trends in Neurosciences*, **21**, 181–8.

Gustafsson, B. and Wigstrom, H. (1986). Hippocampal long-lasting potentiation produced by pairing single volleys and brief conditioning tetani evoked in separate afferents. *Journal of Neuroscience*, **6**, 1575–82.

Gustafsson, B., Wigstrom, H., Abraham, W. C., and Huang, Y. Y. (1987). Long-term potentiation in the hippocampus using depolarizing current pulses as the conditioning stimulus to single volley synaptic potentials. *Journal of Neuroscience*, **7**, 774–80.

Hanse, E. and Gustafsson, B. (1994). TEA elicits two distinct potentiations of synaptic transmission in the CA1 region of the hippocampal slice. *Journal of Neuroscience*, **14**, 5028–34.

Häusser, M. and Clark, B. A. (1997). Tonic synaptic inhibition modulates neuronal output pattern and spatiotemporal synaptic integration. *Neuron*, **19**, 665–78.

Häusser, M., Parésys, G., and Denk, W. (1997). Coupling between dendritic spines and shafts in cerebellar Purkinje cells. *Society for Neuroscience Abstracts*, **23**, 2006.

Hebb, D. O. (1949). *The Organization of Behavior*. Wiley, New York.

Hoffman, D. A. and Johnston, D. (1998). Downregulation of transient K^+ channels in dendrites of hippocampal CA1 pyramidal neurons by activation of PKA and PKC. *Journal of Neuroscience*, **18**, 3521–8.

Hoffman, D. A. and Johnston, D. (1999). Neuromodulation of dendritic action potentials. *Journal of Neurophysiology*, **81**, 408–11.

Hoffman, D. A., Magee, J. C., Colbert, C. M., and Johnston, D. (1997). K^+ channel regulation of signal propagation in dendrites of hippocampal pyramidal neurons. *Nature*, **387**, 869–75.

Holmes, W. R. and Levy, W. B. (1990). Insights into associative long-term potentiation from computational models of NMDA receptor-mediated calcium influx and intracellular calcium concentration changes. *Journal of Neurophysiology*, **63**, 1148–68.

Holmes, W. R. and Levy, W. B. (1997). Quantifying the role of inhibition in associative long-term potentiation in dentate granule cells with computational models. *Journal of Neurophysiology*, **78**, 103–16.

Huang, Y. Y. and Kandel, E. R. (1998). Postsynaptic induction and PKA-dependent expression of LTP in the lateral amygdala. *Neuron*, **21**, 169–78.

Huang, Y. Y. and Malenka, R. C. (1993). Examination of TEA-induced synaptic enhancement in area CA1 of the hippocampus: the role of voltage-dependent Ca^{2+} channels in the induction of LTP. *Journal of Neuroscience*, **13**, 568–76.

Jaffe, D., Johnston, D., Lasser-Ross, N., Lisman, J. E., Miyakawa, H., and Ross, W. N. (1992). The spread of Na^+ spikes determines the pattern of dendritic Ca^{2+} entry into hippocampal neurons. *Nature*, **21**, 244–6.

Jester, J. M., Campbell, L. W., and Sejnowski, T. J. (1995). Associative EPSP-spike potentiation induced by pairing orthodromic and antidromic stimulation in rat hippocampal slices. *Journal of Physiology*, **484**, 689–705.

Johnston, D., Williams, S., Jaffe, D., and Gray, R. (1992). NMDA-receptor-independent long-term potentiation. *Annual Review of Physiology*, **54**, 489–505.

Jung, H. Y., Mickus, T., and Spruston, N. (1997). Prolonged sodium channel inactivation contributes to dendritic action potential attenuation in hippocampal pyramidal neurons. *Journal of Neuroscience*, **17**, 6639–46.

Katz, L. C. and Shatz, C. J. (1996). Synaptic activity and the construction of cortical circuits. *Science*, **274**, 1133–8.

Kelso, S. R. and Brown, T. H. (1986). Differential conditioning of associative synaptic enhancement in hippocampal brain slices. *Science*, **232**, 85–7.

Kelso, S. R., Ganong, A. H., and Brown, T. H. (1986). Hebbian synapses in hippocampus. *Proceedings of the National Academy of Sciences USA*, **83**, 5326–30.

Kirkwood, A. and Bear, M. F. (1995). Elementary forms of synaptic plasticity in the visual cortex. *Biol. Res.*, **28**, 73–80.

Koch, C. and Zador, A. (1993). The function of dendritic spines: devices subserving bio-chemical rather than electrical compartmentalization. *Journal of Neuroscience*, **13**, 413–22.

Koester, H. J. and Sakmann, B. (1998). Calcium dynamics in single spines during coincident pre- and postsynaptic activity depend on relative timing of backpropagating action potentials and subthreshold excitatory postsynaptic potentials. *Proceedings of the National Academy of Sciences USA*, **95**, 9596–601.

Kombian, S. B. and Malenka, R. C. (1994). Simultaneous LTP of non-NMDA- and LTD of NMDA-receptor-mediated responses in the nucleus accumbens. *Nature*, **368**, 242–6.

Korngreen, A., Bergling, S., and Sakmann, B. (1999). Voltage gated potassium channels and back propagation of the action potential in Layer V pyramidal neurons. *Biophysical Society Abstracts*, 290.

Korogod, S., Bras, H., Sarana, V. N., Gogan, P., and Tyc-Dumont, S. (1994). Electrotonic clusters in the dendritic arborization of abducens motoneurons of the rat. *European Journal of Neuroscience*, **6**, 1517–27.

Kossel, A., Bonhoeffer, T., and Bolz, J. (1990). Non-Hebbian synapses in rat visual cortex. *Neuroreport*, **1**, 115–18.

Kullmann, D. M., Perkel, D. J., Manabe, T., and Nicoll, R. A. (1992). Ca^{2+} entry *via* postsynaptic voltage-sensitive Ca^{2+} channels can transiently potentiate excitatory synaptic transmission in the hippocampus. *Neuron*, **9**, 1175–83.

Larson, J. and Lynch, G. (1986). Induction of synaptic potentiation in hippocampus by patterned stimulation involves two events. *Science*, **232**, 985–8.

Levy, W. B. and Steward, O. (1979). Synapses as associative memory elements in the hippocampal formation. *Brain Research*, **175**, 233–45.

Levy, W. B. and Steward, O. (1983). Temporal contiguity requirements for long-term associative potentiation/depression in the hippocampus. *Neuroscience*, **8**, 791–7.

Lisman, J. (1989). A mechanism for the Hebb and the anti-Hebb processes underlying learning and memory. *Proceedings of the National Academy of Sciences USA*, **86**, 9574–8.

Lynch, G., Larson, J., Kelso, S., Barrionuevo, G., and Schottler, F. (1983). Intracellular injections of EGTA block induction of hippocampal long- term potentiation. *Nature*, **305**, 719–21.

Maccaferri, G., Toth, K., and McBain, C. J. (1998). Target-specific expression of presynaptic mossy fiber plasticity. *Science*, **279**, 1368–70.

MacDermott, A. B., Mayer, M. L., Westbrook, G. L., Smith, S. J., and Barker, J. L. (1986). NMDA-receptor activation increases cytoplasmic calcium concentration in cultured spinal cord neurones. *Nature*, **321**, 519–22.

Magee, J. C. and Johnston, D. (1997). A synaptically controlled, associative signal for Hebbian plasticity in hippocampal neurons. *Science*, **275**, 209–13.

Magee, J., Hoffman, D., Colbert, C., and Johnston, D. (1998). Electrical and calcium signaling in dendrites of hippocampal pyramidal neurons. *Annual Review of Physiology*, **60**, 327–46.

Mainen, Z. F., Zador, A. M., Claiborne, B. J., and Brown, T. H. (1990). Hebbian synapses induce feature mosaics in hippocampal dendrites. *Society for Neuroscience Abstracts*, **16**, 492.

Mainen, Z. F., Malinow, R., and Svoboda, K. (1999). Synaptic $[Ca^{2+}]$ transients in single spines indicate NMDA receptors are not saturated. *Nature*, **391**, 151–5.

Malenka, R. C., Kauer, J. A., Zucker, R. S., and Nicoll, R. A. (1988). Postsynaptic calcium is sufficient for potentiation of hippocampal synaptic transmission. *Science*, **242**, 81–4.

Malenka, R. C., Lancaster, B., and Zucker, R. S. (1992). Temporal limits on the rise in postsynaptic calcium required for the induction of long-term potentiation. *Neuron*, **9**, 121–8.

Malinow, R. (1991). Transmission between pairs of hippocampal slice neurons: quantal levels oscillations, and LTP. *Science*, **252**, 722–4.

Malinow, R. and Miller, J. P. (1986). Postsynaptic hyperpolarization during conditioning reversibly blocks induction of long-term potentiation. *Nature*, **320**, 529–30.

Malinow, R. and Tsien, R. W. (1990). Presynaptic enhancement shown by whole-cell recordings of long-term potentiation in hippocampal slices. *Nature*, **346**, 177–80.

Markram, H., Lübke, J., Frotscher, M., and Sakmann, B. (1997). Regulation of synaptic efficacy by coincidence of postsynaptic APs and EPSPs. *Science*, **275**, 213–15.

Martinez, J. L., Jr. and Derrick, B. E. (1996). Long-term potentiation and learning. *Annual Review of Psychology*, **47**, 173–203.

Mayer, M. L. and Westbrook, G. L. (1987). Permeation and block of N-methyl-D-aspartic acid receptor channels by divalent cations in mouse cultured central neurones. *Journal of Physiology*, **394**, 501–27.

Mayer, M. L., Westbrook, G. L., and Guthrie, P. B. (1984). Voltage-dependent block by Mg^{2+} of NMDA responses in spinal cord neurones. *Nature*, **309**, 261–3.

McBain, C. J. and Mayer, M. L. (1994). N-Methyl-D-aspartic acid receptor structure and function. *Physiological Reviews*, **74**, 723–60.

McKernan, M. G. and Shinnick-Gallagher, P. (1997). Fear conditioning induces a lasting potentiation of synaptic currents *in vitro*. *Nature*, **390**, 607–11.

McNaughton, B. L., Douglas, R. M., and Goddard, G. V. (1978). Synaptic enhancement in fascia dentata: cooperativity among coactive afferents. *Brain Research*, **157**, 277–93.

Mel, B. W. (1993). Synaptic integration in an excitable dendritic tree. *Journal of Neurophysiology*, **70**, 1086–101.

Mel, B. W., Ruderman, D. L., and Archie, K. A. (1998). Translation-invariant orientation tuning in visual 'complex' cells could derive from intradendritic computations. *Journal of Neuroscience*, **18**, 4325–34.

Mickus, T., Jung, H., and Spruston, N. (1999). Properties of slow, cumulative sodium channel inactivation in rat hippocampal CA1 pyramidal neurons. *Biophysical Journal*, **76**, 846–60.

Montague, P. R. (1996). The resource consumption principle: attention and memory in volumes of neural tissue. *Proceedings of the National Academy of Sciences USA*, **93**, 3619–23.

Montague, P. R., Gally, J. A., and Edelman, G. M. (1991). Spatial signaling in the development and function of neural connections. *Cerebral Cortex*, **1**, 199–220.

Monyer, H., Burnashev, N., Laurie, D. J., Sakmann, B., and Seeburg, P. H. (1994). Developmental and regional expression in the rat brain and functional properties of four NMDA receptors. *Neuron*, **12**, 529–40.

Muller, W. and Connor, J. A. (1991). Dendritic spines as individual neuronal compartments for synaptic Ca^{2+} responses. *Nature*, **354**, 73–6.

Neher, E. (1998). Vesicle pools and Ca^{2+} microdomains: new tools for understanding their roles in neurotransmitter release. *Neuron*, **20**, 389—99.

Neveu, D. and Zucker, R. S. (1996a). Postsynaptic levels of $[Ca^{2+}]_i$ needed to trigger LTD and LTP. *Neuron*, **16**, 619–29.

Neveu, D. and Zucker, R. S. (1996b). Long-lasting potentiation and depression without presynaptic activity. *Journal of Neurophysiology*, **75**, 2157–60.

Nicoll, R. A. and Malenka, R. C. (1995). Contrasting properties of two forms of long-term potentiation in the hippocampus. *Nature*, **377**, 115–18.

Nowak, L., Bregestovski, P., Ascher, P., Herbet, A., and Prochiantz, A. (1984). Magnesium gates glutamate-activated channels in mouse central neurones. *Nature*, **307**, 462–5.

Otmakhov, N., Shirke, A. M., and Malinow, R. (1993). Measuring the impact of probabilistic transmission on neuronal output. *Neuron*, **10**, 1101–11.

Pacelli, G. J., Su, W., and Kelso, S. R. (1989). Activity-induced depression of synaptic inhibition during LTP-inducing patterned stimulation. *Brain Research*, **486**, 26–32.

Paré, D., Shink, E., Gaudreau, H., Destexhe, A., and Lang, E. J. (1998). Impact of spontaneous synaptic activity on the resting properties of cat neocortical pyramidal neurons *in vivo*. *Journal of Neurophysiology*, **79**, 1450–60.

Patneau, D. K. and Mayer, M. L. (1990). Structure-activity relationships for amino acid transmitter candidates acting at N-methyl-D-aspartate and quisqualate receptors. *Journal of Neuroscience*, **10**, 2385–99.

Pearlmutter, B. A. (1995). Time-skew Hebb rule in a nonisopotential neuron. *Neural Computation*, **7**, 706–12.

Perkel, D. J., Petrozzino, J. J., Nicoll, R. A., and Connor, J. A. (1993). The role of Ca^{2+} entry *via* synaptically activated NMDA receptors in the induction of long-term potentiation. *Neuron*, **11**, 817–23.

Quinn, W. G. (1998). Reductionism in learning and memory. *Novartis Found Symp.*, **213**, 117–21.

Raastad, M., Enriquez-Denton, M., and Kiehn, O. (1998). Synaptic signaling in an active central network only moderately changes passive membrane properties. *Proceedings of the National Academy of Sciences USA*, **95**, 10251–6.

Regehr, W. G. and Tank, D. W. (1992). Calcium concentration dynamics produced by synaptic activation of CA1 hippocampal pyramidal cells. *Journal of Neuroscience*, **12**, 4202–23.

Rogan, M. T. and LeDoux, J. E. (1995). LTP is accompanied by commensurate enhancement of auditory-evoked responses in a fear conditioning circuit. *Neuron*, **15**, 127–36.

Rogan, M. T., Staubli, U. V., and LeDoux, J. E. (1997). Fear conditioning induces associative long-term potentiation in the amygdala. *Nature*, **390**, 604–7.

Sandler, V. M. and Ross, W. N. (1999). Serotonin modulates spike backpropagation and associated $[Ca^{2+}]_i$ changes in the apical dendrites of hippocampal CA1 pyramidal neurons. *Journal of Neurophysiology*, **81**, 216–24.

Scharfman, H. E. and Sarvey, J. M. (1985). Postsynaptic firing during repetitive stimulation is required for long- term potentiation in hippocampus. *Brain Research*, **331**, 267–74.

Schiller, J., Schiller, Y., and Clapham, D. E. (1998). NMDA receptors amplify calcium influx into dendritic spines during associative pre- and postsynaptic activation. *Nature Neuroscience*, **1**, 114–18.

Schultz, W., Dayan, P., and Montague, P. R. (1997). A neural substrate of prediction and reward. *Science*, **275**, 1593–9.

Schuman, E. M. and Madison, D. V. (1994). Locally distributed synaptic potentiation in the hippocampus. *Science*, **263**, 532–6.

Selig, D. K., Lee, H. K., Bear, M. F., and Malenka, R. C. (1995). Reexamination of the effects of MCPG on hippocampal LTP, LTD, and depotentiation. *Journal of Neurophysiology*, **74**, 1075–82.

Spruston, N., Jonas, P., and Sakmann, B. (1995a). Dendritic glutamate receptor channels in rat hippocampal CA3 and CA1 pyramidal neurons. *Journal of Physiology* **482**, 325–52.

Spruston, N., Schiller, Y., Stuart, G., and Sakmann, B. (1995b). Activity-dependent action potential invasion and calcium influx into hippocampal CA1 dendrites. *Science*, **268**, 297–300.

Stevens, C. F. (1998). A million dollar question: does LTP = memory? *Neuron*, **20**, 1–2.

Stuart, G., Schiller, J., and Sakmann, B. (1997a). Action potential initiation and propagation in rat neocortical pyramidal neurons. *Journal of Physiology*, **505**, 617–32.

Stuart, G., Spruston, N., Sakmann, B., and Häusser, M. (1997b). Action potential initiation and backpropagation in neurons of the mammalian CNS. *Trends in Neurosciences*, **20**, 125–31.

Svoboda, K., Tank, D. W., and Denk, W. (1996). Direct measurement of coupling between dendritic spines and shafts. *Science*, **272**, 716–9.

Thomas, M. J., Watabe, A. M., Moody, T. D., Makhinson, M., and O'Dell, T. J. (1998). Postsynaptic complex spike bursting enables the induction of LTP by theta frequency synaptic stimulation. *Journal of Neuroscience*, **18**, 7118–26.

Tomasulo, R. A., Ramirez, J. J., and Steward, O. (1993). Synaptic inhibition regulates associative interactions between afferents during the induction of long-term potentiation and depression. *Proceedings of the National Academy of Sciences USA*, **90**, 11578–82.

Tsubokawa, H. and Ross, W. N. (1996). IPSPs modulate spike backpropagation and associated $[Ca^{2+}]_i$ changes in the dendrites of hippocampal CA1 pyramidal neurons. *Journal of Neurophysiology*, **76**, 2896–906.

Tsubokawa, H. and Ross, W. N. (1997). Muscarinic modulation of spike backpropagation in the apical dendrites of hippocampal CA1 pyramidal neurons. *Journal of Neuroscience*, **17**, 5782–91.

Turrigiano, G. G. and Nelson, S. B. (1998). Thinking globally, acting locally: AMPA receptor turnover and synaptic strength. *Neuron*, **21**, 933–5.

Turrigiano, G. G., Leslie, K. R., Desai, N. S., Rutherford, L. C., and Nelson, S. B. (1998). Activity-dependent scaling of quantal amplitude in neocortical neurons. *Nature*, **391**, 892–6.

Wathey, J. C., Lytton, W. W., Jester, J. M., and Sejnowski, T. J. (1992). Computer simulations of EPSP-to-spike (E–S) potentiation in hippocampal CA1 pyramidal cells. *Journal of Neuroscience*, **12**, 607–18.

White, G., Levy, W. B., and Steward, O. (1988). Evidence that associative interactions between synapses during the induction of long-term potentiation occur within local dendritic domains. *Proceedings of the National Academy of Sciences USA*, **85**, 2368–72.

White, G., Levy, W. B., and Steward, O. (1990). Spatial overlap between populations of synapses determines the extent of their associative interaction during the induction of long-term potentiation and depression. *Journal of Neurophysiology*, **64**, 1186–98.

Wickens, J. (1988). Electrically coupled but chemically isolated synapses: dendritic spines and calcium in a rule for synaptic modification. *Progress in Neurobiology*, **31**, 507–28.

Wigstrom, H., Gustafsson, B., Huang, Y. Y., and Abraham, W. C. (1986). Hippocampal long-term potentiation is induced by pairing single afferent volleys with intracellularly injected depolarizing current pulses. *Acta Physiologica Scandanavica*, **126**, 317–19.

Yang, S. N., Tang, Y. G., and Zucker, R. S. (1999). Selective induction of LTP and LTD by postsynaptic $[Ca^{2+}]_i$ elevation. *Journal of Neurophysiology*, **81**, 781–7.

Yuste, R. and Denk, W. (1995). Dendritic spines as basic functional units of neuronal integration. *Nature*, **375**, 682–4.

Yuste, R., Majewska, A., Cash, S. S., and Denk, W. (1999). Mechanisms of calcium influx into hippocampal spines: heterogeneity among spines, coincidence detection by NMDA receptors, and optical quantal analysis. *Journal of Neuroscience*, **19**, 1976–87.

Zador, A., Koch, C., and Brown, T. H. (1990). Biophysical model of a Hebbian synapse. *Proceedings of the National Academy of Sciences USA*, **87**, 6718–22.

Zhang, L. I., Tao, H. W., Holt, C. E., Harris, W. A., and Poo, M. (1998). A critical window for cooperation and competition among developing retinotectal synapses. *Nature*, **395**, 37–44.

Zukin, R. S. and Bennett, M. V. (1995). Alternatively spliced isoforms of the NMDAR1 receptor subunit. *Trends in Neurosciences*, **18**, 306–13.

14

Structural plasticity of dendrites

Catherine S. Woolley
Northwestern University

Summary

Many theories of learning have proposed that structural changes in synaptic connections between neurons can underlie long-term information storage in the adult brain. However, the fact that circuits encoding learned information are likely to be distributed within and across brain regions, coupled with the inability to identify individual cells and synapses involved in learning, has made it difficult to test this hypothesis directly. Despite these obstacles, a number of experiments have demonstrated experience- or learning-dependent structural changes in dendrites and synapses of cortical structures in mammalian brains. A better appreciation of the prevalence and rapidity of structural plasticity of dendrites can be gained from studying systems with relatively simple circuitry in which the majority of cells are dedicated to a particular function. This approach has shown that physiological stimuli such as hormonal fluctuations induce remarkable plasticity of dendritic structure and synaptic connectivity in multiple hypothalamic regions. Similar changes are also observed in hippocampal neurons, which are known to be involved in learning, offering the opportunity to study at the physiological and molecular level how structural plasticity produced by systemic physiological stimuli is related to learning. Comparison of dendritic structural plasticity in these various systems reveals similarities that may be generalizable to dendrites in many brain regions.

Introduction

The wiring of the adult central nervous system (CNS) classically has been viewed as fixed and structurally stable. Indeed, it has been presumed that stability in the synaptic connectivity within our brains is necessary for continuity of memory and personality. However, such a rigid picture of neural circuitry is contradicted by over 30 years of research demonstrating plasticity in the physical structure of brain circuitry. Numerous studies have shown structural changes in axonal and dendritic arborization in response to lesions or aberrant activity, differential experience, or systemic factors such as hormones.

The most dramatic examples of dendritic structural plasticity occur following lesion-induced deafferentation. Lesion studies have shown that neurons in a wide range of adult brain regions (e.g. neocortex, cerebellum, hippocampus, hypothalamus, striatum, septal nuclei) are capable of retracting, extending or forming new branches of their dendrites. Lesion-induced changes can result in new and sometimes aberrant synaptic connections. Study of neuronal responses to deafferentation is important not only for understanding brain pathologies, but also to define limits for structural changes that are possible and to determine the functional consequences of structural changes. Such studies point to a dependence of dendritic structure on activity within afferent pathways and show that the adult CNS can rewire itself when challenged. However, it is uncertain to what extent lesion-induced structural plasticity is exclusively a consequence of injury or may also reflect processes that occur as a part of normal brain function.

Much of the interest in dendritic structural plasticity in normal (i.e. non-pathological) adult brain function historically has been centered on the idea that the process of learning involves the formation of associations between particular cells or groups of cells through physical changes in the synapses that connect them. Although such ideas are very appealing to many neuroscientists who are interested in understanding the basis of information storage in the brain, several factors complicate the search for learning-induced structural plasticity. First, it is likely that learning involves a refinement of synaptic connectivity, rather than a net increase or decrease in synapse number. Second, it is also likely that learned information is recorded and stored in distributed circuits, so that representation of an individual task or event may alter only a small number of cells (and synapses on those cells) in widespread locations. Since it is virtually impossible to identify individual cells or synapses involved in a learning event, or even to know what synaptic changes to expect, the study of learning-induced structural plasticity is quite difficult.

Nevertheless, two main approaches have produced results consistent with the idea that structural plasticity of dendrites is involved in learning. One approach has been to house animals in very different environments. The hypothesis in these experiments is that experience can alter synaptic connectivity, so large and continuous differences in the activity of multiple motor and sensory pathways might produce measurable differences in parameters of dendritic and synaptic morphology. A second approach has been to train animals in specific tasks for which there is a reasonable understanding of the neural pathways involved, and then to look for structural changes specifically within those pathways. In each case, multiple studies have demonstrated modest but reliable structural differences in dendrites, particularly of cortical neurons, that can be induced with non-pathological stimuli. Currently however, the relationship of these structural changes to altered neuronal function or behavior can only be inferred.

An alternative strategy for understanding the involvement of structural dendritic plasticity in brain function and behavior is to focus on simpler brain areas made up of cells primarily devoted to functions less complex than learning. In this way, physiological stimuli can be used to activate reliably a more homogeneous population of neurons than in studies of learning-related plasticity. This approach has revealed considerable structural plasticity of dendrites in several hypothalamic nuclei. Robust examples include the changes in oxytocin and vasopressin neurons in the supraoptic and paraventricular nuclei in response to dehydration or during late pregnancy and lactation, as well as ovarian hormone induced plasticity in several types of hypothalamic neurons during the estrous cycle. A considerable advantage in the study of structural plasticity of hypothalamic neurons is that changes in dendrites and their associated synapses can more readily be related to function than can changes associated with experience. A key element in structural plasticity in these hypothalamic systems is the withdrawal of astrocytic processes from between neurons, allowing increased dendritic apposition and new synapse formation. This observation has guided the search for cellular and molecular mechanisms of structural changes by pointing to glial cells as active participants in neuronal plasticity.

A third approach, which bridges the two mentioned above, has demonstrated structural plasticity of dendrites in brain areas that are associated with learning, but in response to systemic factors such as hormones. My colleagues and I have published a series of studies examining estradiol and progesterone induced fluctuation in the density and number of dendritic spines and spine synapses on hippocampal pyramidal cells. The well-characterized circuitry of the hippocampus makes study of the functional consequences of dendritic changes for individual cells quite feasible. Further, since these changes occur in a brain region known to be important for learning, hormone-induced structural plasticity of hippocampal dendrites may provide an opportunity to test the relationship of dendritic structural plasticity to learning. The cellular and molecular mechanism(s) by which ovarian hormones regulate hippocampal dendritic plasticity has been studied in detail *in vitro*.

This chapter begins with an historical perspective on structural plasticity and then reviews findings of non-pathological structural plasticity of dendrites in the adult mammalian brain using the three approaches outlined above. The last section summarizes our current understanding of the capacity of adult neurons for structural plasticity and attempts to extract some generalizable themes from comparison of structural changes across multiple brain areas.

Historical perspective on structural plasticity

There is a long history to the idea that structural change in neuronal circuits might underlie changes in adult neural function and thus alter behavior. Even before the elaborate axonal and dendritic structure of neurons was revealed, there was speculation about growth of cells in the brain as a means of developing associations between ideas. One of the earliest references to the concept of structural plasticity comes from Alexander Bain (1872). Previously, the philosopher and physician David Hartley had combined theories of associationism (Locke 1690) and neural 'vibrations' (Newton 1687) in a physiological theory of memory published in 1749. Bain proposed structural plasticity as a mechanism for Hartley's ideas. This showed remarkable intuition given that it was suggested at a time when the detailed structure of neurons was still unknown. Bain wrote:

For every act of memory, every exercise of bodily aptitude, every habit, recollection, train of ideas, there is a specific grouping or coordination of sensations and movements, by virtue of specific growths in the cell junctions.

The development of the Golgi stain, together with improved methods of tissue fixation and the use of achromatic compound microscopes and later apochromatic lenses, revolutionized neurocytology in the late 19th century. The Golgi stain revealed dendrites clearly for the first time, and provided the first evidence of the astounding morphological diversity of neurons. A new picture of the cellular organization of the brain emerged from this work, and provoked new questions and ideas about the functional and structural relationships between neurons (reviewed by Shepherd 1991).

One concept that emerged with a fuller understanding of neuronal morphology was that axonal and dendritic branches of neurons might grow and retract to either enhance or inhibit communication between cells. During the 1890s, there was a great deal of speculation on the possibility of movement of neuronal processes. The concept of the synapse was in its earliest stages, and some envisioned neuronal growth occurring quite rapidly. 'Neural amoeboidism' was a theory originally proposed by Hermann Rabl-Ruckhard and later developed by Mathias Duval. Neural amoeboidism purported that neurons stretched, relaxed and could rapidly move their processes to various locations. Some ideas were fairly extreme. For example, Duval (1895) applied the amoeboid theory to sleep and awakening:

...in man when sleeping, the central arborizations are retracted like pseudopods of an anesthetized leukocyte... the impulse, on passing to the cortical cells, leads to awakening, the successive phases of which clearly suggest the reestablishment of a series of [connections] previously interrupted by retraction and withdrawal of pseudopodial arborizations.

Eugenio Tanzi (1893) considered this theory in relation to learned habits and skills. He hypothesized that passage of nervous impulses could cause lengthening of neuronal arborizations, thus reducing the distance between cells and resistance to passage of impulses between them, thereby altering the functional connection between neurons. Santiago Ramón y Cajal (1894) further suggested that such a mechanism could account for the improvement of existing skills, while learning new skills might require the formation of entirely new connections:

...it can be admitted as very probable that mental exercise leads to a greater development of the dendritic apparatus and of the system of axonal collaterals in the most utilized cerebral regions. In this way, associations already established among certain groups of cells could be notably reinforced by means of multiplication of small terminal branches of the dendritic appendages and axonal collaterals; but in addition, some completely new intercellular connections could be established thanks to the new formation of [axonal] collaterals and dendrites.

These excerpts testify to early enthusiasm for a role of structural plasticity in adult neural function. The initial excitement waned however, particularly with regard to the possibility that structural changes were involved in adult learning. Several observations argued against structural plasticity as an important feature in the adult brain:

(1) critical periods were determined for the development of certain behaviors and later for neural circuitry;

(2) adult neural tissue showed relatively poor capacity for regeneration; and

(3) structural changes in neural circuitry appeared to be too slow to account for the speed with which learning can take place.

The dichotomy between development and adulthood became a dominant model during the first half of the 20th century. Development was viewed as a time of intense structural change, during which proliferation and migration of neurons as well as extensive growth of axonal and dendritic arborizations take place. The adult brain, having completed these developmental processes, appeared relatively structurally stable. The concept of critical or sensitive periods came to the fore; limited time windows in development were described during which an individual's adult characteristics could be modified by differential experience. This idea originated from embryology and was applied to the development of certain behaviors initially by Lorenz (1935) for imprinting and later by Scott and Marston (1950) for socialization of dogs. These behavioral concepts were translated to the development of neural circuitry when Hubel and Wiesel (1963) demonstrated that occluding one eye in the kitten led to a reduction in the number of cortical cells responding to that eye, and later defined a critical period for the cortical effects of visual input (Hubel and Wiesel 1970). Another, related observation that appeared to reduce the likelihood that structural plasticity is a major influence in adult brain function was that neural tissue from mature animals is less able than young tissue to recover from injury (Ramón y Cajal 1928).

A third argument against structural plasticity, particularly as a mechanism involved in learning, was that neuronal growth was simply too slow to account for the rapidity with which some learning can take place (Loeb 1902; Lashley 1929). To be fair, however, it must be noted that the type of learning suggested by early investigators to involve structural changes in the brain was the gradual development of skills (i.e. 'practice makes perfect') as opposed to the potentially more rapid commitment of facts or events to memory. Donald Hebb (1949) proposed a 'dual trace mechanism' to resolve the apparent conflict between near instantaneous learning and the time presumably required for structural changes to take place as a central feature of his now famous neuropsychological theory:

There are memories which are instantaneously established, and as evanescent as they are immediate... Also, some memories are both instantaneously established and permanent. To account for the permanence, some structural change seems necessary, but structural growth presumably would require an appreciable time. If some way can be found of supposing that a reverbatory trace might cooperate with the structural change, and *carry the memory until the growth change is made*, we should recognize the theoretical value of the trace which is an activity only, without having to ascribe all memory to it.

In Hebb's theory, some structural change in neural circuitry is necessary for permanent memory storage, but only when established over time through repetitive or persistent activity in appropriate pathways. This proposal was very appealing from a theoretical standpoint, but it was more than 10 years before experimental evidence supported the notion of experience-dependent structural plasticity.

Experience-dependent structural plasticity of dendrites

Enriched environment—neocortex

In a series of studies published in the early 1960s, Rosenzweig, Bennett, Diamond and colleagues reported the first examples of experience-dependent structural plasticity induced in the brains of adult mammals. Littermate rats were housed as adults in either an isolated, standard or enriched condition. Rats in the enriched housing condition had a variety of visual and tactile stimuli (e.g. toys to play with), in addition to the social interactions available to the standard-condition rats, but not the isolated ones. Initially, these authors reported increased cortical weight and acetylcholinesterase activity in the enriched housing *versus* isolated rats (Rosenszweig *et al.* 1962; Bennett *et al.* 1964). Subsequently it was shown that that the increase in cortical weight was paralleled by increased cortical thickness (Diamond *et al.* 1972), increased dendritic field size of cortical pyramidal cells (Uylings *et al.* 1978) and differences in axodendritic synapse size and density (Diamond *et al.* 1975). Housing 112-day-old rats for 30 days in the enriched condition significantly increased cortical thickness in frontal and visual areas by up to 7% when compared to standard housing (Uylings *et al.* 1978). The same study found that enriched housing also significantly increased the length of terminal dendritic segments of the basal dendrites of layer II and III pyramidal cells by 10–28% when compared with standard housing. Since this time, many other studies have found qualitatively similar, though smaller, housing-induced differences in cortical neurons of aged rats as well as young adults (e.g. Connor *et al.* 1980; Green *et al.* 1983; Greenough *et al.* 1986).

Study of the effects of an enriched environment on synaptic connectivity in the visual cortex has shown a selective increase in the number of multiple synapse boutons—individual presynaptic boutons that form synapses with more than one postsynaptic element (Jones *et al.* 1997). This finding suggests that new synapses formed in adult cortex involve recruitment of preexisting presynaptic elements by new postsynaptic elements.

Enriched environment—cerebellar cortex

Housing-induced changes in dendritic structure also have been reported in adult cerebellar Purkinje cells. For example, Greenough *et al.* (1986) showed that 4.5 months exposure to an enriched compared to standard housing condition produced significantly more (but smaller) Purkinje cell spiny branchlets in rats that were over 2 years old at the beginning of the study. Comparison with a control group suggested that this was partially prevention of an age-related decrease and partially new dendritic growth. The difference between enriched and standard housed animals in number of spiny branchlets per neuron was approximately 16%.

Taken together, findings like these show that various types of neurons in adult and even aged animals retain the capacity for structural change and that increased activity in sensory and motor pathways in adult animals housed under enriched conditions can produce dendritic proliferation and changes in synaptic connectivity.

Behavioral training—neocortex

A different experimental approach specifically directed at determining whether increased use of particular pathways results in structural plasticity of dendrites has been to compare dendritic and synaptic morphology in animals trained on certain tasks to those in naive or activity-matched controls. Greenough and colleagues have been successful in utilizing this approach to study the effects of motor learning on adult neurons in the neocortex and cerebellum.

Early studies from this group demonstrated that training adult rats to reach for a food reward results in altered dendritic morphology of layer V pyramidal cells in the contralateral motor/somatosensory cortex (Greenough *et al.* 1985). Reach training resulted in increased total dendritic length, number of oblique branches and length of terminal dendritic segments in the apical tree. Later, somewhat smaller changes were also observed in the basal dendritic tree of layer II/III pyramidal cells (Withers and Greenough 1989). More recently, Greenough's group has applied unbiased stereological methodology to analyze changes in synaptic connectivity in motor cortex following learning of a more complex motor coordination task.

To study learning-induced synaptic remodeling, adult rats are trained to traverse an obstacle course of rope ladders, narrow beams, etc., which requires refined coordination of limb and body movement for successful navigation. Rats show motor skill learning in that, with practice, they are able to complete the task more rapidly and with fewer errors than in initial attempts. Depending on training conditions and the age of animals used, it takes 5–10 days for animals to plateau in their performance (Kleim *et al.* 1996, 1997, 1998). Controls for this type of behavioral training include animals that perform as much or more general motor activity than those who learn the obstacle course and inactive animals with no opportunities for extra-cage exercise. In an experiment in which 3-month-old animals learned the task in 5 days, stereological examination of synaptic connectivity in layers II/III of motor cortex revealed a significant, training-induced increase in synapse to neuron ratio that occurred during the 5-day learning period (Kleim *et al.* 1996). The increase was approximately 13% and remained unchanged for up to 20 days of continued performance of the task.

Behavioral training—cerebellar cortex

Structural changes in the synaptic connections onto cerebellar Purkinje cells produced by the motor skill learning paradigm described above have been studied extensively. Both imaging (Seitz *et al.* 1990) and lesion (Nasher and Grimm 1978; Weiner *et al.* 1983) data from humans as well as electrophysiological data from experimental animals (Gilbert and Thach 1977; Marple-Horvat and Stein 1987; Ojakangas and Ebner 1992, 1994) suggest involvement of the cerebellar cortex in motor learning. Furthermore, our detailed knowledge of cerebellar synaptic connectivity, in conjunction with theoretical and electrophysiological analyses of cerebellum-dependent learning, provides a framework for relating learning-induced structural plasticity of Purkinje cell dendrites to function.

Purkinje cells are inhibitory and are the sole output neurons of the cerebellar cortex. Excitatory input to Purkinje cells comes from two sources, the parallel fibers and climbing fibers. Each Purkinje cell receives over 100 000 parallel fiber inputs to the spiny branchlets, but only a single climbing fiber input that forms synaptic contacts with the larger caliber primary dendrites. Parallel fiber inputs produce small postsynaptic potentials that can sum to produce a 'simple spike', whereas activation of a single climbing fiber input results in a 'complex spike', consisting of a cluster of high-frequency action potentials (Eccles *et al.* 1967). Models of cerebellum-dependent learning (Marr 1969; Albus 1971; Eccles 1977; Ito 1984) postulate a reduction in the efficacy of the parallel fiber to Purkinje cell synapse mediated by concurrent activation of parallel fibers and climbing fibers. However, there is still controversy about the contribution of changes in effectiveness of this synapse to learning involving the cerebellum (reviewed by Mauk *et al.* 1998 and Raymond 1998).

Indications that structural plasticity may take place at the parallel fiber synapse is provided by experiments showing that motor skill learning results in enduring changes in movement-related simple spike activity (Gilbert and Thach 1977; Ojakangas and Ebner 1992, 1994). To examine this possibility, Greenough and colleagues have used their motor skill learning task to study structural changes in the cerebellar cortex. Thirty days of motor skill training results in altered synaptic connectivity between Purkinje cells and their parallel fiber afferents in a region of cerebellar cortex known to be involved in limb movement (Santori *et al.* 1986). An approximately 24% increase in the number of parallel fiber to Purkinje cell synapses is observed in trained animals compared to controls that were allowed running wheels and so had as much or more motor activity; the increase is 34% compared to controls housed in isolation with no running wheel (Kleim *et al.* 1998). Interestingly, this effect appears to be specific for the parallel fiber input to Purkinje cells as climbing fiber input is structurally unchanged (Kleim *et al.* 1998, but see Andersen *et al.* 1996).

Motor skill learning also increases the dendritic arborization of stellate local circuit neurons in the cerebellar cortex (Kleim *et al.* 1997). Five-month-old rats were trained for 10 days on an obstacle course similar to that used above. Analysis of dendrites of stellate interneurons in the cerebellar cortex showed a 15% increase in dendritic arborization in the trained animals compared to motor activity controls. Since the vast majority of synapses on these cells are from parallel fibers, this finding is consistent with the idea that parallel fiber synapses are an important site of learning-induced structural plasticity in the cerebellar cortex.

However, there are also studies demonstrating that climbing fiber input plays an important role in regulating parallel fiber innervation. Removal of climbing fiber afferents by lesion of the inferior olive results in formation of many aberrant dendritic spines in the proximal dendrites of Purkinje cells; these spines are innervated by parallel fibers (reviewed in Strata *et al.* 1997). It has recently been shown that silencing neuronal activity in the cerebellar cortex by infusion of tetrodotoxin also results in a massive induction of new dendritic spines on Purkinje cell proximal dendrites (Bravin *et al.* 1999). Within 6 days of treatment, proximal dendrites become densely covered with dendritic spine-like structures. Dendritic spine density in large caliber proximal dendrites increases almost 33-fold while the density of spines in the spiny branchlets remains unchanged. These findings not only reveal a remarkable degree of structural plasticity, but also support the suggestion that certain afferents may exert an activity-dependent, repressive influence on the growth of dendritic spines (Strata *et al.* 1997). Thus, hypertrophy of synaptic connections can, in some systems, result from a decrease in network activity.

Structural plasticity of dendrites induced by physiological stimuli

Late pregnancy, lactation, dehydration—supraoptic nucleus

One of the most striking examples of structural plasticity in the adult mammalian brain is observed in the magnocellular neurons of the supraoptic and paraventricular nuclei. Since these regions have simpler circuitry and are largely dedicated to a particular function, it is easier to detect and potentially understand structural plasticity here than in learning-related systems. Supraoptic and paraventricular neurons are responsible for the production and release of oxytocin and vasopressin in response to osmotic challenges as well as during late pregnancy and the period of lactation. The supraoptic nucleus consists almost entirely of magnocellular oxytocin and vasopressin neurons as opposed to the paraventricular nucleus, which also contains several populations of parvocellular neurons. Given the relative neuronal homogeneity of the supraoptic nucleus, structural plasticity in this region has been better characterized, but similar changes occur in the paraventricular nucleus as well (Theodosis and Poulain 1989; Hatton 1997).

Supraoptic neurons are densely packed and usually have 2 to 3 branched dendrites. Axons may project to various sites within the CNS, but all of the neurons have axons terminating in the neural lobe of the pituitary where oxytocin and vasopressin are released. Astrocytes are the predominant type of glial cell; typical stellate astrocytes are scattered throughout, but the majority of glia lie near the base of the brain and extend processes up into the neuropil where they are insinuated between neuronal cell bodies and dendrites. Under basal conditions, only approximately 1–2% of the total neuronal membrane is in direct apposition without intervening glial processes, and the vast majority of synapses are formed between single pre- and postsynaptic elements (Tweedle and Hatton 1977, 1984; El Majdoubi *et al.* 1997). Supraoptic neurons normally have a slow and irregular firing pattern *in vivo*. Under conditions of high hormonal demand, such as at parturition or during lactation, these neurons fire characteristic phasic bursts sufficient to release oxytocin or vasopressin into the blood (Hatton 1997). *In vitro*, oxytocin and vasopressin neurons can be distinguished by their responses to direct current injection (Stern and Armstrong 1998).

Physiological challenges to this system, including dehydration or events associated with motherhood, result in dramatic and reversible changes in dendritic morphology and synaptic connectivity within the supraoptic nucleus. Rearrangement of the physical relationship between neurons and glial cells is key to plasticity of both axosomatic and axodendritic innervation. Only the dendritic changes will be described in detail here.

Robust dendritic plasticity in the supraoptic nucleus occurs during motherhood, both at parturition and during lactation. In the last days of pregnancy, glia withdraw from between neuronal dendrites, resulting in 'dendritic bundling'. The number of dendrites per bundle is further increased at postpartum day 1 and remains high during lactation (Perlmutter *et al.* 1984; Theodosis and Poulain 1984). This change is associated with increased neuronal dye-coupling suggesting up-regulation of gap junctions (Hatton *et al.* 1987; Hatton and Yang 1994). In addition to dendritic bundling, late pregnancy and lactation are associated with a significant increase in the number of synapses formed between single presynaptic and multiple postsynaptic dendritic elements, i.e. an increase in multiple synapse boutons (Perlmutter *et al.* 1984; Theodosis and Poulain 1984). Although such multiple synapse boutons are relatively rare in the unstimulated state, they may increase in frequency 2–4 fold from the 19th to 21st day of gestation and increase still further during lactation (Theodosis and Poulain 1993). These synapses are a mixed population, some γ-amino-butyric acid (GABA)ergic and some glutamatergic (El Majdoubi *et al.* 1997). Both dendritic bundling and formation of multiple synapses are reversible; the basal condition returns within one month following weaning of the young, and a second pregnancy repeats the process (Theodosis and Poulain 1984).

A recent comparison of the dendritic trees of oxytocin and vasopressin neurons in non-pregnant and lactating rats showed profound changes in overall dendritic morphology. In rats that had been lactating for 8–10 days, the total dendritic length of oxytocin neurons was reduced by approximately 41% (Fig. 14.1) whereas the dendritic length of vasopressin neurons was increased by approximately 48% (Stern and Armstrong 1998). These differences in the dendritic tree were due largely to changes in number of dendritic branches at certain distances from the cell body rather than a difference in maximal dendritic extension. Thus during lactation, the dendritic trees of vasopressin neurons proliferate while the dendritic trees of oxytocin cells are pruned, each in specific regions.

Although dendritic changes in supraoptic neurons following an osmotic challenge are less dramatic than with pregnancy and lactation, analysis of changes in the axosomatic innervation of these cells demonstrate how very rapidly synaptic rearrangements can occur. Beagley and Hatton (1992) reported that within 5 h of intraperitoneal injection of a hypertonic saline solution, the frequency of axosomatic multiple synapses in the supraoptic nucleus doubled. This change occurred in parallel with significant increases in somatic membrane appositions and soma size.

Because activating stimuli and physiological outputs of the neurohypophysial system are well characterized, it is feasible to incorporate structural changes in dendritic and synaptic connectivity in the supraoptic and paraventricular nuclei into an understanding of their functional significance. Pregnancy and parturition or challenges to osmotic homeostasis activate the system. Release of oxytocin and vasopressin into the blood represent distinct and quantifiable outputs. Further, known changes in the firing patterns of oxytocin and vasopressin neurons can be correlated with structural changes. When hormonal demand is high, such as during lactation, oxytocin neurons transform from slow and irregular firing to coordinated, phasic bursting. These coordinated bursts produce a bolus of oxytocin sufficient to cause contraction of the myoepithelial cells in the mammary glands and result in milk ejection (Wakerley and Ingram 1993).

Structural changes in the dendrites of supraoptic neurons may be the basis of coordinated firing during lactation (Theodosis *et al.* 1981). One can envision that an increase in direct neuronal apposition through dendritic bundling, possibly with the

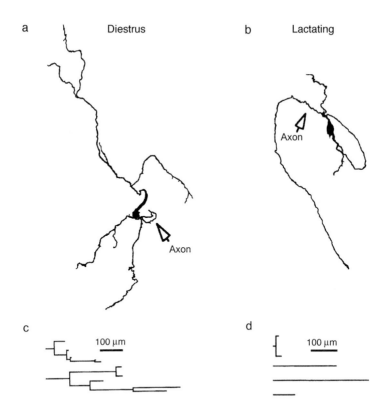

Fig. 14.1 The dendritic tree of oxytocin neurons in the supraoptic nucleus is larger and more highly branched during diestrus than during lactation. (a,b) Camera Lucida drawings of representative oxytocin neurons in the supraoptic nucleus from a diestrus female rat (a) or a lactating rat (b). (c,d) Dendrograms displaying the dendritic structure of each cell shown directly above. Modified from Stern and Armstrong (1998).

formation of dendrodendritic gap junctions, and increased frequency of multiple synaptic contacts could facilitate the coordinated bursts characteristic of lactation. Additionally, it is possible that decreased dendritic arborization of supraoptic oxytocin neurons during the period of lactation makes these cells more electrotonically compact, allowing signals from distal dendritic inputs to be more efficiently propagated to the cell body (Stern and Armstrong 1998). Any of these structural changes can be envisioned to facilitate the efficient, synchronous firing that is essential for appropriate lactation. Although the true relationship(s) between structural, electrophysiological and functional changes in supraoptic neurons is not yet understood, the fact that so many pieces of the puzzle are known makes this a very promising system in which to explore the functional consequences of structural dendritic plasticity.

Additionally, because structural changes on the neurohypophysial system are so dramatic, this system provides a good opportunity to probe the cellular and molecular events involved in structural remodeling of dendrites. In this context, it is especially important to note that retraction of glial processes appears to precede structural changes in neurons. Both astrocytes and neurons in the supraoptic nucleus show high levels of the immature form (containing polysialic acid, PSA) of neural cell adhesion molecules (NCAMs; Bonfanti *et al.* 1992) that are normally associated with the development of neural circuitry. Supraoptic glial also express vimentin, an intermediate filament protein normally associated with immature astrocytes (Bonfanti *et al.* 1993). The involvement of PSA–NCAM or vimentin in dendritic remodeling is not established, but these molecules are also expressed in other regions of the adult brain known to undergo structural remodeling and as such, may act as permissive factors in dendritic structural plasticity (Theodosis and Poulain 1993).

The molecular signals responsible for induction of dendritic remodeling in the neurohypophysial system currently are not known. There is heavy noradrenergic input to this region and osmotic challenges have been shown to induce an upregulation of β-adrenergic receptors in parallel with changes in astrocytic structure (Lafarga *et al.* 1992). As such, activation of β-adrenergic receptors on glia has been suggested to be a signal that could initiate structural plasticity in the dendrites of supraoptic neurons (Hatton 1997).

Ovarian hormone fluctuations—arcuate nucleus

It is well recognized that estrogen is a powerful regulator of synaptic connectivity in the adult as well as developing brain. In the adult, structural changes in synaptic connectivity of a wide variety of brain regions occur in response to fluctuating levels of estradiol: in the preoptic area (Witkin *et al.* 1991; Langub *et al.* 1994), arcuate (Garcia-Segura *et al.* 1986; Olmos *et al.* 1989) and ventromedial nuclei (Carrer and Aoki 1982) of the hypothalamus; lateral septum (Miyakawa and Arai 1987); mid-brain central gray (Chung *et al.* 1988); and hippocampus (e.g. Gould *et al.* 1990; see next section).

In the rat hypothalamus, the effects of estrogen on afferent input to arcuate neurons have been particularly well characterized by Garcia-Segura and colleagues. Although changes in axosomatic input to arcuate neurons are more thoroughly understood than dendritic changes, estrogen has been shown to affect both axosomatic and axodendritic input to these neurons (Matsumoto and Arai 1979; Garcia-Segura *et al.* 1986). Very similar effects are observed in the preoptic area as well, though the timing is somewhat different. Parallels with structural changes in the supraoptic nucleus and the remarkable rapidity with which synapses are formed and eliminated in the arcuate and preoptic nuclei make it worthwhile to briefly outline the effects of estrogen on synapses in these areas.

The arcuate nucleus is a cell group in the mediobasal hypothalamus that is involved in regulation of pituitary luteinizing hormone release. Garcia-Segura and colleagues have analyzed synaptic remodeling in the arcuate nucleus that is associated with fluctuating estradiol levels during the female reproductive cycle (estrous cycle). Elevated estradiol, either from exogenous hormone treatment (Perez *et al.* 1993) or during the estrous cycle (Olmos *et al.* 1989) induces a retraction of GABAergic (Parducz *et al.* 1993) inhibitory inputs to arcuate neurons. Although changes in synaptic input have not been quantified with stereological methods, conventional analyses indicate very robust effects. During the estrous cycle, the density of axosomatic synapses decreases by 50% between the morning and afternoon of proestrus, remains low during estrus and increases again during diestrus (Olmos *et al.* 1989; Garcia-Segura *et al.* 1994*a*). A single estradiol injection to ovariectomized rats produces an approximately 50% decrease in axosomatic synapse density within 24 h, which returns to baseline values by 48 h following hormone treatment (Perez *et al.* 1993). In the preoptic area, axosomatic synapse density increases by 39% in the 24 h between proestrus and estrus (Langub *et al.* 1994). These hormone-induced changes in the density of axosomatic innervation of arcuate neurons most likely reflect changes in the number of axosomatic inputs per cell, since bouton or cell body size were shown not to change.

As in the supraoptic and paraventricular nuclei, synaptic changes in the arcuate are paralleled by structural changes in glial cells. The retraction of inhibitory inputs that occurs between the morning and afternoon of proestrus or following estradiol is paralleled by an increase in glial fibrillary acidic protein immunoreactivity and apposition of glia to neuronal cell bodies (Garcia-Segura *et al.* 1994*b*). Thus it appears that estradiol mediates an exchange of inhibitory synaptic input for glial ensheathment of arcuate neurons.

Because the hypothalamic brain areas in which estrogen regulates synaptic connectivity are known to be important in female reproductive function (e.g. gonadotropin secretion or female sexual behavior), proposals for the functional significance of estrogen-induced structural plasticity in these regions center upon their potential effects on reproductive physiology. For example, in the arcuate nucleus it has been suggested that a retraction of inhibitory inputs results in disinhibition and increased excitatory drive on neurons, the activity of which is necessary for gonadotropin secretion and the consequent preovulation luteinizing hormone surge (Garcia-Segura 1994*a*).

As in the supraoptic nucleus, glia have been suggested to play a prominent role in initiating neuronal structural plasticity in the arcuate nucleus. PSA–NCAM is highly expressed in the arcuate and there is evidence from *in vitro* studies that PSA–NCAM plays a permissive role in structural plasticity in the neurohypophysial system. In arcuate cell cultures, estradiol normally promotes extension of glial processes, as it does *in vivo*. When PSA is specifically removed from these cultures using a bacterial endoneuramidase, the effect of estradiol in astrocytic morphology is blocked (Garcia-Segura 1994*a*).

Glial expression of several growth factors also has been suggested to be important in regulating neuronal structural plasticity, although currently this has not been directly demonstrated. Glial cells in the mediobasal hypothalamus express transforming growth factor-α (TGF-α) and insulin like growth factor-1 (IGF-1) both of which can stimulate release of gonadotropin releasing hormone (Ma *et al.* 1992), the proposed functional consequence of structural changes in circuitry. The expression of these growth factors is regulated by estradiol (during development, Ma *et al.* 1992; and during the estrous cycle, Garcia-Segura 1994*a*). During the estrous cycle, the surface density of IGF-1 immunoreactive glia in the arcuate fluctuates. Highest levels are observed on the afternoon of proestrus, following the peak in estradiol, whereas ovariectomy decreases the density of IGF-1 positive glial profiles (Garcia-Segura 1994*a*). These observations are consistent with a role for such growth factors in regulating structural plasticity in hypothalamic neurons.

Ovarian hormone fluctuations—hippocampus

Ovarian hormones also regulate the synaptic connectivity of hippocampal neurons. However, both the timing of synaptic changes and the type of synapses shown to be affected by estradiol differ between the arcuate and hippocampus. The hippocampal synapses shown to be regulated by estradiol are excitatory synapses formed on dendritic spines.

My colleagues and I have demonstrated in a series of studies that the density and number of dendritic spines and excitatory synapses on hippocampal CA1 pyramidal cells are sensitive to changes in circulating levels of estradiol and progesterone. In contrast, CA3 pyramidal cells and dentate gyrus granule cells in young adult females do not appear to be affected by estradiol. Gould *et al.* (1990) initially demonstrated that ovariectomy decreases the density of dendritic spines on the lateral branches of CA1 pyramidal cell dendritic trees over a 6-day period. This decrease could either be prevented (Gould *et al.* 1990) or reversed (Woolley and McEwen 1993) by estradiol treatment. Reported spine density changes range from 24% (Washburn *et al.* 1997) to 45% (Gould *et al.* 1990) in Golgi-impregnated cells to 22% in biocytin-filled cells (Fig. 14.2; Woolley *et al.* 1997). Importantly, estradiol-induced changes in *density* of dendritic spines occurs without changes in overall dendritic length or number of dendritic branches (Woolley and McEwen 1993), indicating the hormone-induced differences in spine density reflect differences in spine *number* rather than extension and shrinkage of the dendritic tree.

When ovariectomized animals are treated with estradiol, spine density begins to increase within 2 days, remains elevated for the next 1–2 days and then declines gradually over a period of about one week (Woolley and McEwen 1993). Treatment with progesterone subsequent to estradiol initially augments the effect of estradiol over a 2–6-h period (Gould *et al.* 1990; Woolley and McEwen 1993) and then results in a more rapid decrease in spine density than is observed with estradiol alone. By 18 h after sequential estradiol and progesterone treatment, spine density returns to low values similar to those seen in ovariectomized animals (Woolley and McEwen 1993).

The hormonal sensitivity of CA1 pyramidal cell dendritic spines leads to fluctuation in spine density during the estrous cycle that is consistent with the roles that estradiol and progesterone each have been shown to play (Woolley *et al.* 1990). The density of spines is lowest during the estrus phase of the cycle. Spine density builds up as estradiol levels gradually rise during 2–3 days of diestrus. On the evening of proestrus, after 3–4 days of estradiol secretion and shortly after a surge of progesterone, spine density is greatest. Estradiol and progesterone levels then drop overnight and by the end of the following day, back in estrus, spine density has returned to low values. The difference in spine density between late proestrus and late estrus is approximately 30% in Golgi-impregnated tissue.

Both during the estrous cycle and following treatment of ovariectomized rats with estradiol, changes in spine density are paralleled by changes in the density of axospinous synapses (Woolley and McEwen 1992). Importantly, no differences are seen in the density of synapses formed on dendritic shafts. The specificity of estradiol's effect for axospinous synapses is a further indication that hormone-induced changes in synapse density are not an artifact of fluctuation in hippocampal volume,

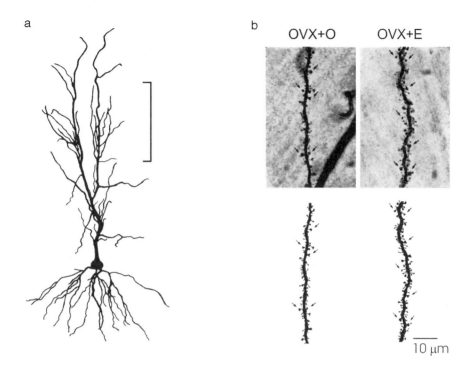

Fig. 14.2 Estradiol increases the density of dendritic spines in the lateral branches of the apical dendritic tree in hippocampal CA1 pyramidal cells. (a) Camera Lucida drawing of a CA1 pyramidal cell showing the region in the apical tree where estradiol has its greatest effect (bracket). (b) Representative photomicrographs (top panels) and Camera Lucida drawings (bottom panels) from an ovariectomized rat treated only with oil vehicle (OVX + O; left panels) or an ovariectomized rat treated with estradiol (OVX + E; right panels). Some dendritic spines are indicated by arrows. Note the estradiol-induced increase in dendritic spine density. Panel (b) is modified from Woolley *et al.* (1997).

since such generalized changes would be expected to affect both spine and shaft synapses.

Serial electron microscopic reconstruction of dendritic spines and presynaptic boutons from estradiol-treated and control ovariectomized rats strongly suggests that new spines induced by estradiol form synapses with preexisting boutons transforming some previously single synapse boutons into multiple synapse boutons (Woolley *et al.* 1996). Thus, in a manner similar to the addition of synapses to visual cortex and supraoptic neurons, new synapses in the hippocampus result in an increase in frequency of multiple synapse boutons.

Similar to what has been observed in the supraoptic and arcuate nuclei, there appears to be a reciprocal relationship between numbers of spine synapses in CA1 and glial hypertrophy. An analysis of glial volume in CA1 across the estrous cycle showed that glia occupy a greater fraction of neuropil during the estrus phase of the estrous cycle than during the proestrus phase (Klintsova *et al.* 1995). Thus, when spine and synapse numbers are lower and bouton volume would also be lower, glial volume is greater. The complementary relationship between glial and neuronal elements may serve to maintain stability in hippocampal and extracellular space volume.

There has been considerable headway made in understanding the physiological consequences of additional spine synapses on hippocampal pyramidal cells. Receptor binding autoradiography initially demonstrated that estrogen treatment produces an increase in binding to NMDA receptors with no effect on binding to non-NMDA glutamate receptors (Weiland 1992; Woolley *et al.* 1997). The increase in NMDA receptor binding was shown to be an effect on the number of binding sites (B_{max}) rather than a change in receptor affinity (Weiland 1992). In line with the binding results, several studies using *in vitro* hippocampal slices have shown electrophysiological effects of estradiol that suggest an up-regulation of NMDA receptor function. First, Wong and Moss (1992) demonstrated that estradiol treatment results in an increase excitatory postsynaptic potential duration and repetitive firing in CA1 pyramidal cells. Second, a cell-by-cell comparison of spine density on cells from ovariectomized control or estrogen treated rats with measures of sensitivity to synaptic input showed a significant association between spine density and sensitivity to NMDA, but not non-NMDA, receptor mediated input (Woolley *et al.* 1997). The suggestion that estradiol up-regulates NMDA receptor expression is further corroborated by the observation that estradiol treatment increases immunofluorescence for NMDA-R1, the obligatory subunit of the NMDA receptor complex (Gazzaley *et al.* 1996)

Several studies of the effects of estradiol on hippocampal electrophysiology recorded *in vivo* also support an effect of estrogen on NMDA receptor physiology. First, the threshold for induction of epileptiform activity is decreased at proestrus and by estradiol treatment (Terasawa and Timiras 1968). Second, the potential for synaptic potentiation in the CA1 region is enhanced at proestrus (Warren *et al.* 1995) and by estradiol treatment (Cordoba-Montoya and Carrer 1997). Baseline synaptic responses in CA1 were unchanged by estradiol or during the estrous cycle. Thus, the estradiol-induced increase in numbers of dendritic spines and spine synapses on CA1 pyramidal cells are tightly correlated with enhancement of two different NMDA receptor-dependent measures of synaptic function.

Since the hippocampus is a brain structure thought to be important for learning and memory, the observation that estradiol regulates structural and functional measures of excitatory input to hippocampal pyramidal cells suggests a means of achieving a long sought after goal—demonstration of a link between structural dendritic plasticity and learning. As such, a number of studies have attempted to relate hippocampus-dependent learning (e.g. spatial learning, contextual fear conditioning) to stages of the estrous cycle or estradiol treatment. The results of these studies, however, have been equivocal. Several studies have demonstrated poorer performance in hippocampus-dependent tasks during proestrus (Galea *et al.* 1995 in voles; Markes and Zecevic 1997; Warren and Juraska 1997) or with estradiol treatment (Korol *et al.* 1994). Other studies have found no difference (Berry *et al.* 1997; Stackman *et al.* 1997). Still other studies report improved performance in aged rats in a relatively difficult version of the radial arm maze (Williams 1996) or with estradiol treatment times longer than those which have been shown to affect hippocampal spine synapses (e.g. Singh *et al.* 1994 and Daniel *et al.* 1997). Thus, a correlation between structural changes and behavioral differences induced by estradiol has not yet been established. However, these results do suggest that exposure to elevated estradiol on the time course of the estrous cycle has a negative, if any, effect on hippocampus-dependent behavior while sustained elevation of estradiol can positively influence hippocampus-dependent behavior.

Taken together, results from a variety of behavioral studies have thus far demonstrated no obvious relationship between increased hippocampal spine synapse numbers and performance on hippocampus-dependent tasks. There are several points to consider in the interpretation of these findings. First, it could be that tests of hippocampal function currently used (e.g. radial arm mazes, water mazes, contextual conditioning) are not sufficiently sensitive to detect the functional consequences of increased numbers of spine synapses on CA1 pyramidal cells. This might be particularly true if spine synapse changes result in a selective increase in NMDA receptor function, as receptor binding and electrophysiological analyses suggest. Second, it should not be assumed that *more versus fewer* CA1 spine synapses will lead to *better versus worse* hippocampal function. In fact, it is possible that during a period of high spine synapse number such as during proestrus, rapid synapse turnover actually impairs hippocampal function. This suggestion is consistent with the studies that report a deficit in hippocampus dependent learning at proestrus.

All of these considerations have lead to several suggestions for the behavioral significance of hormone-induced structural plasticity of hippocampal dendrites. One hypothesis speculates that the hippocampus is optimized for different functions at different times in the estrous cycle; during proestrus (when females are sexually receptive), increased numbers of excitatory synapses on hippocampal pyramidal cells might facilitate appropriate mate selection (Desmond and Levy 1997). Another possibility is that the hormonal sensitivity of hippocampal dendrites is related more to pregnancy and maternal behavior than to the estrous cycle itself (Woolley 1998). It is not yet known whether either of these proposals truly represents the functional significance of hormone-induced changes in hippocampal synaptic connectivity or whether there is some as yet unknown behavioral significance of the identified structural changes. Nevertheless, the fact that estrogen induces structural plasticity in the dendrites of hippocampal neurons, which are known to be involved in cognitive functioning, provides a valuable opportunity to explore how differences in neuronal connectivity affect cognitive function.

Use of dissociated hippocampal cultures has been valuable in addressing cellular and molecular mechanisms by which estradiol increases dendritic spine density. Murphy, Segal and colleagues have performed a series of studies examining the effects of estradiol on spine density in cultured hippocampal neurons. Treatment of hippocampal cultures with estradiol results in a 2-fold increase in dendritic spine density, which is associated with an increased intensity of synaptophysin staining and increased calcium responses to glutamate, and therefore likely represents an increase in functional synaptic contacts (Murphy and Segal 1996).

There are several parallels between estradiol regulation of hippocampal connectivity *in vivo* and *in vitro*. In both cases, the effect of estradiol is delayed; the estradiol-induced increase in spines on cultured neurons is observed 2 days following exposure to the hormone (Murphy and Segal 1996). Also similar to regulation of hippocampal spines *in vivo* (Woolley and McEwen 1994), estradiol regulation of spine density on cultured neurons requires NMDA receptor activation (Murphy and Segal 1996).

These investigators' studies have directly linked estradiol-induced changes in GABAergic inhibition to spine formation in cultured hippocampal neurons. *In vivo*, cells in the CA1 region of the hippocampus that contain classical estradiol receptors are inhibitory interneurons (Loy *et al.* 1988; Weiland *et al.* 1997), suggesting that estradiol might act directly on inhibitory function in the hippocampus. Inhibitory neurons in hippocampal cultures also contain classical estradiol receptors (Murphy *et al.* 1998*a*). Estradiol treatment of hippocampal cultures induces a biphasic response in the GABAergic neurons. Initially, at 12 and 24 h after estradiol exposure, glutamic acid decarboxylase (GAD, the rate-limiting enzyme in GABA synthesis) immunoreactivity is decreased by approximately 50% (Murphy *et al.* 1998*a*). A reduction in the amplitude and frequency of GABAergic miniature inhibitory postsynaptic currents (mIPSCs) and an increase in miniature excitatory postsynaptic currents (mEPSCs) in pyramidal cells parallel this decrease. Thus during the period in which new spines are forming, a decrease in GAD immunoreactivity is accompanied by increased excitatory drive on spiny cells. By 48 h after estradiol exposure, spine density is significantly increased and GAD immunoreactivity overshoots above initial values.

Several further experiments support the suggestion that estradiol regulates spine density by decreasing GABAergic activity and thereby increasing spine density on pyramidal cells in an activity-dependent fashion (i.e. through disinhibition). Murphy and colleagues (Murphy *et al.* 1998*a*) have shown that treatment of cultures with mercaptopropionic acid (MA), an inhibitor of GABA synthesis, mimics the effect of estradiol on spine density and the effects of MA and estradiol are not additive suggesting that they could share a common mechanism. These investigators also showed that treatment of cultures with tetrodotoxin, which would block Na^+ action potential discharge, also blocks the estradiol-induced increase in spine density, a further indication of an activity-dependent mechanism of spine formation *in vitro*.

Estradiol induction of dendritic spines in cultured hippocampal neurons appears to be linked to activation of cAMP response element binding protein (CREB) and CREB binding protein (CBP). Estradiol produces an increase in CBP and phosphorylated CREB that precedes the increase in dendritic spine density (Murphy and Segal 1997). Similar to the effect on spines, blockade of NMDA receptors also inhibits the increase in CBP and phosphorylation of CREB. Two further pieces of evidence from this study corroborate a cAMP-dependent effect of estradiol on spines. First, inhibition of cAMP-dependent protein kinase A with H89 blocks both the estradiol-induced increase in spine density and its effects on CBP and CREB. Second, treatment of cultures with a cAMP analog at least partially mimics the effect of estradiol.

Finally, recent studies suggest that regulation of neurotrophin expression is key to the effects of estradiol on inhibitory function and subsequently on hippocampal dendritic spine density. Murphy *et al.* (1998*b*) have demonstrated that estradiol treatment of hippocampal cultures decreases levels of brain derived neurotrophic factor (BDNF). This decrease in BDNF results in disinhibition of pyramidal cells allowing the activity-dependent increase in dendritic spine density. To demonstrate the role of BDNF in regulation of spine density, Murphy *et al.* (1998*b*) showed that exogenous BDNF can block the estradiol-induced increase in dendritic spine density, whereas BDNF depletion with a selective antisense oligonucleotide or addition of function blocking BDNF antibodies mimics the effect of estradiol.

In vivo studies have demonstrated that expression of BDNF mRNA in hippo-campal neurons is regulated by estradiol and fluctuates during the estrous cycle (Gibbs 1998) suggesting a further parallel with estradiol-induced spine formation *in vitro*. Future studies will undoubtedly determine whether estradiol regulation of dendritic spine density *in vivo* also involves BDNF or possibly other growth factors.

Concluding remarks

A variety of approaches have demonstrated structural plasticity in adult mammalian brain circuitry, particularly in dendrites and their associated synapses. Theories of learning have long postulated that structural change in synaptic connectivity underlie long-term information storage. However, the fact that circuits encoding learned information are likely to be distributed within and between brain regions and our inability to identify individual cells and synapses involved in learning make it difficult to test this hypothesis directly. Even so, a number of experiments have demonstrated consistent experience- or learning-dependent structural changes in dendrites and synapses of neurons of the neocortex and cerebellar cortex.

If one sets aside the issue of learning and one focuses instead on simpler systems dedicated to specific physiological functions, robust structural plasticity in adult dendrites and synapses can be found. The neurohypophysial system and gonadal hormone-sensitive areas of the hypothalamus have been most studied in this context. Because these circuits are less complex, observations of structural plasticity in the hypothalamus are more readily incorporated into an understanding of their func-tional consequences. The observation of hormone-induced structural plasticity in the dendrites of hippocampal neurons, which are known to be important in learning, may be a means to bridge these two approaches. Although initial attempts to relate structural changes in hippocampal synaptic connectivity to learning have been equivocal, future studies will likely reveal the behavioral, and possibly learning-related, consequences of this form of dendritic structural plasticity.

Several generalizable themes emerge from comparison of the structural changes that occur in various brain regions. First, structural plasticity in synaptic connectivity occurs specifically in certain synapse types on a cell rather than a generalized up- or down-regulation of synapse numbers. Thus, in the cerebellum, parallel fiber to Purkinje cell synapses are increased in number by motor skill learning, but climbing fiber synapses are unchanged. In the hippocampus, numbers of synapses formed on dendritic spines are increased by estradiol, while synapses formed on dendritic shafts are unchanged. Recent imaging studies in hippocampal cultures have also shown that rapid NMDA-receptor dependent spine growth is restricted to dendritic regions which have undergone synaptic plasticity (Engert and Bonhoeffer 1999; Miletic-Savatic *et al.* 1999). This suggests that structural changes are dependent on activity within particular pathways.

A second theme is that new synapses in the adult brain appear to involve presynaptic boutons in contact with multiple postsynaptic elements—dendrites or cell bodies. These multiple synapse boutons may result from the addition of new postsynaptic sites to preexisting presynaptic boutons leading to a transformation of single to multiple synapse boutons. New multiple synapses are observed in the visual cortex, supraoptic nucleus and hippocampus. This may explain the lack of axonal growth cones or degenerating axonal terminals associated with non-pathological synapse formation or elimination in the adult.

A third observation that is consistent across multiple brain areas is that structural plasticity of neurons involves dynamic changes in the relationship between neurons and glial cells. Structural changes in neuronal/glial relationships are associated with dendritic plasticity in cortical and hypothalamic areas as well as in the hippocampus. Although perhaps intuitive, the observation that structural change in glial elements occurs in parallel or even before structural change in neurons suggests that glia play an active role in structural modification of neurons. Glial initiation of neuronal structural plasticity has been proposed in the supraoptic nucleus (Hatton 1997), arcuate nucleus (Garcia-Segura 1994*b*) and hippocampus (Desmond and Levy 1997).

Although structural plasticity in adult brain circuitry was demonstrated over 30 years ago, there are still many unanswered questions. For example, it is unknown how prevalent structural plasticity is as a mechanism of normal adult brain function. Nor is it known how rapidly structural changes in dendrites and synapses can or do occur normally. The fact that quite rapid structural changes in the innervation of hypothalamic neurons are observed with fluctuating ovarian hormone levels suggests that structural plasticity could be a more prevalent factor in brain function than we currently appreciate. It could be that changes are detectable in these regions in part because a large proportion of cells responds to an activating stimulus. It is at least *possible* that some synapses are equally rapidly formed and eliminated in many parts of the brain, but a greater variety of inputs and distribution of activated circuits impedes detection. A primary limitation in our current understanding of the prevalence and rapidity of structural plasticity is the inability to view neurons *in vivo* with sufficient resolution to observe real time structural changes in dendrites and synapses. A full appreciation of structural plasticity awaits advances in high-resolution *in vivo* imaging technology that will allow us to observe structural changes in individual neurons taking place in the living brain (see Lendvai *et al.* 1998).

References

Albus, J. S. (1971). A theory of cerebellar function. *Mathematical Biosciences*, **10**, 25–61.

Anderson, B. J., Alcantara, A. A., and Greenough, W. T. (1996). Motor skill learning: changes in synaptic organization of the rat cerebellar cortex. *Neurobiology of Learning and Memory*, **66**, 221–30.

Bain, A. (1872). *Mind and body: the theories of their relation.* H. S. King, London.

Beagley, G. H. and Hatton, G. I. (1992). Rapid morphological changes in the supraoptic nucleus and posterior pituitary induced by a single hypertonic saline injection. *Brain Research Bulletin* **28**, 613–18.

Bennett, E. L., Diamond, M. C., Krech, D., and Rosenzweig, M. R. (1964). Chemical and anatomical plasticity of brain. *Science*, **164**, 610–19.

Berry, B., McMahan, R., and Gallagher, M. (1997). Spatial learning and memory at defined points of the estrous cycle: Effects on performance of a hippocampal dependent task. *Behavioral Neuroscience*, **111**, 267–74.

Bonfanti, L., Olive, S., Poulain, D. A., and Theodosis, D. T. (1992). Mapping of the distribution of polysialylated neural cell adhesion molecule throughout the central nervous system of the adult rat: an immunohistochemical study. *Neuroscience*, **49**, 410–36.

Bonfanti, L., Poulain, D. A., and Theodosis, D. T. (1993). Radial glia-like cells in the supraoptic nucleus of the adult rat. *Journal of Neuroendocrinology*, **5**, 1–6.

Bravin, M., Morando, L., Vercelli, A., Rossi, F., and Strata, P. (1999). Control of spine formation by electrical activity in the adult rat cerebellum. *Proceedings of the National Academy of Science USA*, **96**, 1704–9.

Carrer, H. F. and Aoki, A (1982). Ultrastructural changes in the hypothalamic ventromedial nucleus of ovariectomized rats after estrogen treatment. *Brain Research*, **240**, 221–33.

Chang, Fen-Lei F. and Greenough, W. T. (1982). Lateralized effects of monocular training on dendritic branching in adult split-brain rats. *Brain Research*, **240**, 221–33.

Chung, S. K., Pfaff, D. W., and Cohen, R. S. (1988). Estrogen-induced changes in synaptic morphology in the midbrain central gray. *Experimental Brain Research*, **69**, 522–30.

Conner, J. R., Diamond, M. C., and Johnson, R. E. (1980). Aging and environmental influences on two types of dendritic spines in the rat occipital cortex. *Experimental Neurology*, **70**, 371–9.

Cordoba Montoya, D. A. and Carrer, H. F. (1997). Estrogen facilitates induction of long-term potentiation in the hippocampus of awake rats. *Brain Research*, **778**, 430–8.

Daniel, J. M., Fader, A. J., Spencer, A. L., and Dohanich, G. P. (1997). Estrogen enhances performance of female rats during acquisition of a radial arm maze. *Hormones and Behavior*, **32**, 217–25.

Desmond, N. L. and Levy, W. B. (1997). Ovarian steroidal control of connectivity in the female hippocampus: an overview of recent experimental findings and speculation on its functional consequences. *Hippocampus* **7**, 39–45.

Diamond, M. C., Ingham, C. A., Johnson, R. E., Bennett, E. L., and Rosenzweig, M. R. (1976). Effects of environment on morphology of rat cerebral cortex and hippocampus. *Journal of Neurobiology*, **7**, 75–85.

Diamond, M. C., Lindner, B., Johnson, R., Bennett, E. L., and Rosenzweig, M. R. (1975). Differences in occipital cortical synapses from environmentally enriched, impoverished, and standard colony rats. *Journal of Neuroscience Research*, **1**, 109–19.

Diamond, M. C., Rosenzweig, M. R., Bennett, E. L., Linder, B., and Lyon, L. (1972). Effects of environmental enrichment and impoverishment on rat cerebral cortex. *Journal of Neurobiology*, **3**, 47–64.

Duval, M. (1895). Hypothèse sur la physiologie des centres nerveux: théorie histologique du sommeil. In *Cajal on the cerebral cortex*, (trans. J. DeFelipe and E. Jones), p. 480. Oxford University Press, New York.

Eccles, J. C. (1977). An instruction selection theory of learning in the cerebellar cortex. *Brain Research*, **127**, 327–52.

Eccles, J. C., Ito, M., and Szentagothai, J. (1967). *The cerebellum as a neuronal machine*. Springer, New York.

El Majdoubi, M., Poulain, D. A., and Theodosis, D. T. (1997). Lactation-induced plasticity in the supraoptic nucleus axodendritic and axosomatic GABAergic and glutamatergic synapses: an ultrastructural analysis using the disector method. *Neuroscience*, **80**, 1137–47.

Engert, F. and Bonhoeffer, T. (1999). Dendritic spine changes associated with hippocampal long-term synaptic plasticity. *Nature*, **399**, 66–70.

Galea, L. A. M., Kavakiers, M., Ossenkopp, K. P., and Hampson, E. (1995). Gonadal hormone levels and spatial learning performance in the Morris water maze in male and female meadow voles, *Microtus pennsylvanicus*. *Hormones and Behavior*, **29**, 106–25.

Garcia-Segura, L. M., Chowen, J. A., Parducz, A., and Naftolin, F. (1994*a*). Gonadal hormones as promoters of structural plasticity: cellular mechanisms. *Progress in Neurobiology*, **44**, 279–307.

Garcia-Segura, L. M., Luquín, S., Párducz, A., and Naftolin, F. (1994*b*). Gonadal hormone regulation of glial fibrillary acidic protein immunoreactivity and glial ultrastructure in the rat neuroendocrine hypothalamus. *Glia*, **10**, 59–69.

Garcia-Segura, L. M., Baetens, D., and Naftolin, F. (1986). Synaptic remodeling in arcuate nucleus after injection of estradiol valerate. *Brain Research*, **366**, 131–6.

Gazzaley, A. H., Weiland, N. G., McEwen, B. S., and Morrision, J. H. (1996). Differential regulation of NMDAR1 mRNA and protein by estradiol in the rat hippocampus. *Journal of Neuroscience*, **16**, 6830–8.

Gibbs, R. B. (1998). Levels of trkA and BDNF mRNA, but not NGF mRNA, fluctuate across the estrous cycle and increase in response to acute hormone replacement. *Brain Research*, **787**, 259–68.

Gilbert, F. C. and Thach, W. T. (1977). Purkinje cell activity during motor learning. *Brain Research*, **128**, 309–28.

Gould, E., Woolley, C. S., Frankfurt, M., and McEwen, B. S. (1990). Gonadal steroids regulate dendritic spine density in hippocampal pyramidal cells in adulthood. *Journal of Neuroscience*, **10**, 1286–91.

Green, E. J., Greenough, W. T., and Schlumph, B. E. (1983). Effects of complex or isolated environments on cortical dendrites of middle-aged rats. *Brain Research*, **264**, 233–40.

Greenough, W. T., Larson, J. R., and Withers, G. S. (1985). Effects of unilateral and bilateral training in a reaching task in dendritic branching of neurons in the rat sensory-motor forelimb cortex. *Behavioral and Neural Biology*, **44**, 301–14.

Greenough, W. T., McDonald, J. W., Parnisari, R. M., and Camel, J. E. (1986). Environmental conditions modulate degeneration and new dendrite growth in cerebellum of senescent rats. *Brain Research*, **380**, 136–43.

Hatton, G. I. (1997). Function-related plasticity in hypothalamus. *Annual Review of Neuroscience*, **20**, 375–97.

Hatton, G. I. and Yang, Q. Z. (1994). Incidence of neuronal coupling in supraoptic nuclei of virgin and lactating rats: estimation of neurobiotin and Lucifer yellow. *Brain Research*, **650**, 63–9.

Hatton, G. I., Yang, Q. Z., and Cobbett, P. (1987). Dye coupling among immunocytochemically identified neurons in the supraoptic nucleus: increased incidence in the lactating rat. *Neuroscience*, **21**, 923–30.

Hebb, D. O. (1949). *The organization of behavior*, p. 62. Wiley, New York.

Hubel, D. H. and Weisel, T. N. (1963). Receptive fields of cells in striate cortex of very young, visually inexperienced kittens. *Journal of Neurophysiology*, **26**, 994–1002.

Hubel, D. H. and Wiesel, T. N. (1970). The period of susceptibility to the physiological effects of unilateral eye closure in kittens. *Journal of Physiology*, **206**, 419–36.

Ito, M. (1984). *The cerebellum and neural control*. Raven Press, New York.

Jones, T. A., Klintsova, A. Y., Kilman, V. L., Sirevaag, A. M., and Greenough, W. T. (1997). Induction of multiple synapses by experience in the visual cortex of adult rats. *Neurobiology of Learning and Memory*, **68**, 13–20.

Kleim, J. A., Lussnig, E., Schwarz, E. R., Comery, T. A., and Greenough, W. T. (1996). Synaptogenesis and Fos expression in the motor cortex of the adult rat after motor skill learning. *Journal of Neuroscience*, **16**, 4529–35.

Kleim, J. A., Swain, R. A., Czerlanis, C. M., Kelly, J. L. Pipitone, M. A., and Greenough, W. T. (1997). Learning-dependent dendritic hypertrophy of cerebellar stellate cells: plasticity of local circuit neurons. *Neurobiology of Learning and Memory*, **67**, 29–33.

Kleim, J. A., Swain, R. A., Armstrong, K. A., Napper, R. M. A., Jones, T. A., and Greenough, W. T. (1998). Selective synaptic plasticity within the cerebellar cortex following complex motor skill learning. *Neurobiology of Learning and Memory*, **69**, 274–89.

Klintsova, A., Levy, W. B., and Desmond, N. L. (1995). Astrocytic volume fluctuates in the hippocampal CA1 region across the estrous cycle. *Brain Research*, **690**, 269–74.

Korol, D. L., Unick, K., Goosens, K., Crane, C., Gold, P., and Foster, T. C. (1994). Estrogen effects on spatial performance and hippocampal physiology in female rats. *Society for Neuroscience Abstracts*, **20**, 1436.

Lafarga, M., Berciano, M. T., Del Olmo, E., Andres, M. A., and Pazos, A. (1992). Osmotic stimulation induces changes in the expression of β-adrenergic receptors and nuclear volume of astrocytes in supraoptic nucleus of the rat. *Brain Research*, **588**, 311–16.

Langub, Jr., M. C., Maley, B. E., and Watson, R. E. (1994). Estrous cycle-associated axosomatic synaptic plasticity upon estrogen receptive neurons in the rat preoptic area. *Brain Research*, **64**, 303–10.

Lashley, K. S. (1929). Learning I: Nervous mechanisms in learning. In *The foundations of experimental psychology* (ed. C. Murchinson). Clark University Press, Worcester.

Lendvai, B., Burbach, B. J., and Svoboda, K. (1998). Long-term 2-photon imaging neuronal morphology in the rat neocortex *in vivo*. *Society for Neuroscience Abstracts*, 24, 632.

Locke, J. (1690). *An essay concerning human understanding*. T. Basset, London.

Loeb, J. (1902). *Comparative physiology of the brain and comparative psychology*. Putnam, New York.

Lorenz, K. (1935). Der Kumpan in der Umwelt des Vogels. *Journal of Ornithology*, **83**, 137–213; 289–413.

Loy, R., Gerlach, J. L., and McEwen, B. S. (1988). Autoradiographic localization of estradiol-binding neurons in the hippocampal formation and entorhinal cortex. *Developmental Brain Research*, 39, 245–51.

Ma, Y. J., Junier, M. P., Costa, M. E., and Ojeda, S. R. (1992). Transforming growth factor-α gene expression in the hypothalamus is developmentally regulated and linked to sexual maturation. *Neuron*, **9**, 657–70.

Maletic-Savatic, M., Malinow, R., and Svoboda, K. (1999). Rapid dendritic morphogenesis in CA1 hippocampal dendrites induced by synaptic activity. *Science*, **283**, 1923–7.

Mano, N., Kanazawa, I., and Yamamoto, K. (1989). Voluntary movements and complex spike discharges of cerebellar Purkinje cells. *Experimental Brain Research*, **17**, 265–80.

Markes, E. and Zecevic, M (1997). Sex differences and estrous cycle changes in hippocampus dependent fear conditioning. *Psychobiology*, 25, 246–52.

Marple-Horvat, D. E., and Stein, J. F. (1987). Cerebellar neuronal activity related to arm movements in trained rhesus monkeys. *Journal of Physiology*, **394**, 351–66.

Marr, D. (1969). A theory of cerebellar cortex. *Journal of Physiology*, **202**, 437–70.

Matsumoto, A. and Arai, Y. (1979). Synaptogenic effect of estrogen on the hypothalamic arcuate nucleus of the adult female rat. *Cell and Tissue Research*, **198**, 427–33.

Mauk, M. D., Garcia, K. S., Medina, J. F., and Steele, P. M. D. (1998). Does cerebellar LTD mediate motor learning? Toward a resolution without a smoking gun. *Neuron*, **20**, 359–62.

Miyakawa, M. and Arai, Y. (1987). Synaptic plasticity to estrogen in the lateral septum of adult male and female rats. *Brain Research*, **436**, 184–8.

Murphy, D. D. and Segal, M. (1996). Regulation of dendritic spine density in cultures of rat hippocampal neurons by steroid hormones. *Journal of Neuroscience*, **16**, 4059–68.

Murphy, D. D. and Segal, M. (1997). Morphological plasticity of dendritic spines in central neurons is mediated by activation of cAMP response element binding protein. *Proceedings of the National Academy of Science USA*, **94**, 1482–7.

Murphy, D. D., Cole, N. B., Greenberger, V., and Segal, M. (1998a). Estradiol increases dendritic spine density by reducing GABA neurotransmission in hippocampal neurons. *Journal of Neuroscience*, **18**, 2550–9.

Murphy, D. D., Cole, N. B., and Segal, M. (1998b). Brain-derived neurotrophic factor mediates estradiol-induced dendritic spine formation in hippocampal neurons. *Proceedings of the National Academy of Science USA*, **95**, 11412–7.

Nashner, L. M. and Grimm, K. L. (1978). Analysis of multitop dyscontrols in standing cerebellar patients. In *Cerebral motor control in man: long loop mechanisms*, (ed. J. E. Desmond). Karger, Basel.

Newton, I. (1697). Philosophie naturalis principa mathematica. In, *Origins of neuroscience*, (ed. S. Finger). Oxford University Press, New York.

Ojakangas, C. L. and Ebner, T. J. (1992). Purkinje cell complex and simple spike changes during a voluntary arm movement learning task in the monkey. *Journal of Neurophysiology*, **68**, 2222–36.

Ojakangas, C. L. and Ebner, T. J. (1994). Purkinje cell complex spike activity during voluntary motor learning: relationship to kinematics. *Journal of Neurophysiology*, **72**, 2617–30.

Olmos, G., Naftolin, F., Perez, J., Tranque, P. A., Garcia-Segura, L. M. (1989). Synaptic remodeling in the rat arcuate nucleus during the estrous cycle. *Neuroscience*, **32**, 663–7.

Parducz, A., Pérez, J., and Garcia-Segura, L. M. (1993). Estradiol induces plasticity in GABAergic synapses in the hypothalamus. *Neuroscience*, **53**, 295–401.

Perez, J., Luquin, S., Naftolin, F., and Garcia-Segura, L. M. (1993). The role of estradiol and progesterone in phased synaptic remodeling of the rat arcuate nucleus. *Brain Research*, **608**, 38–44.

Perlmutter, L. S., Tweedle, C. D., and Hatton, G. I. (1984). Neuronal/glial plasticity in the supraoptic dendritic zone: dendritic bundling and double synapse formation a parturition. *Neuroscience*, **13**, 769–79.

Ramón y Cajal, S. (1894). The Croonian lecture: la fine structure des systèmes nerveux. *Proceedings of the Royal Society of London*, **55**, 444–67.

Ramón y Cajal, S. (1928). *Degeneration and regeneration of the nervous system*, (trans. R. M. May). Oxford University Press, London.

Raymond, J. L. (1998). Learning in the oculomotor system: from molecules to behaviour. *Current Opinion in Neurobiology*, **8**, 770–6.

Rosenzweig, M. R., Krech, D., Bennet, E. L., and Diamond, M. C. (1962). Effects of environmental complexity and training on brain chemistry and anatomy: a replication and extension. *Journal of Comparative and Physiological Psychology*, **55**, 429–37.

Santori, E. M., Der, T., and Collins, R. C. (1986). Functional metabolic mapping during forelimb movement in rat. II Stimulation of forelimb muscles. *Journal of Neuroscience*, **6**, 463–74.

Scott, J. P. and Marston, M.-V. (1950). Critical periods affecting the development of normal and maladjustive social behavior of puppies. *Journal of Genetics and Psychology*, **77**, 25–60.

Seitz, R. J., Roland, E., Bohm, C., Greitz, T., and Stone-Elander, S. (1990). Motor learning in man: a positron emission topographic study. *Neuroreport*, **1**, 57–60.

Shepherd, G. M. (1991). *Foundations of the neuron doctrine*. Oxford University Press, New York.

Singh, M., Meyer, E. M., Millard, W. J., and Simpkins, J. W. (1994). Ovarian steroid deprivation results in a reversible learning impairment and compromised cholinergic function in female Sprague–Dawley rats. *Brain Research*, **644**, 305–12.

Stackman, R. W., Blasberg, M. E., Langan, C. J., and Clark, A. S. (1997). Stability of spatial working memory across the estrous cycle of Long–Evans rats. *Neurobiology of Learning and Memory*, **76**, 167–71.

Stern, J. E. and Armstrong, W. E. (1998). Reorganization of the dendritic trees of oxytocin and vasopressin neurons of the rat supraoptic nucleus during lactation. *Journal of Neuroscience*, **18**, 841–53.

Strata, P., Tempia, F., Zagrebelski, M., and Rossi, F. (1997). Reciprocal trophic interactions between climbing fibres and Purkinje cells in the rat cerebellum. *Progress in Brain Research*, **114**, 263–82.

Tanzi, E. (1873). *I fatti e le induzioni nell'odierna istologia del sistema nervoso*, In, *Cajal on the cerebral cortex*, (trans. J. DeFelipe and E. Jones) Oxford University Press, New York, 484.

Terasawa, E. and Timiras, P. S. (1968). Electrical activity during the estrous cycle of the rat: cyclical changes in limbic structures. *Endocrinology*, **83**, 207–16.

Theodosis, D. T. and Poulain, D. A. (1984). Evidence for structural plasticity in the supraoptic nucleus of the rat hypothalamus in relation to gestation and lactation. *Neuroscience*, **11**, 183–93.

Theodosis, D. T. and Poulain, D. A. (1989). Neuronal-glial and synaptic plasticity in the adult paraventricular nucleus. *Brain Research*, **484**, 361–6.

Theodosis, D. T. and Poulain, D. A. (1993). Activity-dependent neuronal-glial and synaptic plasticity in the adult mammalian hypothalamus. *Neuroscience*, **57**, 501–35.

Theodosis, D. T., Poulain, D. A., and Vincent, J. D. (1981). Possible morphological bases for synchronisation of neuronal firing in the rat supraoptic nucleus during lactation. *Neuroscience*, **6**, 919–29.

Tweedle, C. D. and Hatton, G. I. (1977). Ultrastructural changes in rat hypothalamic neurosecretory cells and their associated glia during minimal dehydration and rehydration. *Cell Tissue Research*, **181**, 59–72.

Tweedle, C. D. and Hatton, G. I. (1984). Synapse formation and disappearance in adult rat supraoptic nucleus during different hydration states. *Brain Research*, **309**, 373–6.

Uylings, H. B. M., Kuypers, K., Diamond, M. C., and Veltman, W. A. M. (1978). Effects of differential environments on plasticity of dendrites of cortical pyramidal neurons in adult rats. *Experimental Neurology* **62**, 658–77.

Wakerly, J. B. and Ingram, C. D. (1993). Synchronisation of bursting in hypothalamic oxytocin neurons: possible coordinating mechanisms. *News in Physiological Science*, 129–33.

Warren, S. G. and Juraska, J. M. (1997). Spatial and non-spatial learning across the rat estrous cycle. *Behavioral Neuroscience*, **111**, 259–66.

Warren, S. G., Humphreys, A. G., Juraska, J. M., and Greenough, W. T. (1995). LTP varies across the estrous cycle: enhanced synaptic plasticity in proestrus rats. *Brain Research*, **703**, 26–40.

Washburn, S. A., Lewis, C. E., Johnson, J. E., Voytko, M. L., and Shively, C. A. (1997). 17α-Dihydroequilenin increases hippocampal dendritic spine density of ovariectomized rats. *Brain Research*, **758**, 241–4.

Weiland, N. G. (1992). Estradiol selectively regulates agonist binding sites on the N-methyl-D-aspartate receptor complex in the CA1 region of the hippocampus. *Endocrinology*, **131**, 662–8.

Weiland, N. G., Orikasa, C., Hayashi, S., and McEwen, B. S. (1997). Distribution and hormone regulation of estrogen receptor immunoreactive cells in the hippocampus of male and female rats. *Journal of Comparative Neurology*, **388**, 603–12.

Weiner, M. J., Hallett, M., and Funkenstein, H. (1983). Adaptation to lateral displacement of vision in patients with lesions of the central nervous system. *Neurology*, **33**, 766–72.

Williams, C. L. (1996). Short-term but not long-term estradiol replacement improves radial arm maze performance of young and aging rats. *Society for Neuroscience Abstracts*, **22**, 1164.

Withers, G. S. and Greenough, W. T. (1989). Reach training selectively alters dendritic branching in subpopulations of layer II/III pyramids in rat motor-somatosensory forelimb cortex. *Neuropsychologia*, **27**, 61–9.

Witkin, J. W., Ferin, M., Popilskis, S. J., and Silverman, A. J. (1991). Effects of gonadal steroids on the ultrastructure of GnRH neurons in the rhesus monkey: synaptic input and glial apposition. *Endocrinology*, **129**, 1083–92.

Wong, M. and Moss, R. L. (1992). Long-term and short-term effects of estradiol on the synaptic properties of hippocampal CA1 neurons. *Journal of Neuroscience*, **12**, 3217–25.

Woolley, C. S. (1998). Estrogen-mediated structural and functional synaptic plasticity in the female rat hippocampus. *Hormones and Behavior*, **34**, 140–8.

Woolley, C. S. and McEwen, B. S. (1992). Estradiol mediates fluctuation in hippocampal synapse density during the estrous cycle in the adult rat. *Journal of Neuroscience*, **12**, 2549–54.

Woolley, C. S. and McEwen, B. S. (1993). Roles of estradiol and progesterone in regulation of hippocampal dendritic spine density during the estrous cycle in the rat. *Journal of Comparative Neurology*, **336**, 293–306.

Woolley, C. S. and McEwen, B. S. (1994). Estradiol regulates hippocampal dendritic spine density via an *N*-methyl-D-aspartate receptor dependent mechanism. *Journal of Neuroscience*, **14**, 7680–7.

Woolley, C. S., Gould, E., Frankfurt, M., and McEwen, B. S. (1990). Naturally-occurring fluctuation in dendritic spine density on adult hippocampal pyramidal neurons. *Journal of Neuroscience*, **10**, 4035–9.

Woolley, C. S., Wenzel, H. J., and Schwartzkroin, P. A. (1996). Estradiol increases the frequency of multiple synapse boutons in the hippocampal CA1 region of the adult female rat. *Journal of Comparative Neurology*, **373**, 108–17.

Woolley, C. S., Weiland, N. G., McEwen, B. S., and Schwartzkroin, P. A. (1997). Estradiol increases the sensitivity of hippocampal CA1 pyramidal cells to NMDA receptor-mediated synaptic input: correlation with dendritic spine density. *Journal of Neuroscience*, **17**, 1848–59.

15

Conclusion: the future of dendrite research

Michael Häusser
University College London

Nelson Spruston
Northwestern University

Greg Stuart
Australian National University

Dendrites have delighted the eye and captivated the imagination since their discovery over a century ago. This book documents the great progress that has been made in understanding dendrites since that time. Our appreciation of the structure of neurons has moved, with the help of the electron microscope, down to the level of dendritic and synaptic ultrastructure (Chapters 1 and 4). More recently, molecular biological techniques have enabled us to map the distribution and track the fate of individual molecules in the dendritic tree (Chapters 3 and 4). Thanks to new electrophysiological and imaging techniques we can now record electrical (Chapters 5, 6, 10 and 12) and chemical (Chapter 7) signals in remote dendritic regions, even within the living animal. Our picture of dendritic structure and function also is no longer static, but encompasses the dramatic changes that can occur during plasticity (Chapters 13 and 14) and development (Chapter 2). Finally, modeling has continued to be an essential tool for gaining insights into dendritic function (Chapters 8, 9 and 11). In summary, our knowledge of dendrites has reached a level of richness and complexity unimaginable even a few years ago.

Despite this tremendous progress, the most exciting times in dendrite research lie ahead of us. Much of the knowledge we have accumulated to date has been descriptive. Although we have amassed a detailed catalogue of structural features and molecular machinery, and discovered a wide repertoire of functional effects imparted by the dendritic tree, how these features enable neuronal networks to generate behavior remains elusive. The questions that need to be addressed at this stage are: what computations does each neuron perform within its neuronal network, and which features of dendrites are most relevant to how the neuron performs these computations?

In search of answers to these questions, there are several key areas where substantial progress is expected over the next few years:

1. We need a deeper understanding of the relationship between dendritic form and function. The incredible diversity of dendritic structure (Chapter 1), which makes

neurons a more heterogeneous population of cells than any other cell type in the body, has been appreciated since the days of Cajal, and it begs functional explanation. Wilfrid Rall pioneered the analysis of the electrical behavior of neurons in relation to their structure, and formalized simplifications for passive propagation of potentials in complex geometries (see Chapters 8 and 9). We need to develop analogous simplifications for electrogenesis and spread of potentials in active dendrites, for uniform and non-uniform distributions of voltage-gated channels (Chapter 6). Such an analysis should also be extended to integration and compartmentalization of chemical signals (Chapter 7), which are also likely to be closely linked to dendritic structure. Making simplified, or 'reduced' models of these different processes is an integral step in defining principles which relate geometry to computation, and might also reveal optimization principles which underlie the distribution and function of channels in different dendritic trees. These simplified models will also make it easier to incorporate realistic neurons into large-scale neural-network models (see below). Ultimately, in the spirit of Cajal, it might be possible to look at a dendritic tree and predict how it will function.

2.   We require more insight into the transformation of synaptic input into neuronal output. As described in this book, dendrites have been shown to display a wide range of behavior in response to synaptic input. For example, supralinear, linear, and sublinear summation of inputs have all been observed when combining multiple excitatory inputs. Furthermore, simulations and experiments have shown that dendritic voltage-gated channels can make the response of the neuron either exquisitely sensitive to the spatial pattern of its input, or act as a normalizing influence to reduce the location-dependence of the somatic response (Chapters 9 to 12). We urgently need to formulate rules that clearly define the relationship between input and output under different conditions. These rules should define the input patterns precisely (e.g. distribution in time and space of active synapses, kinetics of synaptic conductances, etc.) and predict patterns of axonal output (e.g. probability of single action potentials with a given timing; probability of bursts of action potentials; probability of calcium spikes) under a given set of background conditions (e.g. level of tonic inhibition; density of available Na^+ channels).

Experimental approaches that will be helpful in defining these rules include simultaneous recordings from multiple sites, either electrically or *via* imaging techniques, and activation of defined numbers/sets of synaptic inputs at known locations on the dendritic tree. As the parameter space available for defining different conditions is potentially very large, we need to be constrained wherever possible by information from *in vivo* recordings in unanesthetized animals. Combining experiments with simulations in detailed compartmental models of the same neurons will be necessary to formalize the rules and help us design experiments to test them further. While the goal is to create a relatively small but comprehensive set of rules that will cover the range of states of the neuron and the network, we must also take into account the variability that exists at various levels. For example, the contribution of noise, arising from synaptic variability and from intrinsic sources, such as voltage-activated channels, must be quantified and incorporated. Also, while neurons of the same type (e.g. Purkinje cells) are likely to perform similar computational tasks, and therefore obey the same input-output rules, variability between individual neurons within a neuronal subtype will have to be considered. Once we have a complete set of such rules and are aware of their limitations, we should be able to predict how each neuron is likely to respond to a given input pattern, and thereby understand the computation performed by the neuron on its input. Understanding these rules and the computations underlying them will be essential to understanding neural network function.

3.   We need to elucidate how the combination of genetic programs and environ-mental influences determines the properties of individual dendritic trees (see Chapters 2, 3, 13 and 14). What makes a cerebellar granule cell so different from a neocortical pyramidal neuron? To what extent is dendritic structure and the distribution of channels in the dendritic tree the result of a predetermined genetic program, or a consequence of the local physical and chemical environment and the pattern and activity of synaptic inputs? The focus should not only be on dendritic structure, but also on how particular inputs are mapped onto the tree, as the spatial pattern of active synapses can have important consequences for neuronal function. Are synaptic contacts made randomly onto dendrites, or can specific inputs be targeted to particular regions of the tree? An understanding of the processes that shape dendritic development can help us to better understand and manipulate the changes occurring during synaptic plasticity in the adult animal, and might enable us to design dendrites with specific features (see below).

4.   Finally, and most importantly, we need a better understanding of the relationship between individual features of dendrites and higher-level function. Defining the role of dendrites in neuronal behavior requires an understanding of the function of the network. Until we understand what computations a particular network does, it will be impossible to determine which properties of individual neurons are necessary for the network to perform these computations. Thus, as outlined in Chapter 9, one of the biggest challenges of the next century will be connect the function of the single neuron to the global operations of the network. There are several approaches that promise to be fruitful. One is to investigate dendritic function in systems, such as those in invertebrates, where neurons are more accessible in the behaving animal, and where the signals of individual neurons can be more closely linked to behavior. This approach has already begun to yield significant results (see Chapter 12) that can help us understand analogous computations in higher animals.

As computers become ever more powerful, another important approach will be to test which features of dendrites confer computational advantages from the point of view of network performance. Real neurons are vastly more complex than the simple, isopotential units currently employed in most large-scale neural network models. The challenge is to identify what level of complexity to incorporate into more realistic neuronal models for use in network simulations. This will require testing both simplified models, incorporating individual computational features, as well as highly detailed models in which multiple features interact, to identify which features (or combination of features) can substantially enhance computation on the network level.

To verify the predictions of these models (and to help generate more accurate predictions), it is essential to be able to record and manipulate electrical and chemical signals in dendrites in awake mammals, thus enabling direct correlation between behavior and specific dendritic signals. Several technical advances promise to make this possible within the next decade. Molecular biological techniques, coupled with an increased knowledge of protein targeting in dendrites, will enable us to selectively remove specific cell types, manipulate densities of specific proteins, and deliver molecules to (or activate drugs in) specific regions of neurons. Using these techniques it might, for example, be possible to modify the density of functional calcium channels in distal regions of the dendritic tree of particular neuronal types, or engineer neurons with different dendritic morphologies. In conjunction with these molecular biological tools, the current rapid progress in imaging and recording techniques should eventually enable both electrical and chemical signals to be recorded from dendrites in behaving animals. Advances in non-invasive imaging techniques might some day even enable comparable measurements to be conducted in man. Ultimately, increased knowledge of dendritic function should help us bridge the gap between single neurons and behavior, which is essential for a deeper understanding of how our brains work.

Index